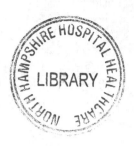

# Outcome-Based Massage

## Massage *From Evidence to Practice*

SECOND EDITION

# Outcome-Based Massage

## From Evidence to Practice

### SECOND EDITION

**Carla-Krystin Andrade, PhD, PT**

Associate Clinical Professor and Course Coordinator
University of California–San Francisco/San Francisco State
    University Graduate Program in Physical Therapy
Department of Physical Therapy and Rehabilitation Sciences,
    School of Medicine, University of California–San Francisco
Private Practice: Stress Free Zone, San Francisco, California

**Paul Clifford, BSc, RMT**

Professor, Massage Therapy Program
School of Health and Wellness
Sir Sandford Fleming College
Peterborough, Ontario, Canada

**Photographs by Marc Boulay, BFA, MA**

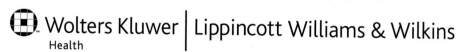
Wolters Kluwer | Lippincott Williams & Wilkins
Health

Philadelphia • Baltimore • New York • London
Buenos Aires • Hong Kong • Sydney • Tokyo

*Acquisitions Editor:* Emily J. Lupash
*Managing Editor:* Linda G. Francis
*Marketing Manager:* Missi Carmen
*Production Editor:* Paula C. Williams
*Designer:* Teresa Mallon
*Compositor:* Circle Graphics

Second Edition

351 West Camden Street          530 Walnut Street
Baltimore, MD 21201             Philadelphia, PA 19106

Printed in China

9 8 7 6 5 4 3 2 1

**Library of Congress Cataloging-in-Publication Data**

Andrade, Carla-Krystin, 1962–
  Outcome-based massage : from evidence to practice / Carla-Krystin Andrade, Paul Clifford
; photographs by Marc Boulay. — 2nd ed.
        p. ; cm.
  Includes bibliographical references and index.
  ISBN-13: 978-0-7817-6760-6 (alk. paper)
  ISBN-10: 0-7817-6760-1 (alk. paper)
  1. Massage. 2. Massage—Decision making. I. Clifford, Paul, MT. II.
Title.
  [DNLM: 1. Massage—methods. 2. Patient Care Planning. 3. Treatment Outcome. WB 537
A553o 2008]
  RA780.5.A53 2008
  615.8′22—dc22
                                        2007042315

DISCLAIMER

Care has been taken to confirm the accuracy of the information present and to describe generally accepted practices. However, the authors, editors, and publisher are not responsible for errors or omissions or for any consequences from application of the information in this book and make no warranty, expressed or implied, with respect to the currency, completeness, or accuracy of the contents of the publication. Application of this information in a particular situation remains the professional responsibility of the practitioner; the clinical treatments described and recommended may not be considered absolute and universal recommendations.

The authors, editors, and publisher have exerted every effort to ensure that drug selection and dosage set forth in this text are in accordance with the current recommendations and practice at the time of publication. However, in view of ongoing research, changes in government regulations, and the constant flow of information relating to drug therapy and drug reactions, the reader is urged to check the package insert for each drug for any change in indications and dosage and for added warnings and precautions. This is particularly important when the recommended agent is a new or infrequently employed drug.

Some drugs and medical devices presented in this publication have Food and Drug Administration (FDA) clearance for limited use in restricted research settings. It is the responsibility of the health care provider to ascertain the FDA status of each drug or device planned for use in their clinical practice.

*The publishers have made every effort to trace the copyright holders for borrowed material. If they have inadvertently overlooked any, they will be pleased to make the necessary arrangements at the first opportunity.*

To purchase additional copies of this book, call our customer service department at **(800) 638-3030** or fax orders to **(301) 223-2320**. International customers should call **(301) 223-2300**.

Visit Lippincott Williams & Wilkins on the Internet: http://www.lww.com. Lippincott Williams & Wilkins customer service representatives are available from 8:30 am to 6:00 pm, EST.

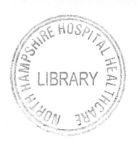

Life is short, the art long, opportunity fleeting, experience treacherous, judgment difficult.

*Hippocrates, Aphorisms I.I.*

*To Our Parents*
*Monique Rey Andrade*
*Margaret Helen (Edwards) Clifford*
*Edmond Patrick Andrade*
*Ernest Ambrose Clifford*

# Contributors

**Trish Dryden, MEd, RMT**
Director, Applied Research Centre
Centennial College
Toronto, Ontario, Canada
(Evidence-Based Practice for Chapter 2)

**Pamela Fitch, BA, RMT**
Professor, Massage Therapy Program
School of Health and Community Studies
Algonquin College
Ottawa, Ontario, Canada
(Ethical and Interpersonal Issues for Chapter 4)

**Paula Tanksley, BA, MPT**
Private Practice: Tanksley Physical Therapy
Oakland, California
(Client Examination Techniques for Chapter 5)

# Subject Matter Experts

**Stephen Goring, BSc, MA, RMT**
Private Practice
Toronto, Ontario, Canada
(Client's emotional response to massage treatment)

**Teresa Randall, MPT**
Staff Physical Therapist
Alameda County Medical Center–Fairmont Campus
San Leandro, California
(Strategies to enhance client adherence)

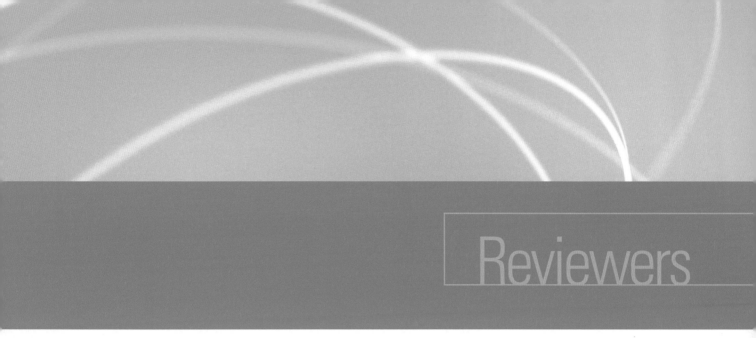

# Reviewers

The authors wish to extend their sincerest thanks to the following individuals who reviewed portions of the manuscript and provided constructive feedback during critical stages of the development of the second edition of this text. Their thought-provoking comments prompted much discussion and helped us refine the final content.

**Rosalyn Pitt, PT, EdD, SPE**
Physical Therapy Department
Tennessee State University
Nashville, Tennessee

**Amanda Baskwill, RMT**
Massage Therapy Program
School of Community and Health Studies
Centennial College
Toronto, Ontario, Canada

**Julianne Lepp, CNMT**
Marietta, Georgia

**Lorraine Allen, PT student**
Tennessee State University
Nashville, Tennessee

**Deborah Edmondson, PT, EdD**
Physical Therapy Department
Tennessee State University
Nashville, Tennessee

**Paul Finch, PhD, MSc, DPodM**
Director of Education
Sutherland-Chan School and Teaching Clinic
Toronto, Ontario, Canada

**Nancy Mezick Cavender, MM, LMT, LNMT**
The Sakeena Center
Massage and Neuromuscular Therapies
Atlanta, Georgia

**Kevin K. Chui, PT, PhD, GCS**
Department of Physical Therapy
and Human Movement Science
Graduate Program in Geriatric Health and Wellness
Sacred Heart University
Fairfield, Connecticut

**Everett L. Lohman, DSc, PT, OCS**
Department of Physical Therapy
Loma Linda University
Loma Linda, California

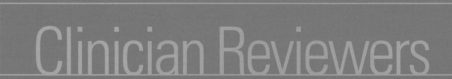

# Clinician Reviewers

The authors are indebted to the following individuals who generously contributed their clinical expertise and feedback during the development of this text.

Benjamin Boyd, MSPT

Bridget Bouyssounouse, BS, PT

Nancy Byl, PT, PhD, FAPTA

Sandi Chan, BS, PT

Tara Detwiler, Certified Advanced Rolfer

Alexandra N. Fallot, BA, MPT

Meghan Gordineer, MPT

Betty Ann Harris, BSc, RMT

Susan Klingaman Estilaei, PT, DPT, OCS

Wendy Katzman, PT, DPTSc, OCS

Shawn Jarman, MPT

Lee Kalpin, RMT

Liz Lester, RMT

Wendy Moore, BA, MSc, MD, FRCP(C)

Gaye Raymond, BS, MS, PT

Kenneth Resznyak, RMT

Rick Ritter, PT, DPT, OCS

Jarek Szymczak, RMT, Certified Lymph Drainage Therapist (Vodder, Germany)

Kimberly Topp, PT, PhD

# FOREWORD BY
# DR. NANCY BYL

I am delighted to write this Foreword for the second edition of *Outcome-Based Massage* written by Carla-Krystin Andrade, PhD, PT, and Paul Clifford, BSc, RMT. Dr. Andrade, Mr. Clifford, and their editor, Linda Francis, along with experienced clinicians and clinical specialists, need to be commended on the rigorous evidence-based content that serves as the foundation for this book. This is the first text I have reviewed on the subject of massage that meets the criteria to promote scientific investigation and evidence-based practice. This book is not only appropriate as a text for an entry-level academic program, but it is also an excellent review and guide for the practicing clinician.

Dr. Andrade and Mr. Clifford provide an excellent conceptual framework for clinicians to understand the different types of massage. They outline the theories about outcome-based assessment, as well as the various models of health, wellness, and disability that need to be considered when applying massage techniques. In addition, they introduce the concept of evidence-based practice and provide guidelines for how to integrate evidence into the clinical use of massage. While providing a structured framework to evaluate outcomes, they also review the concepts of touch and logically categorize the various techniques that have been developed within the framework of massage.

The authors carefully lay the foundation for the client examination needed to provide the basis for treating with massage techniques. The authors highlight the differences in the clinical examination for treatment with massage, as distinguished from the standard clinical examination. In this process, they outline relevant impairments receptive to remediation by massage and wellness goals that clinicians can achieve using massage.

In addition to comprehensive descriptions of massage techniques and their variations, each chapter includes clinical examples that demonstrate how to apply theory to practice and detailed clinical cases that take the reader through the process from diagnosis to discharge, including measurement, treatment planning, and treatment outcomes. In their discussions of treatment planning, the authors make it very clear that massage is one aspect of the client's total treatment. Furthermore, they emphasize that providers must be sensitive to the broad, as well as the specific, issues that challenge recovery, regardless of the impairment. Indeed, their expanded content on ethical and interpersonal issues provides clinicians with tools that they can use to respond to the difficult situations that are often associated with the use of massage in a clinical setting.

Massage is no longer the most common treatment in rehabilitation. Unfortunately, within the current health care environment, many clinicians have moved away from "hands-on" treatment as a regular part of their intervention strategy. In some cases, this is driven by the lack of the provider's time with the client, reimbursement issues, the passive nature of the technique, or the perceived lack of research evidence supporting the specific physiological effects of the different massage techniques. However, we know that touching a person in a safe environment can have measurable benefits. For these reasons, *Outcome-Based*

*Massage* is timely. In this book, the principles of scientific inquiry are meticulously integrated into the technical and humanistic aspects of care. This link between science and practice is not only strong at the beginning of the book, but it is also emphasized throughout every chapter. This book provides a foundation for clinicians to carry out good clinical trials to provide evidence to support the effectiveness of massage as an intervention strategy to enhance the quality of life.

I commend Dr. Andrade, Mr. Clifford, and their team for preparing a rigorous academic text on massage. This is long overdue. I feel confident that clinicians, faculty, students, and even some patients will find this book to be an excellent reference textbook for learning.

**Nancy N. Byl, PhD, PT, FAPTA**
*Professor*
*Department of Physical Therapy and Rehabilitation*
*Science, School of Medicine, University of*
*California–San Francisco*
*University of California–San Francisco/*
*San Francisco State University Graduate Program in*
*Physical Therapy*
*San Francisco, California*

# FOREWORD BY
# DR. JANET KAHN

Some longstanding arguments in the field of therapeutic massage can be settled now, and the good news is that everyone wins. The tension about a presumed competition between the heart and the science of our massage and bodywork has been demonstrated in this second edition of *Outcome-Based Massage* to be a red herring, a distraction, and false at its core. As Andrade and Clifford show us in this invaluable volume, intuition and compassion are not one end of a continuum with purposeful planning and delivery of theory-driven outcome-based treatment on the other end. Rather than being at odds with one another, the heart and science of massage are two different and essential facets of good treatment. They are compatible, and their interplay is in fact the art of massage at its best.

The authors also show us that, while treatments to enhance wellness may not look exactly like treatments to address impaired function, they can and should both be purposefully planned and outcome-oriented. Done well, they each rely upon careful observation, clinical reasoning, and clear goal setting. The goals are different, but the processes are the same. One of the gifts of this second edition of *Outcome-Based Massage* is its direct attention to the similarities and differences in designing massage for both wellness and impairments.

Andrade and Clifford are experienced and skilled educators. They provide in this book not just the idea of becoming more evidence-based and outcome-based in our work, but also the means to do that. They offer a comprehensive approach to assessment, treatment design, and treatment delivery that is meticulously explained in prose, pictures, charts, case studies, and video clips. Whatever kind of learner the reader is, they provide what is needed in order for students and practitioners to give clients the best, which is, after all, what they deserve. The material in this book is as appropriate for advanced practitioners responsible for setting the curriculum for our own continuing education as for the classroom student. This is a welcome resource for educators doing their best to teach skills (e.g., locating relevant research literature) and processes (e.g., clinical reasoning) that were not part of the curriculum when they were being trained. Our field is becoming more sophisticated, and this book helps us all keep pace with the changes.

There are important reasons for us as clinicians and as a profession to hone our skills of clinical reasoning and outcome-based massage. We don't do it to be trendy or to succumb to the medical paradigm. In applying the skills of treatment planning and evaluation of outcome-based massage, the real wisdom of our profession, and of each of us, comes forward. The truth is that all good massage therapists are alert observers with theories about how and why certain treatments work. One of our limitations as a profession has been that we have not encouraged ourselves, or one another, to articulate what we notice and what we think. The word intuition has too often been used in place of slowing down enough to notice and name the signals we are picking up from our clients—postural, palpatory, verbal bits of information that, combined with our past experience, lead us to choose the techniques, the pace, and the encouraging phrases of our treatments. *Outcome-Based Massage* can teach us to name what we are noticing and organize it for the health and well-being of our clients. That is good massage.

It is also the basis of good research. Clinical reasoning and the researcher's mind of inquiry are intimately related, with overlapping skills used for somewhat different purposes. When, as clinicians, we articulate our observations and our theories about how massage works, we are able, as a profession, to identify the research agenda for our field. We can identify the unanswered questions coming from our clinical practice and encourage researchers to investigate these questions. Good practice and good research go hand in hand.

In fact, *Outcome-Based Massage* should be essential reading for researchers of massage who are not practitioners. It delineates the elements of the varied massage techniques in a way that will allow researchers to design more sophisticated protocols for clinical trials. It offers the best current thinking on the effects of specific techniques and mechanisms, both examined and unexamined. The technique-by-technique sections on how massage might work are invaluable.

Personally, I was thrilled when I discovered the first edition of *Outcome-Based Massage* some years ago. It is a user-friendly book too; it is comprehensive yet so well structured and illustrated that it has always been easy to find what I need in it. This second edition retains everything I have always appreciated about *Outcome-Based Massage* and adds to it.

Now there are no excuses left. With the publication of the second edition of *Outcome-Based Massage,* Carla-Krystin Andrade and Paul Clifford have wiped away the excuses some massage therapists have used to avoid staying abreast of the research literature and linking it to their daily practice. They have done away with the excuses of those who claim that their treatments are intuitive (which is good) and therefore can't be planned or thought about (which is wrong). They have erased the excuses of massage educators who emphasize technique (which is good) and neglect teaching clinical reasoning and cultivating the mind of inquiry (which is wrong). In place of our old excuses, Andrade and Clifford have given us everything we need in this volume to think intelligently about massage. This book is an important contribution to the field, a gift to anyone who cares about the development of therapeutic massage and its potential to help people.

**Janet R. Kahn, PhD, NCBMT**
*Director of Research*
*Massage Therapy Research Consortium*
*and Research Assistant Professor,*
*Department of Psychiatry,*
*University of Vermont*
*Burlington, Vermont*

# Acknowledgments

First of all, we cannot begin to express how grateful we are to Linda Francis, our Managing Editor. Linda has been a phenomenal editor who has taken this book to heart and gone beyond the call of duty. In countless ways, this book reflects her dedication and guidance. We would also like to thank the people at Lippincott Williams & Wilkins who have contributed to this project: Peter Darcy for sharing our vision for the second edition; Peter Sabatini, Emily Lupash, and John Goucher for their guidance on the overall direction; Freddie Patane and Mark Flanders for patiently leading us through the steps to an outstanding video; the designers, Terry Mallon and Karen Quigley, who have brought a fresh new look to the book; David Payne who helped guide the early development stages; Paul Montgomery who managed the review process that assisted us in refining the book; and Allison Noplock, Missi Carmen, Katie Schauer, and Christen Murphy whose marketing expertise we value; and Paula Williams and Caroline Define whose production and copyediting expertise made us look amazing in print. In addition, we would like to thank Margaret Biblis and Peg Waltner who championed the first edition.

We would also like to extend our sincere thanks to: the photographer for the first edition, Marc Boulay, for photos that have stood the test of time and the client and therapist models for the first edition: Christopher Alger, Tricia Bachman, Joanne Baker, Dan Boon, Paul Bucciero, Brian Burgess, Melissa Cole, D!ONNE (Francis), Lee Kalpin, Rahima Kassam, Michael Kitney, Amy Knapp, Frank Marincola, Colin Outram, Shahnaz Suteria, Jarek Szymczak, and Jane Wellwood. We are grateful for the patience and assistance of the models for the video: Chanelle Andrade, Etienne Harris, and Chris Lemieux; and we thank Nadeige Andrade, who lent us her home for the shoot. We are truly grateful for our new contributors, Trish Dryden and Pam Fitch, our first edition contributors, Paula Tanksley, Teresa Randall, and Stephen Goring, and the reviewers and clinician reviewers for their wonderful additions to the text.

Paul would like to thank Bill Peacock and Rachel Donovan, for accepting the research for this book as academic renewal; his colleagues at Fleming College—Jennifer Borland Rosin, Annette Doose, Mary Ann Elliott, Kristina Lonsberry, and all the sessional and part time staff—for supportive work "in the trenches" and drafts of some questions; his colleagues at Algonquin College, for conversation; Lee Kalpin, for reading a draft of Chapter 14; many family and friends including members of Affirm United, PARN Men's Group, and Old Men Dancing, for witnessing the ordeal; and Chris Lemieux, for patience plus . . . Om shantih.

Carla-Krystin also wishes to thank her son Alan, her husband Len, and her family members Nadeige, Chanelle, Nikki, Madison, Freddie, Patrick Edmund, and Monique for their love and support, and her colleagues at UCSF/SFSU Graduate Program in Physical Therapy and the Faculty Practice for their guidance.

Finally, we are delighted that our friendship has withstood another edition and trust that our thirst for knowledge and shared vision for an expanded clinical role for massage will continue to guide us.

**C-K and Paul**

## OUTCOME-BASED MASSAGE: FROM EVIDENCE TO PRACTICE

The current health care environment demands that health care practitioners adopt an evidence-based approach to practice and demonstrate the outcomes that they achieve with their massage-based interventions. *Outcome-Based Massage: From Evidence to Practice* shows you how to meet those demands with our unique integration of clinical problem solving, manual skills, evidence-based practice, and interpersonal aspects of massage. This book is for all health care practitioners whose scope of practice permits them to perform massage techniques. We designed it so that entry-level students will find it to be an invaluable textbook and experienced practitioners will use it as an essential clinical reference. Consequently, you do not have to have a prior knowledge of massage to use this book, simply a familiarity with basic scientific language and anatomy.

*Outcome-Based Massage: From Evidence to Practice* is the product of our passionate belief in the importance of massage and the need for a problem-solving approach to using massage in clinical care. We have synthesized the best of the knowledge we have gleaned in almost 50 years of clinical experience in physical therapy, massage therapy, and teaching experience, with physical therapists, massage therapists, nurses, athletic trainers, and occupational therapists. As a result, when you use *Outcome-Based Massage: From Evidence to Practice,* you will learn:

- A practical clinical decision-making process that you can use to examine clients, identify relevant impairments and outcomes, select massage and complementary techniques, design and progress interventions, and discharge clients
- When, why, and how to use massage techniques to achieve 30 categories of outcomes for wellness, the treatment of medical conditions, and palliative care
- Practical skills you need to prepare and position your clients for massage
- Practical skills you need to perform neuromuscular, connective tissue, percussive, passive movement, superficial reflex, and superficial fluid massage techniques using correct manual technique
- How to complement massage with other techniques and homecare
- Therapist self-care and strategies to prevent overuse injuries and "burnout"
- How to successfully manage the unique interpersonal and ethical issues that accompany your use of massage techniques
- How to find, understand, evaluate, and apply current evidence for massage techniques

## WHAT'S NEW IN THE SECOND EDITION

For the second edition of *Outcome-Based Massage,* we have done more than "freshen up" the original content. Instead, we have extended and restructured the content of the book so that it truly reflects its new title, *Outcome-Based Massage: From Evidence to Practice*. Here are some of the changes you will find in this edition:

■ **Content for a Broader Range of Health Care Professions:** We have extended the content to meet the needs of several health care professions that use massage such as physical therapy, massage therapy, occupational therapy, bodywork, chiropractic, athletic training, and naturopathy. We now include content and a level of material that addresses licensure and credentialing requirements in massage for a broader range of health care professions. For example, we cover material that is relevant to (a) the National Certification Examination for Therapeutic Massage and Bodywork: pathology, therapeutic massage and bodywork assessment and application, professional standards, and ethics sections; and (b) the American Physical Therapy Association Required Skills of Physical Therapy Graduates examination: evaluation, plan of care, body mechanics and positioning, interventions–manual therapy techniques, evidence-based practice, and professionalism sections.

■ **Video Clips of Massage Techniques:** We have added a new level of practical instruction with approximately 70 video clips online that show how to perform many of the techniques and sequences illustrated by the photographs in the book. These share the same labels as the photographs in the book, so that readers can cross-reference this material.

■ **Separation of Basic and Advanced Content:** In each chapter, we have sequenced and separated basic material and more advanced content to accommodate the learning needs of readers at different levels. Foundations sections include introductory concepts, basic massage techniques, and common clinical scenarios. Further Study and Practice sections present advanced theoretical frameworks, more demanding clinical techniques, and more complex clinical cases.

■ **Using Massage to Treat Impairments due to Medical Conditions:** We show practitioners how to make the transition from the traditional approach of using standard massage sequences for medical conditions to an outcome-based approach. In particular, we demonstrate how to identify the impairments associated with a client's medical condition and create an intervention that treats those impairments and achieves specific clinical outcomes. We do so by discussing the clinical relevance, treatment considerations, guidelines for using massage techniques, and complementary modalities for 30 impairments related to common musculo-

skeletal, circulatory, respiratory, neurological, and psycho-neuroimmunological conditions.

■ **Sample Sequences of Massage Techniques:** As an adjunct to the principles of designing sequences, we provide step-by-step examples of short regional sequences, long regional sequences, general sequences, and full-body sequences for wellness and the treatment of impairments due to a variety of medical conditions.

■ **Physiological and Psychological Effects of Massage:** We offer more detailed discussions of the possible mechanisms for the physical and psychological effects of massage techniques in the How Techniques Might Work and Outcomes and Evidence sections for each of the techniques.

■ **Comprehensive Overview of Client Examination Techniques:** This unique chapter synthesizes information on a wide range of clinical examination techniques that you can use to assess clients who present with a variety of impairments or wellness goals.

■ **Wellness Massage:** We present a new, holistic model of wellness and demonstrate how to conduct a client examination and treatment planning to create effective massage interventions that achieve a client's wellness outcomes. This provides practitioners with a more flexible alternative to using a standard "full-body wellness massage" sequence for their clients. We also provide step-by-step sample sequences that you can use for wellness interventions.

■ **Expanded Instruction on How to Perform Massage Techniques:** We have enhanced the already exemplary step-by-step instruction on manual technique and approximately 400 illustrations and photographs of massage techniques with several new components that will assist readers in learning manual techniques in, and beyond, the classroom. These include practice sequences for each technique, details of contraindications and cautions to using each technique, and details of how to use the techniques in treatment. We also discuss Eastern and European massage traditions.

■ **Palpation Training:** We introduce the concept of "intelligent touch" and provide extensive instruction on how to use palpation for examination and treatment. Dozens of palpation exercises, which specifically relate to each technique, show you how to use palpation within the context of treatment.

■ **Applying Theory to Practice:** Each chapter contains several examples of ways in which readers can apply the principles introduced in the chapter to real-life clinical situations. In the Foundations sections, Theory in

Practice scenarios include case studies that illustrate how to apply theoretical concepts to basic clinical situations. In the Further Study sections, Clinical Cases show how to apply theory to more complex clinical cases and demonstrate client examination and treatment, clinical decision-making, and methods of charting clinical findings. Critical Thinking Questions on key issues foster clinical decision-making skills for both basic and more advanced content.

- **Evidence-Based Practice:** We introduce the concepts of Evidence-Based Practice and the steps practitioners can use to find, understand, evaluate, and apply current evidence for massage techniques. We also provide an overview of the current state of research and theory on massage and a discussion of the issues related to creating a body of evidence for massage practice.

- **Applying Evidence to Practice:** We show practitioners how to integrate evidence into their daily clinical practice in several ways. For example, Chapters 7 to 12 contain Examining the Evidence sections for each category of techniques that demonstrate how to understand and apply evidence within daily practice. In addition, the How Techniques Might Work sections in Chapters 7 to 12 provide a summary of the current evidence that explains the possible therapeutic effects for each of the massage techniques.

- **Integrated Clinical Decision-Making and Documentation:** We now demonstrate the decision-making process and relevant clinical documentation (using SOAP format) for the Evaluative, Treatment, Treatment Planning, and Discharge phases of the clinical decision-making process using flow charts and an extensive clinical case.

- **Ethical and Interpersonal Issues in Massage:** The physical proximity of massage techniques often generates a heightened level of trust between the practitioner and the client. To address this, we have devoted an entire chapter to ethical and interpersonal issues. This includes details of the therapeutic relationship, a three-phase therapeutic process, an overview of therapists' and clients' rights, and several clinical scenarios to help practitioners understand these issues and the guidelines for practice.

- **Clinical Scope:** We have modified the scope of the book to include wellness and palliative care, as well as to extend the material on the treatment of medical conditions.

- **Extended Glossary:** We have enlarged the glossary to include a larger number of massage-related terms and modalities. We have also cross-referenced the glossary to the text, so that readers can easily identify terms that we define in the glossary.

- **Language:** We recognize that a variety of different health care practitioners will use this book. For the sake of simplicity, we use the terms practitioner, therapist, and clinician interchangeably to refer to the individual who is providing care. Furthermore, practitioners will be treating clients or patients depending on their practice setting. Consequently, we use the terms client and patient interchangeably, to refer to the individual who is receiving care.

# FOR SCHOOLS AND INSTRUCTORS

The second edition of *Outcome-Based Massage* provides a wealth of basic and advanced information on the theory and manual technique of massage. In addition, the book's new structure of separate sections for basic and advanced material allows you to select material that fits the level of your program and the scope of your course. We also provide several online instructional aids to simplify the process of using Outcome-Based Massage as the primary text or an adjunct to your program.

- PowerPoint presentations synthesizing the key information from each chapter, which you can use within lectures or as handouts
- Curriculum guides that illustrate a variety of sequences of chapters and topics for programs of different lengths and levels
- The Test Generator that contains numerous questions on the content
- The extensive set of photographs of manual technique that is available for download
- The video clips of manual techniques that accompany the book are available for download
- The online Student Resource center, which students can access for an interactive quiz bank with additional review questions

# UNIQUE ORGANIZATION AND FEATURES

We base our approach to teaching massage on our observation that practitioners need both clinical decision-making and manual skills, not merely a mechanical "laying on of hands," in order to use massage techniques effectively. Consequently, *Outcome-Based Massage: From Evidence to Practice* guides you through the steps of a four-phase clinical decision-making model: Evaluation, Treatment Planning, Treatment, and Discharge.

**Part I: Client Examination and Treatment Planning.** This section is concerned with the initial stages of clinical decision-making that form the foundation of clinical care.

- Chapter 1, Massage for Wellness and Impairments, outlines frameworks that guide Outcome-Based Massage such as the World Health Organization's International Classification of Functioning, Disability and Health, our Wellness Interactions Model, Donabedian's framework of the components of clinical care, and our framework of Intelligent Touch. This chapter also introduces a classification system for massage techniques that is based on the tissue layers that you treat and the outcomes that you achieve with a technique, rather than the customary division between "traditional" and "modern" techniques.
- Chapter 2, Evidence for Massage, introduces the concepts of evidence-based practice and the steps that practitioners can use to find, understand, evaluate, and apply current evidence for massage techniques.
- Chapter 3, Clinical Decision-Making for Massage, details the book's four-phase clinical decision-making process, using clinical examples to illustrate the application of this process to clinical care. It shows you how to examine the client, analyze and document your examination findings, create a clinical problem list, establish relevant outcomes, select appropriate massage and complementary techniques, create and document a plan of care, progress the intervention, and discharge the client.
- Chapter 4, Interpersonal and Ethical Issues for Massage, addresses the interpersonal aspects of using massage in clinical care, including the client–clinician interaction, the client's emotional response to treatment, and boundary issues. It also examines critical ethical issues that practitioners must attend to when they are using massage techniques.
- Chapter 5, Client Examination for Massage, identifies the unique aspects of the client examination for massage and provides an overview of palpatory and nonpalpatory approaches to assessing body structures and functions, functional activities, and quality-of-life issues that are relevant to the use of massage techniques.

**Part II: Treatment and Discharge.** This section emphasizes psychomotor skills and discusses the clinical decision-making skills used to refine and progress interventions.

- Chapter 6, Preparation and Positioning for Massage, describes what practitioners use to complete their psychological and physical preparation for treatment. It also gives step-by-step procedures for preparing materials and techniques for positioning and draping the client for treatment.
- Chapters 7 through 12 introduce categories of related massage techniques: Superficial Reflex Techniques, Superficial Fluid Techniques, Neuromuscular Techniques, Connective Tissue Techniques, Passive Movement Techniques, and Percussive Techniques. These chapters have a common structure that details the cognitive and psychomotor skills required to apply the 17 massage techniques within a therapeutic intervention. Each chapter contains separate sections for basic and advanced content for each technique.
- Chapter 13, Sequencing Massage Techniques, describes the principles and processes that practitioners can use to design sequences of massage techniques and to progress interventions that incorporate massage techniques from the initial intervention to discharge.
- Chapter 14, Using Massage to Achieve Clinical Outcomes, provides an alternative to the typical application of massage techniques to conditions or special populations. It integrates the material from the technique chapters and shows how to use massage techniques to treat the impairments that accompany common musculoskeletal, neurological, circulatory, respiratory, and psychoneuroimmunological medical conditions.

**Glossary:** The final component of the book is an extensive glossary of terms and additional explanations of clinical concepts that appear in the text.

# THE AUTHORS

A combination of diverse backgrounds is required to do justice to the different, yet complementary, components of clinical decision-making and manual skills that we present in *Outcome-Based Massage: From Evidence to Practice.* Paul, a massage therapist, contributed the approach to massage and treatment planning that he has developed through his extensive manual training, clinical massage practice in varied settings, and experience teaching massage therapists. Carla-Krystin, a physical therapist, developed the approach to using frameworks, outcomes, and clinical decision making to guide treatment planning and the clinical use of massage based on her extensive experience in clinical physical therapy practice, conducting research, and educating physical therapists, massage therapists, nurses, athletic trainers, and occupational therapists.

## A FINAL NOTE

To our knowledge, *Outcome-Based Massage: From Evidence to Practice* is the first massage text that bridges the gap between the traditional approach, which uses standardized massage sequences for medical conditions, and a problem-solving approach of designing sequences of massage techniques to explicitly address impairments or wellness goals. We trust that our approach does justice to the lineage of fine authors of works on massage techniques, physical medicine, and rehabilitation to whom we are in debt. It is our hope that this book contributes to the ongoing restoration of a valuable ancient discipline to a more honored place in modern health care. We welcome your suggestions for refining this approach at ckandrade@yahoo.com or pcliffor@flemingc.on.ca.

# Contents

# Part I Client Examination and Treatment Planning

The chapters in Part I provide the framework for Outcome-Based Massage and cover the first two phases of the clinical decision-making process: the Evaluative Phase and the Treatment Planning Phase. Chapter 1, Massage for Wellness and Impairments, explains outcomes within the context of models of health, disability, and functioning and models of wellness. It also introduces the 30 categories of outcomes that clinicians can use massage techniques to achieve. Chapter 2, Evidence for Massage, presents the principles of evidence-based practice and their application to massage. Chapter 3, Clinical Decision-Making for Massage, details the steps in the four-phase clinical decision-making process that guides the approach to Outcome-Based Massage used throughout the text: Evaluative Phase, Treatment Planning Phase, Treatment Phase, and Discharge Phase. Chapter 4, Interpersonal and Ethical Issues for Massage, introduces the phases of the Therapeutic Process: Building Trust, Exploring Sensation, and Healthy Closure. It also details essential interpersonal and ethical issues that clinicians need to address within the therapeutic relationship throughout the therapeutic process. Chapter 5, Client Examination for Massage, identifies the unique aspects of the client examination for massage. It also provides an overview of palpatory and nonpalpatory approaches to assessing body structures and functions and functional limitations that are relevant to the use of massage techniques.

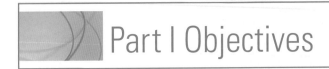

# Part I Objectives

**After studying Part I, the reader will have the information required to:**

1. Describe the World Health Organization's model of health, disability, and functioning.
2. Describe the Wellness Interactions Model.
3. Distinguish between the goals and process for the treatment of clinical conditions and wellness interventions.
4. Identify the components of the structure, process, and outcomes of clinical care.
5. List sources of evidence for clinical practice.
6. Describe methods for locating and evaluating evidence for clinical practice.
7. Define the terms therapeutic relationship, therapeutic contract, and client-centered care.
8. Describe the stages of the therapeutic process.
9. Describe problems that arise in the therapeutic relationship as a result of clients' lack of power in the treatment room, prior experiences of touch, and their emotional response to treatment and the clinician.
10. Recognize the signs of transference and counter-transference in the therapeutic relationship.
11. Describe actions that the clinician can take to enhance the therapeutic relationship by maintaining ethical conduct, addressing clients' emotional responses to touch, and increasing client adherence to treatment regimens.
12. Describe the four phases of the clinical decision-making process for Outcome-Based Massage:

Evaluative Phase, Treatment Planning Phase, Treatment Phase, and Discharge Phase.
13. Describe how to formulate and select tests and measures to confirm a clinical hypothesis about a client's clinical condition.
14. List the steps in synthesizing clinical findings and creating a clinical problem list.
15. List impairments that clinicians can treat with massage techniques and the outcomes that they can achieve by doing so.
16. Formulate outcomes related to impairments and function that are relevant to the use of massage techniques.
17. Outline how to select massage techniques required to remediate impairments, enhance wellness, and achieve identified functional outcomes.
18. Identify the process by which clinicians use the findings from the client re-examinations to modify, refine, and progress interventions.
19. Describe how to identify the client's discharge needs, plan for discharge, and discharge a client.
20. Describe the unique elements of a client examination for massage.
21. Discuss how to perform palpation.
22. Identify the impairments that can be assessed using palpation.
23. Describe a variety of nonpalpatory approaches to assessing the impairments that are relevant to massage.

Therapists can use Outcome-Based Massage to achieve outcomes for wellness and the treatment of impairments. To prepare them for doing so, this chapter uses a clinical scenario to explain the concept of outcomes and to present frameworks that guide therapists' use of massage for wellness and for the treatment of impairments.

## Massage for Wellness and Impairments: Foundations

## OUTCOME-BASED MASSAGE

In the past, massage practice involved the use of massage routines to achieve specific therapeutic effects.[1] **Outcome-Based Massage** builds on that foundation to provide therapists from a variety of health care disciplines with a strategy for integrating the use of massage techniques into their clinical practice. Outcome-Based Massage has several defining features (Box 1-1). First of all, this approach is a problem-solving approach based on the principles of evidence-based practice, outcomes of care, human functioning, and wellness. It also proposes a system of classifying massage techniques on the basis of the tissue layers that they treat and the outcomes they achieve. Finally, Outcome-Based Massage

also involves the use of a systematic clinical decision-making process and a defined process for identifying outcomes, selecting techniques based on the evidence, and applying those techniques using effective psychomotor skills.

## Outcomes for Massage

Outcomes can be the results of a single **intervention** using massage techniques or of all of the interventions in the **plan of care** as a whole.[2] While massage techniques have a multitude of possible outcomes, not all of these outcomes are appropriate for a massage intervention for a given client. Consequently, the therapist needs to use three steps to determine the appropriate treatment outcomes for a

**Defining Features of Outcome-Oriented, Evidence-Informed Massage**

- Guided by the concept of Intelligent Touch.
- Based on models of functioning, disability and health and wellness models.
- Classifies massage techniques on the basis of the tissue layer they treat and the outcomes they achieve
- Uses a systematic clinical decision-making process for identifying treatment outcomes.
- Uses massage techniques to achieve specific treatment outcomes
- Selects massage techniques based on the evidence for their effects
- Modifies interventions to address the client's interpersonal and physical needs
- Integrates massage techniques into interventions using effective practical skills

client. First, the therapist must understand the potential **therapeutic effects** of massage and the evidence for those effects. The therapist must then identify which of the client's **body structures** and functions can appropriately be treated with massage techniques. This commonly goes

hand in hand with the final step of determining whether the therapist is treating the client's impairments or providing a wellness intervention.

## Therapeutic Effects of Massage Techniques

A massage technique can produce multiple therapeutic effects. These may occur locally, only on the site of manipulation, or generally throughout the client's body. The therapeutic effects of massage techniques fall into six categories: mechanical, physiological, psychological, reflex, psychoneuroimmunological, and "energetic" (Table 1-1).[1,3,11] Mechanical effects result from the therapist physically moving the tissues by compression, tension (stretch), shearing, bending, or twisting. In the case of reflex effects, the client's nervous system mediates therapeutic changes. Physiological effects involve a change in biochemical processes in the client's body. Psychological effects, on the other hand, occur in the client's mind, emotions, or behavior. Psychoneuroimmunological effects are those effects in which changes in hormone levels or immune function accompany changes in a client's feeling state. In this case, the term psychoneuroimmunological emphasizes that feeling states, such as relaxation, actually represent complex multisystem phenomena. Finally, energetic effects are direct effects on the client's biomagnetic field and possible secondary effects on the client's body structures and functions.

## Table 1-1    General Therapeutic Effects of Massage Techniques [1,3]

| Effect[a] | Description | Example Outcome |
|---|---|---|
| Mechanical[b] | Effects are caused by physically moving the tissues by compression, tension (stretch), shearing, bending, or twisting | Increased lymphatic return<br>Mobilized bronchial secretions |
| Reflex[b] | Functional change is mediated by the nervous system | Sedation or arousal<br>Facilitation of skeletal muscle contraction |
| Physiological[b] | Involves a change in biochemical body processes | Improved modeling of connective tissue<br>Reduced muscle spasm |
| Psychological | Effect occurs in the mind, emotions, or behavior | Improved social interaction<br>Improved physical self-image |
| Psychoneuroimmunological | Altered feeling state is accompanied by changes in hormone levels or immune function; this term emphasizes that "mere" feeling states like relaxation represent complex multisystem phenomena | Decreased anxiety and cortisol levels<br>Improved T-cell function |
| Energetic | Direct effects on the client's biomagnetic field and possible secondary effects on client's body structures and functions | Improved biomagnetic field pattern<br>Improved energy flow |

[a]Any given massage technique produces multiple effects, and outcomes are usually achieved through several mechanisms operating simultaneously.
[b]Effects may be local, occurring only on the site of manipulation, or general, occurring throughout the body.

## Critical Thinking Question

What issues must therapists consider when creating lists of outcomes for an intervention that will include massage techniques?

### Body Structures and Functions

Outcome-Based Massage distinguishes between the client's body structures and functions. Body structures are the various anatomical structures and systems of the body (Table 1-2).[4,5] **Body functions**, on the other hand, are the physiological

| **Table 1-2** | Summary of Body Structures and Functions from the ICF [4,5] |
|---|---|
| **Body Structure** | **Body Function** |
| Nervous system: brain, spinal cord, and peripheral nerves | ■ Consciousness<br>■ Orientation (time, place, person)<br>■ Intellect<br>■ Energy and drive functions<br>■ Sleep<br>■ Attention<br>■ Memory<br>■ Emotional functions<br>■ Perceptual functions<br>■ Higher level cognitive functions<br>■ Language<br>■ Pain |
| Eye, ear, and related structures | ■ Seeing<br>■ Hearing<br>■ Vestibular (including balance functions) |
| Structures involved in voice and speech: nose, mouth, pharynx, and larynx | ■ Vocalization<br>■ Articulation<br>■ Rhythm and tempo functions |
| Cardiovascular, hematologic, immunologic, and respiratory systems | ■ Heart functions<br>■ Blood pressure<br>■ Hematologic (blood) functions<br>■ Immunologic (allergies, hypersensitivity) functions<br>■ Respiration |
| Digestive, metabolic, and endocrine systems | ■ Digestive functions<br>■ Defecation<br>■ Weight maintenance<br>■ Endocrine gland functions (hormonal changes) |
| Genitourinary and reproductive systems | ■ Urination functions<br>■ Sexual functions |
| Neuromusculoskeletal structures related to movement: head and neck region, shoulder region, upper extremity (arm, hand), pelvis, lower extremity (leg, foot), trunk, and spine | ■ Mobility of joint<br>■ Muscle power<br>■ Muscle tone<br>■ Involuntary movements |
| Skin and related structures (skin glands, nails, hair) | ■ Protective functions<br>■ Repair functions<br>■ Sensation |

---

| Box 1-2 | **Example of Detailed Body Functions** |
|---|---|

### NEUROMUSCULOSKELETAL AND MOVEMENT-RELATED FUNCTIONS

**Functions of the joints and bones**

■ Mobility of joint: Functions of the range and ease of movement of a joint

■ Stability of joint: Functions of the maintenance of structural integrity of the joints

■ Mobility of bone: Functions of the range and ease of movement of the scapula, pelvis, carpal and tarsal bones

**Muscle functions**

■ Muscle power: Functions related to the force generated by the contraction of a muscle or muscle groups

■ Muscle tone: Functions related to the tension present in the resting muscles and the resistance offered when trying to move the muscles passively

■ Muscle endurance: Functions related to sustaining muscle contraction for the required period of time

---

functions of those anatomical systems (Table 1-2 and Box 1-2). Massage techniques are more appropriate for some body structures and functions than others. For this reason, Table 1-3 provides a detailed list of the body structures and functions that massage techniques can address and some of the associated outcomes that therapists can attain through the use of these techniques.

### Interventions for Wellness Versus the Treatment of Impairments

Although interventions for **wellness** and the treatment of **impairments** differ in several ways, the primary distinction is whether or not the focus of **treatment** is on an impairment in the client's body structure or function. This impairment can be any loss or abnormality of the client's body structures or functions that occur as a result of the **pathophysiology** of a medical condition.[6,7] Wellness interventions are not concerned with addressing the client's impairments. Conversely, for the treatment of impairments, the aim is to reduce the impairments associated with medical conditions. Later sections of this chapter will elaborate on the issues related to outcomes that are specific to wellness versus the treatment of impairments.

# MASSAGE FOR IMPAIRMENTS

## Defining Health

Therapists often use massage to change the impairments that stem from medical conditions in order to help an individual return to an optimal state of **health**. Yet the definition of health used by therapists is often unclear. This definition has evolved since the World Health Organization (WHO) stated in 1948 that: "Health is a state of complete physical, mental and social well-being and not merely the absence of disease or infirmity."[8] Therapists now see health as a dynamic process that encompasses multiple domains, including the individual's physical, emotional, social, and intellectual dimensions.[9] In addition, some definitions of health address the individual's ability to fulfill his or her social roles and respond to environmental stressors.[10] Therapists can use these definitions, and the frameworks they support, to understand their clients' health and functioning and to identify how limitations in body structure, body function, activity capacity, and participation occur. These frameworks can also guide therapists in identifying outcomes for different levels of human functioning and determining the most effective approach to intervention.

## The International Classification of Functioning, Disability and Health

The World Health Organization (WHO) developed the International Classification of Functioning, Disability and Health (ICF) to move away from several earlier concepts. First of all, it shifted the focus from people's **disability** to their levels of health. It also eliminated the notions underlying earlier **Disablement Models** that people move along a linear process from health to disability and that disability begins where health ends (discussed in the Models of Health and Disability section of this chapter). Furthermore, the WHO dispensed with the idea that there are separate categories for people with disabilities and those without; instead, every person can experience some degree of decline in health and an accompanying disability. The resulting model presents human function, health, and disability as an interaction between the individual, the disease process, and the environment in which the individual lives (Figure 1-1). This edition of Outcome-Based Massage uses the ICF model to guide massage for impairments.

In the ICF, the emphasis is on health and functioning in society, regardless of the impairments the individual may experience.[4] The model represents the individual at three levels: body structures and functions, activity, and

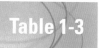

| **Table 1-3** | Body Structures and Functions Amenable to Treatment with Massage and Related Outcomes |
|---|---|

| Impairment in Body Structures and Functions | Outcomes |
|---|---|
| **Musculoskeletal** | |
| ■ Adhesions/scarring | ■ Increased tissue mobility <br> ■ Decreased scarring |
| ■ Impaired connective tissue integrity: fascial restrictions; abnormal connective tissue density; tethering of nerve sheaths and decreased mobility of skin and superficial and deep fascia | ■ Separation and lengthening of fascia <br> ■ Promotion of dense connective tissue remodeling <br> ■ Increased connective tissue mobility |
| ■ Impaired joint integrity: inflammation of joint capsule or ligaments; restrictions of joint capsule and ligaments | ■ Decreased signs of inflammation of joint capsule, tendons, or ligaments <br> ■ Decreased capsular and ligament restrictions <br> ■ Increased joint mobility <br> ■ Increased joint integrity |
| ■ Impaired joint mobility: decreased voluntary range of motion | ■ Increased joint mobility: increased voluntary range of motion |
| ■ Impaired muscle integrity: decreased muscle extensibility; decreased muscle resiliency; tendinopathies; trigger points; muscle strains and tears | ■ Increased muscle extensibility <br> ■ Increased muscle resiliency <br> ■ Decreased signs of inflammation and promotion of healing of tendons <br> ■ Decreased trigger point activity <br> ■ Increased joint mobility <br> ■ Decreased signs of inflammation and promotion of healing of muscle |
| ■ Impaired muscle performance (strength, power, endurance) | ■ Enhanced muscle performance secondary to the enhancement of muscle extensibility, reduction of pain, reduction of muscle spasm, reduction of resting tension, enhancement of joint mobility, normalization of joint integrity, reduction of trigger point activity, etc. <br> ■ Balance of agonist/antagonist muscle function <br> ■ Ease and efficiency of movement |
| ■ Abnormal muscle resting tension and muscle spasm | ■ Decreased muscle spasm <br> ■ Normalized muscle resting tension <br> ■ Increased joint mobility <br> ■ Ease and efficiency of movement |
| ■ Postural malalignment | ■ Normalized postural alignment <br> ■ Increased postural awareness <br> ■ Lengthening of adaptive shortening |
| ■ Swelling: edema, joint effusion, | ■ Decreased joint effusion <br> ■ Decreased edema <br> ■ Increased joint integrity <br> ■ Increased joint mobility |
| **Multisystem** | |
| ■ Impaired sensation secondary to entrapment neuropathy or nerve root compression | ■ Normalized sensation secondary to the reduction of nerve and nerve root compression due to fascial restrictions, postural malalignment, and trigger points |
| ■ Pain | ■ Pain reduction through primary treatment of dysfunction, e.g., active trigger points <br> ■ Counterirritant analgesia <br> ■ Systemic sedation resulting in decreased perception of pain |

*(continued)*

| **Table 1-3** continued | |
|---|---|
| **Impairment in Body Structures and Functions** | **Outcomes** |

**Neurologic**
- Abnormal neuromuscular tone: Spasticity, rigidity, clonus

- Normalized neuromuscular tone
- Alteration of movement responses through proprioceptive and exteroceptive stimulation techniques
- Balance of agonist/antagonist muscle function
- Ease and efficiency of movement

**Cardiovascular**
- Decreased arterial supply
- Decreased venous return
- Increased blood pressure
- Swelling: lymphedema

- Increased arterial supply
- Increased venous return
- Decreased blood pressure
- Increased lymphatic return
- Increased venous return
- Decreased edema
- Increased joint mobility

**Pulmonary**
- Impaired airway clearance

- Increased respiration/gaseous exchange
- Increased airway clearance/mobilization of secretions
- Decreased dyspnea

- Dyspnea

- Decreased dyspnea due to increased airway clearance
- Decreased dyspnea due to increased perceived relaxation

- Decreased rib cage mobility (other than bony abnormality)

- Increased rib cage mobility
- Increased muscle extensibility
- Increased ventilation

**Psychoneuroimmunologic**
- Stress

- Systemic sedation
- Increased perceived relaxation
- Decreased levels of cortisol, epinephrine, and norepinephrine
- Increased levels of serotonin and dopamine
- Increased ability to monitor physical and psychological effects of stress

- Depression

- Improved mood

- Altered body image

- Improved body image and physical self-acceptance

- Immune suppression

- Stimulated immune function

- Altered patterns of sleep

- Improved quantity and quality of sleep

**Gastrointestinal**
- Gastrointestinal immobility secondary to sedentary status

- Stimulated peristalsis

**Central Nervous System**
- Reduced mental focus

- Systemic arousal and enhanced mental focus

- Failure to thrive in high-risk infants

- Promoted weight gain and development through increased vagal activity, sensory organization

- Lethargy

- Sensory arousal and enhanced alertness

**Energetic**
- Less than optimal biomagnetic field pattern
- Reduced energy flow

- Improved biomagnetic field pattern
- Improved energy flow

See references for chapters 6 to 14.

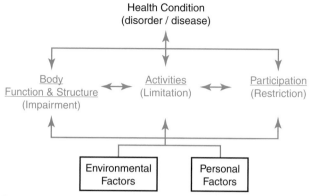

Health Condition
(disorder / disease)

Body
Function & Structure
(Impairment)

Activities
(Limitation)

Participation
(Restriction)

Environmental
Factors

Personal
Factors

**Figure 1-1** ICF: The International Classification of Functioning, Disability and Health. Reprinted from World Health Organization. Towards a common language for functioning, disability and health: ICF: the International Classification of Functioning, Disability and Health. Geneva, Switzerland: World Health Organization; 2002; with permission from the World Health Organization.

participation. As noted previously, body structures are the various anatomical structures and systems of the body (Table 1-2), and body functions are the physiological functions of those anatomical systems (Table 1-2 and Box 1-2). Activity is the individual's execution of a task or action in an ideal situation (Table 1-4). Finally, participation refers to the individual's involvement in a life situation, or his or her ability to execute a task within his environment (Table 1-4). The individual's medical condition, a disease or disorder, affects all three levels of his functioning concurrently. At the same time, the individual's personal and environmental factors, termed here as contextual factors, are all exerting an effect on the individual's body structures and functions, activity, and participation.

The ICF includes a grading system for body structures and functions, activity, participation, and environmental

---

| **Table 1-4** | Activity and Participation Domains from the ICF [4,5] |

**Learning and Applying Knowledge**
- Watching
- Listening
- Learning to read
- Learning to write
- Learning to calculate (arithmetic)
- Solving problems

**General Tasks and Demands**
- Undertaking a single task
- Undertaking multiple tasks

**Communication**
- Communicating with—receiving—spoken messages
- Communicating with—receiving—nonverbal messages
- Speaking
- Producing nonverbal messages
- Conversation

**Mobility**
- Lifting and carrying objects
- Fine hand use (picking up, grasping)
- Walking
- Moving around using equipment (wheelchair, skates, etc.)
- Using transportation (car, bus, train, plane, etc.)
- Driving (riding bicycle or motorbike, driving car, etc.)

**Self-Care**
- Washing oneself (bathing, drying, washing hands, etc.)
- Caring for body parts (brushing teeth, shaving, grooming, etc.)
- Toileting
- Dressing
- Eating
- Drinking
- Looking after one's health

**Domestic Life**
- Acquisition of goods and services (shopping, etc.)
- Preparation of meals (cooking, etc.)
- Doing housework (cleaning house, washing dishes, laundry, ironing, etc.)
- Assisting others

**Interpersonal Interactions and Relationships**
- Basic interpersonal interactions
- Complex interpersonal interactions
- Relating with strangers
- Formal relationships
- Informal social relationships
- Family relationships
- Intimate relationships

**Major Life Areas**
- Informal education
- School education
- Higher education
- Remunerative employment
- Basic economic transactions
- Economic self-sufficiency

**Community, Social, and Civic Life**
- Community life
- Recreation and leisure
- Religion and spirituality
- Human rights
- Political life and citizenship

| Box 1-3 | Grading Criteria for Impairments of Body Structures and Functions [4,5] |
|---|---|

| Grade | Criteria |
|---|---|
| 0 | No impairment; the person has no problem. |
| 1 | Mild impairment; a problem that is present less than 25% of the time with an intensity that a person can tolerate and that happened rarely over the last 30 days. |
| 2 | Moderate impairment; a problem that is present less than 50% of the time with an intensity that is interfering in the person's day-to-day life and that happened occasionally over the last 30 days. |
| 3 | Severe impairment; a problem that is present more than 50% of the time with an intensity that is partially disrupting the person's day-to-day life and that happened frequently over the last 30 days. |
| 4 | Complete impairment; a problem that is present more than 95% of the time with an intensity that is totally disrupting the person's day-to-day life and that happened every day over the last 30 days. |
| 8 | Not specified; there is insufficient information to specify the severity of the impairment. |
| 9 | Not applicable; it is inappropriate to apply a particular code. |

Numbers are as they appear in the original ICF Checklist. Adapted with permission from World Health Organization. *ICF Checklist*. Geneva, Switzerland: World Health Organization; 2003.

factors.[4,8] Impairments in body structure and impairments in body functions are graded separately using a scale (Box 1-3) in which 0 represents an absence of an impairment and 4 represents a complete impairment (8 and 9 are used for unspecified or nonapplicable data). In addition, the ICF assesses problems in body structures on a second dimension—nature of the change—using the 10-point scale shown in Box 1-4. The ICF evaluates activity limitations and participation restrictions across the same domains (Box 1-5) using a scale in which 0 represents no difficulty and 4 represents a complete difficulty (8 and 9 are used for unspecified or nonapplicable data). What differs between the two constructs is the dimension of the task that one assesses. In the case of activity limitations, therapists are concerned with the individual's capacity to execute a task or action without assistance. This represents the highest probable level of functioning for the individual. Participation limitations, on the other hand, reflect how the individual performs the task in her current environment, which can include assistance. Of interest to the therapist is the discrepancy between the individual's capacity for executing the task and her performance in her current environment, a clue to evaluate environmental factors. These environmental factors include: products and technology; natural environment; human changes made to the environment; support and relationships; attitudes of others; and services, systems, and policies. They

receive grades on scales in which 0 represents no barrier or facilitator of an individual's function and 4 represents a complete barrier or facilitator of an individual's function. Finally, the ICF documents personal factors, such as lifestyle, habits, education, and life events, as a means of understanding other factors that could influence the individual's level of functioning.

| Box 1-4 | Additional Grades for Body Structure [4,5] |
|---|---|

| Grade | Criteria |
|---|---|
| 0 | No change in structure |
| 1 | Total absence of structure |
| 2 | Partial absence of structure |
| 3 | Additional part |
| 4 | Aberrant dimensions |
| 5 | Discontinuity |
| 6 | Deviating position |
| 7 | Qualitative changes in structure |
| 8 | Not specified |
| 9 | Not applicable |

Numbers are as they appear in the original ICF Checklist. Adapted with permission from World Health Organization. *ICF Checklist*. Geneva, Switzerland: World Health Organization; 2003.

---

> ## Box 1-5 | Grading Criteria for Activity and Participation[4, 5]
>
> ### Capacity Grade
>
> The degree of difficulty a person has when performing a task or action shows the level of Activity limitation.
>
> ### Performance Grade
>
> The degree of difficulty a person has when performing a task or action in his or her current environment shows the level of Participation restriction.
>
> 0   No difficulty means the person has no problem.
> 1   Mild difficulty means a problem that is present less than 25% of the time with an intensity a person can tolerate and that happened rarely over the last 30 days.
> 2   Moderate difficulty means a problem that is present less than 50% of the time with an intensity that is interfering in the person's day-to-day life and that happened occasionally over the last 30 days.
> 3   Severe difficulty means a problem that is present more than 50% of the time with an intensity that is partially disrupting the person's day-to-day life and that happened frequently over the last 30 days.
> 4   Complete difficulty means a problem that is present more than 95% of the time with an intensity that is totally disrupting the person's day-to-day life and that happened every day over the last 30 days.
> 8   Not specified means there is insufficient information to specify the severity of the difficulty.
> 9   Not applicable means it is inappropriate to apply a particular code.

Numbers are as they appear in the original ICF Checklist. Adapted with permission from World Health Organization. *ICF Checklist.* Geneva, Switzerland: World Health Organization; 2003.

## Client Examination Using the International Classification of Functioning, Disability and Health

Theory in Practice 1-1a clarifies the terminology of the ICF.[4,5]

The client has postural malalignment, which affects her body structures and functions, activity, and participation. The body structures involved are her lumbar spine and her abdominal, hip flexor, and erector spinae muscles. The associated impairments of these body structures are hyperlordosis of the lumbar spine and shortened musculature. The impairments in her body functions, such as pain and muscle weakness, are a consequence of her altered body structure. There are two key contextual factors

---

> ### Theory in Practice 1-1a
> ### Patient with Postural Malalignment
>
> | | |
> |---|---|
> | Patient Profile | ▪ 50-year-old female who is employed as a sales manager has had a recent onset of low back pain following a busy period of traveling. She is overweight because her work and family schedule leave her little time for exercise. She has never been fond of exercising. |
> | Medical Issue | ▪ Postural malalignment (hyperlordosis) and muscular lumbosacral pain |
> | Subjective Findings | ▪ Aching in muscles across her lower back |
> | | ▪ Pain increases with sitting, driving, and standing for >30 minutes |
> | | ▪ Decreased ability to carry out her leisure activities of going to movies and bowling with her children |
> | | ▪ Decreased ability to carry out her role as a sales manager who travels extensively by plane and car |
> | | ▪ Demanding work schedule is necessary because she works partly on commission and has a busy territory |
> | Objective Findings | ▪ Hyperlordotic |
> | | ▪ Tight erector spinae in lumbar region |
> | | ▪ Erector spinae in lumbar region tender on palpation |
> | | ▪ Tight iliopsoas muscles bilaterally |
> | | ▪ Weak abdominal muscles–unable to perform >2 crunches |

affecting this client. The personal factors are her dislike of exercise and her perceived decrease in her **quality of life**. The environmental barrier of a busy schedule of traveling results in increased exposure to activities that aggravate her pain and decreased time for exercise and treatment, which limit the level of function that she may be able to achieve. The result of the interaction among the body structures and functions, medical condition, and contextual factors is that the client has limitations in her capacity to perform work-related activities and leisure activities. Furthermore, she experiences restrictions in her participation in her life situation, namely a decreased ability to perform in and enjoy the activities of her social roles as a sales manager and a parent.

The problem list in Theory in Practice 1-1b summarizes this client's impairments and limitations that will form the basis for determining outcomes for her massage intervention.

## Massage Outcomes for Impairments

The therapist's final step is to determine which outcomes are relevant for the client's needs and the intent of the intervention. In the case of an intervention for the treatment of impairments, the therapist will have a list of impairments in body structures and functions and outcomes that revolve around the treatment of impairments, **recovery**, and the **prevention** of secondary impairments.[11] Theory in Practice 1-1c shows the client's impairments in body structures and functions and some relevant outcomes.

This list of impairments and associated outcomes contains several outcomes that cannot be achieved directly

---

**Theory in Practice 1-1b**

**Patient Problem List Using the International Classification of Functioning, Disability and Health[4,5]**

**1.** Impairments in body structure
- Hyperlordotic
- Tight erector spinae in lumbar region
- Tight iliopsoas muscles bilaterally
- Increased abdominal girth

**2.** Impairments in body function
- Muscular pain in lumbar region
- Weak abdominal muscles

**3.** Activity limitations
- Decreased ability to carry out her role as a sales manager who travels extensively by plane and car
- Decreased ability to carry out her leisure activities of going to movies and bowling with her children

**4.** Participation restrictions
- Inability to perform job of sales manager
- Inability to perform social role as a parent

**5.** Environmental factors
- Demanding work schedule with a lot of traveling

**6.** Personal factors
- Dislike of exercising
- Perceived decreased quality of life and ability to function in and enjoy her social roles as sales manager and parent

---

**Theory in Practice 1-1c**

**Massage Outcomes for the Treatment of Impairments**

| Impairments in Body Structures and Functions | Outcomes |
|---|---|
| Postural malalignment: hyperlordotic | Normalized lumbar spine posture |
| | Improved postural awareness |
| Tight erector spinae muscles in lumbar region | Increased extensibility of erector spinae muscles |
| | Decreased muscle resting tension in erector spinae muscles |
| Tight iliopsoas muscles bilaterally | Increased extensibility of iliopsoas muscles |
| Muscular pain in lumbar region | Decreased muscular pain in lumbar erector spinae muscles |
| | Systemic sedation resulting in decreased perception of pain |
| Weak abdominal muscles | Increased functional strength of abdominal muscles; able to perform abdominal bracing during functional activities and maintain correct pelvic alignment |
| Imbalance of agonist-antagonist muscle function | Enhanced balance of agonist-antagonist muscle function |

| Table 1-5 | Sample Functional Outcomes |
| --- | --- |

| **Activities of Daily Living** | **General Outcomes** |
| --- | --- |
| ■ Increased ability to perform grooming tasks, such as bathing and dressing<br>■ Increased ability to perform work-related tasks, such as lifting and keyboarding<br>■ Increased ability to perform leisure tasks<br>■ Increased ability to perform transfers, such as sit to stand<br>■ Increased ability to perform bed mobility tasks, such as rolling from side to side or scooting<br>■ Increased ability to perform gait and locomotion tasks<br>■ Increased ability to perform functional mobility tasks, such as toilet and bath transfers<br>■ Increased ability to perform cooking tasks<br>■ Improved quality or quantity of movement during functional activity<br>■ Improved safety during functional activity<br>■ Decreased level of supervision required for task performance<br>■ Increased tolerance for positions and activities | ■ Improved self-management of condition<br>■ Decreased risk of recurrence of condition<br>■ Improved decision making regarding health issues<br>■ Reduced utilization and cost of health care services<br>■ Decreased need for adaptive, assistive, supportive, protective, or orthotic equipment or devices<br>■ Ability to recognize and seek intervention for a recurrence of the clinical condition<br>■ Decreased intensity of care required |

Adapted with permission from American Physical Therapy Association. *Guide to Physical Therapist Practice*. 2nd ed. Alexandria, VA: American Physical Therapy Association; 1999. This material is copyrighted, and any further reproduction or distribution is prohibited.

through the use of massage techniques. Consequently, the practitioner needs to select those impairments that are amenable to treatment with massage techniques prior to finalizing the list of desired treatment outcomes. Using Table 1-3 as a guideline will produce the following list of impairments and outcomes for massage.

| Impairments in Body Structures and Functions | Massage Outcomes |
| --- | --- |
| ■ Postural malalignment: hyperlordotic<br>■ Tight erector spinae muscles in lumbar region<br><br><br>■ Tight iliopsoas muscles bilaterally<br>■ Muscular pain in lumbar region<br><br><br><br>■ Imbalance of agonist-antagonist muscle function in lumbar and pelvic regions | ■ Improved postural awareness<br>■ Increased extensibility of erector spinae muscles<br>■ Decreased muscle resting tension in erector spinae muscles<br>■ Increased extensibility of iliopsoas muscles<br>■ Decreased muscular pain in lumbar erector spinae muscles<br>■ Systemic sedation resulting in decreased perception of pain<br>■ Enhanced balance of agonist-antagonist muscle function in lumbar and pelvic regions |

Based on this list of outcomes for massage, the therapist can select massage techniques whose therapeutic effects will achieve the desired outcomes. The chapters on massage techniques include tables that document possible outcomes for individual massage techniques to guide your clinical decision making.

Finally, the therapist is also wise to consider the changes in the client's levels of activity and participation expected from a treatment approach. These are functional outcomes (Table 1-5) that provide meaningful changes for the client and justification for reimbursement for services. Theory in Practice 1-1d shows a sample of relevant functional

### Theory in Practice 1-1d

## Functional Outcomes to Address Limitations in Activity and Participation

■ Patient initiates functional activity readily without fear of pain.

■ Patient is able sit for >30 minutes while traveling in a car or plane without complaints of pain.

■ Patient is able to walk carrying a briefcase >20 minutes without complaints of pain.

■ Patient is able to bowl for >30 minutes without complaints of pain.

outcomes for the client with postural malalignment and muscular low back pain. Note that functional outcomes are an indirect result of the use of massage techniques, rather than outcomes that are specific to the individual massage techniques.

### Critical Thinking Question

What steps can a therapist take to ensure that he can achieve the outcomes he has established for his client using a given set of massage techniques?

## MASSAGE FOR WELLNESS

It is a common misconception that "wellness massage" does not require a sound foundation of clinical reasoning and a systematic outcome-based approach to intervention. Therapists working in the area of wellness are better able to help their clients achieve optimal wellness when they provide massage interventions that are directed at achieving outcomes for wellness, rather than "back rubs." Clear definitions and models of wellness can provide the foundation for the effective use of massage to achieve wellness outcomes.

### Definition of Wellness

Health care professionals now define wellness as encompassing both a balance of "mind, body, and spirit" and individuals' self-perception of their well-being, which is distinct from their state of "health."[10,12] In other words, a person can consider himself as having a high level of wellness, even though he has a medical condition that leaves him with suboptimal health in one or more of the domains of health. For example, people who are living with chronic illnesses, disabilities, or medical conditions associated with age are still capable of experiencing high levels of wellness. Further-more, treatment of their medical conditions can contribute to an increase in their overall level of wellness.

### The Wellness Interactions Model

The distinction between wellness and health has become less well defined as the definition of health has expanded. Nevertheless, there are models of wellness that provide a different perspective on treatment than those models associated with the treatment of impairments.

The **Wellness Interactions Model** (WIM) created for Outcome-Based Massage is based on the ICF.[4] It does not have a continuum or progression through varying levels of disease and health to wellness. Instead, it shows an ongoing interaction between a person, wellness, and his or her environment (Figure 1-2). In this model, an individual's level of wellness can affect any aspect of his or her person at any point in life, and vice versa. At the same time, that individual exists within an environment in which the barriers and facilitators to wellness will influence his or her level of wellness.

In the WIM, a person has multiple dimensions: spirit, brain and body structures and function, activity capacity, ability to participate in society, and wellness behaviors. Spirit, a concept that is not part of traditional models of health, refers to that part of a person's nonphysical being that embodies his or her drive to transcend the physical world.[12-14] As in the ICF, body and brain structures are the various anatomical structures and systems of the body and brain. Body and brain functions, on the other hand, are the physiological functions of the anatomical systems (Table 1-2). In the case of wellness, however, the relevant body structures and functions are those that are free of impairments—grade 0 (Box 1-3). Activity capacity is the individual's ability to execute a task or action in an ideal situation (Table 1-4). In addition, ability to participate in society refers to the individual's performance of those tasks in his or her environment (Table 1-4). Wellness behaviors are personal factors

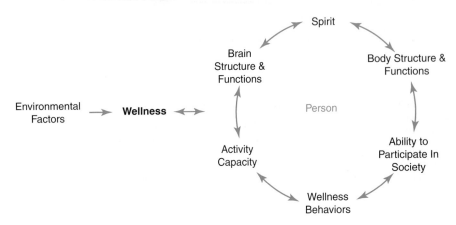

**Figure 1-2** The Wellness Interactions Model.

that play a central role in wellness, such as self-nurturance, healthy lifestyles, readiness for change, and perceived health.[11,15,16] Finally, the WIM highlights the importance of environmental factors: facilitators and barriers to wellness that the individual encounters in his or her social setting. The factors that can affect wellness are many and varied and can include social attitudes, available wellness services, education, and the individual's financial status.[4]

## Critical Thinking Question

What are the differences between health and wellness?

## Client Examination Using the Wellness Interactions Model

In this case, the client does not present with impairments in body structures and function that are secondary to a medical condition. Instead, the client has several body structures and functions that will become the focus of a wellness intervention (Theory in Practice 1-2a). The therapist will examine these structures and functions to ensure that they are free of impairments prior to embarking on a wellness intervention that targets these areas.

| Relevant Body Structures | Relevant Body Functions |
|---|---|
| Structure of the nervous system<br>▪ Brain | Mental functions<br>▪ Energy and drive functions<br>▪ Emotional functions |
| Neuromusculoskeletal and movement-related structure<br>▪ Spine<br>▪ Pelvis | Neuromusculoskeletal and movement-related functions<br>▪ Mobility of joints<br>▪ Stability of joints |
| Muscles of the upper and lower extremities and trunk | ▪ Muscle power functions<br>▪ Muscle resting tension |

## Massage Outcomes for Wellness

In the absence of impairments that stem from a medical condition, the therapist will have a list of relevant body structures and functions and associated outcomes for wellness. These outcomes are directed at optimizing the client's body structures and functions. Theory in Practice 1-2b identifies outcomes for the use of massage for wellness.

### Theory in Practice 1-2a

#### Patient Examination Using the Wellness Interactions Model

| Examination Component | Details |
|---|---|
| Patient Profile | ▪ 65-year-old retired male. He prides himself on being in good shape; he runs daily and regularly does weight training and yoga. |
| Subjective Findings | ▪ He has several wellness goals:<br>  ▪ Prevent stress-related symptoms<br>  ▪ Improve his postural awareness<br>  ▪ Promote faster recovery from exercise<br>  ▪ Maintain muscle strength |
| Objective Findings | ▪ Musculoskeletal system within normal limits |

### Theory in Practice 1-2b

#### Patient Outcomes for Wellness

| Body Structure or Function | Outcomes for Optimizing Wellness |
|---|---|
| ▪ Energy and drive functions | ▪ Increased systemic sedation<br>▪ Increased perceived relaxation<br>▪ Decreased levels of cortisol, norepinephrine, and epinephrine |
| Neuromusculoskeletal and movement-related structures<br>▪ Spine<br>▪ Pelvis<br>▪ Muscles of the upper and lower extremities and trunk | ▪ Enhanced postural awareness<br>▪ Normalized muscle resting tension<br>▪ Enhanced muscular performance<br>▪ Increased ease and efficiency of movement |

Consultation with Table 1-3 shows that all of these outcomes for the client in Theory in Practice 1-2b can be achieved using massage techniques. Therefore, the final step of determining the outcomes for this client's wellness intervention is complete.

### ? Critical Thinking Question

How can a therapist determine if a body structure or function is appropriate for a wellness intervention or for the treatment of impairments?

## COMPARISON OF MASSAGE FOR WELLNESS AND THE TREATMENT OF IMPAIRMENTS

There are several similarities and differences between the use of massage for the treatment of impairments and the use for wellness (Table 1-6). Of critical importance are the similarities in clinical reasoning, client examination, and outcome setting. Massage for both the treatment of impairments and wellness requires a clinical reasoning process in which therapists perform a systematic client examination and establish outcomes to guide the intervention. As noted earlier in this chapter, the primary distinction between interventions for the treatment of impairments and those for wellness is the presence or absence of impairments. Treatment of impairments takes place after an individual has experienced a medical condition and addresses those impairments in body structures and functions (grades 1 to 4) that are the result of that medical condition (Theory in Practice 1-1). The therapist creates a list of impairments and a list of outcomes that are focused on the treatment of impairments, **recovery**, and the prevention of **secondary impairments**. This is in contrast to wellness, which focuses on body structures and functions that are free of impairments (Theory in Practice 1-2). In this case, the therapist creates a list of body structures and functions and outcomes for optimizing these structures and function. Despite this distinction between the treatment of impairments and wellness interventions, in day-to-day practice, many therapists call the treatment of stress-related disorders "wellness." By definition, this treatment of stress-related disorders, such as anxiety or increased muscle tension, is "the treatment of impairments," whereas stress-management inter-

| **Table 1-6** | Comparison of Interventions for Treating Impairments and Wellness Interventions | |
|---|---|---|
| | **Treatment of Impairments** | **Wellness Interventions** |
| Timing of intervention | ■ After the medical condition occurs | ■ At any time in the individual's life |
| Focus of intervention | ■ Signs and symptoms of the medical condition<br>■ Impairments in body structures and functions with grades 1 to 4 | ■ Body structures and functions with impairments of grade 0 (no impairment) |
| Client examination | ■ Examine body structures and functions<br>■ Identify impairments resulting from the medical condition | ■ Examine body structures and functions<br>■ Identify body structures and functions that are relevant to the individual's goals for wellness |
| Overall goal of intervention | ■ Identify and manage impairments resulting from the medical condition | ■ Optimize well-being across physical, mental, spiritual, and social domains |
| Clinical reasoning process | ■ Complete clinical reasoning process | ■ Complete clinical reasoning process |
| Outcomes | ■ Specified outcomes related to identified impairments in body structures and functions<br>■ Based on specific therapeutic effects of massage | ■ Specified outcomes related to identified body structures and functions<br>■ Based on specific therapeutic effects of massage |

ventions that prevent impairments and optimize function are "wellness" interventions.

### Critical Thinking Question

How will the list of clinical issues and associated outcomes differ if the therapist is planning an intervention for wellness versus an intervention for the treatment of impairments?

# CLINICAL FRAMEWORKS FOR OUTCOME-BASED MASSAGE

Two frameworks guide the clinical application of massage techniques in Outcome-Based Massage. First, Intelligent Touch defines the skills that therapists need for successful application of massage techniques. Second, the taxonomy of massage techniques, presented in this chapter, is a novel approach to categorizing massage techniques that is consistent with the aims of Outcome-Based Massage.

## Intelligent Touch

The framework of "Intelligent Touch" defines six skills that we believe therapists must master before they can use massage techniques successfully. These skills are attention and concentration, discrimination, identification, inquiry, and intention. The premise of this model is that therapists who lack, or are deficient in their ability to perform, any of these skills may be unable to achieve the identified outcomes of the techniques consistently. Consequently, we suggest that an effective therapist should not only learn these skills but also practice them continuously.

### Attention and Concentration

Attention and concentration refer to therapists' capacity to focus on the sensory information that they receive primarily, but not exclusively, through their hands. Therapists must learn to focus their awareness on selected aspects of the sensory field at hand and to constantly analyze and organize the many types of information that they obtain. Tissue temperature, texture, and tension are the most basic characteristics that therapists can sense and compare through multiple tissue layers and in different anatomical structures. Massage that therapists perform mechanically or mindlessly, without continuous attention to a broad spectrum of sensory information that is available, produces less than optimal results.

### Discrimination

Discrimination, within the context of Outcome-Based Massage, refers to therapists' ability to distinguish fine gradations of sensory information. With practice, therapists can begin to identify more refined types of sensory information such as tissue characteristics and responses to movement or applied force. Discriminative ability varies widely among novice therapists and can improve with education. Furthermore, although discriminative ability is a fairly common gift, novice therapists may require numerous hours of practice performing massage techniques before their discriminative ability is adequate for independent clinical practice.

### Identification

Therapists must be able to distinguish between healthy and dysfunctional tissue states. In addition, they must be able to identify structures and their response to applied forces. Identification is the component of intelligent touch that benefits the most from formal training in anatomy including: the examination of skeletons, palpation of live bodies, and, ideally, the exploration of cadavers while referencing a well-illustrated anatomical atlas.

### Inquiry

Intelligent touch is inquiring touch. Good therapists are constantly asking questions. The use of massage is no exception to this requirement. Using inquiring touch does not imply that the therapist's touch feels tentative to the client or that it lacks firmness. Instead, it reflects the never-ending set of questions that inform intelligent touch such as: What is this tissue? How does the feel of this tissue relate to the client's history? How does this relate to the client's symptoms? How does this compare to the feel of this type of tissue in other places in the client's body? How does this compare to other healthy and dysfunctional tissues that I have palpated in the past? The process of inquiry requires that therapists make a constant comparison among the tissues they are palpating, other tissues in the client's body, and their memory of other tissues they have palpated.

### Intention

The final element of intelligent touch is intention. Intention refers to the therapist's aim of using massage techniques to produce a more normalized response of the client's tissues or other structures. Consequently, intention depends on the therapist having a clear notion of the feel of improvements in the function of tissue and other structures that can arise during the application of any given massage technique. Therapists also need to understand how this improved feel relates to outcomes for body structures and functions, as well as functional outcomes. Therapists who have clear intentions know how both healthy and dysfunctional tissues respond to massage. In addition, they work to produce as close to the ideal tissue response as possible, given the constraints of the client's characteristics and the clinical setting.

## Taxonomy of Massage Techniques

Several systems name classical (Swedish) massage techniques in reference to the motions of the therapist: gliding, kneading, rubbing, shaking, and hitting. Therapists have added many "modern" terms to these basic terms, which often reference an originator's name or a foreign language descriptor. We believe that the final effect is incongruous and without a sound clinical rationale. The classification system retained from the first edition of *Outcome-Based Massage* seeks to avoid some of the limitations of these two approaches to classification.

This text intentionally avoids the division into "classical" and "modern" service-marked methods. In doing so, we recognize that several innovative massage or "body work" methods have influenced the contemporary practice of massage substantially and give these methods their due acknowledgement. Nevertheless, we can organize almost all modern and classical techniques into six clusters of related techniques (Box 1-6), to which we have applied names that we trust make sense to readers.

Therapists apply the structured touch of massage in a specific manner in order to achieve selected therapeutic outcomes. Consequently, the therapeutic effects or possible outcomes of techniques are important when classifying massage techniques. Techniques cannot, however, be classified based solely on their therapeutic effects because a given technique can produce multiple outcomes. For this reason, we base our taxonomy for massage techniques on anatomy, operational requirements, and outcomes. First, we present those techniques that are directed towards superficial tissues. Second, we present those techniques that affect deeper tissues. Third, we present those techniques that affect multiple tissue layers. In addition, we group methods that require the therapist to palpate and observe similar phenomena together. Finally, we place those techniques that require therapists to acquire simpler skills before those techniques that require complex skills.

We use these criteria to define four broad categories of massage techniques that engage particular types of tissue: superficial reflex techniques, superficial fluid techniques, neuromuscular techniques, and connective tissue techniques. These criteria also produce two categories of techniques that engage multiple tissue layers: passive movement techniques and percussive techniques. Techniques in each of these six categories have specific therapeutic effects. In addition, the techniques in the first five categories may produce psychoneuroimmunological effects, such as the reduction of stress.[14]

### Superficial Reflex Techniques

These techniques engage only the skin and may produce reflex effects, such as hyperstimulation analgesia, but no mechanical effects.

### Superficial Fluid Techniques

These techniques engage skin, superficial fascia, and subcutaneous fat down to the investing layer of the deep fascia. They produce mechanical effects on superficial lymphatics and possibly the venous circulation.

### Neuromuscular Techniques

These techniques engage muscle and the tissues it contains. They affect the function of the contractile element, connective tissue hydration, and lymphatic return. They may also produce complex reflex effects.

### Connective Tissue Techniques

These techniques engage superficial and deep layers of connective tissue. They mechanically affect the hydration,

| Box 1-6 | **Categories of Massage Technique** |
| --- | --- |

Superficial reflex techniques
Superficial fluid techniques
Neuromuscular techniques
Connective tissue techniques
Passive movement techniques
Percussive techniques

extensibility, and modeling of connective tissue. They may also produce complex reflex effects.

## *Passive Movement Techniques*

These techniques produce substantial tissue or joint motion without effort on the part of the client. They engage multiple tissues and structures and have wide-ranging effects on fluid flow, connective tissue, and the neural control of muscle tone.

## *Percussive Techniques*

These techniques deform and release tissues quickly. They engage different tissues depending on the force with which therapists apply them. Therapists use them primarily in cardiopulmonary rehabilitation to assist bronchial drainage and airway clearance mechanically. They may also produce useful reflex neuromuscular effects.

## REVIEWING THE BASICS

The International Classification of Functioning, Disability and Health and the Wellness Interactions Model, the principles of **evidence-based medicine**, and the concept of

**Intelligent Touch** combine to provide the theoretical framework for Outcome-Based Massage. In Outcome-Based Massage, therapists evaluate a client's body structures and functions, levels of activity and participation, and contextual factors and use this information to define which body structures and functions need to be addressed in their interventions. Whenever relevant, they use findings on the client's limitations in activity and participation to define functional outcomes that they can reasonably expect to achieve through the intervention. Within the model for treating impairments, therapists treat the client's impairments in body structures and functions as a means of enhancing the client's level of activity and participation and decreasing the client's impairments. In wellness interventions, therapists direct their interventions towards the client's body structures and functions as a means of optimizing wellness. In both treatment approaches, therapists re-evaluate the client's body structures and functions to refine their selection of treatment techniques from the taxonomy of six types of techniques. Finally, they re-evaluate the client's body structures and functions and levels of activity and participation to determine when to terminate based on the client's achievement of identified outcomes.

## Massage for Wellness and Impairments: Further Study and Practice

## STRUCTURE, PROCESS, AND OUTCOMES OF MASSAGE INTERVENTIONS

Earlier sections introduced the concept of outcomes of **clinical care**. Clinicians provide clinical care to their clients as they conduct their examinations and interventions. Although the outcomes of massage interventions have generated much excitement, outcomes are but one of the three components of clinical care defined by Donabedian.[2] The other two components, which are equally important, are the structure and process of clinical care (Figure 1-3). This section will discuss each of these components of clinical care in greater detail using Theory in Practice 1-3a to illustrate key points.

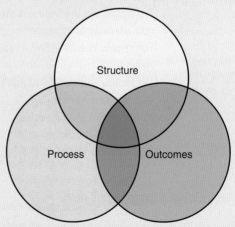

**Figure 1-3** Components of clinical care. Adapted from Donabedian A. Evaluating the quality of medical care. *Milbank Q.* 1966;3:166–206; with the permission of *Milbank Quarterly.*

## Theory in Practice 1-3a

### Patient with Carpal Tunnel Syndrome

| | |
|---|---|
| Patient Profile | 30-year-old male, who is employed as a data entry clerk, has long-standing carpal tunnel syndrome on the right side as a result of long periods of keyboarding. |
| Medical Condition and Pathophysiology | Carpal tunnel syndrome |
| | Inflammation of the wrist and finger flexor tendons in the region of the carpal tunnel |
| | Inflammation results in pressure on the median nerve as it passes through the carpal tunnel |
| Subjective Findings | Pain in fingers and hand |
| | Inability to perform customary job-related activities, especially typing, filing, and writing |
| | Inability to perform leisure activity of playing racquetball |
| | Inability to perform activities of daily living, especially grooming and household tasks that involve lifting |
| | Fear of experiencing pain during functional activity |
| | Inability to carry out social roles as a data entry clerk and a member of a racquetball club |
| | Limited health insurance to cover the cost of treatment for carpal tunnel syndrome |
| Objective Findings | Edema in the region of the carpal tunnel |
| | Paresthesia in the fingers in the median nerve distribution |
| | Decreased wrist and finger range of motion |
| | Weakness and atrophy of thenar muscles and lumbricals |
| | Weakness of wrist muscles |
| | Wears a wrist splint |

## Structure of Care

According to Donabedian,[2] the **structure of care** is the human, physical, and financial resources available for delivering care. This includes the staff, the clinical environment, and the organization's financing, among other resources. Often, despite the clinician's best intentions, the structure in which she provides care has an impact on her approach to treatment. Consider the situation of the clinician treating the client with carpal tunnel syndrome (Theory in Practice 1-3a and b) in a busy outpatient setting with restrictions on reimbursement for services, 20-minute treatment sessions, and a high proportion of aides assisting with treatment delivery. This setting presents different constraints and benefits than those that the clinician would encounter in an on-site occupational injury center with 45-minute treatment sessions, few adjunct personnel, and a flexible reimbursement structure. A clinician treating clients with industrial injuries in the busy outpatient setting is less likely to have time for extensive use of hands-on massage techniques and will have a greater component of education in self-care than the clinician treating the client in the on-site occupational rehabilitation setting. For this reason, clinicians need to be aware of the context in which they treat their clients, even though this will not be an explicit component of treatment planning.

## Theory in Practice 1-3b

### Examples of Structure of Clinical Care

**Human Resources**

| | |
|---|---|
| Organization of staff | Interdisciplinary team |
| Number and distribution of staff | 6 clinicians, 1 aide, 2 administrative staff |
| Qualifications and training of staff | 1 MD, 1 physical therapist, 1 occupational therapist, 1 massage therapist, 1 rehabilitation aide |

**Physical and Financial Resources**

| | |
|---|---|
| Size of facility | 6 rooms on a single floor |
| Geographic location of facility | On-site at large software company |
| Organization of facility | Central gym, reception area, and 4 treatment rooms |
| Equipment available | Fully equipped treatment rooms |
| Formal financing | Software company contracts with occupational rehabilitation company |

## Process of Care

The **process of care** is the manner in which the clinician delivers care.[2] It refers to how the activities between the clinician and the client take place. There are two aspects to the process of care: the technical aspects of how the clinician provides care and the interpersonal aspects of the client–clinician interaction. The importance of the process of care cannot be emphasized enough. Clinicians need to understand the process by which they deliver care to their clients in order to improve their interventions. This understanding can also enable them to identify whether they can improve the outcomes they achieve by changing the process of care—the manner in which they deliver care.

### Technical Aspects of the Process of Care

The appropriateness and adequacy of the examination performed, the clinician's evaluation of the client's presenting problems, the intervention plan outlined, and the interventions selected and provided by the clinician are the technical aspects of the process of care that are most relevant to the practicing clinician.[2] Examination, evaluation, treatment planning, and intervention are interdependent processes within the clinical decision-making process. For example, a clinician's failure to evaluate the relevant impairments related to the client's medical condition adequately will lead to an intervention that does not effectively address the client's impairments. As a result, it is less likely that the client's functional limitations that result from these impairments will improve with treatment. In the case of a client with carpal tunnel syndrome (Theory in Practice 1-3a), if the clinician evaluated only strength and paresthesia, the intervention he or she provided would fail to address the pain that could be limiting his ability to perform functional activities and contributing to his other symptoms. As later chapters will discuss, a clinician can use regular re-examination of the client's status to monitor the adequacy of the intervention he or she is providing. This will provide the clinician with several opportunities for refining the intervention and for enhancing the technical process of care delivery.

### Interpersonal Aspects of the Process of Care

The client and the clinician are typically the central players in the process of clinical care.[2] They engage in a clinical relationship, which is often referred to as the **therapeutic relationship**. The list of interpersonal aspects of the process of care in Theory in Practice 1-3c can serve as a reminder

---

**Theory in Practice 1-3c**

### Aspects of the Process of Clinical Care

**Technical Aspects**

- Utilization patterns
- Appropriateness of referrals
- Completeness of diagnosis
- Appropriateness of examinations and evaluations performed by practitioners
- Adequacy of interventions selected and provided by practitioners
- Relevance of treatment goals set by practitioners
- Patterns of treatment by practitioners

**Interpersonal Aspects**

Patient
- Patient's physical and psychological characteristics
- Patient's expectations of treatment
- Level of patient participation in care

Practitioner
- Practitioner's interpersonal skills
- Practitioner's skill as an educator
- Patient–practitioner interaction
- Patient–practitioner communication
- Level of patient adherence to plan of care

---

of the importance of the therapeutic relationship and the impact that it can have on clinical outcomes.

Three components make up the interpersonal aspects of the delivery of care.[2] At the heart of clinical care lies the client and all of the things that he brings into treatment, such as physical and psychological characteristics, family history, lifestyle, work and home environment, and belief systems. In addition, the client enters treatment with expectations for treatment and outcomes that will affect the treatment process whether or not the clinician inquires about these expectations. The clinician's interpersonal manner is the second component. A clinician's primary purpose is not merely to implement treatment plans. In reality, the clinician's ability to engage, educate, motivate, and support the client throughout the treatment process is as important as the clinician's technical skill. The interaction between client and clinician is the third component. The quality of this interaction can shape the level of client adherence, client motivation, and in many ways, the results of the plan of care. Therefore, the clinician is wise to engage the client

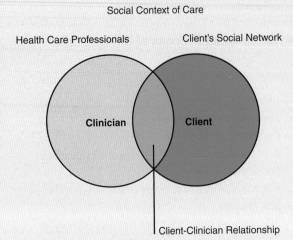

Figure 1-4  Social context of care.

in the therapeutic process, to solicit and respect the client's input on the plan of care and treatment outcomes, to consider the context in which the client lives and works, and to seek the client's feedback throughout the course of treatment. This is particularly true in the clinical use of massage techniques because the use of touch can raise issues related to personal vulnerability, emotional responses to treatment, and the need to set appropriate boundaries between the client and clinician.

Rarely is the interpersonal process of clinical care limited to the interactions that occur between the client and clinician; typically, this process occurs within a larger social context (Figure 1-4).[2] First, the health care setting may include a variety of health care professionals with whom both clinician and client may interact. In addition, the client has a social network of caregivers, relatives, and others who may participate in, or have an impact on, the process of clinical care. The complexity of the interactions will vary with the clinical setting, the client, and the client's presenting medical condition. For example, a clinician who is treating a geriatric client with a stroke in a rehabilitation setting will have to manage numerous interactions over the course of treatment. These may include interactions with the client, the client's family, the other members of the health care team in the rehabilitation setting, and possibly some community-based resources for the family. On the other hand, the clinician who is treating the client with carpal tunnel syndrome (Theory in Practice 1-3a) in the on-site occupational injury center will only have to interact with the client, the referring physician, and, perhaps, the client's supervisor.

## Critical Thinking Question
What are the differences between the structure and the process of care?

## Outcomes of Care

As noted earlier in this chapter, outcomes can be the result of a single intervention using massage techniques or of all of the interventions in the care plan as a whole.[2] There are a number of ways to measure **outcomes of care**. Administrators may be more concerned with cost-effectiveness, the efficiency of care, and client satisfaction. Clinicians, on the other hand, may look at the short-term and long-term effects of care on the client's body structures and function, levels of activity and participation, and overall wellness. Clients, in turn, bring their own perspective on the relevant effects of care on their impairments, functional limitations, and quality of life.

Regardless of the type of outcome selected, the clinician needs to be cautious not to overemphasize outcomes and ignore the structure and process of care. In reality, a clinician needs to understand and evaluate the structure and process of care to determine why the intervention was successful or not. Furthermore, the danger always exists that a clinician may discard a potentially effective intervention because the outcomes achieved were poor when, in fact, the problem lay in the manner in which the intervention was delivered (process of care). A holistic, client-centered intervention will, therefore, consider the structure, process, and outcomes of clinical care.

## Critical Thinking Question
What are the components of care that can affect the outcomes achieved by a clinician?

# MODELS OF HEALTH AND DISABILITY

Earlier sections of this chapter introduced the International Classification of Health, Disability and Functioning (ICF). There are several other theoretical frameworks of health and disability that preceded that model. This section will examine the Disablement Models that clinicians use to guide interventions in health care.

## Disablement Models

Prior to the emphasis on models of disablement, clinicians used the **Medical Model**, which focused on measuring and treating the client's presenting impairments without a specific consideration of the client's other personal factors. This approach evolved as the models of disablement provided a

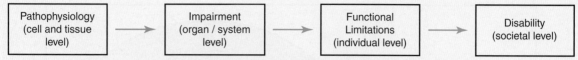

Figure 1-5 Modified Nagi model of disablement. Reprinted with adaptations from Pope A, Tarlov A, eds. *Disability in America: Toward a National Agenda for Prevention.* Washington, DC: National Academy Press; 1991:9; with the permission of the National Academy Press.

new perspective from which to view clinical care. This perspective broadened the clinician's approach to examination, evaluation, and treatment to encompass the client's functional limitations and disability, as well as his or her presenting impairments.[6,7] In addition, there was also a greater acknowledgment of the impact of society as a whole on a client's potential level of function. For example, a clinician who used the Medical Model in the treatment of a client would address the client's physical impairments in the clinical treatment planning. By contrast, a clinician who was treating the client using the Disablement Models would also assess the client's functional and societal limitations and address these in treatment planning as appropriate.

The modified Nagi model (Figure 1-5) is one of the earlier Disablement Models.[6] The National Center for Medical Rehabilitation Research (NCMRR)[7] Model of Disablement (Figure 1-6) incorporates the International Classification of Impairments, Disabilities, and Handicaps (ICIDH) and the Nagi Functional Limitations Model.[6,7] The modified Nagi model and the NCMRR model define four basic components of the process of disablement: pathophysiology, impairment, **functional limitations**, and disability. The NCMRR

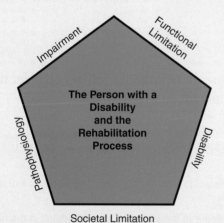

Figure 1-6 National Center for Medical Rehabilitation Research's model of components of the disablement process. Reprinted with permission from the National Institute of Child Health and Human Development. Research plan for the National Center for Medical Rehabilitation Research. Public Health Service NIH Publication No. 93-3509. Bethesda, MD: National Institutes of Health, US Department of Health and Human Services; 1993.

model includes a fifth component, societal limitations, and places the person with the disability and the rehabilitation process at the center of the model to emphasize their importance.

Jette[17] added health-related quality of life to the Disablement Model. He defined health-related quality of life as individuals' ability to function in and derive satisfaction from their social roles when their health status is impaired. For the sake of completeness, he included both the objective and subjective aspects of experience. In the resulting model (Figure 1-7), health-related quality of life is related to both functional limitations and disability.

In these Disablement Models, used in the first edition of *Outcome-Based Massage* and the second edition of the *Guide to Physical Therapist Practice*, the disablement process follows a linear course, with some bidirectional relationships.[6,7,17,18] The pathophysiology occurs at the cellular level. It is the disease, syndrome, or lesion that interferes with the body's normal processes or structures. An impairment, loss, or abnormality of the affected individual's physiological, anatomical, cognitive, or emotional structure or function occurs as a result of the initial or subsequent pathophysiology. Physical and psychological impairments lead to a functional limitation: a restriction of the individual's ability to perform actions or activities within the range considered normal for the organ or organ system. A disability occurs when an individual is unable to perform his or her socially defined tasks, activities, or roles to the expected level. At this point, one considers the societal limitations: those limitations to an individual's level of function that result from physical or attitudinal barriers in society. Finally, health-related quality of life explains how the functional limitations and disability experienced by the individual may lead him to perceive that he has a decreased quality of life or decreased ability to function in and enjoy his social roles.

## Client Examination Using the Disablement Models

Application of the Disablement Model to the clinical scenario of a data entry clerk with carpal tunnel syndrome (Theory in Practice 1-3a) yields the following components. In the

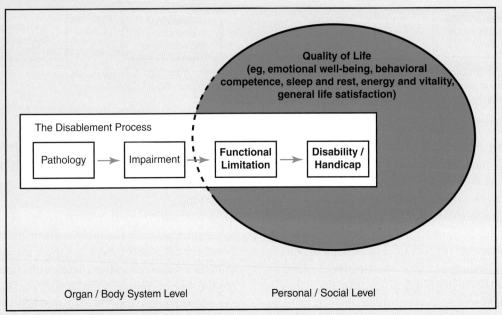

Figure 1-7  Conceptual model of quality of life. Reprinted from Jette AM. Using health-related quality of life measures in physical therapy outcomes research. *Phys Ther.* 1993;73:528–537; with the permission of the American Physical Therapy Association.

case of carpal tunnel syndrome, the pathophysiology involves the inflammation of the wrist and finger flexor tendons in the region of the carpal tunnel. This inflammation results in pressure on the median nerve as it passes through the carpal tunnel. In turn, the pressure on the median nerve leads to the **primary impairments** of pain, paresthesia, weakness, and atrophy of the thenar muscles and lumbricals. These primary impairments can contribute to the development of secondary impairments, such as decreased joint range of motion at the wrist and weakness of wrist and hand muscles secondary to disuse. As a consequence of the primary and secondary impairments outlined, this client is unable to perform work-related activities, leisure activities, and activities of daily living with hand and wrist joint range of motion and strength that are within normal limits. When an individual is unable to perform his socially defined tasks, activities, or roles to the expected level, this is considered a disability. The client is unable to perform his socially defined roles as a data entry clerk and a member of a racquetball club. In addition, the societal limitation of reduced health insurance restricts the amount of rehabilitation that the data entry clerk can obtain, thereby limiting the level of function that he may be able to achieve. Finally, health-related quality of life explains how the functional limitations and disability experienced by the data entry clerk may lead him to perceive that he has a decreased quality of life or decreased ability to function in and enjoy his social roles as a data entry clerk and a member of a racquetball club.

## Comparison of the Disablement and ICF Models

In contrast to the Disablement Models, the ICF does not suggest that the individual progresses from having an impairment to a functional limitation to a disability and a handicap.[6,7] Theory in Practice 1-3d shows the similarities and differences between the clinical problem lists stemming from the Disablement Model and ICF model. Al-

**Theory in Practice 1-3d**

## Comparison of Patient Problem Lists for the Disablement and ICF Models

| Problems for the Disablement Model | Problems for the ICF Model |
|---|---|
| 1. Impairments<br> Pain<br> Edema in the region of the carpal tunnel<br> Paresthesia<br> Decreased joint range of motion of wrist and fingers | 1. Impairments in body structure<br> Edema in the region of the carpal tunnel<br> Pressure on the median nerve<br> Decreased joint range of motion of wrist and fingers |

Decreased strength of hand and wrist muscles
2. Functional limitations
   Inability to perform customary job-related activities, especially typing, filing, and writing
   Inability to perform leisure activity of playing racquetball
   Inability to perform activities of daily living, especially grooming and household tasks that involve lifting
   Fear of exacerbating pain limits initiation of functional activity
3. Disability
   Inability to perform job of data entry clerk
   Inability to perform social role as a member of a racquetball club
4. Societal limitation
   Limited health insurance
5. Quality of life
   Perceived decreased ability to function in and enjoy his social roles of data entry clerk and member of a racquetball club

2. Impairments in body function
   Pain
   Paresthesia
   Decreased strength of hand and wrist muscles
3. Activity limitations
   Inability to perform customary job-related activities, especially typing, filing, and writing
   Inability to perform leisure activity of playing racquetball
   Inability to perform activities of daily living, especially grooming and household tasks that involve lifting
4. Participation restrictions
   Inability to perform job of data entry clerk
   Inability to perform social role as a member of a racquetball club
5. Environmental factors
   Limited health insurance
6. Personal factors
   Fear of exacerbating pain limits initiation of functional activity
   Perceived decreased ability to function in and enjoy his social roles of data entry clerk and member of a racquetball club

---

**Box 1-7**  **Comparison of Terminology from the Disablement and International Classification of Functioning, Disability and Health Models**

| Disablement Models | ICF Model |
| --- | --- |
| Disease and pathophysiology | Medical condition |
| Impairments | Body structures and functions: Impairments grades 0 to 5 |
| Functional limitations/ disability | Activity: Limitations in capacity for activity |
| Handicap | Participation: Limitations in performance of activity in environment |
| No comparable term | Personal factors |
| No comparable term | Environmental factors: Barriers or facilitators |

though, at first glance, it may seem to be simply using new terms for existing concepts (Box 1-7), the ICF offers more than a mere renaming of constructs.[4,5] The ICF model provides a broader foundation for models of wellness than the Disablement Models. Of primary importance in this regard is the change from a linear progression from disease to handicap to an interactive model that highlights the impact of environmental factors and personal factors. The classification of impairments by body structures and functions and the associated grading system allow the clinician to identify body structures and functions where the impairments have a score of 0, or no impairment. At the same time, the ICF accommodates existing notions of functional limitations and functional outcomes within its concept of limitations in activity and participation. The comparison of an individual's capacity for executing a task and her performance of that task in her environment focuses clinicians on the ways in which they can address environmental barriers through their interventions. Finally, the inclusion of personal factors supports the analysis of the role of healthy lifestyles and perceived health that are important aspects of wellness.

## Critical Thinking Question

What are the differences between Disablement Models, the Wellness Interactions Model, and the ICF model?

# WELLNESS MODELS

## Continuum-Based Models of Wellness

There are a variety of wellness models supported by different ways of understanding health and disease. These models range from Travis's original Wellness Model,[19] based on the continuum of health and disease, to the Wellness Interactions Model, which uses the ICF, developed for Outcome-Based Massage. This section describes the wellness models that preceded the Wellness Interactions Model described earlier in this chapter.

Travis and Ryan[19] initially conceptualized wellness as a state of optimal health and well-being. They depicted wellness on a continuum from premature death at one end, through differing levels of disease, to high-level wellness at the other end (Figure 1-8). In this model, an individual progressed to high-level wellness via the stages of awareness, education, and growth. Furthermore, interventions for health fell within the medical treatment model, whereas those for wellness were in the realm of wellness, with a neutral zone between the two. Theorists have added to this model of wellness by presenting the levels of interventions for wellness and illness in different forms.[10] In all of these models, as in the Disablement Models discussed earlier, the individual moves through a linear progression from death to high-level wellness.

## Wellness Outcomes in the Presence of a Medical Condition

The Wellness Interactions Model addresses the fact that individuals with medical conditions can also have body structures and functions that are free of impairments and, therefore, appropriate for wellness interventions. The 30-year-old with carpal tunnel syndrome still has body structures and functions for which the clinician can establish outcomes for wellness, despite the impairments and limitations in activity and participation that stem from his medical condition. For example, his sleep pattern, energy levels, and resting tension in his shoulder and neck muscles are within normal limits. Consequently, he can have wellness goals for optimizing these body structures and functions, as illustrated in Theory in Practice 1-3e.

---

**Theory in Practice 1-3e**

### Wellness Outcomes for the Patient with Carpal Tunnel Syndrome

| Relevant Body Structures | Relevant Body Functions |
|---|---|
| Structure of the nervous system | Mental functions |
| ▪ Brain | ▪ Energy and drive functions |
| | ▪ Sleep |
| Structure of the respiratory system | Function of the respiratory system |
| ▪ Respiratory system | ▪ Respiration |
| Neuromusculoskeletal and movement-related structures | Neuromusculoskeletal and movement-related functions |
| ▪ Head and neck region | ▪ Muscle resting tension |
| ▪ Shoulder region | |

---

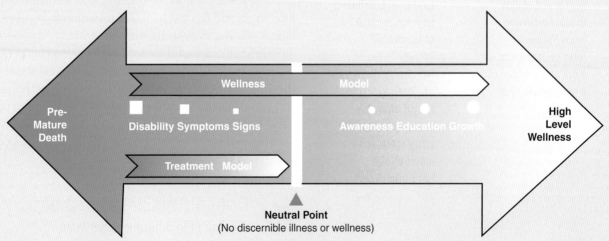

**Figure 1-8** The Wellness Continuum. Reprinted with permission from Travis J, Ryan R. *Wellness Workbook: How to Achieve Enduring Health and Vitality.* 3rd ed. Berkeley, CA: Celestial Arts; 2004.

| Body Structure or Function | Wellness Outcome |
|---|---|
| Brain | Increased quality and quantity of sleep |
| | Increased energy |
| Respiratory system | Increased ventilation |
| Muscles of the head, neck, and shoulder region | Normalized muscle resting tension |

**Critical Thinking Question**

In which situations is it inappropriate to establish wellness outcomes for a client?

## References

1. Field TM. Massage therapy effects. *Am Psychol.* 1998;53:1270–1281.
2. Donabedian A. Evaluating the quality of medical care. *Milbank Q.* 1966;3:166–206.
3. Oschman JL. *Energy Medicine: The Scientific Basis.* Edinburgh: Churchill-Livingston; 2000.
4. World Health Organization. Towards a common language for functioning, disability and health: ICF: the International Classification of Functioning, Disability and Health. Geneva, Switzerland: World Health Organization; 2002.
5. World Health Organization. ICF Checklist. Geneva, Switzerland: World Health Organization; 2003.
6. Nagi S. Disability concepts revisited: implications for prevention. Executive summary. In: Pope A, Tarlov A, eds. *Disability in America.* Washington, DC: National Academy Press; 1991:1.4.
7. National Institute of Child Health and Human Development. Research plan for the National Center for Medical Rehabilitation Research. Public Health Service NIH Publication No. 93-3509. Bethesda, MD: National Institutes of Health, US Department of Health and Human Services; 1993.
8. World Health Organization. Preamble to the Constitution of the World Health Organization as adopted by the International Health Conference. International Health Conference, New York, June 19–22, 1946.
9. O'Donnell MP. Definition of health promotion. *Am J Health Promot.* 1989;3:5.
10. Schuster T, Dobson M, Jauregui M, Blanks R. Wellness lifestyles I: a theoretical framework linking wellness, health lifestyles, and complementary and alternative medicine. *J Altern Complement Med.* 2004;10:349–356.
11. Tappan FM, Benjamin P. *Tappan's Handbook of Healing Massage Techniques.* 3rd ed. Stamford, CT: Appleton & Lange; 1998.
12. Nemcek MA. Self nurturance: research trends and wellness model. *AAOHN J.* 2003;51:260–266.
13. Oxford University Press. *Oxford English Dictionary.* Oxford: Oxford University Press; 2006.
14. Hillman J. *A Blue Fire.* New York: Harper Paperbacks; 1991.
15. Moore T. *Care of the Soul.* New York: Harper Paperbacks; 1994.
16. Prochaska JO, DiClemente CC. Transtheoretical therapy: toward a more integrative model of change. Psychother Theory Res Pract. 1982;19:276–288.
17. Jette AM. Using health-related quality of life measures in physical therapy outcomes research. *Phys Ther.* 1993;73:528–537.
18. American Physical Therapy Association. *Guide to Physical Therapist Practice.* 2nd ed. Alexandria, VA: American Physical Therapy Association; 1999.
19. Travis J, Ryan R. *Wellness Workbook: How to Achieve Enduring Health and Vitality.* 3rd ed. Berkeley, CA: Celestial Arts; 2004.

# Chapter 2
## Evidence for Massage

Evidence is information on clinical care that researchers and therapists collect in a systematic manner. Evidence is typically about the outcomes and, occasionally, the process of clinical care. As both providers and consumers of health care information and services, therapists are bombarded daily with evidence in a variety of forms, ranging from professional journals to the Internet and public discussion. Clients also deal with the same bewildering array of opinions and information. Rather than answering questions, this information often raises new questions such as: "What is good evidence?" and "What constitutes best evidence when making clinical decisions?" This chapter will address these questions. It will also describe how evidence helps therapists to serve their clients better. Finally, it will introduce concepts related to the steps of finding, understanding, critically evaluating, and applying best evidence to clinical practice.

## Evidence for Massage: Foundations

### WHY THERAPISTS NEED EVIDENCE

Menard,[1] suggests that an evidence-based approach is essential in health care and provides several reasons for using evidence to inform clinical practice. First and foremost, therapists need evidence in order to provide the best possible care to their clients. **Evidence** supports the theoretical foundation of a discipline and helps therapists to be critical thinkers. It also helps them to distinguish between useful and safe practices and those that might be harmful to clients. Furthermore, it assists them in educating themselves and their clients about what massage and other health care interventions can and cannot do. Second, evidence fosters public acceptance of massage and other complementary health care techniques and provides a common language that facilitates communication about massage techniques. Third, evidence enables therapists to stay current, to be lifelong learners, and to be better consumers of health care resources themselves.

Increasingly, as massage becomes more widely accepted,[2,3] consumers, health care practitioners, government agencies, professional associations, and researchers are asking important questions about the safety and effectiveness of massage as a health care intervention.[4,5] Furthermore, increased use of and reimbursement for massage interventions brings an increased requirement for accountability. Consequently, therapists need to know which massage techniques work best for which clients and under which conditions.

On a more personal level, therapists are also ethically committed to being lifelong learners who participate in self-reflection and the continuous development of skills, knowledge, and attitudes in professional practice. In this arena, evidence can guide clinical decision making and professional growth.

# EVIDENCE-BASED PRACTICE OR EVIDENCE-BASED MEDICINE

The systematic use of evidence in clinical decision making is the basis of evidence-based practice or evidence-based medicine. Sackett et al.[6(p1)] define **evidence-based medicine (EBM)** as ". . . the integration of best research evidence with clinical expertise and client values." Within this definition, **best research evidence** means the best available clinical, client-centered research that examines the accuracy, safety, and efficacy of diagnostic and assessment tests, prognosis markers, and therapeutic interventions. **Clinical expertise** is the therapist's ability to use her clinical skills and past experience to identify each client's unique health status and the potential risks and benefits of interventions that she could use in each case. **Client values** refer to the unique preferences, goals, and expectations that each client brings to the therapeutic relationship. Sackett et al. propose that therapists need to integrate all of these components in order to become proficient in evidence-based practice.

Greenhalgh,[7] further defines evidence-based medicine as ". . . the enhancement of a therapist's traditional skills in diagnosis, treatment, prevention, and related areas through the systematic framing of relevant and answerable questions and the use of mathematical estimates of probability and risk." This adds two important concepts to

Sackett's definition. The first is that therapists need to learn how to ask clinical questions that are answerable, something that is not as straightforward as it initially sounds. Second, therapists have to understand the basic concepts of designing and conducting research.

Critics of evidence-based practice offer several reasons why it is difficult to base clinical decision making on "best evidence."[8,9] They maintain that, at times, there is very little evidence and, at other times, there is too much of it. In addition, they suggest that therapists do not have enough time to find research papers, read them, and distinguish the bad papers from the good. Finally, they point out that interpreting how to put the new information into clinical practice can also seem daunting. Notwithstanding these obstacles, Outcome-Based Massage considers the adoption of evidence-based practice to be an important goal for therapists.

## Initiating Evidence-Based Practice

For students and therapists, the first step in engaging in evidence-based practice can be to develop their ability to use evidence from different sources. The four essential competencies for research literacy are the ability to find, understand, critically evaluate, and apply research evidence to practice (Box 2-1).[1] Although it is beyond the scope of this book to provide comprehensive information on how to develop research literacy skills, we will use this list of essential competencies and Theory in Practice 2-1 to 2-5 to guide the introduction to evidence-based practice.

### Critical Thinking Question
What are the arguments for and against a therapist adopting an evidence-based approach to practice?

## FINDING THE EVIDENCE FOR PRACTICE

Evidence can come from primary or secondary sources.[1,10] The **primary source** directly documents the **primary research**, which is the original research conducted by therapists or researchers. Types of primary research include: clinical trials, surveys, ethnographies, and a variety of other research designs. Primary sources are typically professional journals, conference presentations, and, occasionally, text books. A **secondary source** is a summary of the information presented in a primary source. Secondary sources can include **secondary research** studies, which summarize and

Dryden T, Achilles R. Research Literacy for Complementary and Alternative Health Care Practitioners: An Online Course. Accessed February 18, 2007. Available at http://www.centennialcollege.ca/.

## Box 2-1   Research Literacy Competencies

1. Ability to find the evidence for practice:
   - Distinguish between refereed journals and other published sources of information.
   - Demonstrate the ability to access information through the Internet to conduct a literature search.
2. Ability to understand research evidence:
   - Describe the nature, variety, and value of different kinds of research and evidence.
   - Distinguish between kinds of methodological designs in research.
   - Identify and understand basic statistical concepts.
3. Ability to critically evaluate research evidence:
   - Identify and understand underlying assumptions and biases in varying forms of research and evidence.
   - Identify and understand underlying assumptions and biases in varying forms of statistical methods.
4. Ability to apply research evidence in clinical practice:
   - Create researchable questions to apply to practice.
   - Confirm, modify, or alter practice based on best evidence.
   - Disseminate information and research findings to clients and others in various forms to increase shared knowledge and informed choice.

draw conclusions from primary studies, such as nonsystematic literature reviews, systematic literature reviews, and meta-analyses. There are also a wide variety of other secondary sources, such as textbooks, the popular media, the Internet, professional courses, and professional journals.

## Theory in Practice 2-1

### Initiating Evidence-Based Practice

A practitioner in an outpatient setting noticed that he had been seeing a growing number of patients with pain secondary to osteoarthritis (OA) of the knees and hips. This attracted his attention because he had been treating these patients on a case-by-case basis. He wondered if he could make his intervention more effective by incorporating some new information on OA and the management of that condition.

## Evidence from Secondary Sources

Secondary sources of evidence are often easier to locate than primary sources. Consequently, searching the Internet and popular media is often the first step a student or therapist who is new to evidence-based practice will take in finding the evidence for practice. Unfortunately, one cannot assume that these secondary sources accurately report the original findings. As a result, there are several cautions to using secondary sources. First, therapists must read information in the popular media, such as newspapers and magazines, carefully because the findings of the original research study can be manipulated or distorted by publication bias and reporting techniques. Second, although the Internet is the fastest growing public repository of information, it requires knowledge of good search techniques to find relevant resources. There is a common myth that all information on the Internet is one keyword and one click away. Anyone who has tried to find quality research on massage on the Internet by typing the key word "massage" into a search engine will understand how challenging it can be to find good evidence on the Internet. Furthermore, the quality of information on the Internet varies from researchers' own accounts of their work to members of the general public posting information that is of personal interest. Therefore, therapists are encouraged to examine Internet content to identify the source and reputation of the information. Finally, although selected groups of peers review textbooks with greater rigor than the popular media is reviewed, there is no standard for judging the evidence textbooks present and the accuracy with which they quote primary sources. The same issue applies to secondary sources in professional journals and professional courses.

## Evidence from Primary Sources

Regardless of the ease with which one can access secondary sources, therapists will find that the most accurate representation of the evidence is the researcher's original documentation of his or her work. Therapists can locate primary sources through databases for scientific and health-related information (Box 2-2). Even within primary sources, there is a hierarchy of quality of information. The peer-reviewed professional journal is the gold standard. Peer review is a prior-to-publication process in which a group of experts from a profession independently review research articles for scientific merit, participant safety, ethical considerations, and other rigorous criteria. They then make recommendations on whether or not the articles meet the criteria for

---

**Box 2-2**     **Examples of Databases of Health and Scientific Journals**

---

## PRIVATE

### Alt-HealthWatch

Content: Alt-HealthWatch is a full-text database of periodicals, peer-reviewed journals, academic and professional publications, magazines, consumer newsletters and newspapers, research reports, and association newsletters focused on complementary, alternative, and integrated approaches to health care and wellness.

### CINAHL (Cumulative Index to Nursing and Allied Health Literature)

Content: Comprehensive index to nursing literature and selective index in allied health areas; includes 500+ journals and selected dissertations, proceedings, media, and standards of professional practice.

### AMED

Content: AMED is a unique bibliographic database produced by the Health Care Information Service of the British Library. It covers a selection of journals in allied health professions, complementary medicine, and palliative care.

### PsycARTICLES

Content: PsycARTICLES is a database of full-text articles from (43+) journals published by the American Psychological Association (APA), the APA Educational Publishing Foundation, the Canadian Psychological Association, and Hogrefe and Huber. The database includes all material from the print journals.

### Hooked on Evidence

Content: The American Physical Therapy Association's Hooked on Evidence website is a database containing current research evidence on the effectiveness of physical therapy interventions.

The website has a searchable database of article extractions relevant to the field of physical therapy, lists of useful Web resources, and clinical practice guidelines based on systematic reviews of the literature.

## PUBLIC AND/OR FREE

### PubMed

Content: PubMed (http://pubmed.gov) is a specialized public access database managed by the U.S. National Library of Medicine that includes over 16 million citations from MEDLINE and other life science journals, links to some full text articles, and related resources back to the 1950s.

### ERIC

Content: The Education Resources Information Center (ERIC) is a digital library of education-related resources sponsored by the Institute of Education Sciences of the U.S. Department of Education. The collection consists of electronic bibliographic records describing journal and nonjournal literature selected by ERIC from 1966 to 2003 and full-text articles.

### CHID

Content: CHID is a bibliographic database produced by agencies of the National Institutes of Health. This database provides titles, abstracts, and availability information for health information and health education resources.

### PEDro

Content: PEDro is the Physiotherapy Evidence Database. It has been developed by the Centre for Evidence-Based Physiotherapy to give rapid access to bibliographic details and abstracts of randomized controlled trials, systematic reviews, and evidence-based clinical practice guidelines in physical therapy.

---

publication. Peer-reviewed journals state their criteria for inclusion, thereby enabling therapists to make informed choices about some of the underlying assumptions or potential biases a publication may have. Although peer review increases the likelihood that the research information published is of high quality, it is still useful for therapists to read all publications with a thoughtful and critical eye. By contrast, the review process is less rigorous for journals without peer review, conference presentations, and professional courses.

## Critical Thinking Question

What are (a) the similarities and differences and (b) the advantages and disadvantages of primary and secondary sources?

### Finding the Evidence for Practice

The practitioner began by consulting his clinical textbooks (secondary sources) to increase his understanding of the pathophysiology and clinical issues related to OA. Then he read about different therapeutic approaches for pain due to OA. He was surprised to see that there were contradicting approaches to using massage techniques for these patients. As a result, he decided to explore the research literature. Since he was not familiar with database searches, he first found some of the articles cited in the reference sections of the textbooks. These were somewhat dated, and none were specifically on the use of massage techniques for pain due to OA. As a result, he decided to venture into database searches. For this, he selected PubMed as a starting point since he could access it from his computer at work. Using combinations of the keywords "massage," "soft tissue techniques," "osteoarthritis," "pain," "alternative medicine," and "complementary medicine," he found several articles. He sifted through these until he found a few current studies on massage interventions for people with OA.

# UNDERSTANDING THE EVIDENCE FOR PRACTICE

Understanding evidence requires that therapists gain a basic understanding of research and evaluate the underlying assumptions and biases of research studies. There are two primary approaches to conducting research: quantitative and qualitative.[1,10] Quantitative research methods evolved from basic science research and use the collection and analysis of numerical data. Qualitative research methods, from the social sciences research tradition, use the collection and analysis of word-based experiential and observational data, rather than numbers.

## Assumptions of Quantitative and Qualitative Research

Qualitative and quantitative research differ on five basic assumptions (Table 2-1).[11] The first assumption relates to the nature of reality. The underlying assumption in **quantitative research** is that there is a reality that exists independently of people. This is in sharp contrast to **qualitative research**, which assumes that people define reality. The relationship between the researcher and the subject of research is the basis of the second assumption. Quantitative research is based on the belief that researchers can stand back from reality in order to observe and measure it using "objective" instruments. On the other hand, qualitative researchers consider themselves to be part of the reality they are studying. Consequently, they propose that there is no distinction between the observer and what he or she observes and acknowledge that researchers change reality as they study it.

These key differences provide the foundation for what quantitative and qualitative researchers consider to be the "truth," the relationship between facts and values, and the goal of investigation.[11] The cornerstone of quantitative

| **Table 2-1** | Assumptions of Quantitative and Qualitative Research | |
| --- | --- | --- |
| | **Quantitative Research** | **Qualitative Research** |
| Nature of reality | Reality is independent of people. | Reality is defined by people. |
| Relationship between investigator and research subject | Investigator is independent of the subject of the research. | Investigator affects the subject of research during the research process. |
| Nature of truth | Truth is whatever comes the closest to "reality." | There is no single "truth" since everyone has his or her own opinion. |
| Relationship between fact, values, and research | Objectivity on the part of the researcher is the gold standard. | What the investigator studies and learns reflects his values and interests. |
| Goal of research | To produce laws about reality that he or she can generalize to other situations. | Verstehen: an interpretive understanding of the group or phenomenon being observed. |

Adapted with permission from Lincoln Y, Guba E. *Naturalistic Inquiry.* Newbury Park: Sage; 1985; and Smith JK. Quantitative versus qualitative research: an attempt to clarify the issue. *Educational Res.* 1983;12:6–13.

research is that there is a single "truth" or accurate representation of reality. This is the opposite of the assumption in qualitative research that there can be multiple theories on the phenomenon being studied, each of which is equally acceptable. In quantitative research, the quality of the researcher's methodology is the test to determine which theory comes the closest to approximating the "truth." Furthermore, quantitative researchers use specified scientific methods to rule out bias and show that their results did not occur by chance. These techniques include manipulating the clinical setting and participants, measuring phenomena, controlling the environment as much as possible, and using statistical analyses. This strategy supports their principle that researchers can reproduce results of other studies if they use the same objective procedures. On the other hand, since qualitative researchers are not attempting to document a single "truth" about a phenomenon, they observe phenomena in their natural setting and document their insights about their observations. Their data include interviews, direct observations, and artifacts such as journals. Furthermore, qualitative researchers do not use "objectivity," or the test of reproducing others' findings by duplicating their methods, as a standard for their work. These assumptions about truth and the relationship between facts and values lead us to the goal of research.

The goal of quantitative researchers is to discover laws about the causes and effects of phenomena that they can then generalize to other situations. In light of the fact that qualitative researchers embrace the notion of multiple coexisting theories, they do not search for generalizable laws. Instead, the goal of qualitative researchers is a deep understanding of the subject that they are observing. These differing assumptions of quantitative and qualitative research result in different methods for collecting and analyzing data.

## Quantitative and Qualitative Research Designs

There are many types of quantitative research study designs.[1,10] Descriptive studies provide a record or description of events or activities. Researchers can use these designs to form hypotheses or statements that researchers can show to be true or false by collecting and analyzing data. Descriptive study designs include: case reports, case series, and correlational studies. On the other hand, explanatory studies try to explain the connections between events or variables and examine cause and effect. Researchers use these studies to test hypotheses. Explanatory study designs

are either experimental or quasi-experimental. Experimental studies include randomized clinical trials and other variations on designs with randomization and control groups. By contrast, quasi-experimental studies are those that lack randomization and control groups, such as studies in which an individual acts as his own control. Textbooks on research methods[1,10,12,13] contain a more detailed discussion of terminology, procedures, and statistics associated with quantitative research designs for massage and allied health care.

There are also many types of qualitative studies, the most common of which are grounded theory, ethnography, and phenomenology.[1,10,11] Data collection most often takes place in the natural environment where the behaviors or phenomena that are the subject of the research actually take place, rather than in the laboratory or the highly controlled clinical environment, as is the case in quantitative research. Grounded theory, developed by Glaser and Strauss,[14] involves the generation of theory from participants' responses. In other words, researchers transcribe, categorize, and sort participants' responses to identify patterns and develop theory. An ethnography describes and interprets the activities of a group of people who have a common feature. Finally, phenomenologic studies are those that describe a specific aspect of a group's experiences and are concerned with how individuals interpret and make sense of their experiences, as opposed to simply describing those experiences. Textbooks on the methods and terminology of qualitative research include those by Lincoln and Guba[11] and Glaser and Strauss.[14]

## Designs for Massage Research

Massage is a complex intervention with physiological, psychological, social, and spiritual components. It is challenging to try to separate the specific effects of massage, such as neurological or cardiovascular effects, from the nonspecific effects, including the therapeutic relationship and environment. So which research method is more appropriate for research on massage techniques: qualitative or quantitative? That depends on the research question one is asking. Some research questions benefit from one method or the other; however, we can best answer some research questions using a combination of qualitative and quantitative research methods. Consider the research question about the effectiveness of a particular massage intervention for a particular population: "Do daily interventions of massage improve the gestational date achieved of women with high-risk pregnancies who are on bed rest?" Researchers could answer this question best using a quantitative design.

**Theory in Practice 2-3**

**Understanding the Evidence for Practice**

The practitioner decided to begin with the randomized clini-cal trial (RCT) "Massage Therapy for Osteoarthritis of the Knee" in the *Archives of Internal Medicine* because he had heard that RCTs were more rigorous. He chose not to discard the survey and the case report on a single patient because he felt that they might also have important information to offer.

Before reading the article, he took a look at pointers for reading research in one of his textbooks. He noted that RCTs were, among other things, intended to test a hypothesis and use randomization and control to decrease the likelihood that the findings were due to chance.

Perlman A, Sabina A, Williams A, Njike V, Katz D. Massage therapy for osteoarthritis of the knee. Arch Intern Med. 2006;166:2533–2538.

Whereas, researchers can answer a research question about the meaning of the massage experience for the client (such as: "What are the perceptions and experiences of daily massage interventions of women with high-risk pregnancies who are on bed rest?") better using qualitative research methods. More and more, individuals conducting research on massage techniques are recognizing that existing research methodologies fail to address critical aspects of massage. For this reason, researchers are devel-oping new research methods for research on massage. **Whole systems research**, for example, is an approach for examining the complex interrelationship between the spe-cific and nonspecific effects of a massage intervention or a massage practice as a whole.[15]

## Critical Thinking Question

What are examples of research questions that can best be answered using (a) quantitative designs, (b) qualitative designs, and (c) whole systems designs?

# EVALUATING THE EVIDENCE FOR PRACTICE

When asked, "What is good evidence?" a wise person replied, "It depends on who is asking." By this, she meant that evidence is not neutral or unbiased. People under spe-cific historical and social conditions generate evidence on massage techniques. Consequently, like all other forms of knowledge, this information is not entirely free of biases or errors. Knowing that real people, under real and often less-than-ideal circumstances, generate evidence does not mean that therapists cannot rely on evidence to help them make sound clinical decisions. It does mean, however, that they need to use evidence in an educated and critical man-ner. To do so, therapists need to go beyond evaluating the methodology used to obtain the evidence. They should also consider how research questions get asked and why, how evidence is obtained and by whom, who funds and conducts research, and who stands to benefit from research. This weighing of the relative strengths, weaknesses, and biases of evidence is a critical component in the clinical decision-making process.

## Evidence Levels and Evidence Houses

Guidance on how to evaluate evidence comes from multiple sources. Sackett et al.[6] have created a hierarchy of research designs, called **levels of evidence**, and a systematic approach for evaluating evidence (Box 2-3). This hierarchy ranks sev-eral different types of studies.[6,16] **Systematic reviews** evaluate findings from individual studies and combine these find-ings using statistical techniques. **Randomized controlled trials** use control groups and the random assignment of partici-pants into experimental or control groups. In **cohort studies**, researchers follow the outcomes of a group of participants who they identify as having received the intervention and a group with similar characteristics who did not. **Case-control studies** are those in which researchers identify individuals who have similar outcomes and examine their history to determine if they received the same intervention. A **case series** is a summary of findings on a group of participants with similar characteristics or who received the same inter-vention without reference to findings on a control group. Studies at the top of Sackett's hierarchy provide the strong-est evidence of a cause-and-effect relationship between the intervention and the outcome and vice versa.

Critics of this approach point out that the hierarchy of research designs in the levels of evidence favors quanti-tative research methods.[7-9] They note that at the top of Sackett et al.'s[6] levels of evidence is the randomized con-trolled trial (RCT), which is considered the most rigorous of the experimental designs because of its level of experi-mental control and randomization of participants. At the bottom of the hierarchy is descriptive research, which lacks a high degree of control and randomization. This tra-ditional hierarchy of evidence is a concern for research on massage techniques because it suggests that much of the evidence for massage comes from traditions of research that rank lower on the levels of evidence and are, thus, less

| Box 2-3 | Sample of Sackett's Levels of Evidence | |
|---|---|---|
| **Grade of Recommendation** | **Level of Evidence** | **Type of Study** |
| A | 1a | Systematic reviews of randomized controlled trials (RCTs) |
| | 1b | Individual RCTs with a narrow confidence interval |
| | 1c | All or none case series |
| B | 2a | Systematic reviews of cohort studies |
| | 2b | Individual cohort studies and low-quality RCTs |
| | 2c | Outcomes research |
| | 3a | Systematic reviews of case-control studies |
| | 3b | Individual case-controlled studies |
| C | 4 | Case series and poor-quality cohort and case-control studies |
| D | 5 | Expert opinion without explicit critical appraisal, or based on physiology, bench research, or "first principles" |

Adapted with permission from Sackett D, Straus SE, Richardson WS, Rosenberg W, Haynes B. *Evidence-Based Medicine: How to Practice and Teach EBM.* Edinburgh: Churchill Livingstone; 2000:7–8; and Glaros S. All evidence is not created equal: a discussion of levels of evidence. *PT Magazine.* 2003;11:42–49, 52.

rigorous. To address this issue, Jonas[9] proposes building an "**evidence house**" that includes many kinds of rigorous research methods, rather than a hierarchical model, as Sackett does. He suggests that including a variety of research methodologies, such as qualitative research methods, can provide a more balanced and complete picture of what constitutes massage and how it works.

## Reading and Evaluating Research Articles

The sheer volume of research evidence available can be daunting. Some professional journals attempt to collect, summarize, and comment on recent articles to make it easier for therapists to stay current. Some forms of this secondary research, such as meta-analyses, use rigorous criteria to evaluate all related studies on a particular subject and can be a useful way for therapists to review the conclusions of a number of related studies simultaneously. In addition, Sackett et al.[6] provides guidelines for a systematic analysis of research articles to determine their rigor.

Therapists must resist the temptation to read the Introduction and then skip to the Discussion and Conclusions of a research article. A systematic assessment of the credibility of the conclusions of a research study enables therapists to determine the degree to which it is appropriate for them to apply that evidence to their own clinical

practices. How to Read a Research Article Critically, in the advanced section of this chapter, outlines a basic process that can provide a starting point for using the evidence in the research literature for Outcome-Based Massage. Although an in-depth treatment of the process for analyzing research articles is beyond the scope of this book, the chapters on treatment techniques will introduce brief analyses of samples of evidence to illustrate this approach.

### Theory in Practice 2-4

### Evaluating the Evidence for Practice

The practitioner was relieved to see that the article was only six pages long. On reading the Introduction, he saw that the researchers' purpose was to evaluate the effectiveness of massage therapy for OA. He reviewed the Methods and learned that the study had 66 subjects, men and women aged 35 and up, who received care for OA on an outpatient basis. He was pleased to see that the researchers had eliminated people who had had recent steroid use or confounding health conditions such as fibromyalgia or cancer. This made it easier for him to judge the effects of the massage techniques on the OA pain.

The practitioner reviewed the procedures and saw that the researchers had randomly assigned participants into one of two groups. The treatment group received 8 weeks of weekly hour-long full-body Swedish massage interventions by certified massage therapists. The control group went on a waiting list to receive the same intervention after the first 8-week period. The study included several measures. The first was the WOMAC, a questionnaire that assessed pain, stiffness, and functional limitations. The other measures were the Visual Analog Scale (VAS) for pain, joint range of motion, and time to walk 50 feet.

When he moved on to the Results, the practitioner found that all of the participants completed the study and that, at the beginning of the study, both groups were the same on all baseline measures except pain (the treatment group reported higher levels of pain). He had some difficulty following the statistics, but he did figure out that the treatment group showed a statistically significant difference on range of motion, WOMAC score (pain, stiffness, and function), VAS pain reports, and the time to walk 50 feet. After they received the 8-week intervention, the control group showed similar changes.

The researchers, physicians, and physician's assistants attributed the decrease in perceived pain and stiffness and increases in range of motion, perceived functional level, and ability to walk 50 feet to the Swedish massage interventions. The practitioner noted that they had selected Swedish massage techniques of petrissage, tapotement, and effleurage because they were commonly used techniques. He was disappointed to see that the authors did not offer any physiological explanation for their findings. Furthermore, they did not give a rationale for delivering a 1-hour full-body massage to individuals who presented with knee pain or for allowing the therapists to choose the massage techniques at their discretion. He recognized that the fact that it was an RCT did not guarantee that it would provide sound evidence for his clinical practice.

### Critical Thinking Question

What are some situations or ways in which randomized clinical trials fail to provide sound evidence for the use of massage techniques?

## APPLYING EVIDENCE TO PRACTICE

Applying best evidence to practice is one set of threads in the complex tapestry of professional practice. Sackett et al.[6] outline how an evidence-based approach to practice integrates best research evidence, clinical expertise, and client values. Adopting an evidence-based approach to practice is a process that requires that a therapist becomes aware

of her own assumptions, biases, and knowledge base.[17] An ethical therapist continuously examines and develops her knowledge, skills, and attitudes throughout her professional career. She seeks out and critically evaluates the best evidence for practice and then applies relevant information to confirm, modify, or alter her approach to practice. Since she recognizes that future research may show that some of today's accepted practices are ineffective, she feels comfortable challenging conventional wisdom and thinking for herself. Finally, she understands that acquiring research literacy and developing an evidence-based practice is not about learning a specific set of skills for a single use. Instead, it is about integrating critical thinking into all aspects of her professional life and using evidence to enhance her own sense of professional accomplishment and her clients' well-being. Box 2-4 outlines some activities

| **Box 2-4** | **Activities That Facilitate Evidence-Based Practice** |

- Pose specific questions of practical value to clients
- Search for best evidence
- Critically evaluate best evidence
- Take action guided by that evidence
- Reflect
- Formulate thoughtful questions
- Read critically
- Discuss and learn with others
- Confirm, alter, or modify practice
- Continuously learn and self-evaluate
- Set aside time to journal and reflect on practice
- Set aside time to search the Internet; set up "Alerts" for new information
- Subscribe to journals/newsletters
- Join a peer supervision group
- Join your professional association
- Take professional development courses in research literacy and research capacity
- Find professional supervision or a mentor
- Join an evidence-based professional group
- Critically evaluate your own performance
- Commit to lifelong learning
- Create an evidence-based newsletter for clients
- Give talks/information-sharing sessions in your community
- Write and publish case reports and critiques of best evidence
- Get involved with research initiatives by collaborating with established academic researchers

Adapted with permission from Gibbs LE. *Evidence-Based Practice for the Helping Professions: A Practical Guide with Integrated Multimedia.* Pacific Grove, CA: Thompson, Brooks, Cole; 2003:19.

that therapists can use to facilitate their development of an evidence-based approach to practice.

## ? Critical Thinking Question

Which of the activities in Box 2-4 can you reasonably initiate within the next month? Write out the steps you need to take to implement one of these activities and put that plan into action.

---

### Theory in Practice 2-5

### Applying Evidence to Practice

The practitioner pondered what he had just learned and tried to identify how this information would assist him in treating his patients with OA. He listed the guidelines for management from his clinical textbooks and his own clinical experience:

**Key Impairment in Body Structures and Functions for Massage**

1. Pain–acute nociceptive and chronic pain
2. Decreased muscle extensibility
3. Muscle spasm
4. Decreased joint mobility, complaints of morning stiffness
5. Increased muscle resting tension
6. Trigger points
7. Postural malalignment
8. Altered sleep patterns secondary to chronic pain
9. Altered body image

**Key Functional Limitations**

1. Gait problems
2. Pain with functional activities, such as walking, standing, and transfers
3. Decreased activity tolerance secondary to pain, muscle weakness, and compensatory movements

**Key Clinical Outcomes for Massage Techniques**

1. Effleurage
   - Sedation
   - Reduced perception of pain
2. Petrissage
   - Reduced muscle resting tension
   - Sedation
   - Increased muscle extensibility
   - Marginal effect on trigger point reduction resulting in pain reduction
3. Tapotement
   - Not indicated for the key impairments for OA pain
   - Increased alertness

4. Stripping
   - Reduction of trigger point activity resulting in pain reduction
5. Specific Compression
   - Reduction of trigger point activity
6. Joint Play/Mobilization Techniques
   - Low-grade techniques for pain reduction resulting in pain reduction
7. Complementary Techniques to Include:
   - Stretching
   - Ice or heat
   - Therapeutic exercise
   - Functional activity

The practitioner then listed the effects of massage techniques that this research study proposed:

1. Tapotement
2. Effleurage
3. Petrissage
   - Increased range of motion
   - Pain reduction
   - Increased perceived function
   - Reduced perceived stiffness
   - Improved gait

The practitioner's first decision based on his evaluation of the evidence, clinical experience, and his patients' needs was not to provide 1-hour full-body Swedish massage interventions since his patients had one or two affected joints. He also thought that he could use his treatment time more effectively with a more localized treatment that incorporated other massage and complementary techniques.

The practitioner's next decision was to ensure that his clinical examination addressed the key impairments in body structures and functions for OA to provide him with a better framework for selecting massage and other complementary techniques. The practitioner's quandary was that the research study had combined three massage techniques with differing clinical effects without specific guidelines for applying them. Based on his clinical knowledge, he chose petrissage as the most useful of the three techniques for treatment, since tapotement was primarily for stimulation and effleurage was more useful as an introductory technique. In addition, he chose to add stripping, specific compression, joint play/mobilization techniques, and complementary techniques to the interventions depending on his patients' presenting impairments in body structures and functions. The practitioner's final decision was to go back to the research literature to get more information on the effects of petrissage, stripping, specific compression, and joint play techniques in general and for patients with OA.

## REVIEWING THE BASICS

Massage is known for its integration of body, mind, and spirit. Does integrating best evidence into clinical practice undermine the importance of a therapist's ability to feel and use his intuition? Thinking and feeling in attunement with the unique needs and preferences of clients is both the art and science of massage. One enhances the other. Many brilliant and creative solutions arise from hunches, intuition, and feelings. Evidence-based practice works best when therapists develop their capacity to think critically, to feel, and to follow their intuition simultaneously. For these reasons, therapists are wise to develop the ability to find, understand, critically evaluate, and apply research to practice.[18-27] They must select research from primary and secondary sources with a critical eye. When consuming that research, they must familiarize themselves with research methodologies from qualitative, quantitative, and whole systems approaches and consider the contributions of levels of evidence and evidence houses. Finally, they must be lifelong learners who continue to apply new evidence to their clinical practices throughout their careers.

## Evidence for Massage: Further Study and Practice

This section outlines some advanced issues in the areas of the research methodology and trends in massage research.

## TRENDS IN THE EVIDENCE ON MASSAGES

Research on massage is in its infancy. Nevertheless, the volume of high-quality research on massage has increased in recent years. For the greater part, these studies have investigated the safety and benefits of massage. Most of this work focuses on pain relief, psychological effects, and effects on the immune system. Consequently, there are fewer rigorous studies on other physiological effects of massage techniques such as muscle tension, connective tissue integrity, or fluid. Finally, researchers have also used meta-analyses and other systematic reviews of massage research to identify the most commonly reported and substantiated effects of massage techniques.

### Massage and Pain

A small, but growing, number of clinical trials suggest that massage can reduce pain in people with headaches,[28,29] low back and other orthopedic pain,[30-33] osteoarthritis,[34] pregnancy and labour,[35] and adult and pediatric cancer.[36-40] In addition, Furlan et al.[33] offer several conclusions in their Cochrane systematic review on massage and low back pain. They note that there is moderate evidence that massage reduces the intensity and quality of pain, compared with a placebo, in clients in the earlier stages of chronic low back pain. They also found moderate evidence that massage may reduce pain intensity and improve function in clients with chronic low back pain. In general, they state that massage interventions may save money by reducing the number of health care provider visits, the use of pain medications, and the costs of back care services.[41] Furthermore, they report that the beneficial effects of massage are long-lasting (at least 1 year postintervention) for clients with chronic low back pain. Finally, the effects of massage interventions improve when they are delivered by a licensed clinician and are combined with exercise and education.[42]

### Psychological Effects of Massage

There is increasing evidence that massage techniques may produce significant psychological benefits such as the reduction of stress, depression, and anxiety in many different populations.[43-47] Moyer et al.[47] take an innovative approach in their meta-analysis of massage research by adopting a psychotherapy perspective in light of the limitations of using a medical model for massage research. They conclude that multiple applications of massage may reduce perceived pain. In addition, they point out that trait anxiety and depression are among the best documented psychological effects of massage, with a course of interventions using massage techniques providing benefits similar in magnitude to those of psychotherapy.

### Massage and Immune Function

Many research studies have found a significantly positive effect of massage on the various indices of immune function, but this finding has not been uniform.[45-63] For example, there is an ongoing debate on whether biochemical indicators of stress, such as cortisol, serotonin, and dopamine levels, change following massage therapy. Several studies from the University of Miami's Touch Research Institute have shown that cortisol levels decrease following massage, whereas other studies have not demonstrated these findings, suggesting that further research is needed in this area.

## Other Physiological Effects of Massage

The following is a selection of other possible physiological effects of massage techniques on which there is a limited amount of research. First of all, several recent studies have reported a positive effect of massage on fatigue and the quality and quantity of sleep in people with a variety of conditions.[64–98] In addition, some research suggests that massage techniques may improve venous and lymphatic return, but much more research is needed to support this.[94–103] This is similar to the situation for the use of massage to increase arterial flow; the body of research is small and contradictory.[87,104–111] Furthermore, a small amount of recent research tends to confirm the traditional use of percussion for airway clearance,[112–116] although mechanical devices are probably equally effective. Oddly enough, there are no readily available studies on the effect of massage on reducing the resting tension of healthy muscle, which is a commonly quoted reason for intervention in the general population. This may be due to a poor understanding of what physiological processes contribute to resting tension in healthy muscle and the problems inherent in reliably assessing resting tension.[117] Finally, there is limited evidence to support the use of massage to reduce elevated tone associated with some neurological conditions.[118–120]

As the following section, Issues in Massage Research, suggests, a lack of evidence for the effects of massage are more of a reflection of methodological limitations than of a lack of potential treatment effectiveness. Clinicians can still benefit from reading the existing research on massage as long as they are aware of its strengths and limitations.

## ISSUES IN MASSAGE RESEARCH

Many of the same methodology issues faced by research on complementary and alternative health, and by health care research in general, currently plague the research on the effects of massage techniques. The issues include:

■ A lack of relevant outcome measures
■ Weak research methods
■ Poorly defined procedures for interventions
■ Heterogeneous or small samples

However, these limitations should not deter progress in this area. Instead, an understanding of the current limitations can fuel advances in research on massage techniques. Furthermore, clinicians should note that there is an ever-increasing number of well-designed studies, including randomized clinical trials, that systematically document the positive effects of massage techniques.

## Issues in Current Research Methodologies

The Cochrane Systematic Review by Haraldsson et al.[121] of the effects of massage for people with mechanical neck disorders illustrates some of the current limitations of massage research. First of all, they found that the methodological quality of the studies was low and classified 12 of the 19 studies as low-quality studies. In addition, the heterogeneity of the participants in the studies prevented statistical pooling of results across studies. On the positive side, the characteristics of participants in the studies were well reported. By contrast, the studies had poor descriptions of the massage intervention and the experience of the treating clinicians. Descriptions of interventions often combined multiple techniques and omitted descriptions of the specific interventions and their rationale. Some studies included massage interventions that many clinicians would not consider appropriate for the conditions under investigation. In addition, only 11 of the 19 studies provided sufficient detail to determine who was actually delivering the intervention. Finally, the variations in the massage techniques and research methods made it impossible for these authors to draw conclusions about the effectiveness of massage for improving neck pain and function.

## Directions in Designing and Reporting Research for Massage

In acknowledgement of the existing limitations in the research, there is a movement underway to develop clearer guidelines for designing and reporting research on massage. Several of these efforts are intended to cross disciplines and journals with the aim of enhancing the overall quality of evidence on massage techniques.

In the realm of research design, several key issues are targeted for improvement. These include:

■ Increasing the number of studies on effectiveness
■ Providing clear definitions of massage protocols or interventions that include the dosage and frequency of interventions

- Evaluating specific massage techniques, rather than using global interventions that combine multiple techniques
- Outlining the qualifications of treating clinicians and other study personnel
- Examining the complex nonspecific effects of massage such as the therapeutic relationship and clinical setting
- Creating and using outcome measures that can measure the potential effects of massage
- Increasing the number of participants in studies or using methodologies that are appropriate for studies with small sample sizes
- Using more systematic and rigorous research designs for qualitative, quantitative, or whole systems studies

Peer-reviewed journals provide guidelines for reporting research. In addition, some organizations are developing standards that apply to multiple journals and disciplines. The CONSORT Statement, for example, takes an evidence-based approach to improving the quality of reports of randomized trials.[122] This statement is available in several languages and has been endorsed by prominent medical journals such as *The Lancet, Annals of Internal Medicine,* and *Journal of the American Medical Association.* CONSORT is comprised of a checklist and flow diagram to offer researchers a standard way to report trials. The checklist includes items, based on evidence, that researchers need to address in their reports. To supplement this, the flow diagram provides researchers with a clear picture of the progress of research participants in the trial, from the time of randomization to groups until the end of their involvement in the project. The intent is to make reports of the experimental process more clear so that users of the data can evaluate it effectively.

As stated previously in this chapter, ethical clinicians continuously examine and develop their knowledge, skills, and attitudes throughout their professional careers. Critically evaluating the methodology we use in massage studies is another key component that is necessary for enhancing the quality of research studies on massage techniques and the evidence to support the use of massage techniques in clinical practice.

# HOW TO READ A RESEARCH ARTICLE CRITICALLY

Clinicians can assess the relative strengths and weaknesses of a research study for themselves by asking good questions while reading research articles.[1,6,9,37,38,121,123] Table 2-2 includes some questions that clinicians can use to guide their reading.

## The Introduction

Clinicians can glean the purpose of the study from the Introduction. This is also the section in which quantitative studies will outline the hypothesis the study is testing. In reading the Introduction, clinicians can determine if there is a clear clinical problem or gap in the research that provides a sound rationale for the study. In addition, they can examine the clinical population and clinical issues that the study addresses and decide if they are relevant for their own clinical practice.

## Research Methods

Whether the study is qualitative or quantitative, the Methodology section often holds the key to the credibility of the study. There are several important issues for novice clinicians to consider. First, clearly defined procedures for interventions, and the training of the clinicians providing interventions, will assist clinicians in determining (a) whether the interventions are relevant for their clinical populations, (b) whether researchers delivered them correctly, and (c) whether they could reproduce them in their own clinical practice. Second, clinicians can consider the characteristics of the study sample and judge whether they are a good representation of the clinical population or if researchers selected them in a manner that may distort the results. Third, clinicians can peruse the research procedures to identify if they are well-described, logical, and enable the researchers to answer the question or purpose they stated in the Introduction. Finally, clinicians need not shy away from the data analysis section. Even without advanced statistical knowledge, clinicians can make sense of the basic intent of the analysis and evaluate whether the researchers analyzed the relevant data. For example, did the researchers use some means of determining a correlation between scores if they claim to be identifying relationships? Or, did they use tests that show differences between the scores of groups if they state that they are comparing the performance of those groups?

## Research Results

Whether results are in a narrative, tables, charts, or other diagrams, they must be well organized and easily understood. The main issue for clinicians is whether the researchers could have reasonably obtained their results using the procedures they described. From there, clinicians can locate the positive and negative findings the researchers report. Clinicians are wise to return to the Results section as they read

## Introduction

- Is the clinical issue/problem or gap in the research clearly stated?
- Do the authors provide a complete and up-to-date literature review?
- Did the authors examine other studies that focus on similar designs, populations, and outcomes?
- Does the literature review provide support for clinical problem or research gap?
- Is the problem clinically relevant?
- Do the authors provide a stated model or paradigm that forms the theoretical basis for the study?
- Are the purposes or research questions clearly stated and supported by the literature?
- Does the quantitative study provide an identified hypothesis or expectation?

## Methods—Quantitative Studies

- Are the participants well described and a good representation of the clinical population?
- Do the authors give sufficient information on the sample and sampling approach for you to determine whether there is any bias in recruiting?
- Do the research methods allow the researcher to address the purpose of the study?
- Does the research design address threats to internal validity such as history, maturation, or testing?
- Are the interventions (independent variables) and anticipated response or outcomes (dependent variables) clearly described so you know what the authors are trying to measure?
- Do the authors describe the measures clearly and provide information on their reliability, validity, and other psychometric properties?
- Is it clear what questions the authors are answering with each measure?
- Do the authors control or deliver the intervention (independent variable) systematically?
- Are the treatment procedures and training of the people delivering the intervention described clearly enough so that you could reproduce them?
- Do the authors describe the research procedures clearly so that you can evaluate whether they are logical and reproducible?
- Do the authors analyze all of the important data?
- Does the data analysis match the design and purposes of the study?

## Methods—Qualitative Studies

- Are the participants and the context in which they live well described?
- Are the researchers qualified to use the methods described in their study? For example, are they experienced interviewers?

- Do the authors clearly describe their sample and sampling approach for you to determine whether there is any bias in recruiting?
- Are the treatment procedures and training of the people delivering the intervention described clearly enough so that you could reproduce them?
- Do the research methods allow the researcher to address the purpose of the study?
- Do the researchers use rigorous and appropriate methods for collecting high-quality data?
- Do the researchers describe techniques they use to increase the quality of their results and interpretations?
- Have the researchers accounted for all of the participants, or did some of them leave the study?
- Does the data analysis match the design and purposes of the study?

## Results

- Do the authors clearly report key findings from data analysis, or are there missing data?
- Are the findings consistent with the stated purpose and procedures?
- For quantitative studies, do the authors state whether their results are statistically significant or clinically significant?
- Could the researcher have reasonably obtained the reported results using the procedures they outline?
- For quantitative studies, do you believe that changes in outcomes or response (dependent variables) are due to the intervention (independent variable)?
- For qualitative studies, are the results credible, given the question and the methods?

## Discussion/Conclusions

- Are the conclusions what you would expect from the authors' stated results and purposes?
- In quantitative studies, do the authors state whether the hypothesis was rejected or accepted?
- Do the authors relate their findings to existing literature and clinical practice when explaining their conclusions?
- Do the authors provide a logical explanation for their results or lack of results?
- Do the authors outline limitations of their design and suggested improvements?
- Do the authors provide directions for future research suggested by their study?
- Would you change the way you practice based on this study?

## General Questions

- Is it a peer-reviewed journal with blinded reviewers?
- Are the background and experience of the researchers appropriate for the study?
- Is there any bias resulting from the agencies that funded the study?

Adapted from Menard MB. *Making Sense of Research: A Guide to Research Literacy for Complementary Practitioners.* Toronto: Curties-Overzet; 2003; and Dumholdt E, Malone T. Evaluating research literature: the educated clinician. *Phys Ther.* 1984;65:487–491.

the Discussion and Conclusions to see if the researchers' findings do, in fact, support their conclusions.

## Discussion and Conclusions

Armed with a basic analysis of the study, clinicians can review the researchers' conclusions with a critical eye. Do the authors give logical explanations for their findings or lack of findings? Do they use the existing literature to support their arguments? Are there gaps in the logic of their conclusions or limitations to the study design? These are some of the questions clinicians can consider at this point. Finally, they can focus on identifying the relevance of the study's findings for their own clinical practice.

### References

1. Menard MB. *Making Sense of Research: A Guide to Research Literacy for Complementary Practitioners.* Toronto: Curties-Overzet; 2003.
2. Eisenberg DE, Davis RB, Ettner SL, Appel S, Wilkey S, Van Rompay M, Kessler RC. Trends in alternative medicine use in the United States, 1990–1997: Results of a follow-up national survey. *JAMA.* 1998;280:1569–1575.
3. Ramsey SD, Spencer AC, Topolski TD, Belza B, Patrick DL. Use of alternative therapies by older adults with osteoarthritis. *Arthritis Rheum.* 2001;45:222–227.
4. Dryden T, Achilles R. Massage Therapy Research Curriculum Kit. Evanston, IL: American Massage Therapist Foundation; 2004.
5. Dryden T, Findlay B, Boon H, Verhoef M, Mior S, Baskwill A. Research requirement: literacy amongst complementary and alternative health care (CAHC) practitioners. Ottawa: Natural Health Products Directorate, Health Canada; 2004.
6. Sackett D, Straus SE, Richardson WS, Rosenberg W, Haynes B. *Evidence-Based Medicine: How to Practice and Teach EBM.* Edinburgh: Churchill Livingstone; 2000.
7. Greenhalgh T. How to read a paper. *BMJ.* 2001;322:3–5.
8. Lewith GT, Jonas W, Walach H. *Clinical Research in Complementary Therapies: Principles, Problems and Solutions.* Edinburgh: Churchill Livingstone; 2001.
9. Jonas WB. The evidence house: something we can all live in. *West J Med.* 2001;175:79–80.
10. Portney L, Watkins M. *Foundations of Clinical Research: Applications to Practice.* Norwalk, CT: Appleton & Lange; 1993.
11. Lincoln Y, Guba E. *Naturalistic Inquiry.* Thousand Oaks, CA: Sage Publications; 1995.
12. Hymel G. *Research Methods for Massage and Holistic Therapies.* St. Louis: Elsevier, Mosby; 2005.
13. Guyatt G, Rennie D. *User's Guide to the Medical Literature: Essentials of Evidence-Based Clinical Practice.* Chicago: American Medical Association Press; 2001.
14. Glaser BG, Strauss AL. *The Discovery of Grounded Theory: Strategies for qualitative research.* New York: Aldine de Gruyter; 1967.
15. Ritenbaugh C, Verhoef MJ, Fleishman S. Whole systems research: a discipline for studying complementary and alternative medicine. *Altern Ther Health Med.* 2003;9:32–36.
16. Glaros S. All evidence is not created equal: a discussion of levels of evidence. *PT Magazine.* 2003;11:42–49, 52.
17. Gibbs LE. *Evidence-Based Practice for the Helping Professions: A Practical Guide with Integrated Multimedia.* Pacific Grove, CA: Thompson, Brooks, Cole; 2003:19.
18. Benjamin BE, Piltch C. Ben Benjamin's corner. Massage therapists need to embrace research. *Massage Ther J.* 2005;44:32–35.
19. Cassidy CM. Methodological issues in investigations of massage bodywork therapy. Part IV: experimental research designs. *J Bodywork Movement Ther.* 2003;7:240–250.
20. Cassidy CM. Methodological issues in investigations of massage/bodywork therapy. Part III: qualitative and quantitative designs for MBT and the bias of interpretation. *J Bodywork Movement Ther.* 2003;7:136–141.
21. Cassidy CM. Methodological issues in investigations of massage/bodywork therapy. Part II: making research designs and data credible: model fit validity, combining scientific soundness with the explanatory model of massage and bodywork therapies. *J Bodywork Movement Ther.* 2003;7:71–79.
22. Cassidy CM. Methodological issues in the scientific investigation of massage and bodywork therapy. Part I. *J Bodywork Movement Ther.* 2003;7:2–10.
23. Hymel GM. Integrating research competencies in massage therapy education. *J Bodywork Movement Ther.* 2005;9:43–51.
24. Hymel GM. Advancing massage therapy research competencies: dimensions for thought and action. *J Bodywork Movement Ther.* 2003;7:194–199.
25. Richardson J. Developing and evaluating complementary therapy services. Part 1: establishing service provision through the use of evidence and consensus development. *J Altern Complement Med.* 2001;7:253–260.
26. Stuttard P. Working in partnership to develop evidence-based practice within the massage profession. *Complement Ther Nurs Midwifery.* 2002;8:185–190.
27. American Physical Therapy Association. *Guide to Physical Therapist Practice.* 2nd ed. Alexandria, VA: American Physical Therapy Association; 1999.
28. Quinn C, Chandler C, Moraska A. Massage therapy and frequency of chronic tension headaches. *Am J Public Health.* 2002;92:1657–1661.
29. Hernandez-Reif M, Dieter J, Field T, Swerdlow B, Diego M. Migraine headaches are reduced by massage therapy. *Intern J Neurosci.* 1998;96:1–11.
30. Tsao J. Effectiveness of massage therapy for chronic, nonmalignant pain: a review. *eCAM Advance Access.* Published online on February 5, 2007. Available at http://ecam.oxfordjournals.org/cgi/content/full/nel109v1.

31. Dryden T, Baskwill A, Preyde M. Massage therapy for the orthopaedic patient: a review. *Orthop Nurs.* 2004;23:327–332.

32. Cherkin D, Eisenberg D, Sherman K, Barlow W, Kaptchuk T, Street J, et al. Randomized trial comparing traditional Chinese medical acupuncture, therapeutic massage, and self-care education for chronic low back pain. *Arch Intern Med.* 2001;161: 1081–1088.

33. Furlan A, Brosseau L, Imamura M, Irvin E. Massage for low-back pain: a systematic review within the framework of the Cochrane Collaboration Back Review Group. *Spine.* 2002;27: 1896–1910.

34. Perlman AI, Sabina A, Williams L-A, Njike JV, Katz D. Massage therapy for osteoarthritis of the knee: a randomized controlled trial. *Arch Intern Med.* 2006;116:2533–2538.

35. Chang M, Wang S, Chen C. Effects of massage on pain and anxiety during labour: a randomized controlled trial in Taiwan. *J Adv Nurs.* 2002;38:68–73.

36. Gecsedi R. Massage therapy for patients with cancer. *Clin J Oncol Nurs.* 2002;6:52–54

37. Cassileth B, Vickers A. Massage therapy for symptom control: outcome study at a major cancer centre. *J Pain Symptom Manage.* 2004;28:244–249.

38. Fellowes D, Barnes K, Wilkinson S. Aromatherapy and massage for symptom relief in patients with cancer. *Cochrane Database Syst Rev.* 2004;2:CD002287.

39. Post-White J, Hawks R. Complementary and alternative medicine in pediatric oncology. *Semin Oncol Nurs.* 2005;21: 107–114.

40. Phipps S, Dunavant M, Gray E, Rai SN. Massage therapy in children undergoing hematopoietic stem cell transplant: results of a pilot trial. *J Cancer Integr Med.* 2005;3:62–70.

41. Cherkin D, Sherman K, Deyo R, Shekelle P. A review of the evidence for the effectiveness, safety, and cost of acupuncture, massage therapy, and spinal manipulation for back pain. *Ann Intern Med.* 2003;138:898–906.

42. Preyde M. Effectiveness of massage therapy for subacute low-back pain: a randomized controlled trial. *Can Med Assoc J.* 2000;162:1815–1820.

43. Hanley J, Stirling P, Brown C. Randomised controlled trial of therapeutic massage in the management of stress. *Br J Gen Pract.* 2003;53:20–25.

44. Field T, Pickens J, Prodromidis M, et al. Targeting adolescent mothers with depressive symptoms for early intervention. *Adolescence.* 2000;35:381–414.

45. Field T, Diego MA, Hernandez-Reif M, Schanberg S, Kuhn C. Massage therapy effects on depressed pregnant women. *J Psychosom Obstet Gynaecol.* 2004;25:115–122.

46. Bost N, Wallis M. The effectiveness of a 15 minute weekly massage in reducing physical and psychological stress in nurses. *Aust J Adv Nurs.* 2006;23:28–33.

47. Moyer C, Rounges J, Hannum J. A meta-analysis of massage therapy research. *Psychol Bull.* 2004;130:3–18.

48. Shor-Posner G, Hernandez-Reif M, Miguez M, et al. Impact of a massage therapy clinical trial on immune status in young Dominican children infected with HIV-1. *J Altern Complement Med.* 2006;12:511–516.

49. Boylan M. Massage boosts immunity in breast cancer patients. *J Aust Trad Med Soc.* 2005;11:59–62.

50. Hernandez-Reif M, Ironson G, Field T, et al. Breast cancer patients have improved immune and neuroendocrine functions following massage therapy. *J Psychosom Res.* 2004;57: 45–52.

51. Shor-Posner G, Miguez MJ, Hernandez-Reif M, Perez-Then E, Fletcher M. Massage treatment in HIV-1 infected Dominican children: A preliminary report on the efficacy of massage therapy to preserve the immune system in children without antiretroviral medication. *J Altern Complement Med.* 2004;10: 1093–1095.

52. Goodfellow LM. The effects of therapeutic back massage on psychophysiologic variables and immune function in spouses of patients with cancer. *Nurs Res.* 2003;52:318–328.

53. Lovas JM, Craig AR, Raison RL, Weston KM, Segal YD, Markus MR. The effects of massage therapy on the human immune response in healthy adults. *J Bodywork Movement Ther.* 2002;6:143–150.

54. Diego MA, Field T, Hernandez-Reif M, Shaw K, Friedman L, Ironson G. HIV adolescents show improved immune function following massage therapy. *Int J Neurosci.* 2001;106:35–45.

55. Field T, Cullen C, Diego M, et al. Leukemia immune changes following massage therapy. *J Bodywork Movement Ther.* 2001; 5:271–274.

56. Birk TJ, McGrady A, MacArthur RD, Khuder S. The effects of massage therapy alone and in combination with other complementary therapies on immune system measures and quality of life in human immunodeficiency virus. *J Altern Complement Med.* 2000;6:405–414.

57. Field T, Hernandez-Reif M, Diego M, Schanberg S, Kuhn C. Cortisol decreases and serotonin and dopamine increase following massage therapy. *Int J Neurosci.* 2005;115:1397–1413.

58. HernandezReif M, Field T, Krasnegor J, Theakston H, Hossain Z, Burman I. High blood pressure and associated symptoms were reduced by massage therapy. *J Bodywork Movement Ther.* 2000;4:31–38.

59. Hart S, Field T, Hernandez-Reif M, et al. Anorexia nervosa symptoms are reduced by massage therapy. *Eating Disorders.* 2001;9:289–299.

60. Furlan AD, Brosseau L, Imamura M, Irvin E. Massage for low-back pain: a systematic review within the framework of the Cochrane Collaboration back review group. *Spine.* 2002;27: 1896–1910.

61. McRee LD, Noble S, Pasvogel A. Using massage and music therapy to improve postoperative outcomes. *AORN J.* 2003;78: 433–442, 445–447.

62. Taylor AG, Galper DI, Taylor P, et al. Effects of adjunctive Swedish massage and vibration therapy on short-term postoperative outcomes: a randomized, controlled trial. *J Altern Complement Med.* 2003;9:77–89.

63. Okvat HA, Oz MC, Ting W, Namerow PB. Massage therapy for patients undergoing cardiac catheterization. *Altern Ther Health Med.* 2002;8:68–70, 72, 74–75.

64. Hernandez-Reif M, Field T, Krasnegor J, Theakston H. Lower back pain is reduced and range of motion increased after massage therapy. *Int J Neurosci.* 2001;106:131.

65. Tiffany Field. Fibromyalgia pain and substance P decrease and sleep improves after massage therapy. *J Clin Rheumatol.* 2002;8:72–76.

66. Smith MC, Kemp J, Hemphill L, Vojir CP. Outcomes of therapeutic massage for hospitalized cancer patients. *J Nurs Scholarsh.* 2002;34:257–262.

67. Escalona A, Field T, Singer-Strunck R, Cullen C, Hartshorn K. Brief report: improvements in the behavior of children with autism following massage therapy. *J Autism Dev Disord.* 2001;31:513–516.

68. Tsay SL, Rong JR, Lin PF. Acupoints massage in improving the quality of sleep and quality of life in patients with end-stage renal disease. *J Adv Nurs.* 2003;42:134–142.

69. Field T, Hernandez-Reif M, Diego M, Feijo L, Vera Y, Gil K. Massage therapy by parents improves early growth and development. *Infant Behav Dev.* 2004;27:435–442.

70. Williams AF, Vadgama A, Franks PJ, Mortimer PS. A randomized controlled crossover study of manual lymphatic drainage therapy in women with breast cancer-related lymphoedema. *Eur J Cancer Care (Engl).* 2002;11:254–261.

71. Cullen LA, Barlow JH. A training and support programme for caregivers of children with disabilities: an exploratory study. *Patient Educ Couns.* 2004;55:203–209.

72. Field T. Massage and aroma therapy. *Int J Cosmetic Sci.* 2004;26:169–170.

73. Shen P. Two hundred cases of insomnia treated by otopoint pressure plus acupuncture. *J Tradit Chin Med.* 2004;24:168–169.

74. Soden K, Vincent K, Craske S, Lucas C, Ashley S. A randomized controlled trial of aromatherapy massage in a hospice setting. *Palliat Med.* 2004;18:87–92.

75. Weze C, Leathard HL, Stevens G. Evaluation of healing by gentle touch for the treatment of musculoskeletal disorders. *Am J Public Health.* 2004;94:50–52.

76. Dieter JN, Field T, Hernandez-Reif M, Emory EK, Redzepi M. Stable preterm infants gain more weight and sleep less after five days of massage therapy. *J Pediatr Psychol.* 2003;28:403–411.

77. Wang XH, Yuan YD, Wang BF. Clinical observation on effect of auricular acupoint pressing in treating sleep apnea syndrome. *Zhongguo Zhong Xi Yi Jie He Za Zhi.* 2003;23:747–749.

78. Barlow J, Cullen L. Increasing touch between parents and children with disabilities: preliminary results from a new programme. *J Fam Health Care.* 2002;12:7–9.

79. Ferber SG, Laudon M, Kuint J, Weller A, Zisapel N. Massage therapy by mothers enhances the adjustment of circadian rhythms to the nocturnal period in full-term infants. *J Dev Behav Pediatr.* 2002;23:410–415.

80. Field T. Massage therapy. *Med Clin North Am.* 2002;86:163–171.

81. HernandezReif M, Field T, Largie S, et al. Parkinson's disease symptoms are differentially affected by massage therapy vs. progressive muscle relaxation: a pilot study. *J Bodywork Movement Ther.* 2002;6:177–182.

82. Tsay SL, Chen ML. Acupressure and quality of sleep in patients with end-stage renal disease: a randomized controlled trial. *Int J Nurs Stud.* 2003;40:1–7.

83. Agarwal KN, Gupta A, Pushkarna R, Bhargava SK, Faridi MM, Prabhu MK. Effects of massage & use of oil on growth, blood flow & sleep pattern in infants. *Indian J Med Res.* 2000;112:212–217.

84. Shen P. Two hundred cases of insomnia treated by otopoint pressure plus acupuncture. *J Tradit Chin Med.* 2004;24:168–169.

85. Deng G, Cassileth BR, Yeung KS. Complementary therapies for cancer-related symptoms. *J Support Oncol.* 2004;2:419–429.

86. Ironson G, Field T, Scafidi F, Hashimoto M, Kumar M, Kumar A, et al. Massage therapy is associated with enhancement of the immune system's cytotoxic capacity. *Intern J Neurosci.* 1996;84:205–217.

87. Williams AF, Vadgama A, Franks PJ, Mortimer PS. A randomized controlled crossover study of manual lymphatic drainage therapy in women with breast cancer-related lymphedema. *Eur J Cancer Care (Engl).* 2002;11:254–261.

88. Cassar M. The application of massage in psychogenic disorders. *Positive Health.* 2004;24:45–45.

89. Richards K, Nagel C, Markie M, Elwell J, Barone C. Use of complementary and alternative therapies to promote sleep in critically ill patients. *Crit Care Nurs Clin North Am.* 2003;15:329–340.

90. Cho YC, Tsay SL. The effect of acupressure with massage on fatigue and depression in patients with end-stage renal disease. *J Nurs Res.* 2004;12:51–59.

91. Yang JH. The effects of foot reflexology on nausea, vomiting and fatigue of breast cancer patients undergoing chemotherapy. *Taehan Kanho Hakhoe Chi.* 2005;35:177–185.

92. Cassileth BR, Vickers AJ. Massage therapy for symptom control: outcome study at a major cancer center. *J Pain Symptom Manage.* 2004;28:244–249.

93. Deng G, Cassileth BR, Yeung KS. Complementary therapies for cancer-related symptoms. *J Support Oncol.* 2004;2:419–426.

94. Kohara H, Miyauchi T, Suehiro Y, Ueoka H, Takeyama H, Morita T. Combined modality treatment of aromatherapy, footsoak, and reflexology relieves fatigue in patients with cancer. *J Palliat Med.* 2004;7:791–796.

95. Post-White J, Kinney ME, Savik K, Gau JB, Wilcox C, Lerner I. Therapeutic massage and healing touch improve symptoms in cancer. *Integr Cancer Ther.* 2003;2:332–344.

96. Rexilius SJ, Mundt C, Erickson Megel M, Agrawal S. Therapeutic effects of massage therapy and handling touch on caregivers of patients undergoing autologous hematopoietic stem cell transplant. *Oncol Nurs Forum.* 2002;29:E35–E44.

97. Offenbacher M, Stucki G. Physical therapy in the treatment of fibromyalgia. *Scand J Rheumatol Suppl.* 2000;113:78–85.

98. Field T, Quintino O, Henteleff T, Wells-Keife L, Delvecchio-Feinberg G. Job stress reduction therapies. *Altern Ther Health Med.* 1997;3:54–56.

99. McNeely ML, Magee DJ, Lees AW, Bagnall KM, Haykowsky M, Hanson J. The addition of manual lymph drainage to compression therapy for breast cancer related lymphedema: a randomized controlled trial. *Breast Cancer Res Treat.* 2004;86:95–106.

100. Harris SR, Hugi MR, Olivotto IA, Levine M, Steering Committee for Clinical Practice Guidelines for the Care and Treatment of Breast Cancer. Clinical practice guidelines for the care and treatment of breast cancer: 11. Lymphedema. *CMAJ.* 2001;164:191–199.

101. Andersen L, Højris I, Erlandsen M, Andersen J. Treatment of breast-cancer-related lymphedema with or without manual lymphatic drainage: a randomized study. *Acta Oncol.* 2000;39:399–405.

102. Badger C, Preston N, Seers K, Mortimer P. Physical therapies for reducing and controlling lymphedema of the limbs. *Cochrane Database Syst Rev.* 2004;4:CD003141.

103. Johansson K, Albertsson M, Ingvar C, Ekdahl C. Effects of compression bandaging with or without manual lymph drainage treatment in patients with postoperative arm lymphedema. *Lymphology.* 1999;32:103–110.

104. Shoemaker JK, Tiidus PM, Mader R. Failure of manual massage to alter limb blood flow: measures by Doppler ultrasound. *Med Sci Sports Exerc.* 1997;29:610–614.

105. Tiidus PM, Shoemaker JK. Effleurage massage, muscle blood flow and long-term post-exercise strength recovery. *Int J Sports Med.* 1995;16:478–483.

106. Sabir'ianov AR, Sabir'ianova ES, Epishev VV. Trends in slow wave variability of the central circulation in healthy individuals in response to massage of the collar cervical region. *Vopr Kurortol Fizioter Lech Fiz Kult.* 2004;6:13–15.

107. Liu Y, Xu S, Yan J, et al. Capillary blood flow with dynamical change of tissue pressure caused by exterior force. *Sheng Wu Yi Xue Gong Cheng Xue Za Zhi.* 2004;21:699–703.

108. Tsarev AI, Ezhova VA, Kunitsyna LA, Slovesnov SV, Chukreeva LN, Kolesnikova EI. Aromamassage of the cervical collar region in the combined treatment of patients with atherosclerotic dyscirculatory encephalopathy. *Vopr Kurortol Fizioter Lech Fiz Kult.* 2004;5:6–7.

109. Drust B, Atkinson G, Gregson W, French D, Binningsley D. The effects of massage on intra muscular temperature in the vastus lateralis in humans. *Int J Sports Med.* 2003;24:395–399.

110. Sabir'ianov AR, Shevtsov AV, Sabir'ianova ES, et al. Effect of reflex-segmental massage on central hemodynamics in healthy people. *Vopr Kurortol Fizioter Lech Fiz Kult.* 2004;2:5–7.

111. Prilutsky B. Medical massage and control of arterial hypertension. *Massage Bodywork.* 2003;18:62.

112. Varekojis SM, Douce FH, Flucke RL, et al. A comparison of the therapeutic effectiveness of and preference for postural drainage and percussion, intrapulmonary percussive ventilation, and high-frequency chest wall compression in hospitalized cystic fibrosis patients. *Respir Care.* 2003;48:24–28.

113. Oermann CM, Sockrider MM, Giles D, Sontag MK, Accurso FJ, Castile RG. Comparison of high-frequency chest wall oscillation and oscillating positive expiratory pressure in the home management of cystic fibrosis: a pilot study. *Pediatr Pulmonol.* 2001;32:372–377.

114. Fink JB. Positioning versus postural drainage. *Respir Care.* 2002;47:769–777.

115. Maa SH, Sun MF, Hsu KH, et al. Effect of acupuncture or acupressure on quality of life of patients with chronic obstructive asthma: a pilot study. *J Altern Complement Med.* 2003;9:659–670.

116. Hess DR. The evidence for secretion clearance techniques. *Respir Care.* 2001;46:1276–1293.

117. Simons DG, Mense S. Understanding and measurement of muscle tone as related to clinical muscle pain. *Pain.* 1998;75:1–17.

118. Hernandez-Reif M, Field T, Largie S, et al. Cerebral palsy symptoms in children decreased following massage therapy. *Early Child Dev Care.* 2005;175:445–456.

119. Duval C, Lafontaine D, Hérbert J, Leroux A, Panisset M, Boucher JP. The effect of Trager therapy on the level of evoked stretch responses in patients with Parkinson's disease and rigidity. *J Manipulative Physiol Ther.* 2002;25:455–464.

120. Siev-Ner I, Gamus D, Lerner-Geva L, Achiron A. Reflexology treatment relieves symptoms of multiple sclerosis: a randomized controlled study. *Mult Scler.* 2003;9:356–361.

121. Haraldsson BG, Gross AR, Myers CD, Ezzo JM, Morien A, Goldsmith C, Peloso PM, Bronfort G, Cervical Overview Group. Massage for mechanical neck disorders. *Cochrane Database Syst Rev.* 2006;3:CD004871.

122. CONSORT Statement. Accessed February 18, 2007. Available at http://www.consort-statement.org/.

123. Dumholdt E, Malone T. Evaluating research literature: the educated clinician. *Phys Ther.* 1984;65:487–491.

# Chapter 3

## Clinical Decision-Making for Massage

The clinical decision-making process guides the therapist through the examination, treatment, and discharge of the client. The decision-making process proposed for Outcome-Based Massage addresses issues that are specific to the integration of massage techniques into clinical practice. This chapter discusses clinical decision making over four phases: the Evaluative Phase, the Treatment Planning Phase, the Treatment Phase, and the Discharge Phase. It provides guidelines for therapists to use to enhance the appropriateness and adequacy of the client examinations, plans of care, and interventions they plan and provide.

*Note that the numbers of the steps in Figures 3-1, 3-2, 3-3, and 3-4 correspond to the step numbers that appear in Theory in Practice 3-1 through 3-27 and in many of the headings in this chapter.*

## Clinical Decision-Making for Massage: Foundations

### THE CLINICAL DECISION-MAKING PROCESS

The terms clinical decision making, clinical reasoning, and clinical problem solving are used to describe the process by which therapists analyze client information and formulate and progress therapeutic regimens for their clients.[1–6] The **clinical decision-making model** for Outcome-Based Massage discussed in this chapter integrates clinical reasoning models with the frameworks for massage discussed in the earlier chapters.

Although we present this model graphically as a series of numbered steps, we do not intend therapists to use it in a linear, sequential manner. In reality, as research indicates, therapists who are engaged in the clinical decision-making process often perform several steps of the process concurrently.[4] In addition, therapists use an iterative decision-making process, rather than a linear process. In other words, they cycle through the same steps of the decision-making process several times, and each time that they repeat the steps, they expand on their information and refine their hypotheses.

## Phases in Clinical Decision-Making

This clinical decision-making model has four phases: the **Evaluative Phase**, the **Treatment Planning Phase**, the **Treatment Phase**, and the **Discharge Phase**; each of the phases has a distinct purpose and procedures. Together, these phases lead the therapist through a systematic process that enhances the fit between the client's presenting issues and treatment techniques. This will ultimately improve the quality of care that therapists deliver, their clients' outcomes, and client satisfaction.

The Evaluative Phase provides the foundation of the clinical treatment process. The steps in the Evaluative Phase revolve around formulating and confirming a **clinical hypothesis** about the client's clinical problem or wellness goals. This phase begins with data gathering through the **client examination** and also involves confirming the **clinical problem** or articulating the **wellness goals**, creating a summary of clinical findings, and deciding whether to pursue treatment.

The steps in the Treatment Planning Phase involve identifying body structures and functions that are appropriate for treatment and selecting treatment techniques that will produce improvements in the client's impairments in body structures and functions, functional limitations, or overall wellness.[5] The Treatment Planning Phase for Outcome-Based Massage begins with the summary of clinical findings from the Evaluative Phase and ends with a written **plan of care**.

The Treatment Phase is an ongoing cycle of treatment, **re-examination**, and treatment progression that begins after the therapist completes the plan of care. The end of this phase is not clearly delineated; instead, there is a gradual transition from Treatment Phase to Discharge Phase.

The final phase is the Discharge Phase. **Discharge** involves the transition of the client from the therapist's care to self-care or to treatment by another therapist. The Discharge Phase begins before the client's discharge date; it spans the period from the initiation of discharge planning to the actual discharge date.

### Clinical Decision-Making for Wellness Interventions

Therapists will use this four-phase clinical decision-making process for both the treatment of impairments in body structures and functions and wellness **interventions**. The primary distinction between clinical decision making for the treatment of impairments and wellness is the need to address impairments in body structures and functions. These impairments can be any loss or abnormality of the client's body structures or functions that occurs as a result of the pathophysiology of a medical condition.[1] Treatment of impairments takes place after an individual has experienced a medical condition and addresses those impairments in body structures and functions (grades 1 to 4) that are the result of that medical condition. In the Evaluative Phase, the therapist creates a list of impairments and a list of outcomes that focus on the **treatment of impairments**, recovery, and the prevention of secondary impairments. This is in contrast to clinical decision-making for wellness, which focuses on body structures and functions that are free of impairments. In this case, the therapist creates a list of body structures and functions and outcomes for optimizing these during the Evaluative Phase. The Theory in Practice clinical scenario of the client with neck pain will illustrate the steps in the clinical decision-making process for Outcome-Based Massage in the treatment of impairments. Readers can apply the information on the distinction between clinical decision-making for treatment of impairments versus wellness interventions to arrive at the guidelines for the latter.

## EVALUATIVE PHASE

We cannot emphasize the importance of the Evaluative Phase enough. When a client presents for clinical care, it is often because he or she has a problem. Through the client examination and the **evaluation** of the clinical findings, the therapist clarifies the client's clinical problem and identifies the client's relevant impairments and functional limitations.

### Theory In Practice Scenario
#### Patient with "Neck Pain"

The patient is a 28-year-old woman who works as a cashier in a supermarket with a 2-month history of neck pain of gradual onset. Her referral states "Neck Pain."

*We have written a clinical scenario that is broad enough to apply to multiple professions. Readers need to use the scope of practice for their professions to guide their use of the examination and treatment techniques noted in this scenario.*

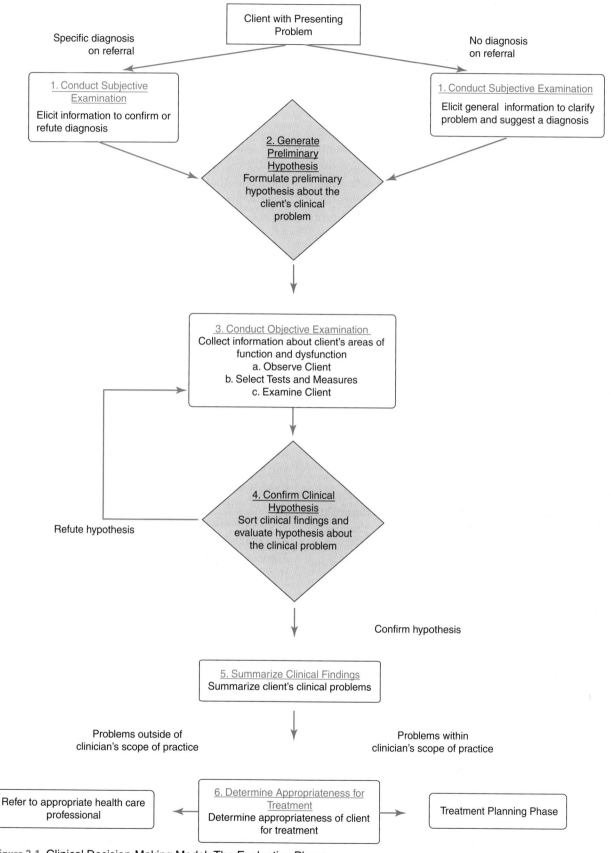

**Figure 3-1**  Clinical Decision-Making Model: The Evaluative Phase.

She will then use this information for outcome identification and treatment planning. Consequently, an appropriate, accurate, and comprehensive Evaluative Phase can enhance the potential effectiveness of an intervention.

## Client Examination

The Evaluative Phase begins with the client examination, which involves collecting information on the client's health status and clinical condition through history taking, a general systems review, and tests and measures.[7] Therapist and client characteristics can influence the scope of the examination a therapist performs. Relevant therapist characteristics include: her scope of practice, her area of specialization, and the type of examination she selects. Client characteristics include: the client's diagnosis and general health status, the nature of the clinical setting, and the acuity, severity, complexity, and stability of the client's condition (Table 3-1). The initial multidisciplinary neurological examination for a geriatric client with Parkinson's disease in an inpatient setting, for example, would be broader in scope and cover the issues in more detail than an interim examination of an adolescent with chondromalacia patellae in an outpatient orthopedic clinic.

### Conduct Subjective Examination (Step 1)

Prior to taking the client history, the therapist identifies whether or not there is a specific diagnosis on the client's referral. If there is a specific diagnosis, then the therapist's **history taking** and **subjective examination** will include questions relating to that diagnosis and will focus on eliciting information to confirm or refute the client's presenting diagnosis. If, on the other hand, the client has a referral without a **medical diagnosis**, the therapist begins by eliciting general information that will serve to clarify the client's presenting problem and suggest a clinical diagnosis. Chapter 5, Client Examination for Massage, provides suggestions for issues to consider in history taking for massage. Therapists can document the client's history within the written plan of care or separately.

### Generate Preliminary Clinical Hypothesis (Step 2)

Existing clinical decision-making models all include some form of data gathering and the formulation and testing of a clinical hypothesis.[1-5] In the current model, the therapist forms a preliminary clinical hypothesis about the client's key clinical problems based on the diagnosis on the client's referral and the information she has gathered from the history and subjective examination.

### Conduct Objective Examination (Step 3)

#### Observe Client

Once the therapist has formed her preliminary clinical hypothesis, she observes the client to identify observational cues that may support her hypothesis. At this early stage of the examination, the therapist needs to avoid having too narrow a focus. The observation of the client should be general enough to provide data that may suggest an alternative hypothesis, yet still enable the therapist to identify specific clinical signs that are consistent with her hypothesis. This observation can include postural alignment, muscle bulk and contours, and other areas outlined in this chapter and the individual techniques chapters. Based on her observations, the therapist may be able to refine her hypothesis about the client's clinical problem.

#### Select Tests and Measures

The therapist then proceeds to the next step in gathering data to confirm or refute her clinical hypothesis: the selection and application of **tests and measures**. The types of tests and measures and the order in which the therapist conducts them will differ with the client's characteristics and condition. In other words, therapists use different examination approaches for clients with neurological, musculoskeletal, cardiopulmonary, or psychoneuroimmunological conditions. For example, a musculoskeletal examination in physical therapy may consist of postural analysis, visual inspection, range of motion testing, muscle performance testing, and palpation. By contrast, a cardiopulmonary examination in physical therapy may consist of visual inspection, palpation, percussion, and auscultation. Additional modifications exist for examinations for adult, pediatric, and geriatric clients.

The selection of appropriate tests and measures is one of the most difficult components of the examination. The problem lies not in a lack of information but in the possibility of being overwhelmed by the considerable number of possible special tests and clinical signs. The therapist faces the challenge of recalling appropriate examination techniques, noting the client's response, and making a correct interpretation of the findings. Having one or two hypotheses about the client's problem can assist the therapist in refining her choice of examination techniques.

| Table 3-1 | Scope and Content of Client Examinations | | | |
|---|---|---|---|---|
| | **Initial Examination** | **Interim Examination or Re-Examination** | **Discharge Examination** | **Follow-Up Examination** |
| Scope | ■ Detailed exploratory examination | ■ Focused examination related to the identified outcomes related to impairments and functional limitations | ■ Detailed examination related to the intervention provided and the outcomes related to impairments and functional limitations the client has achieved | ■ Focused examination related to (a) the maintenance of previously achieved outcomes related to impairments and functional limitations or (b) the identification of ongoing treatment needs |
| Timing | ■ Performed prior to the initiation of treatment | ■ Performed at intervals following the initiation of treatment | ■ Performed at the end of the intervention period and prior to discharge of the client | ■ Performed following discharge from an episode of care |
| Objectives | ■ Confirm or refute the client's presenting diagnosis<br>■ Identify and measure the client's impairments, functional limitations, and functional areas to provide a basis for treatment planning and a baseline for interim examinations<br>■ Identify and measure the client's prior and presenting level of function to provide a basis for identifying reasonable functional outcomes | ■ Identify and measure changes in the client's impairments and functional level from the baseline established at the initial examination<br>■ Determine the client's achievement of outcomes<br>■ Determine the client's readiness for treatment progression<br>■ Determine the need to modify the plan of care or outcomes | ■ Determine the client's readiness for discharge through measurement of progress on outcomes<br>■ Identify and measure client's discharge needs<br>■ Identify and measure changes in the client's impairments and functional level from the baseline established at the initial examination. | ■ Identify and measure changes in the client's health status, impairments, and functional level from the baseline established at the most recent discharge examination<br>■ Determine client's level of safety and adaptation to their environment<br>■ Determine client's ongoing treatment needs |
| Components | ■ History to elicit information to confirm or refute the presenting diagnosis or to establish a diagnosis if none is given<br>■ Tests and measures to (a) confirm or refute the presenting diagnosis or to establish a diagnosis if none is given and (b) identify and measure impairments and functional limitations | ■ Tests and measures to determine changes in impairments and functional limitations | ■ History to summarize treatment<br>■ Discussion of the client's perceived discharge needs<br>■ Tests and measures to determine client's impairments and functional level at discharge | ■ History to elicit information on changes in health status, safety, and adaptation to the environment<br>■ Tests and measures to determine changes in impairments and functional limitations |

---

### Theory In Practice 3-1

#### Conduct Subjective Examination

Since the referral does not provide a specific diagnosis, the practitioner includes questions aimed at clarifying whether the patient has a radiculopathy or a soft-tissue injury. These questions include:

■ Radiation of pain
■ 24-hour pain behavior
■ Effect of position on pain
■ Presence of paresthesia

The patient's responses about her neck pain do not include radiating pain below the elbow, paresthesia, or pain increasing with cervical extension or lateral flexion.

The patient reports:

■ An insidious onset of localized neck and shoulder pain
■ Stiffness and decreased active cervical range of motion
■ Neck muscle tightness
■ Neck muscle spasm
■ Transient headaches

---

### Examine the Client

To keep data at a manageable level, the therapist may find it effective to first select and carry out a few tests that therapists commonly use to confirm or refute a given condition. If the findings are positive, the therapist can then collect more gen-

---

### Theory In Practice 3-2

#### Generate Preliminary Clinical Hypothesis

Based on the findings of the history and subjective examination, the practitioner hypothesizes that the patient's symptoms are due to the presence of active myofascial trigger points.

A myofascial trigger point is a hyperirritable spot within a skeletal muscle that is associated with a hypersensitive palpable nodule in a taut band.[8] Trigger points may refer pain, create nerve entrapment, contribute to muscle weakness, and significantly limit range of motion. Active trigger points, which are painful even when they are not being palpated, contribute to the following:

■ Decreased muscle flexibility and muscle strength
■ Increased referred pain during compression. In this case, they will produce referred pain in a pain pattern specific to that trigger point and can produce referred motor and autonomic responses.
■ Local twitch response in the muscle fibers in the area of the active trigger point when stimulated

---

### Theory In Practice 3-3a

#### Observe Client

The practitioner gathers observational data to initiate his identification of whether the patient has myofascial neck pain, rather than a radiculopathy.

His observations include:

■ No neck or shoulder girdle muscle wasting
■ Forward head posture
■ Visible muscle spasm in the region of the right upper trapezius

Using this information, the practitioner refines his clinical hypothesis to state that the patient has active myofascial trigger points in the right upper trapezius and possibly levator scapula muscles.

---

eral information about the client's impairments, functional limitations, and areas of function. If the findings from these confirmatory tests are negative, the therapist can decide whether she needs additional tests or needs to change her hypotheses. In situations in which the therapist does not have a clear clinical hypothesis, scanning examinations provide a means of quickly determining the integrity of several systems and assessing the nature of the client's symptoms.[9] Chapter 5, Client Examination for Massage, provides information on some examination techniques for massage that the reader can use to guide his or her selection of examination techniques.

## Evaluation of Findings

### Confirm the Clinical Hypothesis (Step 4)

At the conclusion of her client examination, the therapist analyzes the impairments stemming from the client's clinical condition and either confirms or refutes her clinical

---

### Theory In Practice 3-3b

#### Select Tests and Measures

The practitioner selects tests and measures that will provide information that will confirm or refute the presence of myofascial trigger points. These include:

■ Palpation of trapezius and levator scapulae muscles
■ Cervical range of motion
■ Upper extremity dermatomes
■ Upper extremity myotomes
■ Cervical compression and distraction
■ Performance of functional activities

---

**Theory In Practice 3-3c**

### Examine the Client

1. The practitioner examines the patient for signs of trigger points through palpation of the patient's trapezius and levator scapulae muscles for:
   - The presence of taut bands or nodules
   - The occurrence of a twitch response
   - Specific patterns of pain referral
2. The practitioner examines the patient's cervical spine with the following tests:
   - Range of motion: He notes that the patient presents with decreased active cervical range of motion.
   - Strength: He documents decreased strength of the right scapular elevation and retraction (trapezius and levator scapulae).
3. The practitioner rules out the presence of a radiculopathy by testing:
   - Upper extremity dermatomes and myotomes
   - Cervical compression
   - Cervical distraction
   He records the negative findings on these tests.
4. The practitioner assesses the patient's functional level since he can use the patient's functional areas to compensate for areas of dysfunction. In doing so, he notes the patient's difficulty performing the functional tasks associated with her job as a cashier, including:
   - Driving to work
   - Lifting and transferring objects with her right arm
   - Reaching objects above her head

---

**Theory In Practice 3-4**

### Confirm the Clinical Hypothesis

The practitioner identifies the critical impairments stemming from the patient's medical condition. He also confirms his clinical hypothesis that the following clinical signs are secondary to active myofascial trigger points in the right upper trapezius and right levator scapulae muscles:
- Neck pain and headaches
- Spasm
- Muscle tightness
- Decreased range of motion
- Decreased strength
- Inability to lift and reach

---

hypothesis. Some health care professions call the process and result of analyzing and organizing the findings from the client examination into clusters or syndromes the **therapy diagnosis**.[7] If the findings from the client examination do not support the therapist's clinical hypothesis, she will have to reformulate her hypothesis and repeat the process of selecting and carrying out appropriate tests and measures. There are situations in which the client may not present with a clearly defined clinical condition. In that case, it may be appropriate for the therapist to focus the treatment planning process on the general goal of improving the client's presenting impairments and functional limitations, rather than on identifying and treating a specific clinical condition.[7]

### Summarize Pertinent Clinical Findings (Step 5)

Once the therapist confirms her clinical hypothesis, she produces a summary of the impairments and functional limitations with which the client presents. This summary can be documented within the written plan of care or separately. In Outcome-Based Massage, as with other clinical approaches, failure to identify the impairments that are contributing to the client's functional limitations can lead to the development of an intervention that is not effective in achieving the established **functional outcomes**. In the clinical example, had the therapist assumed that the client was presenting with functional limitations secondary to a radiculopathy, he would have provided a regimen that would not have relieved the client's symptoms or improved the client's functional level.

### Determine Appropriateness for Treatment (Step 6)

Not all clients who receive a referral for treatment will actually require treatment. Therefore, therapists must review the findings from the client examination and determine whether the client would benefit from treatment such as the direct application of treatment techniques, education, or coordination of services. Once the therapist has confirmed that treatment is appropriate, and before she begins treatment planning, she needs to determine whether she has a **legal right to treat** and the **clinical competence to treat** the client's clinical condition.

In addition to legal issues related to right to treat, the therapist also has to make an ethical decision regarding her competence to treat the client's presenting clinical problems. This is a subjective decision that requires a balance of confidence in one's clinical skills and an objective assessment of the limitations of one's clinical expertise. In other words, it is not sufficient that the therapist's practice act permits the provision of interventions for a condition or the application of selected techniques; the therapist must also have sufficient training to administer this care appropriately, safely, and effectively.

## Theory In Practice 3-5: Items to Chart

### Summarize Pertinent Clinical Findings

Subjective     Pain:
- Neck pain at rest, at end of range of motion, and during functional activity; reported pain intensity of 8/10 on a visual analog scale
- Reported inability to drive or check out groceries at the cash register for > 10 minutes secondary to increased neck pain
- Tightness of neck muscles on waking and with fatigue
- Transient headaches (temporal region)

Functional Limitations:
- Inability to drive for > 10 minutes secondary to increased neck pain
- Inability to perform repetitive upper extremity movements in standing using the right arm for > 10 minutes (as required for checking out groceries at the cash register) secondary to neck pain
- Inability to perform lifting and transferring tasks required for her job

Objective     Observation:
- Forward head posture

Palpation:
- Palpable muscle spasm in the right trapezius
- Palpable taut bands in trapezius and levator scapulae
- Reported positive pattern of pain referral on palpation of the right trapezius trigger point
- Reported positive pattern of pain referral on palpation of the right levator scapulae trigger point
- Twitch response on palpation of trigger point locations in upper trapezius and levator scapulae muscles

Range of Motion:
- Decreased active cervical range of motion: flexion 50%, extension 75%, right rotation 75%, left lateral flexion 50%
- Tightness of the right trapezius and the right levator scapulae muscles
- Range of motion of shoulder, elbow, wrist, and hand within normal limits

Strength:
- Decreased strength: right levator scapulae—scapular elevation = grade 4−, right trapezius—scapular elevation, scapular retraction = grade 4−
- Strength of other shoulder, forearm, and hand muscles = 5/5

Functional Activities
- Inability to reach objects placed 1 foot above head with the right arm (as required for retrieving items from overhead shelves) secondary to neck pain
- Inability to lift a 5-lb object above shoulder level using the right arm (as required for placing boxes of dried goods on overhead shelves) secondary to neck pain
- Inability to lift and transfer a 15-lb object using the right arm (as required for placing customers' purchases into shopping carts) secondary to neck pain
- Inability to perform > 3 repetitions of lifting and transferring a 3-lb object at waist level using the right arm (as required for checking out customers' groceries and placing them in shopping bags) secondary to neck pain.

## Critical Thinking Question

Your client presents with a referral stating "Back Pain" after a recent fall. During your history taking, you suspect that he may have both a back injury and a hamstring strain. What are the steps that you would follow in the Evaluative Phase to address these two issues?

## Theory In Practice 3-6

### Determine Appropriateness for Treatment

The practitioner in this clinical scenario has training in trigger point therapy and considers the treatment of this patient with myofascial neck pain to be within his professional scope of practice and clinical competence. If this patient with neck pain had signs of an underlying metabolic disorder, significant radiculopathy, or any unusual clinical findings, it would be appropriate for the practitioner to refer the patient to a physician for further examination and treatment.

# TREATMENT PLANNING PHASE

## Analyze Findings and Generate the Clinical Problem List (Step 7)

Before the therapist can begin selecting treatment techniques, she needs to organize the clinical findings on the client's impairments and functional limitations into a **clinical problem list** to guide treatment planning. First of all, it is important for the therapist to distinguish between the client's areas of function and dysfunction or those areas that will respond to the direct application of treatment techniques and those that will not. Rather than dismissing areas of function because they do not require treatment, the therapist is wise to identify which of these areas she can use to compensate for impairments that are not amenable to active treatment. An example of this strategy occurs later in this chapter.

Once the therapist has identified the areas of dysfunction, it is important for her to differentiate between the client's impairments and functional limitations. Impairment can be any loss or abnormality of the client's body structures or functions, whereas functional limitations refer to the individual's ability to execute tasks within his or her environment.[1] The strategy used in treatment planning for Outcome-Based Massage will be to select treatment techniques to treat the identified impairments and to use the identified functional limitations as a baseline for setting functional outcomes. Once the therapist completes these tasks, she can compile the clinical problem list.

## Identify Functional Outcomes (Step 8)

The therapist can now focus on identifying relevant functional outcomes in collaboration with the client and predicting the amount of time needed to achieve these outcomes. These outcomes should be consistent with the functional limitations that she documented during the client examination. Table 1-5 (Chapter 1) gives examples of functional outcomes. The therapist will base the outcomes and the time needed to achieve them on several factors:

- The client's current and prior level of function
- The severity, complexity, stability, and acuity of the client's condition
- The client's discharge destination
- The literature on the prognosis for an individual with that condition
- The therapist's judgment, from clinical experience, of what the client has the potential to achieve[7]

In addition, therapists can seek guidance from articles on clinical practice and research in professional journals, clinical texts, general practice guidelines for professions, or the numerous practice guidelines that are available for specific clinical conditions. In some health care professions, this process of predicting the client's level and timing of improvement is know as the **therapy prognosis**.[7]

It is not sufficient to identify the long-term functional outcomes for the client; the therapist must also identify short-term outcomes and predict what level of improvement the client can achieve in a given time frame. This is necessary because, although long-term functional outcomes are useful for gauging the client's readiness for discharge, they are of little value in evaluating the client's immediate and ongoing response to treatment. A short-term outcome that the client can achieve within a few sessions provides a useful early benchmark of the effectiveness of the intervention and can be an invaluable aid to the ongoing modification and progression of treatment. The time period for achieving these short-term outcomes will vary with the acuity, severity, complexity, and stability of the client's condition; the expected rate of change in the client's functional level; the frequency of interventions; the anticipated duration of the treatment; and the clinical setting. The therapist's goal is to set outcomes in measurable and meaningful increments that the client can reasonably achieve in the allocated time period. It may be appropriate, for example, to set weekly, or even daily, outcomes for a client in an acute care or outpatient setting who the therapist expects to have significant functional gains over a short course of treatment. By contrast, monthly outcomes may be more meaningful for a geriatric client in a skilled nursing setting who receives treatment for a chronic condition.

A common question is: "How can the therapist determine whether the functional outcomes are appropriate for massage?" In reality, the issue is whether the impairments that the therapist must address in order to achieve the functional outcome are appropriate for treatment with the use of massage as the primary treatment technique. This decision about the relevance of the impairments for massage comes later in this phase of the decision-making process.

## Identify Treatable Impairments and Relevant Outcomes (Step 9a)

Once the therapist has established functional outcomes, she works backwards to identify:

- Which impairments need to be treated to facilitate the achievement of the functional outcomes

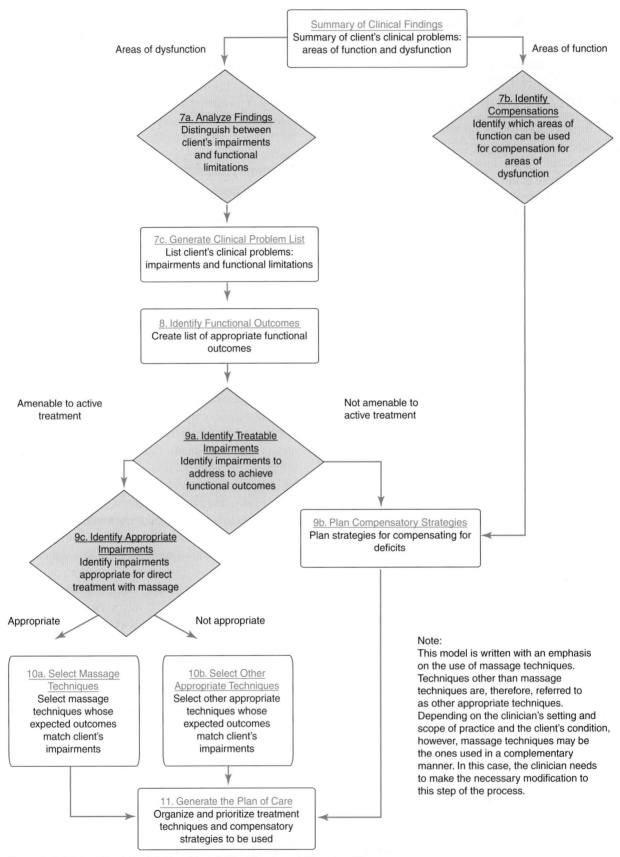

**Figure 3-2** Clinical Decision-Making Model: The Treatment Planning Phase.

## Analyze Findings and Generate the Clinical Problem List

Impairments
- Pain: Neck pain and temporal headaches
- Decreased muscle extensibility: Tightness of trapezius and levator scapulae muscles
- Postural malalignment: Forward head posture
- Muscle resting tension: Muscle spasm in the right trapezius
- Decreased active cervical range of motion
- Decreased muscular performance: Decreased right trapezius and right levator scapulae strength and endurance
- Decreased muscle integrity: Active trigger points in the right upper trapezius and levator scapulae

Functional Limitations
- Inability to drive for > 10 minutes secondary to increased neck pain
- Inability to perform repetitive upper extremity movements in standing using the right arm for > 10 minutes secondary to neck pain
- Inability to reach objects placed 1 foot above head with the right arm secondary to neck pain
- Inability to lift a 5-lb object above shoulder level using the right arm secondary to neck pain
- Inability to lift and transfer a 5-lb object using the right arm secondary to neck pain
- Inability to perform > 3 repetitions of lifting and transferring a 3-lb object at waist level using the right arm secondary to neck pain

## Identify Functional Outcomes

The practitioner identifies the functional outcomes outlined below based on (a) the patient's presenting functional limitations and (b) the observation that the patient is a young woman who is in good health, besides the myofascial neck pain, and who had normal functional ability before the onset of pain 2 months prior to the examination.

**Functional Limitations**

1. Inability to drive for > 10 minutes secondary to increased neck pain
2. Inability to perform repetitive upper extremity movements in standing using the right arm for > 10 minutes (as required for checking out groceries at the cash register) secondary to neck pain
3. Inability to reach objects placed 1 foot above head with the right arm (as required for retrieving items from overhead shelves) secondary to neck pain
4. Inability to lift a 5-lb object above shoulder level using the right arm (as required for placing boxes of dried goods on overhead shelves) secondary to neck pain
5. Inability to lift and transfer a 15-lb object using the right arm (as required for placing customers' purchases into shopping carts) secondary to neck pain
6. Inability to perform > 3 repetitions of lifting and transferring a 3-lb object at waist level using the right arm (as required for checking out customers' groceries and placing them in shopping bags) secondary to neck pain

**Functional Outcomes**

Short-Term Outcomes (2 weeks)
1. Able to drive for ½ hour without complaints of pain
2. Able to work checking out groceries at the cash register for ½ hour, with appropriate breaks, without complaints of pain
3. Able to lift a 5-lb object and place it on shelf at shoulder level—1 repetition without complaints of neck pain
4. Able to reach objects placed 1 foot above head with the right arm without complaints of neck pain
5. Able to lift and transfer an 8-lb object at waist level with the right arm without complaints of pain
6. Able to perform 5 repetitions of transferring a 5-lb object at waist level using the right arm without complaints of pain.

Long-Term Outcomes (Discharge: 4 weeks)
1. Able to drive for 1.5–2 hours without complaints of neck pain
2. Able to work checking out groceries at the cash register for 2 hours, with appropriate breaks, without complaints of pain
3. Able to lift an 8-lb object and place it on shelf at shoulder level—5 repetitions without complaints of neck pain
4. Able to reach objects placed 2 feet above head with the right arm without complaints of neck pain.
5. Able to lift and transfer a 15-lb object at waist level with the right arm without complaints of neck pain
6. Able to perform 15 repetitions of transferring a 5-lb object at waist level using the right arm without complaints of neck pain

- Which of these impairments are amenable to active treatment
- Which impairments require compensations because they are not amenable to active treatment
- The **impairment-related outcome** for each impairment that she will treat

Traditionally, therapists established treatment goals and selected treatment techniques based solely on the impairments that they observed during the client examination. The adoption of models of functioning, disability, and health in health care has expanded this focus to include the impact of treatment on clients' body structures, body functions, level of activity, and functional limitations.[1] Therapists now identify and treat clients' underlying impairments and address their level of activity and functional limitations.[5] What remains unclear is whether there is a direct relationship between improved impairments and improvements in functional level. A balanced approach to treatment planning is to identify and treat the client's impairments as a means of facilitating the achievement of the functional outcomes, rather than focusing solely on impairments or functional limitations.

---

**Theory In Practice 3-9a**

### Identify Treatable Impairments and Relevant Outcomes

| Functional Limitation | Associated Impairments |
|---|---|
| Inability to perform driving tasks | ■ Pain: Neck pain and temporal headaches<br>■ Postural malalignment: Forward head posture<br>■ Decreased active cervical range of motion<br>■ Muscle spasm in the right trapezius<br>■ Decreased muscle integrity: Active trigger points in the right upper trapezius and levator scapulae |
| Inability to perform repetitive upper extremity movements in standing | ■ Pain: Neck pain and temporal headaches<br>■ Postural malalignment: Forward head posture<br>■ Decreased active cervical range of motion |
| | ■ Muscle spasm in the right trapezius<br>■ Decreased muscular performance: Decreased right trapezius and right levator scapulae strength and endurance<br>■ Decreased muscle integrity: Active trigger points in the right upper trapezius and levator scapulae<br>■ Decreased muscle extensibility: Tightness of trapezius and levator scapulae |
| Inability to perform lifting tasks | ■ Pain: Neck pain and temporal headaches<br>■ Decreased muscle extensibility: Tightness of trapezius and levator scapulae<br>■ Muscle spasm in the right trapezius<br>■ Decreased muscular performance: Decreased right trapezius and right levator scapulae strength and endurance<br>■ Decreased muscle integrity: Active trigger points in the right upper trapezius and levator scapulae |

---

Although the therapist will use the identified functional outcomes as the primary means of judging the client's progress, it is still beneficial for her to identify outcomes related to impairments. The therapist can then use the client's progress, or lack thereof, on the outcomes related to the client's impairments as a basis for determining whether the client is responding to the treatment techniques that she is applying. Table 13-1 (Chapter 13) contains some examples of outcomes related to impairments.

## Plan Compensatory Strategies (Step 9b)

The therapist also distinguishes between the impairments that are amenable to active treatment and those for which she must plan a means of compensation. The clinical scenario of the client with myofascial cervical pain is admit-

## Identify Treatable Impairments and Relevant Outcomes

| Impairment | Outcome |
| --- | --- |
| ▣ Pain: Neck pain and temporal headaches | ▣ Pain reported is 0/10 on a visual analog scale |
| ▣ Postural malalignment: Forward head posture | ▣ Normalized cervical and head posture |
| ▣ Decreased muscle integrity: Active trigger points in the right upper trapezius and levator scapulae | ▣ No signs of active trigger points on palpation of trapezius and levator scapulae muscles; no palpable taut bands, positive pattern of pain referral, or twitch signs |
| ▣ Decreased active cervical range of motion | ▣ Active cervical range of motion: Flexion 100%, extension 100%, right rotation 100%, left lateral flexion 100% |
| ▣ Muscle spasm in the right trapezius | ▣ No palpable muscle spasm in the right trapezius muscle |
| ▣ Decreased muscular performance: Decreased right trapezius and right levator scapulae strength and endurance | ▣ Muscle strength: Right levator scapulae—scapular elevation = grade 5; right trapezius—scapular elevation, scapular retraction = grade 5 |
| ▣ Decreased muscle extensibility: Tightness of trapezius and levator scapulae muscles | ▣ Normal extensibility of the right trapezius and the right levator scapulae muscles |

tedly a straightforward one in which all of the client's impairments are amenable to active treatment. A more complex case would be, for example, a 65-year-old client who is 3 months post a right-sided cerebrovascular accident. The therapists treating this client have identified a left drop foot, left-sided weakness, primitive movement patterns, increased tone in the trunk and involved extremities, painful left shoulder subluxation, and edema in the left hand as the primary impairments. Of these, the drop foot has shown no further signs of recovery and no longer appears amenable to active treatment. Consequently, the therapists do further examination to rule out a peripheral nerve injury or other localized damage to the tibialis anterior muscle. They then consider the drop foot to be an impairment for which they can use a **compensatory strategy** of an ankle-foot orthosis and ambulatory aids. The therapists can also use one of the client's available functional areas to compensate for this impairment in addition to using external orthoses and devices; for example, gait training in the use of the more functional pelvic and lower extremity muscle groups to compensate for the drop foot during ambulation.

## Identify Impairments Appropriate for Massage Techniques (Step 9c)

In the clinical decision-making model for Outcome-Based Massage, the Treatment Planning Phase also includes the identification of those impairments that are most appropriate for the application of massage techniques. The therapist bases this decision on her knowledge of the expected outcomes of massage techniques and whether massage techniques can have a direct or secondary effect on the impairment. There are three possible options: massage has a **direct effect** on the impairment; massage has a **secondary effect** on the impairment; and massage has no effect on the impairment. Identifying between massage techniques that have a direct effect on the impairment and those that do not assists the therapist in creating an intervention that will result in improved functional outcomes and prioritizing treatment techniques within an intervention. If the massage technique has no documented or demonstrated effect on the impairment, the therapist has little justification for including it in the intervention. A general summary of the expected outcomes of Table 1-5 (Chapter 1) presents massage techniques to assist the therapist in determining when it is appropriate to treat an impairment using massage techniques.

At this point in the decision-making process, as previously mentioned, the therapist is able to determine whether the use of massage techniques is appropriate for the client's impairments.

## Select Treatment Techniques (Steps 10a, 10b)

Once the therapist has identified the impairments for which massage techniques have a direct effect or secondary effect, she can proceed with selecting the techniques she

## Identify Impairments Appropriate for Massage Techniques

| Impairments | Role of Massage |
|---|---|
| Pain: Neck pain and headaches | ▣ Direct effect on pain due to presence of active trigger points |
| Decreased muscle extensibility of trapezius and levator scapulae | ▣ Direct effect on muscle extensibility |
| Postural malalignment: Forward head posture | ▣ Direct effect on the lengthening of shortened anterior neck and trunk muscles |
| | ▣ There will also be a secondary effect resulting from the inactivation of the trigger points since the decrease in pain will minimize the compensatory postural changes that are due to trigger point pain. |
| Spasm in the right trapezius | ▣ Direct effect on muscle spasm |
| Decreased active cervical range of motion | ▣ Direct effect on the lengthening of shortened anterior neck and trunk muscles that contribute to decreased range of motion |
| | ▣ There will also be a secondary effect from the inactivation of the trigger points since the decreased range may be due, in part, to a combination of trigger point pain and compensatory muscle guarding. |
| Decreased muscular performance: Decreased right trapezius and right levator scapulae strength | ▣ Secondary effect since weakness is likely secondary to trigger point pain and disuse. |
| Decreased muscle integrity: Active trigger points in the right upper trapezius and levator scapulae | ▣ Direct effect on the active myofascial trigger points |

will use in the intervention. The therapist matches appropriate massage techniques to impairments by considering three factors:

1. Match of expected outcome, related to impairments, of the massage technique to the client's impairment
2. Identification of **contraindications** or **cautions** in the application of that technique given the client's clinical condition
3. The therapist's legal right and competence to use the technique

The chapters on massage techniques describe the expected outcomes of each massage technique to assist therapists in selecting massage techniques.

Simply matching impairments to the outcomes of massage techniques is not sufficient to guarantee that a technique is appropriate for that client's condition. Before performing any massage technique, the therapist needs to consider the general cautions and contraindications to the application of that technique for the client's clinical condition (Table 3-2).[10–23] The techniques chapters cover the relevant clinical considerations, cautions, and contraindications for specific massage techniques.

While this list is a necessary starting point for the consideration of cautions and contraindications to treatment, the therapist should also use her judgment about the application of massage techniques to the client at hand. A useful rule of thumb is that, if a client's condition requires

## Select Treatment Techniques

| Massage Techniques | Other Appropriate Treatment Techniques |
|---|---|
| ▣ Specific compression | ▣ Moist heat for trigger point pain |
| ▣ Superficial effleurage | ▣ Ice for acute spasm |
| ▣ Superficial stroking | ▣ Specific stretches for trapezius and levator scapulae muscles |
| ▣ Petrissage | ▣ Postural re-education |
| ▣ Broad-contact compression | ▣ Active range of motion exercises |
| ▣ Stripping | ▣ Strengthening exercises |
| ▣ Self-care specific compression with a hand-held massage device | ▣ Self-care education |
| | ▣ Functional activity |

| Table 3-2 | Suggested Cautions and Contraindications for Reflex and Mechanical Massage Techniques[10–23,25,26] |
|---|---|

| **Local Conditions** | **General Conditions** |
|---|---|

**Contraindications**

- Acute flare-up of inflammatory arthritis: rheumatoid arthritis, systemic lupus, Reiter's syndrome, etc.
- Acute neuritis
- Aneurysms
- Areas of altered or impaired sensation
- Baker's cyst
- Ectopic pregnancy
- Esophageal varicosities
- Frostbite
- Local contagious skin condition
- Local infection
- Local irritable skin condition
- Malignancy
- Open wound or sore
- Peripheral neuropathy
- Phlebitis, thrombophlebitis, arteritis
- Post anti-inflammatory injection (24–48 hours)
- Recent burns
- Undiagnosed lump

**Contraindications**

- Acute conditions requiring first aid: anaphylaxis, epileptic seizure, pneumothorax, myocardial infarction, syncope, status asthmaticus, cerebrovascular accident, diabetic coma, insulin shock, appendicitis
- Advanced kidney failure*
- Advanced respiratory failure*
- Anemia (depending on the cause)*
- Diabetes with complications*
- Eclampsia
- Hemophilia*
- Hemorrhage
- Highly metastatic cancers
- Intoxication
- Liver failure*
- Sepsis
- Severe atherosclerosis*
- Shock
- Significant fever (> 101.5°F or 38.3°C)
- Systemic contagious/infectious condition
- Unstabilized cerebrovascular accident
- Unstable hypertension
- Unstable myocardial infarction

**Cautions**

- Acute disk herniation
- Acute inflammatory condition
- Allergies to lubricants and cleansers
- Anti-inflammatory injection site
- Buerger's disease
- Chronic abdominal or digestive disease
- Chronic arthritic conditions
- Chronic diarrhea
- Chronic or longstanding superficial thrombosis
- Contusion
- Endometriosis
- Flaccid paralysis
- Fracture—while casted and immediately after cast removal
- Hernia
- Joint instability or hypermobility
- Kidney infection or stones
- Mastitis
- Minor surgery
- Pelvic inflammatory disease
- Pitting edema
- Portal hypertension
- Presence of pins, staples
- Prolonged constipation
- Recent abortion or vaginal birth
- Trigeminal neuralgia

**Cautions**

- Asthma
- Atherosclerosis
- Cancer
- Chronic congestive heart failure
- Chronic kidney disease
- Client taking medications that alter neurological, cardiovascular, psychological, or kidney function
- Coma
- Drug withdrawal
- Emphysema
- Epilepsy
- Hypertension
- Hypotension
- Immunosuppression
- Inflammatory arthritis
- Major or abdominal surgery
- Multiple sclerosis
- Osteoporosis
- Post cerebrovascular accident
- Post myocardial infarction
- Pregnancy and labor
- Psychiatric conditions
- Recent head injury
- Spasticity or rigidity

*Skilled clinicians with advanced training may consider these to be cautions, rather than contraindications.

ongoing management by another health care professional, then it is appropriate for the therapist to consult that health care professional for guidelines regarding cautions and contraindications to treatment.

The therapist also needs to consider whether there are any anatomical structures that can be damaged during the application of massage techniques.[10–24] For example, the application of friction or specific compression over a peripheral nerve in a location where it is close to the skin may produce a neuropraxia.[25] While some sources describe "**endangerment sites**" (Table 3-3) as areas of the human body over which the use of direct or sustained pressure is contraindicated,[10,26] the therapist may also use her judgment in determining whether these areas are contraindicated for other massage techniques. Students and novice therapists who are not experienced in applying treatment techniques should take a conservative approach to applying massage techniques to endangerment sites and in situations in which there are specific cautions or contraindications to the use of a technique.

## Generate the Plan of Care (Step 11)

It is unlikely that a plan of care will consist only of massage techniques. The therapist must also select other treatment techniques, such as therapeutic exercise, electrotherapeutic modalities, and education and training on functional activity, that she will need to use in order to achieve the identified outcomes. These treatment techniques will vary depending on the scope of practice of the health care professionals.

A list of treatment techniques does not constitute a plan of care; the therapist also needs to specify and document the treatment parameters within the client's written plan of care. The duration of the episode of care (the current treatment period) and the frequency of interventions should be consistent with the severity, stability, complexity, and acuity of the client's clinical condition; the client's treatment tolerance; the client's prognosis; and the identified outcomes. Other factors that can influence the duration of care and frequency of treatment sessions include: the client's cognitive status, pre-existing conditions, potential discharge destination, overall health status, and probability of prolonged impairment.[7] The therapist must also determine the scope, frequency, and duration of the massage techniques in the intervention. The Using Massage to Achieve Clinical Outcomes chapter provides further information about these issues. Finally, the therapist also needs to consider the client's home or work environment, social context, and personal goals for treatment to ensure that the intervention adequately addresses these factors. Failure to do so may have a negative impact on the level of the client's adherence with self-care and participation in the plan of care.

### Critical Thinking Question

Your client is a 16-year-old boy who is nonverbal and fully dependent for all care following a severe head injury. In your examination, you identify multiple impairments, including decreased muscle extensibility, decreased joint range of motion, and decreased skin integrity. On the other hand, you are finding it difficult to identify functional outcomes and compensatory strategies for this client. What process could you use to develop a balanced plan of care for this client, and what might this plan include?

| Table 3-3 | Selected Endangerment Sites[10,11,13] |
| --- | --- |

| Head and Neck | Trunk | Extremities |
| --- | --- | --- |
| ■ Neck, including anterior and posterior triangle<br>■ Eye<br>■ Trachea<br>■ Styloid process of the temporal bone | ■ Axilla<br>■ Xiphoid process<br>■ 12th (floating) rib<br>■ Kidneys in the area of the 12th rib<br>■ Umbilicus<br>■ Linea alba<br>■ Sciatic notch | ■ Ulnar nerve at medial epicondyle<br>■ Femoral artery, nerve, and vein in the area of the inguinal triangle |

| | |
|---|---|
| **Theory In Practice 3-11: Items to Chart** | |

## Generate the Plan of Care

Subjective

Plan of Care

History of Present Illness:

▩ Two months ago, the patient had insidious onset of localized neck and shoulder pain, right side greater than the left, with stiffness, decreased active cervical range of motion, neck muscle tightness, neck muscle spasm, and transient headaches.

▩ Seen by M.D. and given muscle relaxants with little effect

▩ Is right handed

Current Medication: Acetaminophen for pain

Current Functional Status: On reduced hours secondary to neck pain and difficulty performing job-related tasks

Past Medical History: Unremarkable; no prior history of neck or upper extremity injuries; no prior therapy

Pain: Neck pain at rest, at end of range of motion, and during functional activity; reported pain intensity of 8 on a visual analog scale; transient headaches (temporal region)

Muscle Tightness: Tightness of neck muscles on waking and with fatigue

Functional Limitations: Reported inability to drive or check out groceries at the cash register for > 10 minutes secondary to increased neck pain

Prior Functional Level: Full-time cashier at supermarket; able to perform all job-related tasks without difficulty

Objective

Posture: Forward head posture

Palpation:

▩ Palpable muscle spasm in the right trapezius

▩ Palpable taut bands in the right trapezius and levator scapulae

▩ Reported positive pattern of pain referral on palpation of the right trapezius trigger point

▩ Reported positive pattern of pain referral on palpation of the right levator scapulae trigger point

▩ Twitch response on palpation of trigger point locations in the right upper trapezius and the right levator scapulae muscles

Range of Motion:

▩ Decreased active cervical range of motion: flexion 50%, extension 75%, right rotation 75%, left lateral flexion 50% with pain at end of range of motion; other ranges full and painfree

▩ Full and painfree active range of motion of shoulder, elbow, wrist, and hand bilaterally

Muscle Extensibility: Tightness of trapezius and levator scapulae muscles

Strength:

▩ Decreased strength of the right levator scapulae—scapular elevation = grade 4–

▩ Decreased strength of the right trapezius—scapular elevation, scapular retraction = grade 4–

▩ Strength of other shoulder, wrist, and finger motions = grade 5

Functional Limitations:

▩ Inability to drive for > 10 minutes secondary to increased neck pain

▩ Inability to perform repetitive upper extremity movements in standing using the right arm for > 10 minutes (as required for checking out groceries at the cash register) secondary to neck pain

▩ Inability to reach objects placed 1 foot above head with the right arm (as required for retrieving items from overhead shelves) secondary to neck pain

▩ Inability to lift a 5-lb object above shoulder level using the right arm (as required for placing boxes of dried goods on overhead shelves) secondary to neck pain

▩ Inability to lift and transfer a 15-lb object using the right arm (as required for placing customers' purchases into shopping carts) secondary to neck pain

▩ Inability to perform > 3 repetitions of lifting and transferring a 3-lb object at waist level using the right arm (as required for checking out customers' groceries and placing them in shopping bags) secondary to neck pain

| | |
|---|---|
| Analysis | Trigger points in right upper trapezius and levator scapulae muscles with associated muscle tenderness, muscle tightness, and decreased cervical spine range of motion |

Impairments:

- Pain: Neck pain and temporal headaches
- Decreased muscle extensibility: Tightness of trapezius and levator scapulae muscles
- Postural malalignment: Forward head posture
- Muscle resting tension: Muscle spasm in the right trapezius
- Decreased active cervical range of motion
- Decreased muscular performance: Decreased right trapezius and right levator scapulae strength and endurance
- Decreased muscle integrity: Active trigger points in the right upper trapezius and levator scapulae

Functional Limitations:

- Inability to drive for > 10 minutes secondary to increased neck pain
- Inability to perform repetitive upper extremity movements in standing using the right arm for > 10 minutes secondary to neck pain
- Inability to reach objects placed 1 foot above head with the right arm secondary to neck pain
- Inability to lift a 5-lb object above shoulder level using the right arm secondary to neck pain
- Inability to lift and transfer a 5-lb object using the right arm secondary to neck pain
- Inability to perform > 3 repetitions of lifting and transferring a 3-lb object at waist level using the right arm secondary to neck pain

Outcomes (related to impairments):

- Pain reported is 0/10 on a visual analog scale
- Normalized cervical and head posture
- No palpable muscle spasm in the right trapezius muscle
- No signs of active trigger points on palpation of trapezius and levator scapulae muscles: palpable taut bands, positive pattern of pain referral, or twitch signs
- Active cervical range of motion: flexion 100%, extension 100%, right rotation 100%, left lateral flexion 100%
- Normal extensibility of the right trapezius and the right levator scapulae muscles
- Muscle strength: right levator scapulae – scapular elevation = grade 5; right trapezius – scapular elevation, scapular retraction = grade 5

Functional Outcomes

Short-Term Outcomes (2 weeks):

- Able to drive for ½ hour without complaints of pain
- Able to work checking out groceries at the cash register for ½ hour, with appropriate breaks, without complaints of pain
- Able to lift a 5-lb object and place it on shelf at shoulder level—1 repetition without complaints of neck pain
- Able to reach objects placed 1 foot above head with the right arm without complaints of neck pain
- Able to lift and transfer an 8-lb object at waist level with the right arm without complaints of pain
- Able to perform 5 repetitions of transferring a 5-lb object at waist level using the right arm without complaints of pain

Long-Term Outcomes (Discharge: 4 weeks):

- Able to drive for 1.5–2 hours without complaints of neck pain
- Able to work checking out groceries at the cash register for 2 hours, with appropriate breaks, without complaints of pain
- Able to lift an 8-lb object and place it on shelf at shoulder level—5 repetitions without complaints of neck pain
- Able to reach objects placed 2 feet above head with the right arm without complaints of neck pain
- Able to lift and transfer a 15-lb object at waist level with the right arm without complaints of neck pain
- Able to perform 15 repetitions of transferring a 5-lb object at waist level using the right arm without complaints of neck pain
- Independent in self-care and therapeutic exercise program

Plan    Treatment: 2 × week for 4 weeks

Massage Techniques:
- Specific compression
- Superficial effleurage
- Superficial stroking
- Petrissage
- Broad-contact compression
- Stripping
- Self-care specific compression with a hand-held massage device

Therapeutic Exercise:
- Specific stretches for trapezius and levator scapulae muscles
- Postural re-education
- Active range of motion exercises for cervical spine
- Strengthening exercises for cervical and scapular muscles

Modalities:
- Moist heat in the location of the trigger points to reduce trigger point activity and pain
- Ice for acute muscle spasm

Functional Training:
- Functional training in lifting and transferring required for effective job performance as a cashier

Education:
- Self-care education in pain and trigger point management

# TREATMENT PHASE

## Select Treatment and Re-Examination Techniques (Steps 12a, 12b)

The therapist is ready to initiate treatment once she has completed the plan of care. First, she selects a subset of the prioritized massage and **complementary treatment techniques** from the plan of care as a starting point. The aims of the first stage of treatment are to gauge the client's treatment tolerance and to ascertain whether the treatment techniques can affect the client's impairments. It is, therefore, advisable for the therapist to select those techniques that are most likely to have a direct effect. At the outset of the episode of care, the therapist also identifies which subjective and objective examination techniques she can use to determine whether the client is having a positive response to treatment. In doing so, she includes questions that seek the client's perspective on her progress and the intervention. This information is invaluable because these factors can signal problems that the client is having with the intervention and can provide the therapist with guidance on how to improve client adherence to or participation in the plan of care.

## Carry Out Initial Intervention (Step 13)

As mentioned earlier, during the first stage of treatment, the therapist is evaluating the appropriateness of the plan of care and gauging the client's treatment tolerance. She bases the intensity of the interventions on the level of acuity of the client's condition, using less intense treatments for a more acutely ill client and vice versa. In addition, she is cautious not to introduce too many treatment techniques at once because that will make it difficult for her to identify the techniques to which the client had a positive or adverse response. The therapist also conducts formal and informal client examinations to determine the client's response to treatment.

## Conduct Client Re-Examination (Step 14)

The therapist can perform informal client examinations at any time during the interventions. Palpation and the massage techniques themselves can provide information on the client's response to the technique the therapist is applying and to the intervention as a whole (see Chapter 5, Client Examination for Massage). These informal

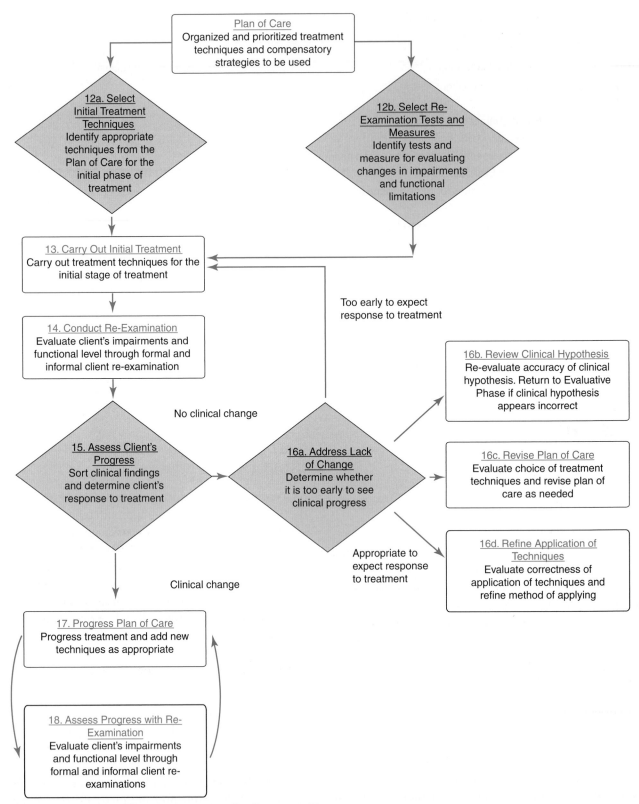

**Figure 3-3** Clinical Decision-Making Model: The Treatment Phase.

<table>
<tr><td colspan="3">

**Theory In Practice 3-12a, 3-12b**

## Select Treatment and Re-Examination Techniques

</td></tr>
<tr><td>

**Massage Treatment Technique**

</td><td>

**Complementary Technique**

</td><td>

**Examination Techniques**

</td></tr>
<tr><td>

- Superficial stroking on the site of the acute spasm
- Broad-contact compression

</td><td>

- Specific stretches for trapezius and levator scapulae muscles
- Ice for spasm
- Self-care education for pain control

</td><td>

Subjective
- Pain reports
- Perceptions of treatment and progress made

Objective
- Muscle spasm
- Trigger point pain referral pattern
- Range of motion

</td></tr>
</table>

<table>
<tr><td colspan="2">

**Theory In Practice 3-13, 3-14, 3-15**

## Carry Out Initial Treatment, Conduct Client Re-Examination, and Assess Client Progress

</td></tr>
<tr><td></td><td>

**Patient's Response to Initial Interventions (1 week)**

</td></tr>
<tr><td>

Treatment Technique

</td><td>

- Superficial stroking on the site of the spasm
- Broad-contact compression on the location of the trigger points and off the site of the spasm
- Petrissage off the site of spasm
- Specific stretches for trapezius and levator scapulae muscles
- Ice on the location of the muscle spasm
- Self-care education for pain control

</td></tr>
<tr><td>

Results of Informal Examination

</td><td>

- Patient had negative response to use of ice for spasm; this exacerbated trigger point pain. Superficial stroking was used for spasm.
- Moist heat applied to the trigger point location may be more effective for pain relief.
- Patient's trigger points were initially too sensitive to tolerate specific compression; broad-contact compression was used.
- Patient was able to perform specific stretches for trapezius and levator scapulae muscles appropriately.

</td></tr>
<tr><td>

Results of Formal Examination

</td><td>

- Decreased reports of pain during functional activity—reported pain intensity of 6.5 on a visual analog scale
- Decreased muscle spasm
- Pattern of pain referral—unchanged

</td></tr>
<tr><td>

Practitioner's Conclusions

</td><td>

Patient is responding to treatment. Trigger point therapy is appropriate.

</td></tr>
</table>

examinations can be interspersed throughout the interventions. Once the client has reached a point at which the therapist can reasonably expect a measurable clinical change, the therapist carries out a more formal re-examination using the tests and measures she selected for this purpose. This re-examination focuses on the identification and measurement of changes in the client's impairments and functional level from the baseline established at the initial examination.

## Assess Client Progress (Step 15)

The therapist uses the re-examination as a means of determining the client's progress towards the achievement of the identified outcomes and the client's readiness for treatment progression. She can also use this information as the basis for her decision on whether to modify the plan of care or the identified outcomes.

## Address Lack of Change (Steps 16a, 16b, 16c, 16d)

If the result of the client re-examination is that the client does not demonstrate any clinical change, the therapist must first determine whether it may be too early to observe a change. If this is the case, she reattempts treatment with

the original set of techniques and may consider the addition of another treatment technique before the next formal re-examination. If, however, the therapist believes that the client has had ample time to demonstrate a clinical change, then the therapist must re-evaluate the appropriateness of the plan of care. Possible causes for the therapist to consider for the client's failure to respond to interventions are an incorrect clinical hypothesis, an inappropriate treatment technique, or an incorrect application of a technique. If the therapist's clinical hypothesis was incorrect, she will need to revisit the Evaluative Phase and repeat the client examination to identify the client's clinical condition. The therapist can remedy the choice of inappropriate treatment techniques by selecting more appropriate techniques and modifying the plan of care. Finally, if the therapist's choice of clinical hypothesis and treatment techniques appears to be accurate, then she needs to refine her application of the treatment techniques.

## Progress Plan of Care and Assess Progress Through Re-Examination (Steps 17, 18)

Once the therapist is confident that the direction of the plan of care is appropriate, then the cycle of treatment progression and informal or formal re-examination begins. Throughout this cycle, the therapist ensures that she assesses both the client's impairments and functional level at appropriate intervals. Ideally, each intervention should incorporate an element of informal examination and progression or modification of either the treatment techniques or client education. The Using Massage to Achieve Clinical Outcomes chapter discusses these issues in greater detail. During the application of each treatment technique, the therapist informally evaluates the client's response and uses this information to fine tune the intervention and her application of treatment techniques. The therapist can also use these informal examinations to identify when the client has a flare-up of her clinical condition that results in an increase in her impairments and functional limitations. The timing of formal examinations of the client's progress on functional outcomes will depend on the timeframes that the therapist has defined for those outcomes.

### Critical Thinking Question

Your objective examination shows that your client is making significant improvements on the outcomes for the key impairments that you selected. Nevertheless, she reports little progress with her functional outcomes. What steps could you use to identify what to correct in your intervention? How might you modify your intervention to improve her progress on her functional outcomes?

## DISCHARGE PHASE

## Identify Post-Discharge Needs (Step 19)

There is, unfortunately, no exact formula to use for determining when to initiate the discharge process. Consequently, the therapist can initiate discharge planning as early as the first session or much later in the treatment process. There are many factors that can influence the therapist's decision on when to begin the Discharge Phase. First of all, the therapist must also consider the client's characteristics, such as the client's progress with her functional outcomes, her psychological and educational readiness for discharge, and the resources needed and available to the client following discharge. In addition, the therapist cannot ignore the constraints to discharge planning imposed by the nature of the clinical setting and the predicted length of the episode of care. For example, in the Theory in Practice clinical scenario, the therapist can begin discharge planning in earlier sessions because of the relative brevity of the client's course of treatment. Although one can argue that every intervention is preparing the client for discharge, there are specific activities that are associated with facilitating an effective discharge.

## Initiate Post-Discharge Education and Referrals (Steps 20, 21)

As the client approaches achievement of 75% of her functional outcomes, the therapist needs to initiate a discussion of the client's discharge concerns and needs. This may occur earlier if the client appears to have complex needs that will require more discharge planning or the clinical setting dictates shorter **episodes of care**. Although the therapist may not be able to address all of the client's discharge needs, a complete list of discharge needs is valuable for planning self-care education, referrals to other health care professionals, and other client resources.

By the time the client is close to achieving her functional outcomes, the therapist should have initiated referrals, identified equipment needs and initiated purchases, finalized the content of home programs, and begun discharge self-care education. The emphasis of the final sessions prior to discharge will shift to include a larger educational component. Chapter 4, Ethical and Interpersonal Issues in Massage, also discusses the psychological preparation of the client for discharge. If the therapist

## Progress Plan of Care and Assess Progress Through Re-Examination

| | Week 2 | Week 3 |
|---|---|---|
| Treatment Techniques | **Massage Techniques**<br>▦ Broad-contact compression<br>▦ Petrissage<br>▦ Specific compression<br>**Other Appropriate Treatment Techniques**<br>▦ Specific stretches for trapezius and levator scapulae muscles<br>▦ Heat to location of trigger points for pain<br>▦ Postural re-education<br>▦ Active range of motion exercises<br>▦ Functional activity<br>▦ Self-care education—add home range of motion and stretching program | **Massage Techniques**<br>▦ Broad-contact compression (decreased duration)<br>▦ Petrissage (decreased duration)<br>▦ Stripping (increased duration and depth)<br>▦ Specific compression (increased duration and depth)<br>**Other Appropriate Treatment Techniques**<br>▦ Specific stretches for trapezius and levator scapulae muscles<br>▦ Heat for preparation for stretching<br>▦ Postural re-education<br>▦ Functional activity<br>▦ Strengthening exercises<br>▦ Self-care education—add self-care specific compression with a hand-held massage device |
| Results of Patient Re-Examination | **Functional Outcomes**<br>▦ Reports being able to drive for 0.5 hours without complaints of neck pain<br>▦ Able to perform repetitive upper extremity movements while standing 0.75 hours without complaints of neck pain<br>▦ Able to lift a 5-lb object and place it on shelf at shoulder level—5 repetitions without complaints of neck pain<br>▦ Able to reach objects placed 1 foot above head with the right arm without complaints of neck pain<br>▦ Able to lift and transfer a 5-lb object at waist level with the right arm without complaints of neck pain<br>▦ Able to perform 10 repetitions of transferring a 5-lb object at waist level using the right arm without complaints of neck pain<br>**Other Examination Findings**<br>▦ Reported recent flare-up of pain following attempts to increase work time<br>▦ Reported pain intensity of 5 on a visual analog scale by end of week<br>▦ Pattern of pain referral—decreased intensity of pain on palpation of trigger points<br>▦ Active cervical range of motion: flexion 75%, extension 90%, right rotation 90%, left lateral flexion 75%<br>▦ Strength: right levator scapulae—scapular elevation = grade 4; right trapezius—scapular elevation, scapular retraction = grade 4 | **Functional Outcomes**<br>▦ Reports being able to drive for 1 hour without complaints of neck pain<br>▦ Able to perform repetitive upper extremity movements while standing 1.25 hours without complaints of neck pain<br>▦ Able to lift a 10-lb object and place it on shelf at shoulder level—1 repetition without complaints of neck pain<br>▦ Able to reach objects placed 1.5 feet above head with right arm without complaints of neck pain<br>▦ Able to lift and transfer a 10-lb object at waist level with the right arm without complaints of neck pain<br>▦ Able to perform 15 repetitions of transferring a 5-lb object at waist level using the right arm without complaints of neck pain<br>**Other Examination Findings**<br>▦ Reported pain intensity of 3.5 on a visual analog scale<br>▦ No pain referral on palpation of upper trapezius trigger point; minimal reports of pain for levator scapulae trigger point<br>▦ Active cervical range of motion: flexion 90%, extension 100%, right rotation 100%, left lateral flexion 75%<br>▦ Strength: right levator scapulae—scapular elevation = grade 4+; right trapezius—scapular elevation, scapular retraction = grade 4+ |

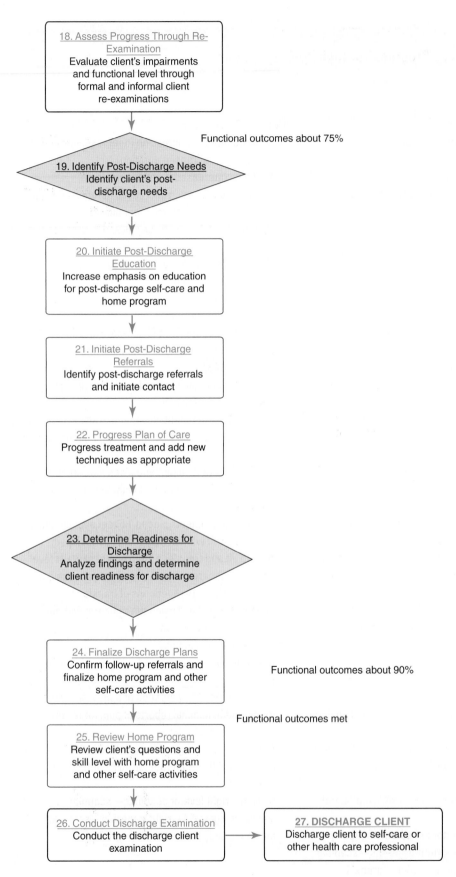

Figure 3-4 Clinical Decision-Making Model: The Discharge Phase.

refers the client to another health care professional, for example a subacute unit or home health care, the discharge process will also include written and verbal communication with the other therapists.

## Progress Plan of Care and Determine Readiness for Discharge (Steps 22, 23)

As the client approaches the final stages of treatment, the therapist ensures that she has appropriately completed the progression of the various components of the plan of care. She uses the results of her ongoing client re-examinations to guide the rate at which she progresses interventions. These clinical findings also indicate when the client has achieved 90% of her functional outcomes.

## Finalize Discharge Plans and Review Home Program (Steps 24, 25)

As the client nears completion of her course of treatment, the therapist ensures that the client is competent in her post-discharge self-care program. She also confirms that she has finalized all post-discharge arrangements.

| Theory In Practice 3-19, 3-20, 3-21 | |
|---|---|
| **Identify Post-Discharge Needs and Initiate Post-Discharge Education and Referrals** | |
| **Impairment/Functional Limitation** | **Post-Discharge Need** |
| ▪ Pain | ▪ Pain management self-care education<br>▪ Self-care specific compression with a hand-held massage device |
| ▪ Difficulty performing job-related activities | ▪ Ergonomic education and work site assessment |
| ▪ Decreased muscle extensibility | ▪ Home stretching program |
| ▪ Decreased range of motion | ▪ Home range of motion program |

| Theory In Practice 3-22, 3-23 | |
|---|---|
| **Progress Plan of Care and Assess Progress Through Re-Examination** | |
| **Week 4** | |
| Treatment Techniques | Massage Techniques<br>▪ Petrissage (decreased duration)<br>▪ Broad-contact compression (decreased duration)<br>▪ Specific compression (increased duration)<br>▪ Stripping (increased duration and depth)<br>Other Appropriate Treatment Techniques<br>▪ Postural re-education<br>▪ Functional activity<br>▪ Strengthening exercises<br>▪ Self-care education—add ergonomics education, review education on identifying and managing flare-ups |
| Results of Patient Re-Examination | Re-Examination Findings<br>Discharge concerns:<br>▪ Cashier station is not ergonomically correct, and this aggravates pain. Patient is concerned about how to manage flare-ups.<br>▪ Patient is able to demonstrate all self-care activities correctly.<br>▪ Reported pain intensity is 1 on a visual analog scale.<br>▪ There is no pain referral on palpation of upper trapezius or levator scapulae trigger points. |

## Conduct Discharge Examination and Discharge Client (Steps 26, 27)

The final, or discharge, client examination provides the therapist with a confirmation of the client's readiness for

---

**Theory In Practice 3-24, 3-25**

### Finalize Discharge Plans and Review Home Program

The practitioner outlines a self-care program that addresses the patient's discharge needs. It contains components that reflect the patient's presenting impairments and functional limitations.

**Week 4: Self-Care Program**

- Pain management
- Ergonomics
- Home stretching
- Home range of motion
- Self-care specific compression with a hand-held massage device

---

discharge. It also is a record of the status of the client's impairments and functional level at the time of discharge.

### Critical Thinking Question

Your client has met all of the functional outcomes and outcomes for impairments that you established for her intervention. She has, however, made little progress with her self-care education and home program. What process can you use to facilitate a timely discharge for this client?

## ONGOING CARE

Therapists must modify the four-phase clinical decision-making process for clients who require ongoing episodes of care because of their clinical condition or the nature of their clinical care. Clients who require ongoing episodes of care include:

- Pediatric clients with developmental disabilities
- Clients with chronic or terminal conditions who are at risk for deterioration of health status
- Geriatric clients who are at risk for falls or deterioration of health status
- Clients who have ongoing disability and health care needs as a result of spinal cord injury, head injury, amputation, or other traumatic injury
- Clients who are receiving wellness interventions

---

**Theory In Practice 3-26, 3-27**

### Conduct Discharge Examination and Discharge Client

The practitioner documents the clinical findings on the discharge examination. These findings indicate that the patient has achieved her outcomes and is ready for discharge.

**Discharge Examination Findings: Functional Outcomes**

- Able to drive for 2.5 hours without complaints of neck pain using stretches and postural checks
- Able to work checking out groceries at the cash register for 2 hours without complaints of neck pain; takes appropriate breaks and uses stretches and postural checks; has had ergonomic adjustments to cashier station; occasional complaints of neck tightness with fatigue
- Able to perform lifting tasks required for work as a cashier:
  1. Able to lift an 8-lb object and place it on shelf at shoulder level—5 repetitions without complaints of neck pain
  2. Able to reach objects placed 2 feet above head with the right arm without complaints of neck pain
  3. Able to lift and transfer a 15-lb object at waist level with the right arm without complaints of neck pain
  4. Able to perform 20 repetitions of lifting and transferring a 5-lb object at waist level using the right arm without complaints of neck pain

**Other Examination Findings**

- Reported pain intensity of 0.5 on a visual analog scale
- Normalized cervical and head posture
- No palpable muscle spasm in the right trapezius muscle
- No signs of active trigger points on palpation of trapezius and levator scapulae muscles: palpable taut bands, positive pattern of pain referral, or twitch signs
- Active cervical range of motion: flexion 100%, extension 100%, right rotation 100%, left lateral flexion 100%
- Normal extensibility of the right trapezius and the right levator scapulae muscles
- Muscle strength: right levator scapulae—scapular elevation = grade 5; right trapezius—scapular elevation, scapular retraction = grade 5

The clinical decision-making process does not end at the Discharge Phase when a client requires ongoing episodes of care. First, the therapist's discharge planning must include organization, or at the very least a discussion, of the follow-up care. Second, the therapist must plan and implement a follow-up client examination and thus initiate the Evaluative Phase once more.

The follow-up examination (see Table 3-1) is a focused client examination in which the therapist determines whether the client has demonstrated a deterioration of impairments or functional level since the prior examination. Based on the clinical findings she obtains from this examination, the therapist identifies whether the client has new treatment needs. If the client does not require ongoing care, the therapist documents this finding and organizes further follow-up if warranted. However, if the client does demonstrate a deterioration in status, the therapist initiates the Treatment Planning Phase of the clinical decision-making process and then moves onto the Treatment and Discharge Phases. In the case of wellness interventions, the therapist does not base the need for ongoing care on a deterioration of health status but on the identification of the client's need for interventions to maintain or improve his or her current level of wellness.

### Critical Thinking Question

How would you modify the steps in the four-phase clinical decision-making process if your client presented with wellness goals, rather than a medical condition?

## REVIEWING THE BASICS

Therapists can use the clinical decision-making process proposed for Outcome-Based Massage as a guide through the Evaluative, Treatment Planning, Treatment, and Discharge Phases of clinical care. The aim of this process is to enable the therapist to integrate massage techniques effectively into clinical care as the primary or complementary treatment technique. Although the steps in this process are presented in a linear sequence, the process is an iterative one in which the therapist may perform several steps concurrently. The decision-making model proposed in this chapter provides guidelines for enhancing the appropriateness and adequacy of the examinations, plans of care, and interventions provided by therapists.

## Clinical Decision-Making for Massage: Further Study and Practice

This section introduces some additional issues that a clinician can consider during the clinical decision-making process.

## LEGAL RIGHT TO TREAT

Legal right to treat refers to whether the clinician's professional scope of practice includes the treatment of the client's clinical problem, the examination techniques, and the treatment techniques that the clinician wishes to use. Professional scope of practice is dictated by the laws of the jurisdiction in which the clinician practices. Health care professions have practice acts that protect public health and safety by regulating the qualifications, registration, and discipline of members of the profession. For each profession, these practice acts outline the qualifications; licensing or registration requirements; treatments that can be applied by the professional; grounds for discipline; and sanctions that will be applied to violators of the prac-

tice act. Legal right to treat can be a gray area where the practice of massage is concerned. Clinicians from a range of health care professions can use some massage techniques within their scope of practice without advanced training or certification, while others cannot. Athletic Trainers, Massage Therapists, Nurses, Occupational Therapists, Physical Therapists, Chiropractors, and other bodyworkers can incorporate superficial reflex techniques, such as stroking applied to facilitate relaxation, into the interventions for clients with a variety of clinical conditions. By contrast, the application of manual lymph drainage techniques for the management of lymphedema may be outside the scope of practice of several of these health care professionals. In addition, the clinician needs to determine whether the client has other therapeutic needs that a clinician from a different health care profession could address more appropriately. This situation would warrant a referral to that health care professional for treatment of those clinical problems that are outside of the clinician's scope of practice. In light of the complexity of issues related to scope of practice, clinicians need to consult the practice acts for their professions to determine their legal right to use massage techniques for the different clinical conditions they encounter in clinical practice.

## COMMON ERRORS IN HYPOTHESIS GENERATION

The research on clinical decision-making can provide some guidance on how to avoid some common errors in hypothesis generation and verification. Comparisons of master and novice clinicians have shown that master clinicians included in their data gathering both objective data and information on their clients' perceptions of their medical condition and functional limitations.[2] This integration of findings from different sources assisted the master clinicians in confirming the clinical hypotheses. Unlike novice clinicians, master clinicians were selective in the data that they gathered and were able to depart from a standard examination framework to seek clarification on issues that arose during the examination. This strategy prevented the problem of becoming overwhelmed by a large amount of irrelevant data, which novice clinicians frequently encountered. Generating a few hypotheses about the client's clinical problem early in the examination appeared to give the clinician more opportunities for refining the hypothesis and arriving at a hypothesis that the clinical findings supported.[3,4] This research also highlights several common errors made by clinicians during an examination. Having too many hypotheses made it difficult for the clinician to use a focused set of tests and measures and resulted in them gathering divergent information. In addition, making hypotheses very general, so that they would fit inconsistent findings, led the clinicians to arrive at incorrect conclusions about the client's clinical condition. Finally, incorrect conclusions also occurred when the clinicians made the error of exaggerating findings to justify an existing hypothesis rather than acknowledging that the existing hypothesis was incorrect and seeking a new hypothesis.

## IDENTIFICATION OF IMPAIRMENTS APPROPRIATE FOR MASSAGE TECHNIQUES

Since the decision regarding the relevance of impairments for massage is a critical one, here are further examples of how clinicians can make this decision. Consider the case of a client who presents with the impairments of pain, adhesions, and decreased muscle extensibility in the later stages of therapy after surgical repair of the Achilles tendon. The clinician can use connective tissue techniques to increase muscle extensibility and promote remodeling of dense connective tissue. Consequently, massage techniques are appropriate as primary treatment techniques for adhesions and decreased muscle extensibility. In this situation, the massage technique will have a direct effect on the impairment, and the clinician can use other techniques in a complementary manner.

There are also circumstances in which massage techniques can have a secondary or indirect effect on an impairment. For example, a client presents with decreased muscle performance secondary to pain, guarding, and muscle spasm following the reduction of a glenohumeral dislocation. In this situation, the clinician can use superficial reflex techniques to reduce pain, guarding, and muscle spasm and thus facilitate improvements in muscle performance. If a massage technique has a secondary effect on the impairment, the clinician may choose to use that technique in a complementary manner within the intervention. In this case, the primary treatment techniques would be therapeutic exercise. Finally, if the client presented with the impairment of muscle weakness secondary to a peripheral neuropathy, then the impairment would not be appropriate for massage because massage techniques do not have a documented effect on neurologically based muscle weakness.

## DISCHARGE ISSUES

Can you discharge a client if he has not met the outcomes defined for his intervention? There is much discussion and controversy about whether clinicians can terminate treatment for reasons other than the clients' achievement of their clinical outcomes, such as the end of reimbursement or the client's request. Ideally, the clinician will use the extent to which the client achieves his clinical outcomes as the guide for discharge. There are circumstances, however, in which the client need not meet the established functional outcomes before discharge. These situations include:

- When the clinician recognizes that the outcomes are not achievable given the client's condition and health status
- When the client's functional level reaches a plateau before achieving the outcomes, but he carries out his daily activities sufficiently to justify discharge

- When the client is unable to progress towards the outcomes because of medical or psychological complications
- When the client refuses ongoing treatment
- When the clinician believes that the client cannot benefit from further treatment[7]

Ultimately, the clinician must use her clinical judgment, input from the client, and examination findings to guide her decisions about the timing of discharge. In all situations, appropriate documentation of the rationale for discharge is necessary.

Another concern is whether you can justifiably continue to treat a client after he has met his identified outcomes. If the client's clinical outcomes were consistent with the severity, complexity, stability, and acuity of his medical condition, then the clinician cannot ethically justify ongoing treatment. If a clinician is uncertain whether treatment should end, she should re-evaluate the client's clinical outcomes within the context of her scope of practice. This will assist her in determining whether the client has ongoing therapeutic needs that she can address or whether she needs to refer the client to another health care professional for care.

## References

1. World Health Organization. Towards a common language for functioning, disability and health: ICF: the International Classification of Functioning, Disability and Health. Geneva, Switzerland: World Health Organization; 2002.
2. Jensen GM, Shepard KF, Gwyer J, Hack LM. Attribute dimensions that distinguish master and novice physical therapy clinicians in orthopedic settings. *Phys Ther.* 1992;72:711–722.
3. May B, Dennis J. Expert decision-making in physical therapy: a survey of practitioners. *Phys Ther.* 1991;71:190–206.
4. Payton O. Clinical reasoning process in physical therapy. *Phys Ther.* 1985;65:924–928.
5. Sullivan P, Markos P. *Clinical Decision-Making in Therapeutic Exercise.* East Norwalk, CT: Appleton & Lange; 1999.
6. Rothstein JM, Echternach JL, Riddle D. The Hypothesis-Oriented Algorithm for Clinicians II (HOAC II): a guide for patient management. *Phys Ther.* 2003;83:455–470.
7. American Physical Therapy Association. Guide to Physical Therapist Practice. Alexandria, VA: American Physical Therapy Association; 2005.
8. Simons DG, Travell JG, Simons LS. *Travell and Simons' Myofascial Pain and Dysfunction: The Trigger Point Manual. Volume 1: Upper Half of Body.* 2nd ed. Baltimore, MD: Williams and Wilkins; 1999.
9. Magee D. *Orthopedic Physical Assessment.* 4th ed. Philadelphia: WB Saunders; 2005.
10. Fritz S. *Fundamentals of Therapeutic Massage.* St. Louis, MO: Mosby-Yearbook; 2004.
11. Tappan FM, Benjamin P. *Tappan's Handbook of Healing Massage Techniques: Classic, Holistic and Emerging Methods.* 4th ed. Upper Saddle River, NJ: Prentice Hall; 2004.
12. Werner RE, Benjamin BE. *A Massage Therapist's Guide to Pathology.* Baltimore, MD: Lippincott Williams & Wilkins; 2002.
13. de Domenico G, Wood EC. *Beard's Massage.* 5th ed. Philadelphia: WB Saunders; 2007.
14. Batavia M. Contraindications for therapeutic massage: do sources agree? *J Bodywork Movement Ther.* 2004;8:48–57.
15. Cohen MH, Kemper KJ. Complementary therapies in pediatrics: a legal perspective. *Pediatrics.* 2005;115:774–780.
16. Grant AC, Wang N. Carotid dissection associated with a handheld electric massager. *South Med J.* 2004;97:1262–1263.
17. Grant KE. Massage safety: injuries reported in Medline relating to the practice of therapeutic massage—1965–2003. *J Bodywork Movement Ther.* 2003;7:207–212.
18. Miesler D. Geriatric massage: assessment and contraindications for the geriatric client. *Massage Bodywork.* 1996;11:66.
19. Ugboma HA, Akani CI. Abdominal massage: another cause of maternal mortality. *Niger J Med.* 2004;13:259–262.
20. Wada Y, Yanagihara C, Nishimura Y. Internal jugular vein thrombosis associated with shiatsu massage of the neck. *J Neurol Neurosurg Psychiatry.* 2005;76:142–143.
21. Walton TH. Exploring contraindications to massage therapy. *J Soft Tissue Manipulation.* 1999;6:5–13.
22. Whitehill W, Gustman B. Massage and skin conditions: indications and contraindications. *Athletic Ther Today.* 2002;7:24–28.
23. Yokoyama T, Shimizu Y. A case of bilateral chylothorax following neck massage. *Nihon Kokyuki Gakkai Zasshi.* 2004;42:1034–1036.
24. National Institute of Child Health and Human Development. Research plan for the National Center for Medical Rehabilitation Research. Public Health Service NIH Publication No. 93-3509. Bethesda, MD: National Institutes of Health, US Department of Health and Human Services; 1993.
25. Herskovitz S, Strauch B, Gordon MJV. Shiatsu-induced injury of the median recurrent motor branch. *Muscle Nerve.* 1992;15:1215.
26. Salvo SG. *Massage Therapy: Principles and Practice.* Philadelphia: WB Saunders; 2005.

# Chapter 4

# Interpersonal and Ethical Issues for Massage

Therapists who use massage are usually not psychotherapists. Yet, good hands-on therapy depends to a large degree on the therapist's ability to listen, observe, help clients be aware of changes, respond to discomfort, modify interventions according to client wishes, and reinforce the changes clients make. Furthermore, regardless of how well a therapist addresses impairments and functional limitations, the client may make little progress without client participation in clinical decision making, ethical behavior on the part of the therapist, and clear communication. For teaching purposes, we often separate the clinical or technical aspects of care from the interpersonal interactions that occur between therapist and client. In reality, the technical and interpersonal aspects of care are closely intertwined. Since interpersonal issues are often more subtle and less easily addressed than direct mechanical problems, the first part of this chapter will provide clear explanations of the therapeutic relationship, the therapeutic process, and problems that may arise in the therapeutic relationship. The second part of the chapter will outline concrete strategies for ethical decision making and enhancing the therapeutic relationship in typical "in the moment" clinical situations.

## Interpersonal and Ethical Issues for Massage: Foundations

## COMPONENTS OF THE THERAPEUTIC RELATIONSHIP

*"At the heart of any treatment encounter is the therapeutic relationship between the practitioner and patient."*

MITCHELL A, CORMACK M.
*The Therapeutic Relationship in Complementary Health Care.*
London: Churchill Livingstone; 1998:37.[1]

## The Therapeutic Relationship

Donabedian's[2] model of clinical care (Figure 4-1) describes the interaction that occurs between the client and the therapist as a critical interpersonal component of the process of clinical care. This **therapeutic relationship** is a trust relationship, rather than a simple interaction between two people, because of the client's vulnerability and the therapist's responsibility not to exploit or harm the client through this vulnerability.[3] It is a rich and dynamic interaction in

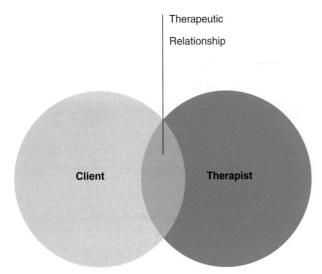

Therapeutic

Relationship

Client

Therapist

**Figure 4-1** Therapeutic relationship.

which a client's spoken and unspoken wishes interact with what the therapist perceives to be feasible, appropriate, and helpful. The therapeutic relationship provides a container for the hopes, expectations, and fears of the client. It provides a zone of safety for the client in which the client can stop, sense, reflect, and change with the help of the therapist.

The therapist sets the tone of the therapeutic relationship based on her willingness to share information, support client goals, and empathize with the client's circumstances or condition.[2,3] Most importantly, the therapist must hold the best interests of the client above all other aspects of the interaction. Consequently, a healthy alliance between the therapist and the client depends on the therapist's awareness and acceptance of the client's needs (Box 4-1). If the therapist is skilled in observation, seeks clarification, and adapts the intervention to the client's abilities or tolerance, then therapeutic outcomes will most likely succeed.[3] If the therapist cannot read the client's desires, body language, and behavioral cues, then the client will not find the therapeutic relationship dependable. If this occurs, the client may feel unsafe and unable to trust the therapeutic process.

## The Therapeutic Contract

The therapeutic relationship provides the framework for negotiating the clinical care that the client will receive. The **therapeutic contract** is the form that this negotiation takes.[2,3] In the process of formulating this contract, the client brings his or her condition, wishes for treatment, and expectations for success to the therapist. The therapist sifts through all the information she can glean from the client's story and an objective client examination and then develops an interven-

---

**Box 4-1** **Clients' Needs in a Therapeutic Relationship**

Safety
- Promotes trust and allows the client to explore sensation and make therapeutic change

Predictability
- Reduces the need to adapt to a new situation
- Further promotes trust in the therapeutic relationship

Patience
- Gives the client permission to feel sensation and pain and to make therapeutic change

Compassion and Empathy
- Helps establish an alliance with the therapist that promotes desired outcomes

Clear Consent Negotiation
- Involves client in making decisions about outcomes

Clear and Explicit Interpersonal Process
- Underscores the integrity of the therapeutic process and the safety of the therapist

Healthy Boundaries
- Contains and establishes the context for the therapeutic experience

Time to Explore Sensation
- Teaches the client to be present in his or her body and aware of sensations and the willingness to change

Responsible Closure
- Prepares the client to move from the therapeutic realm to the outside world

---

tion that she believes will help the client. Although it seems mechanical, the process of developing and working with a therapeutic contract is complex. Sometimes this commitment seems simple and straightforward. At other times, therapists can forget or feel conflicted with their contractual responsibilities—a situation that puts their clients at risk for poor outcomes. In addition, while some aspects of the therapeutic contract are explicit, problems can arise, in part, because many aspects of the contract are unspoken.[4]

## Client-Centered Care

**Client-centered care** is a philosophy of care that underlies the therapeutic relationship for Outcome-Based Massage. This approach to care looks beyond the mere delivery of services to the client to include advocacy, empowerment, respect for the client's autonomy, and the client's participation in decision-making.[5] When a therapist commits to client-centered care, the client and therapist share the decision-making about how the intervention will proceed. Other best practices for client-centered care can encompass recognizing that the clients are experts on their own lives, focusing on the client's goals, and providing timely, responsive, and consistent care.

# THE THERAPEUTIC PROCESS

The therapeutic process parallels the clinical decision-making process outlined in Chapter 3, Clinical Decision Making for Massage (Figure 4-2). It outlines the interpersonal issues and phases in the therapeutic relationship that arise during the course of providing care to a client within an individual session or the overall episode of care. There is always a beginning, middle, and end to the thera-

peutic process.[6] If a therapist acknowledges where she and the client are in the therapeutic process, then she enhances the client's feelings of safety.[7] If therapists are unsure what phase is occurring, then the client may be vulnerable to therapist miscommunication or assumption. This is particularly important when working with clients who have a history of trauma or other emotional challenges.

## Beginning Phase: Building Trust

The first part of the therapeutic process establishes the norms of treatment and helps to clarify the therapeutic relationship for the client.[1,3,6] When clients feel safe and comfortable, they are more likely to participate fully in the intervention. If clients appear unfamiliar with massage techniques, it is important to explain the approach to treatment and how the therapy works. Figure 4-3 outlines some steps that the therapist can follow within the Building

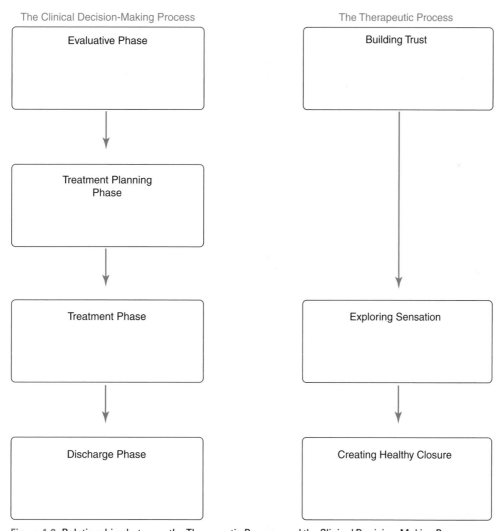

**Figure 4-2** Relationships between the Therapeutic Process and the Clinical Decision-Making Process.

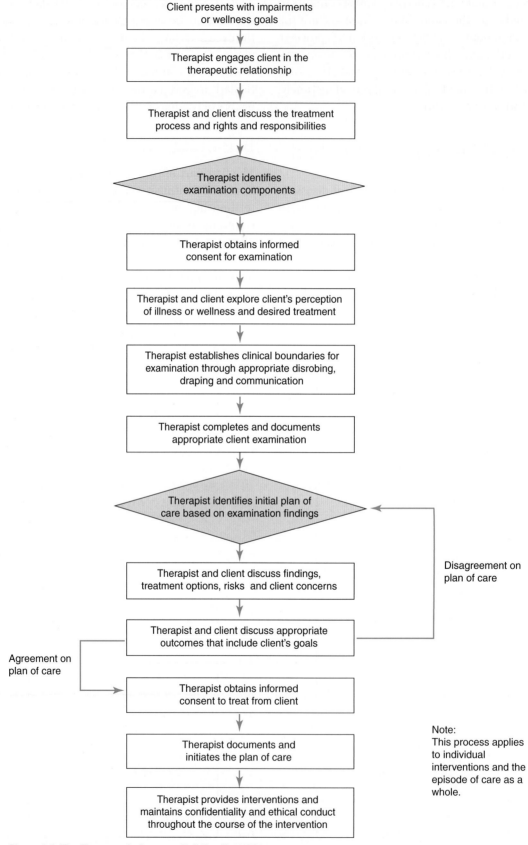

**Figure 4-3** The Therapeutic Process: Building Trust Phase.

Trust phase of the therapeutic process. Trust is an essential cornerstone of the therapeutic relationship, and it may only develop if the client feels safe. Box 4-2 outlines some basic actions that foster trust between the client and therapist.

## Mid Phase: Exploring Physical Sensations

Once the client feels confident in the therapeutic relationship, she may be ready to explore the physical sensations, conditions, or problems that led her to seek treatment using massage.[7] If a client feels emotionally vulnerable regarding the intimacy of touch, exploring her body's sensations in response to treatment may help her change her attitudes towards touch. Exploring physical sensations may be painful, historically significant, pleasurable, or frightening for the client. Therefore, during this part of the therapeutic process, it is essential for the therapist to pay attention to the client's verbal and nonverbal cues so that the client does not progress beyond her level of comfort. If the pace of treatment supports the client's ability to process the sensations she experiences, then she may gain a better understanding of her body and her personal somatic history. Figure 4-4 outlines some steps that the therapist can follow within the Exploring Physical Sensations phase of the therapeutic process. Box 4-3 details some actions that support the client's exploration of physical sensations and the therapeutic process as a whole.

The therapeutic process is not linear; instead, it is a dynamic interaction in which the client can move back and forth among stages depending on her level of comfort,

safety, and health.[1,3,6] At any time, it is possible for the client to lose focus and experience a need to rebuild trust with the therapist if she becomes distressed as a result of an increase in pain or a personal upset. If the therapist is fully aware of what is occurring at any given time and responds appropriately, then the client will feel safe. Furthermore, the therapeutic process can conclude naturally as the client becomes more independent and able to manage her condition

## Final Phase: Creating Healthy Closure

There comes a time in the therapeutic process when clients prepare to complete treatment and take on their own self-care.[1,3,6] This process is easier for some clients than for others. Clients who feel emotionally attached to therapists or appreciate their empathy and compassion may find it painful to leave the therapeutic relationship. Nevertheless, prolonging the therapy beyond its natural course is not helpful for either client or therapist. It is important for clients to understand at the outset of treatment that there is a natural point of closure that will come when they have achieved their outcomes and are ready for independent self-care. Like any good coach, the therapist can prepare her clients for the point of closure by encouraging independence and acknowledging their gains. Regularly re-examining and reviewing client gains can facilitate a positive closure. Figure 4-5 identifies a possible sequence of steps that therapists can use to promote healthy closure.

Therapists are human and may also feel attached to their clients.[1,3,6] It is very important at this stage that therapists not indulge themselves by encouraging clients to continue in a therapeutic relationship past a natural point of closure. This does not mean that clients cannot enter therapy again in the future to address another condition or part of their bodies with massage techniques. It does mean that each therapeutic process needs to have a natural beginning, middle, and ending; otherwise, one or both partners in the therapeutic relationship may find the therapeutic process stagnant.

Clients who have derived satisfaction from the therapist's use of massage techniques may wish to continue on a maintenance or preventative basis.[6] The therapist needs to negotiate this within the limits for intervention that are defined by her profession's scope of practice. Furthermore, it is often important for both parties to openly acknowledge a change in the therapeutic contract. Regardless of how closure occurs, the more open the discussion of the issues, the easier it will be for clients to explore different paths of healing and for therapists to let go and move on.

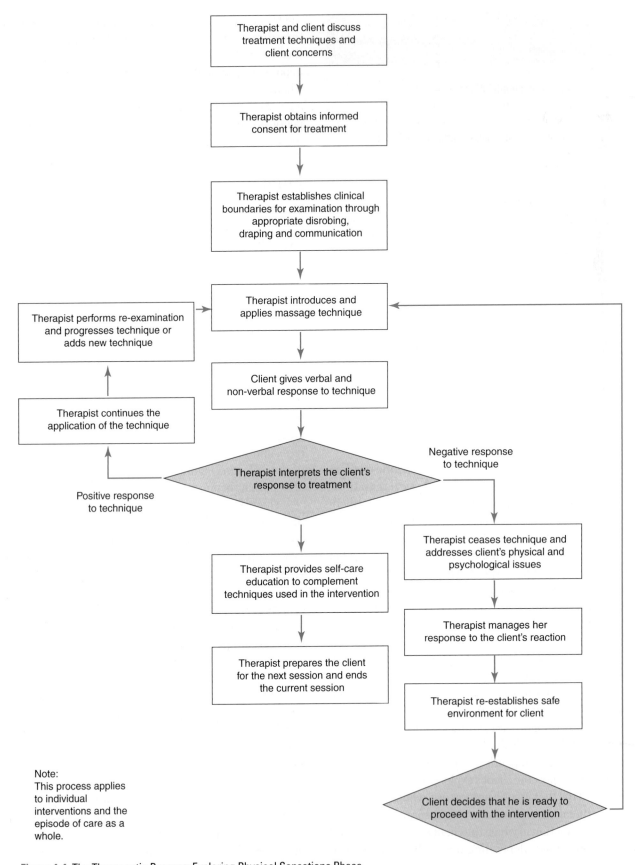

**Figure 4-4** The Therapeutic Process: Exploring Physical Sensations Phase.

**Actions That Enhance the Therapeutic Process**

- Adhere to guidelines for ethical conduct.
- Maintain clinical boundaries during the intervention through appropriate draping and communication with client.
- Perform appropriate preparations of materials for each intervention.
- Use appropriate physical and psychological therapist self-care during the course of interventions.
- Use appropriate body mechanics and manual technique.
- Deliver interventions in a safe manner.
- Demonstrate responsible caring and concern for the client.
- Support client's willingness to explore sensations.
- Assist the client in deepening his or her relaxation and somatic awareness.
- Celebrate client successes and efforts to change.
- Actively listen and watch for cues throughout the intervention that require changing or adapting the course of the intervention.
- Respond appropriately to a client's emotional reaction to treatment.
- Facilitate client participation in and adherence to the intervention.
- Elicit client's ongoing feedback on progress with clinical outcomes.
- Provide the client with appropriate education.
- Encourage client self-care to help build independence.
- Delegate care to and supervise adjunct staff appropriately.
- Maintain updated documentation on the intervention provided and the client's response.
- Maintain communication with referring practitioner, as appropriate.

# CLIENT-RELATED PROBLEMS IN THE THERAPEUTIC RELATIONSHIP

## Client Vulnerability

There are many obstacles to a successful therapeutic relationship. The client–therapist relationship is complicated by the imbalance of power from two sources.[8,9] The first is the therapist's presumed role of "healer" and his possession of information and skills that the client needs. The second is the client's vulnerability and dependence on the therapist. In addition, the use of massage techniques

involves the therapist touching parts of the client's body that are often unclothed. How the client interprets and responds to this form of touch will depend on a variety of factors, such as culture, religion, gender, upbringing, and personal experiences of touch.[10] Finally, changing a person's body structure with massage techniques can evoke emotional responses or trigger tissue memories.[11-16] Clients' responses to touch can be exaggerated or negative if they are emotionally fragile or have had negative past experiences of touch.[6,7,10]

## Lack of Power and Authority in the Treatment Room

The authority of the therapist creates an imbalance of power between therapists and clients.[6,8,9,17] Clients are vulnerable, often fully or partially disrobed, and usually lying prone or supine. Therapists, on the other hand, are dressed, standing, and hold the authority, knowledge, and responsibility for the intervention. Since clients may have little or no awareness of their own physical responses, therapists' professional experience puts clients at a considerable disadvantage. For these reasons, clients may interpret therapists' behavior as that of a friend, a parent, or intimate partner if they do not understand the nature of the imbalance of power in the therapeutic relationship.

Because therapists are in a position of authority, clients' personal history with authority figures may also play into the therapeutic process.[6,8,9,17] Clients who are in the habit of agreeing with authority figures may agree with whatever therapists suggest during the course of treatment, regardless of whether they actually agree. It is, therefore, essential for therapists to acknowledge clients' susceptibility to suggestion and to clearly and unequivocally empower clients to ask questions, stop at any time, or change positions so that they remain safe, comfortable, and able to continue with treatment.[6] In addition, therapists must also ensure that they do not abuse the power they have within the therapeutic relationship by behaving inappropriately towards their clients.[8,9,17]

## Emotional Responses to the Therapist

It is common for clients to project feelings from earlier relationships onto their therapists.[8,17] This occurs because it is human to interpret the present based on one's experience of the past. If the therapist reminds the client of an important person in her past, the client may relate to the therapist

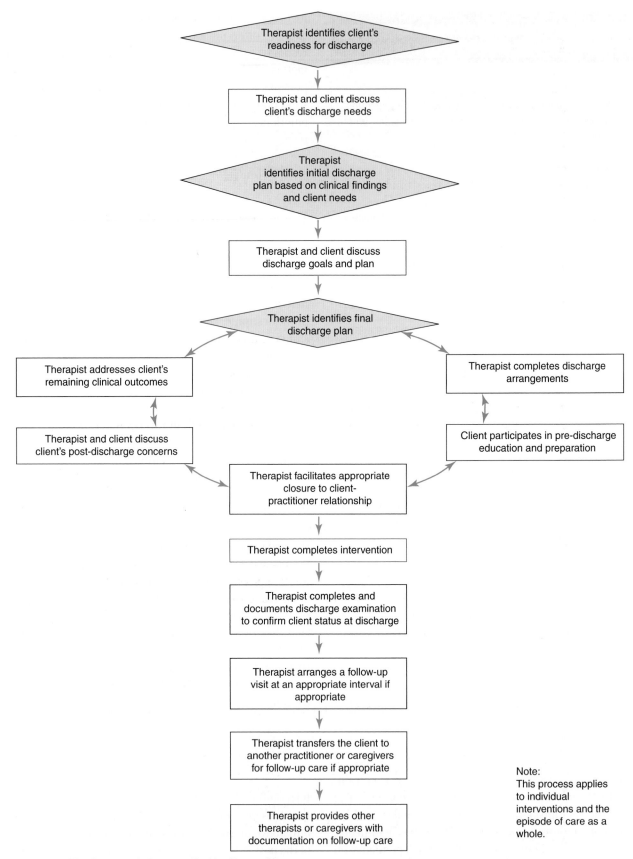

Figure 4-5  The Therapeutic Process: Healthy Closure Phase.

in the same way that she did in the relationship she remembers. This is called **transference**, and it forms an important component of the therapeutic process. Transference is particularly strong when a client receives touch from a person who she perceives to have power and authority.

If the person the client remembers was a positive influence on her, like a coach or a teacher, then the client may be encouraged or motivated to do whatever the therapist asks and follow up with self-care strategies carefully. Unfortunately, it is also possible that the transference may stem from a historically negative relationship, and the client's transferred feelings may seem painful, unpredictable, confusing, and, at times, alarming for a therapist who does not recognize the possibility of transference.

## Emotional Responses to Massage Techniques

Reich, a student of Freud's, identified relationships between chronic muscular tension and psychological disorders.[14,15] He recognized that these patterns of muscular tension were not merely symptoms of his clients' neuroses but actually the means by which they avoided experiencing emotions related to childhood psychological traumas and maintained their psychological disorders. By incorporating bodywork into his psychoanalytic practice, he found that treating patterns of chronic muscular tension resulted in emotional and psychological responses that enabled his clients to become aware of the feelings that they were avoiding. Based on this observation, he formed a theory about the connection between the body and the emotions

Reich proposed that the bodies of all living organisms vibrate or "pulsate" in an ongoing cycle of expansion and contraction.[14,15,18] During normal levels of nervous system activity, these "pulsations" are difficult to observe. The intensity of these "pulsations" will increase, however, with increases in the intensity of an individual's emotional response. For example, an individual will shake when she experiences intense excitement or fear, or her chest will heave when she sobs. Furthermore, Reich theorized that people can learn to control their emotions by learning to control their physical reactions, or "pulsations," even when the reasons for avoiding these emotions are unconscious.

Essentially, individuals can control the "pulsations" in their bodies by tensing groups of opposing muscles around a specific skeletal structure that is related to the emotion that they are trying to control.[19] This controlled tensing of the muscles can be short term in nature or long term and habitual—not even relaxing in sleep. This muscle tension reduces the spontaneous movement in that part of the

body and can result in that skeletal structure being generally held in a stiff and relatively fixed position known as "holding" or emotional structuring. Eventually, the posture of the entire body can reflect a psychological attitude. Not all muscle tension, however, is the result of an attempt to achieve emotional control. An individual's patterns of muscular tension may also be related to genetic predispositions, compensatory changes, injuries, and physical occupational stresses. Furthermore, not only can psychological attitudes affect muscular tension, but the opposite may also be true.

Rolf, and others, maintained that a change in myofascial length or tension that changes the structure of an individual's body will shift the way he or she is in the world.[12,13,16] They believed that individuals become accustomed to a specific way of feeling their bodies and experiencing their usual physical sensations. In addition, during regular states of consciousness, individuals have their usual repertoire of emotional reactions with which they can identify. When the structure of their bodies is changed, they can experience new physical experiences—feelings of warmth and tingling or sensations in areas of which they were previously unaware. New thoughts and feelings, other than the ones that they normally recognize, can also accompany these changes in physical structure. These thoughts and feelings may be so subtle that they are difficult to recognize, such as a delicate feeling of openness or a momentary feeling of vulnerability. On the other hand, the change in their bodies' structure might evoke an emotional response that is so strong that it makes it difficult for them to function socially. Therapists should, therefore, recognize that the application of a massage technique always has the potential to evoke an emotional response that stems from a change in the structure of the client's body. They also need to distinguish between the emotional response to a release of the client's tissues and the usual emotional response to being touched.

## Tissue Memory

Touch may trigger unexplained, odd, or unusual responses that appear to arise more from the client's history than from the actual therapeutic technique.[20] When clients have negative or traumatic personal histories, they may exhibit surprising or disturbing responses to the most benign touch. Without understanding the neurological underpinnings of trauma, therapists may be quite puzzled by the degree of **hyperarousal**, sensitivity, or **dissociation** that can occur with some clients.

It is important for therapists to recognize that **tissue memory** is encoded in the tissue of the body and not in the brain.[21] For example, if a person has a skiing accident that causes an anterior dislocation of the humerus, then each time the person's arm moves quickly into the same pattern as the dislocation, a memory of the injury will surface. This is a body memory or "kindling."[21] Tissue memory may not occur as a conscious, chronologic image of the experience but rather may be felt emotionally or somatically. Apprehension, nausea, anger, pain, or whatever describes the initial response to the injury may surface again when the therapist moves the client's humerus into a pattern that is reminiscent of the initial event.

When a therapist touches a client for the first time, it activates a cascade of neurological responses that help the client to interpret whether or not the touch is safe or threatening.[7,21] Textbooks on neurobiology describe this neurological response to touch in detail. It is essential for the therapist to respect the client's ability to receive touch when he is deciding on a treatment plan. If the client perceives the initial touch by the therapist as a threat, then the entire desired outcome for the intervention may be lost. Furthermore, it is unlikely that hands-on massage techniques will succeed until the client can receive touch without perceiving a threat. Therapists must also bear in mind that client vulnerability can increase the likelihood that a client who has negative history of touch will perceive therapeutic touch to be threatening.

## Negative Past Experiences of Touch

If clients have experienced a painful or difficult past, traumatic injuries, abuse, or a fear of being touched, then they are particularly vulnerable to triggered responses to touch or potential misunderstanding regarding the intentions of the therapist. Clients who seem the most vulnerable or fragile in the therapeutic setting may have some or all of the emotions, conditions, or behaviors outlined in Box 4-4.[7]

How clients bonded with their parents and how they were touched as children create their frame of reference for interpreting the level of safety, pleasure, or fearfulness that accompanies touch experiences. A person who received hugs, love, and security while growing up is more likely to interpret touch in a positive and open way, without fearing for her safety, because her first encounters with touch taught her that she is safe in the world.[6] Since only half to two-thirds of the general population fit into this category,[22] up to half of the people whom therapists encounter may have insecure touch histories. This half of the population may have childhood touch histories that are mixed with neglect, inconsistent caregiving, or frightening and disturbing circumstances that the therapist cannot ignore.[6,22]

| Box 4-4 | **Signs of Fragile Clients** |
| --- | --- |

- Emotionally vulnerable, distant, brittle, edgy, sad, distraught, guarded, or angry
- Exhibit wide arcs and swings of emotion (sad, mad, glad)
- Chronic pain, headaches, insomnia, hyperarousal, flattened affect, depression, anxiety
- Possible history of neglect, trauma, abuse
- Recently experienced deep grief, loss, or profound stress
- Feel anxious with touch and intimacy
- Have little or no frame of reference for positive and healthy touch or interpersonal relationships
- May be distinctly prone to transference
- Hyperaware of seductive or inappropriate behavior or may (mis)read a therapist's intentions

Adapted from Fitch P. Talking Body Listening Hands Workshops, with permission from the author.

If an individual's parents neglected or never touched her as a child, then the experience of massage techniques might seem bizarre or disturbing to her because she has no clear frame of reference for safe touch. On the other hand, if a client's caregiver was present and loving one day but unavailable or rejecting the next, then the client may need considerable reassurance and consistency from the therapist in order to trust the therapeutic process. Finally, if a client has experienced abusive touch, then a therapeutic environment that involves touch is unlikely to feel safe at all. Touch in this circumstance may remind clients of earlier negative and frightening encounters.[6] In all of these situations, the client may not be conscious or aware of the impact of her personal touch history. Reminders from earlier years may emerge as unwelcome sensations, sudden pain, emotional charge, or hypersensitivity, known as traumatic memory.[20]

In each of these circumstances, the client requires a feeling of safety within the therapeutic relationship.[7] Without this feeling of safety, the client cannot trust the process or the therapist. Furthermore, the client is unlikely to be able to relax and focus on the present. She will be drawn back into her unresolved past experiences of touch and may forget the present therapeutic intent.

## Trauma and Anxiety

Some clients have experienced significant trauma that results in posttraumatic stress disorder.[7,23] The primary symptoms include: hyperarousal, **hypersensitivity**, numbness to feelings or parts of the body, dissociation from the

## Box 4-5  Symptoms of Posttraumatic Stress

- Hypervigilance: strong startle response to touch or sound
- Insomnia
- Nightmares
- Anxiety and fearfulness
- Depression
- Despair
- Numbness that manifests either emotionally or physically
- Anger and tactile defensiveness
- Discomfort with pleasurable experiences
- Dissociation from the present
- Amnesia
- Chronic pain and somatization
- Hypersensitivity: fear reaction when startled, touched, or approached
- Inability to relax

Adapted with permission from Dryden T, Fitch P. Recovering body and soul from post-traumatic stress disorder. *Massage Ther J.* 2000;39:41–60.

present, and an inability to relax. Box 4-5 lists some common symptoms to assist therapists in identifying these clients. These clients may find the treatment sessions anxiety provoking.

When faced with a threat, most people respond with a "flight or fight" reaction. On the other hand, when some people are faced with a threat and they cannot figure out how to respond, they will "freeze."[24] Fight, flight, or freeze responses relate to altered limbic pathways and disrupted homeostasis. The therapist may witness all three responses in his clients.

If a therapeutic encounter causes a client to react fearfully, then it may be very difficult for the client to hear instructions, respond appropriately, remain present, or allow the intervention to proceed normally.[24] This occurs because the client is caught in a fight, flight, or freeze response. In an extreme case, the therapist's touch may recall painful personal history that can cause the client to dissociate or disconnect from the intervention, temporarily forget her surroundings, or temporarily lose touch with reality.

### Critical Thinking Question

What steps can you take to determine whether a client's negative response to your application of a massage technique is due to his negative history of touch or your application of the technique?

## THERAPISTS' STRATEGIES FOR ENHANCING THE THERAPEUTIC RELATIONSHIP

Touch demands intimate human contact, interaction, and response.[6,10] The therapist's behavior in response to the client is every bit as important as the examination or massage techniques she uses. One may view the therapist as a "canvas" on which the client paints his or her therapeutic goals, hopes and fears, and abilities and limitations. How well the therapist responds to the client's wishes can influence the outcomes of the intervention. If a therapist believes that success depends wholly on the intervention she provides, then she may ignore one of the most fundamental aspects of manual therapies.

The manner in which a therapist supports the therapeutic relationship depends largely on her awareness of her own morals, values, and beliefs regarding health, illness, and physical dysfunction, as well as her knowledge of her professional role and responsibilities.[6,8,9] In the same way that clients develop a frame of reference about touch and safety based on childhood experiences, therapist attitudes towards illness, health, and physical dysfunction shape their professional responses to clients' needs. When clients present with conditions that are puzzling, disturbing, or remind the therapist of personal experiences, then it becomes more challenging for the therapist to remain present in the therapeutic relationship and accepting of the clients' needs.

## Maintain Ethical Conduct

The need for a discussion of ethical decision-making and conduct stems from the difference in power between therapist and client.[6,8,9] In a therapeutic relationship, the client perceives the therapist as an authority figure with specific knowledge and influence. By consulting with the therapist, the client places a degree of trust in the competence and ability of the therapist to help. In manual therapies, the client may be partially or completely undressed, and the therapist may spend up to an hour touching the client's body. Under these circumstances, the client must trust that the therapist will not exploit her.

Ethical issues are not confined to any particular phase of the therapeutic process; instead, therapists must address these issues at all points during and beyond the therapeutic relationship. Both the client and the therapist have rights and responsibilities that result from their participation in the therapeutic relationship. The importance of these rights and responsibilities is underscored by the fact that health care professions have a clearly articulated set of guidelines for ethical conduct in clinical practice to which they expect all members of their profession to adhere.[25-33] Professional ethical codes are sets of moral principles that promote commonly held values and beliefs that support technical standards of practice.[25-33] These codes of ethics provide a template for making clinical decisions that honor the clients' needs within a moral **framework** that is acceptable for therapists.

In order to respond appropriately to the needs of a client, a therapist must first understand the ethical framework that defines her professional behavior.[25-33] One of the first codes of ethics acknowledged in health care was *primum non nocere* or "first, do no harm." The therapist must first "do no harm." At first glance, this would mean no bruises, increased inflammation, or undue pain as a result of overly vigorous treatment. Clinical experience also suggests that the interaction between therapists and their clients is an aspect of client care that may cause significant concern or injury. Consequently, the therapist must ensure that all aspects of care that she provides promote positive outcomes.

Ethical decision making requires that therapists consider the following factors when planning treatment.[8,9,25-33]

Client Needs
■ What kind of intervention does this client really need?
■ What are this client's expressed and unexpressed outcomes?

Power Imbalance
■ How comfortable is this client with authority?

Setting the Framework
■ How comfortable is this client in this treatment room?

Limits to Care
■ How far are you prepared to go in helping this client?

## Clients' Rights and Responsibilities

The client comes into the client–therapist relationship with rights that exist to protect her from victimization or harm by the therapist, as well as to ensure that she receives a high standard of care. The clients' rights summarized in Box 4-6 revolve around issues of autonomy, privacy, information, confidentiality, and respect.[25-33]

However, the client is not without responsibility in the client–therapist interaction. As the clients' responsibilities outlined in Box 4-7 suggest, the client must bear the respon-

| Box 4-6 | **Clients' Rights** |
|---|---|

■ Accessible and impartial access to care
■ Autonomy: freedom of choice of therapist; right to participate in decision-making during treatment; right to refuse or leave treatment regardless of the therapist's opinion; right to a consultation with another therapist
■ Care in a safe health care environment
■ Confidentiality; specifically, no disclosure of any information about the client without his or her written consent
■ Continuity of care
■ Dignity, including the right not to remain disrobed longer than necessary
■ Privacy, both visual and auditory; this includes not having to disclose any information that is not relevant to the care the client is receiving
■ Respect for client values and cultural beliefs
■ Right to be informed of his or her rights
■ Timely and accurate information on the status or background of the therapist providing care, the intervention provided, risks, side effects, alternatives, whether it is a research study, and post-discharge treatment needs

sibility of acting on his or her rights and must, in turn, treat the therapist with respect.

The following sections provide examples of ethical responses to the client-related problems discussed earlier in this chapter. This list includes potentially harmful behaviors that therapists must avoid in order to keep the therapeutic relationship safe for clients. Therapists and students will find details of the ethical behaviors required by their professions in their professional codes of ethics.

| Box 4-7 | **Clients' Responsibilities** |
|---|---|

■ Provide accurate information to the therapist
■ Accept the consequences of refusing care, altering care, or choosing an alternative option to care
■ Act with consideration and respect for therapists and others in that setting
■ Adhere to instructions provided by the therapist
■ Follow rules of conduct of the health care setting
■ Assure that financial obligations to the therapist or facility are met

# Obtain Informed Consent

## Informed Consent for Treatment

Client-centered care supports the principle of **informed consent** by giving clients the information that they need in order to choose the type of intervention that will suit them best.[25–33] Before the therapist can examine the client or initiate the treatment plan, he requires the client's understanding and consent. Obtaining clear and informed consent for treatment from a client involves ensuring that the client understands the intent and direction of therapy. This process requires that the therapist explain exactly what he is going to do and how he will achieve the specified outcomes. It also requires that the client hears and understands the therapist's explanation, since clients who do not hear the explanation may agree without understanding what the therapist means.

Consent to massage techniques can occur at three levels.[6,7] First, the client may agree "from the head," thinking to themselves, "This seems to make sense. . . ." Second, if the client considers that the intent of the therapist is to help, the client may agree "from the heart" based on her emotional response to the therapist and the environment (for example, "I like Janey, she won't hurt me . . . I guess it's okay . . ."). Finally, in order for a client to agree "from the body," the client must feel safe and prepared for the intervention. The acceptance of the intervention may take a while to register in the client's tissues. When the intervention feels right to the client, the client's muscles will soften and release tension easily, the client will rest deeply, her breathing may slow, and the client will give control of the intervention over to the therapist.

## Informed Consent for Painful or Uncomfortable Procedures

Therapists who use massage techniques may need to cause the client temporary discomfort in order to give the client relief from pain, even as they maintain the client's overall comfort, safety, and trust.[6,7] In addition, although it appears paradoxical, clients who are in pain or uncomfortable with touch may seek a form of therapy that could be painful or intimate. This occurs because the prospect of a pleasurable sensation or relief from pain may be sufficient to entice the client to try an intervention that may be outside of her level of comfort with touch. In light of the pain and/or intimacy associated with massage techniques, the therapist must ensure that the client understands and accepts the responsibilities of the therapeutic relationship and the possible responses to treatment techniques before he proceeds with an intervention that the client may find uncomfort-

able.[6–8,25–33] Otherwise, if the client does not trust the therapist and the therapeutic relationship, she may mistakenly perceive that the therapist intends to inflict pain.

## Critical Thinking Question

In which situations are you unable to obtain informed consent for examination and treatment from a client? What must you do prior to initiating examination or treatment?

# Avoid Highly Emotional or Sexualized Responses to Clients

When the client is experiencing transference in his relationship with the therapist, his ability to succeed in treatment depends on how the therapist responds to his projected feelings. There are a variety of possible responses; the therapist may feel flattered by the client's intense positive regard, have an urge to challenge the client's misconceptions, accept the transference because it feels like the easiest course of action, or discharge the client out of alarm and confusion. If the therapist misinterprets or acts inappropriately toward a client's transference, she may ignore the articulated treatment outcomes or make it impossible to achieve them. This puts the client in the difficult situation of having his unconscious feelings for the therapist interrupt or jeopardize his therapeutic progress.

Countertransference occurs when a therapist allows his unresolved feelings and personal issues about people outside of the therapeutic relationship to influence his relationship with a client.[8,17] If a therapist is experiencing countertransference toward a client, then he may ignore the client's best interests and allow his own needs to direct the intervention. Furthermore, when a therapist engages in sexualized contact with a client, he discards the purpose of the intervention, betrays the client's trust, and either minimizes or completely ignores the client's needs. At the same time, the client in the therapeutic relationship is vulnerable to suggestion and may not realize the harm of the therapist's actions. In these circumstances, clients may feel confused or alarmed by the change in relationship and attention. To avoid the problems associated with transference and countertransference, the therapist needs to remain focused on the treatment goals and providing a healthy therapeutic relationship.

## Sexualized Behavior

It is unethical and abusive for therapists to engage in personal or sexualized contact with clients because of the power imbalance between therapists and their clients. Furthermore, therapists must not sexualize massage techniques because the degree of intimacy inherent in hands-on work, coupled with the authority of their position, makes clients vulnerable to suggestion. When a therapist acts on his fantasies about a client, he has abused the client.[25–34] Some jurisdictions consider comments of a sexual nature, in addition to sexualized touching and intercourse, to be sexual abuse.[25–34]

## Flirtatious or Seductive Behavior

Flirtatious or seductive behavior on the part of the therapist, or client, takes the focus away from the goals of treatment and increases the potential for transference or countertransference.[25–34] In addition, it may compound issues that arise because of the client's personal history of touch and attitudes about intimacy. Moreover, if the flirtatious behavior continues, it could result in negative or abusive consequences. For these reasons, therapists must avoid even flirtatious and seductive behavior and politely discourage these in their clients.

## Specialness

When the therapist treats a client in a special way or gives the impression that the care that the client receives is different from or better than the norm, it enhances the potential for transference and **boundary violations**.[17] Therapists should, therefore, make a conscious effort to avoid behaviors that suggest that a particular client is special in some way.

## Showing Affection Inappropriately

It is predictable that the therapist may find some clients more appealing than others. Acknowledging one's affection for a client is sometimes helpful in facilitating the therapeutic process. Conversely, telling the client repeatedly what a special person she is can only emphasize any existing transference or countertransference and may put the client at risk for abuse. Be sure that if you show affection for a client, that it is in the client's best interests for her to experience this affection.[17]

## Unintentional Touching

The proximity of the therapist's body to a client can convey strong, and possibly unintentional, messages, particularly if the therapist is attracted to the client.[8,17] Brushing the client's body with one's hips or abdomen may occur inadvertently during treatment. If, however, it appears to happen more frequently with one client than with others, there is a distinct possibility that countertransference is at play. In addition, the client may perceive the unintentional touch as an expression of intimacy, affection, or control. No matter how innocuous the therapist's unintentional touch is, there is a possibility that the client may interpret the message incorrectly. The following are some guidelines on the characteristics that people use to interpret touch[8]:

- The part of the other person's body that touches the person
- The part of the person's body that is touched
- How long the touch lasts
- How much pressure is used
- Whether there is movement after contact is made
- If anyone else is present to witness the touch
- The relationship between the person performing the touch and the person receiving the touch
- The verbal exchange that accompanies the touch
- Other nonverbal behaviors that are present
- Prior touch experiences

---

### Theory in Practice 4-1

## Dealing with the Patient's Emotional Response to the Practitioner

#### Situation

A practitioner is treating a patient for a hamstring strain that she sustained while playing badminton. During early sessions, the patient appeared shy and nervous. Over the course of the first four sessions, she began to trust the practitioner's integrity and learned to relax into the massage techniques. Now, midway through the episode of care, the practitioner has become alarmed because the patient told him that he is the first man who has ever made her feel so special.

The patient moans happily when the practitioner applies massage techniques to her leg and shows signs of being attracted to him. As the intervention progresses, she expresses her attraction and appreciation for his therapy more openly.

The practitioner knows that he does not intend to cross any professional boundaries, but he feels increasingly uncomfortable treating the patient and wishes that she would just go away.

It appears that the patient has transferred her feelings about men and intimacy to the practitioner. Whatever her past experience with men, she enjoys the intimacy of the sessions. Consequently, she may be confusing therapeutic intimacy with the kind of closeness that one might have in a personal relationship.

The practitioner is uncomfortable because he is receiving a type of attention that he does not want and does not intend to encourage. He does not appear to understand that her behavior has more to do with her past history with men than specifically with him.

**Resolution**

Baffled by the patient's behavior, the practitioner discusses her case with a **peer supervisor**. He recognizes that the patient may continue to exhibit her attraction and appreciation for him unless he addresses her behavior directly. On the other hand, he also knows that this transference may gradually lessen, and she may be able to see him more clearly for the health care professional that he is. The practitioner decides, for the sake of future sessions, to gently and compassionately explain to the patient that he is pleased she finds the interventions beneficial but that his responsibility to her is strictly professional. Following his discussions with the patient, she gradually begins to respond to him in a more appropriate manner.

## Critical Thinking Question

What actions can you take when you recognize that there is a mutual attraction between you and your client to ensure that you are behaving in an ethical manner?

# Maintain Clear Communication and Boundaries

Despite the therapist's efforts to achieve full informed consent prior to embarking on an intervention, the therapeutic contract may remain implicit or unspoken.[1-3] If a therapist does not communicate clearly, a client may misunderstand the intent of a particular intervention. If a therapist ignores the client's needs or insists on a particular form of treatment, then the client may feel hurt or traumatized by the experience. The responsibility for achieving the desired outcomes rests on the therapist's skill in reading and responding to the client's cues throughout the therapeutic process.

## Unexpressed Expectations and Histories

Clients present with a variety of conditions, perspectives, and experience to therapists. Unfortunately, clients do not share complete personal histories with therapists for a variety of reasons.[4,35-41] This occurs during the clinical interview when either the details seem petty to the client or the client considers them far too significant to share with a stranger. Incomplete histories can lead to problems with treatment planning and the client's response to treatment. In addition, clients do not always articulate their expectations for treatment to therapists, although these are critical for a successful outcome.[4,35-41] Consequently, a therapist may not meet the client's expectations because the therapist is unaware that these unspoken wishes exist. Not fully appreciating the client's reason for seeking treatment using massage techniques can result in misunderstanding, confusion, and hurt. For these reasons, therapists must use active listening, observation, and full investigation of clients' reactions to gain a clear understanding of clients' problems, histories, and expectations for treatment.

## Keeping Secrets

It is important for therapists to ensure confidentiality in order for clients to trust the therapeutic process.[25-41] At the same time, it is essential that therapists refrain from asking their clients to keep secrets about the treatments that they receive.[17] All aspects of treatment and the therapist's comments should be explicit and clear. Asking a client to keep a secret about interventions confers a "special status" to the client that is linked to intimacy and promotes transference. This act also removes any freedom the client has to discuss, process, or question the therapeutic relationship and interventions with other clients or people.

## Comments about Body Size or Appearance

Unconditional positive regard is one of the common factors that supports a therapeutic relationship.[17,36-41] When clients appear inhibited about their body size or appearance, it is not helpful for the therapist to make comments that underscore this discomfort. On the other hand, there are times when body size may contribute to pain, and a responsible therapist should find a tactful way of sharing this perspective so that the client is fully informed.

## Dual Relationships

**Dual relationships** describe situations in which clients and therapists have more than one kind of relationship.[17,36–41] There are very good reasons why therapists are discouraged from engaging in dual relationships. When a therapist is also a brother or sister or friend to a client, then the relationship that came first is likely to determine the therapist's behavior towards the client. For example, a therapist who is treating one of his parents will find it is difficult to remain objective because his parent–child relationship is the most dominant.

---

### Theory in Practice 4-2
### Unexpressed Expectations and Histories

#### Situation

The patient was in a serious car accident over a year ago and her neck has never been the same. She has been seeing the practitioner for more than 3 months. The patient has never had much luck with therapy because the practitioners always seemed to get frustrated with her and discharge her without really addressing her neck pain. She thinks that the present practitioner is the first person who has really stuck by her. One day, she shyly admits to the practitioner that she is the best thing that has happened to her since her car accident.

The practitioner finds the patient's neck pain perplexing. She realizes that the car accident has caused some restriction and pain, but she cannot find any objective examination findings to corroborate the patient's subjective reports. The patient continues to report that her pain is constant, and she appears somewhat depressed. The practitioner recognizes her discomfort, but she cannot understand why the patient continues to come for treatment when there does not seem to be any shift in her pain.

One day, the practitioner discusses her "challenging patient" (without mentioning names) with an insurance adjuster who has been working with accident claims for years. The adjuster tells her that he has seen all this before. He suggests that the patient is just trying to get more treatment and tells her that the insurance industry calls this behavior malingering. He also suggests that the practitioner should discharge the patient because she is just taking advantage of the system.

After her discussion with the adjuster, the practitioner meets with the patient and informs her that she has done all that she can for her and that it is time for her discharge. Much to the practitioner's surprise, the patient bursts into tears and becomes distraught. After calming her down, the practitioner assures her that she does not have to leave therapy if she does not want to.

#### Questions to Consider

1. What just happened here?
2. Which aspect of the therapeutic process has the practitioner negated?
3. What does the practitioner need to do in order to re-establish the therapeutic relationship?
4. What actions of the patient have contributed to the current situation?
5. What else should the practitioner address in the Plan of Care for her patient with chronic pain?

The practitioner and the patient have been living in two different realities. Although the patient has not told the practitioner about all the other therapists, for the first time, she has begun to trust a therapeutic process. The practitioner has been facilitating the patient's trust by simply bearing witness to her pain and treating her over the course of 3 months without questioning the need for discharge. When the practitioner discussed her patient with the insurance adjuster, she heard an industry term "malingering" that made her doubt the patient's integrity. The practitioner didn't reflect further but simply acted on the adjuster's suggestion to discharge her patient on the basis of malingering.

The patient, having just begun to trust the therapeutic process, was dumbfounded when the therapist sought to discharge her. The distressing news removed the patient's fledgling sense of safety, making it difficult, once again, for her to trust a practitioner.

The practitioner was not aware that the patient was still in the phase of Building Trust. She had been intuitively offering a safe environment in which the patient could experience her pain. When the practitioner brought up the idea of discharge, the patient once again experienced the trauma of discharge and punishment for not getting better on a therapist's timetable.

#### Resolution

The practitioner returned to the beginning of the therapeutic process with her patient by completing a full examination and negotiating a plan of care that clearly addresses her impairments and functional limitations. The patient, in turn, disclosed her full history of treatment and medical issues.

Through these activities, both patient and practitioner developed a greater understanding of the limits to care for the patient. In addition, the practitioner involved other health care practitioners in her patient's care for additional physical testing and for psychosocial support, since she could not provide these within her treatment sessions.

At what point will the patient be ready for discharge? The practitioner realized that she should have asked this question early in the intervention so that both parties could be prepared for and agree on the point of closure. To remedy this oversight, they set mutually agreed upon times for re-examination as a team so that they knew where they were in the therapeutic process. When the patient achieved some goal, no matter how small, they celebrated their victory with some form of acknowledgement such as a star on her chart, a handshake, or simply eye contact and a few words of encouragement. The practitioner understood that the patient needed help to get back on track and that she has found the coaching that she needs in the practitioner. She also recognized that, if she ignores these psychosocial concerns now, the patient is at risk of becoming increasingly debilitated by chronic pain. Since the practitioner was able to see her role as an educator, as well as a practitioner who treats patients' physical issues, she was able to assist the patient out of the cycle of chronic pain that she lives with daily.

Once the practitioner re-established the therapeutic process, she helped the patient to understand that there is a beginning, middle, and end to all treatment. In doing so, she communicated to the patient that it is up to her to move forward if she wants and that she would accompany the patient on the journey until she meets her goals.

## Accommodate Negative Experiences of Touch, Trauma, or Posttraumatic Stress Disorder

Clients can overcome the negative aspects of negative experiences of touch or trauma or the symptoms of posttraumatic stress disorder through a harmonious therapeutic process that has clear client–therapist boundaries.[7,36–41] First, the therapist must be able to read and respond to the client's reactions, proceed slowly and carefully with treatment, and modify interventions to prevent further hyperarousal and distress. In response, the client may experience increased comfort within the therapeutic relationship and may learn to accept, and even enjoy, touch and treatment using massage techniques. This can have physiological benefits for the client because the sense of safety and comfort that comes from being soothed can assist in shutting off the limbic response to stress (fight, flight, or freeze) and facilitate the relaxation or parasympathetic response. In this way, treatment using massage techniques can teach clients an alternative response to touch than a perceived threat. In addition, it can help them learn how to receive positive and healthy touch within a relationship that has clear boundaries.

### Theory in Practice 4-3

### Working with Negative Experiences of Touch or Trauma

**Situation**

A 45-year-old man has come to you for treatment. He fatigues easily and moves his body away from even the slightest degree of pressure. In addition, he holds his breath and tenses each time you touch his mid back, slightly arching his lumbar spine and guarding.

You feel frustrated and cannot find a way to treat this patient's low back. You find yourself tensing and sense a building anger towards this "hard to please" patient.

*Questions to Consider*

1. What is going on here?
2. What can you do to change the direction of this therapeutic encounter?
3. What self-care strategies can you use in order to manage your own anger?

This patient is demonstrating the hypersensitivity reaction that occurs when someone has an old injury or trauma. The fact that he has come to you for treatment suggests that he believes that massage and manual techniques can help. His history of trauma is, however, hampering his ability to respond positively to interventions. It can be frustrating when a patient responds in this way because his reactivity requires that you treat him differently than other patients. It may require some creativity on your part to establish a treatment plan that helps the patient without activating his hypersensitivity.

**Resolution**

One way to change your treatment approach would be to acknowledge the patient's discomfort and ask him if there is any way that you could modify your interventions to make him more comfortable. It might be helpful to ask the patient if he has ever injured his back in any way because muscle guarding is a common way that people protect old injuries.

It may also be true that the patient is not that aware of his responses or his own discomfort. The intimacy of the hands-on therapy may feel confusing. Furthermore, his responses may be as much of a surprise to him as they are to you. First principles of "do no harm" suggest that it might be better for you to treat other parts of his body until he is able to receive touch on his back more easily.

The patient would also benefit from some coaching on deep abdominal breathing. You could show him how to breathe through the discomfort before attempting any deeper work on his back. Demonstrating some self-care strategies and acknowledging what isn't working will show him that you have his best interests in mind and do not want to harm him. This can only help to ease any discomfort he may feel. Once he begins to trust you, then he can become an ally in the healing experience.

Being angry or frustrated at this does not help you to provide patient-centered care. In the short term, deep breathing and committing yourself to responding professionally and compassionately are better strategies for managing your feelings. Nevertheless, if a patient like this triggers feelings of anger or discomfort, it is best to discuss the case with a peer or supervisor so that you can better understand what is bothering you. Once you understand and can acknowledge the triggers you are reacting to, this behavior will lose the ability to frustrate you.

# Maintain Privacy

## Appropriate Draping

Using appropriate draping to respect client privacy facilitates the sense of safety that the client feels and promotes a healthy therapeutic relationship.[25-41] At the same time, the therapist should accomplish draping with the least fuss possible. When therapists nervously spend extended periods of time attending to the draping or repeatedly tuck sheets in until the client feels over-bound, they move the emphasis from the desired treatment outcomes to their concerns about exposing the client. This excessive concern may frighten clients into wondering what may happen next or annoy the client because it is taking time away from hands-on treatment.

## Permission for Intrusive Work

There are times during treatment using massage techniques that the therapist must place a finger or a hand in a sensitive location. Intra-oral work, massage on the attach-

ments of the groin or psoas, or breast or abdominal massage may feel invasive to clients who are uncomfortable with the therapist touching them in these locations. In these situations, therapists must carefully negotiate with the client where and how deeply they touch them.[25-41] This clear informed consent is particularly important when the client reports that she feels uncomfortable.

To obtain consent for intrusive work, the therapist must explain the procedure clearly, answer any questions, and ask for the client's permission to perform the techniques he deems appropriate.[25-41] Once the therapist has obtained permission, he must perform exactly the techniques that he said that he would perform. In addition, he must obtain client feedback about her comfort and response to those techniques. After he has completed the intervention, he must review what he did and ask the client for any follow-up questions. This approach will communicate to the client that she is safe with the therapist and can trust the therapeutic process.

## Privacy for History Taking

Clients' words deserve as much privacy as their bodies, a fact that therapists often forget.[25-41] Conducting client interviews in open gyms and asking clients for feedback on their response to treatment in waiting rooms or hallways are among the ways in which therapists inadvertently violate clients' privacy. Clients differ in terms of what they consider to be sensitive topics. Consequently, therapists need to provide clients with as much privacy as possible within their clinical setting during history taking, feedback on response to treatment, and other discussions of client information. Doing so will include ensuring that sensitive discussions with clients do not occur in the presence of administrative staff, adjunct staff, or other clients.

---

**Theory in Practice 4-4**

### Maintaining Client Privacy

**Situation**

Patient A became the practitioner's patient when she was pregnant with her first child. She found treatment with massage techniques helpful in managing her low back pain and swollen ankles, which were especially troublesome in her third trimester. The practitioner even came to the hospital to treat Patient A right after her baby was born. Since Patient A loves everything that the practitioner does in the course of treatment, she suggested that her pregnant best friend (Patient B) see the practitioner.

Patient A discussed this suggestion with the practitioner. In doing so, she explained to the practitioner that this was Patient B's first pregnancy and that she was a little worried about how things were going. Patient A confided that Patient B would need extra support during her pregnancy since her husband was overseas.

A few weeks later, Patient B arrived for her appointment. Patient B was quiet and reluctant to share the details of her situation with the practitioner. The session progressed as a normal introductory session. The practitioner was pleased when Patient B admitted that she felt more relaxed at the end of the session and scheduled another appointment the following week.

A few days later, Patient A arrived for her appointment with the practitioner. She asked her how Patient B had liked her session. The practitioner, not used to discussing one patient with another, reluctantly shared that the friend seemed shy but that she liked the intervention. Patient A asked the practitioner if Patient B had told her that her husband was going to remain overseas for the next 6 months and gave her the details of how her friend was responding. The practitioner was unaware of this and told her so. After listening to Patient A, the practitioner decided to speak to Patient B about how her husband's absence was affecting her.

*Questions to Consider*

1. What is going on here?
2. How would you describe the practitioner's behavior?
3. What actions does the practitioner need to take to ensure that she maintains her patient's friend's (Patient B) right to privacy?

Every therapeutic relationship needs to be founded on patient safety and confidentiality so that the patient may trust the therapeutic process. The patient needs to know that what she says or experiences is not discussed with anyone else, except in very specific confidential situations such as peer supervision.

Health care often mixes physiological responses with personal, social, or emotional information. While individuals' responses to treatment may vary, they are all most definitely private. The confidentiality that cloaks therapeutic encounters is like a boundary around the patient. Only the patient may discuss her experience or health care with friends or family. A practitioner must never share a patient's condition, confidences, responses to treatment, and other personal information, or the patient's trust will be broken.

In this case, Patient A initiated the contact between Patient B and the practitioner. She hopes that her friend will receive the help she needs during her pregnancy, and she shares these hopes and expectations with the practitioner. As a health care professional, the practitioner wants to help Patient B, but she makes a mistake in considering Patient A's perspective.

First, by listening to Patient A talk about Patient B's problems, the practitioner communicates indirectly to her that they are equally responsible for Patient B's health care. The practitioner does not stop Patient A from discussing her friend, and she does nothing to create a boundary between her as the practitioner, who should maintain complete confidentiality for all patients, and Patient B.

Second, the practitioner resolves to discuss the information from Patient A with Patient B. This confirms that there is now a triangle between the three women. This is a breach of trust since it will confirm to Patient B that the practitioner has discussed her with Patient A. This action, although well intentioned, ignores the nature of the friendship between Patient A and Patient B. The practitioner has no knowledge of how their friendship works and may appear to be siding with Patient A against Patient B. This type of triangulating damages the therapeutic process.

Third, by not allowing the therapeutic process to unfold naturally with Patient B, the practitioner has compromised her objectivity and her ability to assess and address Patient B's needs for treatment.

### Resolution

The practitioner stopped all discussions about Patient B with Patient A. She also chose not to mention the information that Patient A gave her because this would enhance the triangle relationship. This was difficult to establish after the fact, but in this case, it was necessary to be direct and truthful. The practitioner used an "I" statement to clarify to Patient A, without pointing fingers, what exactly had to change:

> "When I listened to you the other day as you described your friend's circumstances, I felt uncomfortable because my job as a practitioner is to maintain confidentiality for all my patients. I appreciate your comments, but I will not discuss your friend with you again."

The practitioner also discussed the situation with one of her peers to get guidance on how to ensure Patient B's privacy. Above all else, the practitioner committed to ensuring Patient B's complete confidentiality regarding her health care.

## Seek Further Information on Ethical Conduct

The therapist bears the burden of responsibility in the client–therapist relationship because of the therapist's need to ensure that he does not abuse the power that he holds within this relationship.[25-41] Not only does the therapist have the responsibilities to the client (Box 4-8), but he also has responsibilities to his profession and society as a whole that are beyond the scope of this chapter. Consequently, the therapist needs to seek out and understand the ethical code for his profession.

Under which circumstances can a therapist use his or her own judgement, rather than the professional code of ethics, to guide a questionable clinical situation?

---

### Box 4-8 — Therapists' Responsibilities to Clients

#### ISSUES RELATED TO INTERACTIONS WITH A CLIENT

- Demonstrate responsible caring and concern for the client.
- Do not guarantee a cure or misrepresent the potential effects of the intervention.
- Do not treat clients when under the influence of any substance that would impair the ability to treat safely.
- Listen to and respect client's values, beliefs, and needs.
- Maintain appropriate clinical boundaries and avoid sexual interaction of any sort with clients.
- Provide client-centered, preventative care.
- Provide the client with an opportunity to give voluntary and informed consent.
- Respond appropriately to client's emotional reaction to treatment.
- Use draping to maintain the client's privacy and appropriate clinical boundaries.

#### GENERAL ISSUES

- Act in the client's best interests.
- Act without conflict of interest.
- Assume responsibility for and provide appropriate examination, treatment, progression of care, and discharge planning.
- Communicate information on the client's care to the referring therapist (within restraints of maintaining confidentiality).
- Delegate care to and supervise adjunct staff or students appropriately and take responsibility for the care they provide.
- Document all of the client's findings accurately and appropriately.
- Ensure and maintain a high level of competence.
- Maintain confidentiality of records and information and obtain a signed release prior to disclosure.
- Do not refuse a client care on the basis of race, gender, culture, religion, sexual orientation, age, etc.
- Do not treat the client unless the client's clinical condition (prevention, curative, maintenance, wellness) warrants it, thus avoid the overutilization of services.
- Provide client-centered, preventative care.
- Provide services to meet the client's needs, rather than for financial gain.
- Provide the highest standard of care possible.
- Request consultation from other therapists as appropriate.
- Take responsibility for the care provided to a client.
- Transfer the client to another therapist, as appropriate, when the client–therapist relationship is ended or the client is discharged.
- Use sound judgment.
- Work within the scope of practice and refer to another therapist when the client's condition requires treatment that is beyond your legal scope of practice or level of competence.

Box 4-9 **Therapists' Rights**

- Ability to make independent clinical judgments
- Freedom to decline to treat a client if it would compromise the therapist's ethics, dignity, or values
- Right to work in an environment in which the therapist can practice without coercion, conflict of interest, or undue influence, including being pressured into overutilization of services for the facility's financial gain
- Right to be treated with respect and consideration by clients and colleagues

## Therapists' Rights

Unfortunately, therapists' rights are rarely discussed. With the increasing erosion of the therapist's autonomy in practice, it is important not to lose sight of therapists' right to respect, to exercise their best clinical judgment, and to work in environments in which they can practice without coercion, conflict of interest, undue influence, or inappropriate scheduling demands (Box 4-9). Therapists are wise to familiarize themselves with their rights and ensure that they are being met in their practice settings.

## REVIEWING THE BASICS

The therapeutic relationship, a trust relationship, between the client and the therapist lies at the core of client-centered care. Within this relationship, the client and therapist negotiate a course of treatment that they articulate as the therapeutic contract. The therapeutic process parallels the phases of the clinical decision-making process as the client and therapist move through the stages of Building Trust, Exploring Physical Sensations, and Healthy Closure. The therapeutic process is complicated by a number of factors, including the client's vulnerability, because of the intimacy of touch, the therapist's authority and power in the therapeutic relationship, and the fact that clients do not always fully disclose their expectations and histories. Other client-related obstacles can be their negative experiences of touch, tissue memories, trauma, and anxiety. Strategies that therapists can use to enhance the therapeutic relationship include maintaining ethical conduct and addressing the client's emotional response to massage. Since both technical and interpersonal factors can have an impact on the outcomes of care that the client can achieve, therapists would be wise to attend to both of these aspects in the planning and delivery of care to their clients.

# Interpersonal and Ethical Issues for Massage: Further Study and Practice

This section provides advanced methods for how to address the client's emotional response and enhance client adherence with the therapeutic process.

## ADDRESSING THE CLIENT'S EMOTIONAL RESPONSE

Clinicians are often unprepared for the client's emotional response to the application of massage techniques. The information in this chapter serves as an overview of some basic strategies for responding to the client. The clinician should ensure that she remains within the limits of her professional scope of practice and clinical training when she is addressing the client's emotional needs that arise during an intervention. In particular, the clinician should recognize when it is appropriate to refer the client to a

physician or a health care professional who can provide psychosocial care.

## Recognizing the Client's Emotional Process

Reichian theory suggests that levels of emotional release lie on a continuum from overt to subtle.[14,15,18] In this continuum, signs of overt emotional release are easily recognized, and those of subtle release are less easily recognized. The signs and sensations of the usual vibratory and spontaneous movement in the body that accompany a subtle emotional release in the body include an increase in the rate of breathing; gurgles in the throat and abdomen; swallowing; tearing; the production of sounds, such as sighing or moaning; spontaneous jerking of musculature; itches; sensations of heat and cold; and the movement of energy.

These are usually simply signs and sensations of physical release or the movement from a tense state of sympathetic nervous system activation to a relaxed state of parasympathetic nervous system activation. When clinicians use massage in a clinical setting, the occurrence of these signs and sensations in the client do not lead to anything other than a state of physical relaxation. By contrast, when the client's physical signs and sensations are accompanied by thoughts and beliefs that form an emotion, an emotional release occurs.

The client can also manifest the physical and behavioral signs of limiting or containing, rather than releasing, emotions.[14,15,18] These attempts to limit the vibratory or spontaneous movement in the body lead to reactions such as becoming still and silent, holding one's breath, a rigidity in the musculature, and focusing one's attention on an unrelated situation or distracting conversation. The individual will be able to maintain a distance from emotional content as long as these strategies are successful. The client's need to prevent emotional release can be in conflict with the massage-related treatment outcomes. For example, if a client needs to maintain a certain degree of muscular tension in order to limit the vibratory and spontaneous movement in his body, this may be in conflict with the goal of deep relaxation of his tense musculature. If the clinician is able to see the client's need to prevent emotional release and control his physical reactions as a reflection of his fear of unresolved and difficult emotional terrain, then she may be better able to respect his need for these behaviors.

# Dealing with Emotional Release

The most appropriate response for a clinician without training in working with emotional and psychological issues is to provide an atmosphere in which the client feels comfortable and safe to express his emotions as they arise. This can be achieved by using the strategies outlined in the following sections.

## Encourage the Client to Give Feedback

Clinicians can facilitate open communication with the client by creating an open, accepting environment and encouraging the client to talk about what does not work for him during a session.[15,42–46] In addition, asking the client for his consent to treatment both before and during a session can reaffirm his right to refuse any aspect of the intervention and contribute to his sense of safety.

## Respect the Client's Need to Avoid or Contain His Emotions

There are times when the client needs to use strategies to avoid or contain his emotions and the clinician finds that this need is in conflict with the goal of relaxation.[15,42–46] Paradoxically, acceptance of the client's need to avoid or contain his emotions can reduce the tension associated with his response and allow him to achieve a greater level of relaxation.

## Containment

Unless the clinician has discussed a "contract" with the client that involves the exploration of his emotions, then she must simply deal with whatever arises when the client experiences an emotional release.[15,42–46] Although everyone has his or her own unique way of being with someone who is experiencing intense emotions, within the context of an intervention, this usually involves avoiding any actions that might intensify the client's emotional reaction. For example, engaging in the content of the emotion by asking the client questions can intensify his emotional reaction and lead to difficult interpersonal dynamics if the clinician's questions are not consistent with the client's emotional state and needs. In addition, moving to an area of the client's body where the emotional reaction is focused can also potentially intensify his emotional reaction. Although intensifying the client's emotional reaction may be desirable, asking for the client's consent before doing so allows him to control what he feels is appropriate for him and, in turn, helps him contain the level of his emotional reaction to what is suitable for the situation.

## Know One's Comfort Level with Emotional Expression

Being comfortable with clients' expressions of emotions is a skill that clinicians develop with repeated exposure to clients' emotions.[15,42–46] It is important for the clinician to acquire this skill and to learn her level of comfort with clients' emotions in preparation for a situation in which she encounters a client who starts to express his emotions. When a clinician exceeds her comfort level and pretends to be comfortable with her client's emotional expression, it can erode the client–clinician relationship for several reasons. The client may feel a lack of safety as a result of the clinician's falseness, or the clinician may feel that the client's emotional needs have gone beyond the proper boundaries of the client–clinician relationship.

When the clinician becomes aware that she has passed her acceptable comfort level, she must communicate to the client what level of emotions she can and cannot respond to within the session.[15,42–46] Communicating one's limits appropriately can result in the client feeling good about himself and understanding the limits for emotional expression and processing within a treatment session. This skill not only involves the clinician knowing ways of phrasing the appropriate information, but also requires that the clinician be aware of when she begins to feel discomfort so that she has time to communicate with the client in a calming and accepting manner. Appropriate communication can help to avoid the interpersonal disconnection that can occur when the clinician suddenly feels overwhelmed and withdraws. This is important because these disconnections can leave the client feeling like there is something wrong about his emotions and can result in negative interpersonal dynamics between the client and clinician that are difficult to resolve.

## Being with Emotional Expression

Ideally, the clinician will allow the client's emotions to arise with acceptance, rather than encouragement or discouragement. An excellent way to communicate this acceptance to the client is through "mirroring"[36] or feeding to the client an empathetic understanding or perception of his present emotional state through verbal statements or physical touch. These strategies include rephrasing or repeating the client's communications, applying massage movements that match the client's expression of his emotions, or respectfully stopping the treatment while the client expresses his emotional state. Regardless of the strategy the clinician uses, she needs to ensure that she matches her response to the state and level of intensity of the client's emotional expression, rather than engaging in the actual content of these emotions.[15,16,42–46] This becomes particularly important when the client is in the middle of an intense emotion because problems may arise when the clinician fails to match the client. For example, if the clinician noticeably lowers the intensity of her engagement when the client is increasing the intensity of his emotions, then the client may feel that his emotional expression is not accepted. If, on the other hand, the clinician noticeably raises the intensity of her engagement beyond the intensity of the client's emotional expression, then the client may feel that he should be expressing something more than he is. With practice, it is possible for the clinician to develop a repertoire of phrases that she can use to ask the client what he needs in these situations. While both the timing and phrasing of these statements will improve with practice, it is important for the novice to attempt these communications, even if somewhat awkwardly, so that the client can have open communication with the clinician.

Emotions generally have an intensity that peaks and then passes, followed by a more reflective period.[11,15,42–46] A general rule of thumb is for clinicians to provide clients with a "space" that is free from large amounts of verbal communication and difficult physical manipulations when they are in the intense phase of emotional expression. Clients often appreciate the invitation, even if they choose not to accept it, to share their experience after the intensity of the emotions has passed. This sharing of emotions can help clients to integrate their experiences in the presence of clinicians' empathetic listening and monitoring.

Finally, clinicians always need to be aware of the appropriate roles of the client–clinician relationship.[11,15,42–46] Although a small amount of sharing by the clinician may help reduce a client's sense of isolation, appropriate sharing is perhaps the most difficult art to master. The biggest danger faced by clinicians is the subtle, or not so subtle, reversal of the client–clinician role. Because sharing by the clinician is not required for empathetic attunement, it is better to err on the side of caution and not share anything too personal. When clinicians find that they have an emotional response to something that arises out of a clinical session, it is important for them to seek an appropriate means of dealing with those feelings such as talking with a supportive colleague, supervisor, or mentor.

## STRATEGIES TO ENHANCE CLIENT ADHERENCE

The client's **adherence** to the plan of care is the final component of the interpersonal aspects of the process of clinical care addressed in this chapter. The literature defines adherence in a variety of ways.[47–66] Responsibility is placed on the client in the definition that adherence is the extent to which clients follow the instructions for care that they negotiate with their health care providers. Adherence can also be viewed as being influenced by the clinician when it is defined as a positive behavior that occurs when a client is motivated by the clinician to adhere to the negotiated plan of care because of a perceived positive outcome or benefit. However it is defined, adherence to the prescribed plan of care is necessary for the attainment of positive outcomes. Several models attempt to identify the factors that influence clients' motivation and adherence. For example, Keller's ARCS[51] model suggests that clients' motivation to participate in health care programs reflects several factors including the extent to which therapists gain their attention, the relevance of the information to them, their confidence in their ability to perform the desired task, and their level of satisfaction with their performance. Based on research, various authors have suggested a variety of strategies for increasing clients' adherence to prescribed plans of care that are outlined in this section and in Box 4-10. These strategies revolve around the client's ability to understand the regimen and follow the directions that were provided, the type of instructions provided by the clinician, and the extent to which the clinician tailors the regimen to the client's needs.

Unfortunately, the types of information that clients are least likely to remember are instructions and advice.[47-66] The more information a client receives, the more he is likely to forget. Clients generally remember what clinicians tell them first and what they consider to be the most important. There is no correlation between the amount of information that is remembered and age or intelligence, although clients with more medical knowledge will recall more information. In addition, a myriad of factors can influence a clients' readiness to learn, such as their age, personality, health beliefs, knowledge about their conditions, understanding of the intents and benefits of treatment, and social factors. Furthermore, moderately anxious clients will recall more information than highly anxious clients or clients who are not anxious.

Adherence decreases when clinicians give unclear instructions; conversely, specific advice may increase adherence.[47-66] For this reason, simple, direct, and repetitive instructions are most effective. For example, "You must do this exercise 10 times when you get out of bed every morning" will be recalled more readily than "Do this exercise several times each day." Furthermore, clients have difficulty complying when they are unclear why the various aspects of the regimen are important, even if the regimen is relatively simple. For example, the addition of the explanation "Putting ice on your ankle and elevating it by putting it up on a chair will help relieve the pain and swelling that you have in your ankle . . ." as a precursor to instructions for the application of ice, may clarify for the client why it would be beneficial to adhere to those instructions.

Modification of the characteristics of the prescribed regimen can increase adherence.[47-66] Since adherence decreases with increasing duration of the episode of care and with increasing complexity of the intervention, clinicians should simplify complex interventions by breaking the plan of care into sequential steps. Furthermore, clients are less likely to adhere to interventions that they perceive as intruding into their daily activities, and the simplest intervention that is compatible with the client's lifestyle is most effective. Consequently, clinicians should also tailor self-care programs to clients' activities and lifestyles. Finally, clients respond positively when clinicians appear to accept that problems arise in integrating a regimen into a client's lifestyle and are available to help the client make modifications.

Clients place a high value on information, although clinicians often underestimate the extent to which they do so.[47-66] Consequently, client education can become an intervention, not merely an adjunct to treatment. When a clinician is using client education as a primary intervention, small groups can be an effective approach. A small group format allows clients to hear information repeated several times and provides opportunities for reinforcing that

---

| Box 4-10 | **Examples of Strategies to Increase Client Adherence** |
|---|---|

- Create a collaborative relationship between the client and the therapist.[47-66]
- Provide clients with information about their disease, the rationale and goals for treatment, and the benefits and risks of treatment.
- Whenever possible, simplify and customize programs.
- Prioritize activities and share this information with clients.
- Evaluate clients' comprehension and ability to perform tasks at intervals.
- Provide cues for remembering information.
- Provide clients with strategies for self-monitoring of their programs.
- Use behavioral contracts and positive reinforcement of clients' successes.
- Involve clients' families and significant others in their care, as appropriate.
- Evaluate the level of client compliance at regular intervals during the episode of care.
- Discuss potential barriers to learning or adherence with the client and assist them in removing those barriers.
- Provide challenges and meaningful opportunities for clients to succeed.
- Keep the material you present to clients stimulating but not overstimulating.
- Use familiar concepts, concrete examples, and familiar language to increase clients' receptiveness to new information.
- Provide clients with ongoing opportunities to apply their newly learned skills.

knowledge. Other clients may ask questions that another client may be hesitant to ask either in a group setting or one-on-one with the clinician. Group participation may also contribute to a sense of community by allowing the client to be with others with similar conditions. Small group sessions can also facilitate the client's proficiency in specific skills that she requires for successful self-management of chronic conditions. If skill acquisition is the primary goal of a small group, then clinicians should spend the majority of the time in the sessions on practice and the provision of feedback to the clients. In this context, breaking clients into pairs to practice skills and to develop action plans can be beneficial.

## References

1. Mitchell A, Cormack M. *The Therapeutic Relationship in Complementary Health Care*. London: Churchill Livingstone; 1998.
2. Donabedian A. Evaluating the quality of medical care. *Milbank Q*. 1966;3:166–206.
3. Bachelor A, Horvath A. The therapeutic relationship. In: Hubble M, Duncan B, Miller S, eds. *The Heart and Soul of Change*. Washington, DC: American Psychological Association; 2005.
4. Hubble M, Duncan B, Miller S, eds. *The Heart and Soul of Change*. Washington, DC: American Psychological Association; 2005.
5. Nelligan P. Client centered care: Making the ideal real. *Hosp Q*. 2002;5:70–76.
6. Fitch P. Intimacy and attachment in massage therapy. *Massage Ther J*. 2005;43:113–121.
7. Dryden T, Fitch P. Recovering body and soul from post-traumatic stress disorder. *Massage Ther J*. 2000;39:41–60.
8. Benjamin B, Sohnen-Moe C. *The Ethics of Touch*. Tucson, AZ: SMA Associates; 2004.
9. The College of Chiropractors of Ontario, College of Massage Therapists of Ontario, College of Physiotherapists of Ontario. *Where's My Line?* Toronto: The College of Chiropractors of Ontario, College of Massage Therapists of Ontario, College of Physiotherapists of Ontario; 2005.
10. Nathan B. *Touch and Emotion in Manual Therapy*. London: Churchill Livingstone; 1999.
11. Updledger J. *Somatoemotional Release and Beyond*. Palm Beach Gardens, FL: UI Publishing; 1990.
12. Lowen A. *Bioenergetics*. New York: Penguin Books; 1976.
13. Peirrakos JC. *Core Energetics*. Mendocino, CA: LifeRhythm; 1987.
14. Reich W. *The Function of the Orgasm*. New York: Orgone Institute Press; 1942.
15. Goring S. Relational characterology and embodiment: an interpersonal interpretation of the characterological and somatic theories of Alexander Lowen and Stephen Johnson. Unpublished Masters Thesis. Northfield, VT: Vermont College of Norwich University; 1994.
16. Rolf IP. *Rolfing: The Integration of Human Structure*. New York: Harper and Row; 1977.
17. McIntosh N. *The Educated Heart*. Memphis: Decatur Bainbridge Press; 2004.
18. Reich W. *Character Analysis*. 3rd ed. New York: Simon and Shuster; 1972.
19. Keleman S. *Emotional Anatomy*. Berkeley, CA: Center Press; 1986.
20. van der Kolk B. The body keeps the score: approaches to the psychobiology of posttraumatic stress disorder. In: van der Kolk B, McFarlane A, Weisaeth L, eds. *Traumatic Stress*. New York: Guilford; 1996.
21. Scaer R. *The Trauma Spectrum: Hidden Wounds and Human Resiliency*. New York: Norton; 2005.
22. Benoit D. Attachment and Regulation Seminar. Ottawa, Ontario: Algonquin College; November 2002.
23. American Psychiatric Association. *Diagnostic Criteria from DSM IV*. Washington, DC: American Psychiatric Association; 1994.
24. Levine P. *Waking the Tiger: Healing Trauma*. Berkeley, CA: North Atlantic Books; 1997.
25. Quality Assurance Committee of the College of Massage Therapists of Ontario. *Code of Ethics and Standards of Practice*. Toronto, Ontario: College of Massage Therapists of Ontario; 1999.
26. American Physical Therapy Association. *Code of Ethics and Guide for Professional Conduct*. Alexandria, VA: American Physical Therapy Association; 2004.
27. Canadian Physiotherapy Association. *The Code of Ethics and Rules of Conduct*. Toronto, Ontario: Canadian Physiotherapy Association; 2005.
28. Commission on Standards. *Occupational Therapy Code of Ethics*. Bethesda, MD: American Occupational Therapy Association; 1994.
29. International Chiropractors Association. *ICA Code of Ethics*. Arlington, VA: International Chiropractors Association; 1985.
30. American Association of Drugless Practitioners. *Code of Ethics*. Gilmer, TX: American Association of Drugless Practitioners; 2007.
31. American Massage Therapy Association. *Code of Ethics for Massage Therapists*. Evanston, IL: American Massage Therapy Association; 2005.
32. Nursing Practice Division. *Code of Ethics for Nurses*. Washington, DC: American Nursing Association; 2001.
33. Canadian Association of Occupational Therapists. *Canadian Framework for Ethical Occupational Therapy Practice*. Ottawa, Ontario: Canadian Association of Occupational Therapists; 2006.
34. Government of Ontario. *Regulated Health Professions Act (Ontario). Procedural Code*. Ottawa, Ontario: Government of Ontario; 1999.
35. Moyer CA, Rounds J, Hannum W. A meta-analysis of massage therapy research. *Psychol Bull*. 2004;130:3–18.
36. Benjamin BE, Sohnen-Moe C. The benefits of supervision programs: peer supervision and clinical supervision groups provide therapists with a safe harbor and forum for professional development. *Massage Ther J*. 2003;41:116–121.
37. Fitch P. Nurturance, intimacy and attachment. *J Soft Tissue Manipulation*. 2004;12:6–9.
38. Polseno D. Ethically speaking. Are you safe? *Massage Ther J*. 2004;43:128,130.
39. Polseno D. Ethically speaking. Enabling: the dark side of being helpful (part one). *Massage Ther J*. 2003;42:136–138.

40. Polseno D. Ethically speaking. Enabling: the dark side of being helpful (part two). *Massage Ther J.* 2003;42:124,126–127.

41. Polseno D. Ethically speaking. Say it ethically: language and terminology (part three). *Massage Ther J.* 2004;43:136,138–139.

42. Wolf E. *Treating the Self: Elements of Clinical Self Psychology.* New York: Guildford Press; 1988.

43. Seam M. *Bodymind Energetics: Towards a Dynamic Model of Health.* Rochester, NY: Healing Arts Press; 1989.

44. Smith E. *The Body in Psychotherapy.* Jefferson, IL: McFarland and Company; 1985.

45. Mindell A. *Dreambody: The Body's Role in Revealing the Self.* Boston: Sigo Press; 1982.

46. Kurtz R. *Body-Centered Psychotherapy: The Hakomi Method.* Mendocino, CA: LifeRhythm; 1990.

47. Hulka B. Patient-clinician interactions and compliance. In: Haynes R, Taylor D, Sackett D, eds. *Compliance in Health Care.* Baltimore: The Johns Hopkins University Press; 1979: 62–77.

48. Claxton AJ, Cramer J, Pierce C. A systematic review of the associations between dose regimens and medication compliance. *Clin Ther.* 2001;23:1296–1310.

49. Sluijs EM. A checklist to assess patient education in physical therapy practice: development and reliability. *Phys Ther.* 1991;71: 561–569.

50. Center for Health Promotion and Education and Centers for Disease Control. *Strategies to Promote Self Management of Chronic Disease.* Atlanta: Center for Health Promotion and Education and Centers for Disease Control; 1982.

51. Visser J, Keller JM. The clinical use of motivational messages: an inquiry into the validity of the ARCS model of motivational design. *Instruct Sci.* 1990;19:437–470.

52. O'Donohue W, Levensky E. *Promoting Treatment Adherence: A Practical Handbook for Health Care Providers.* Thousand Oaks, CA: Sage Publications; 2006.

53. Becker MH. Theoretical models of adherence and strategies for improving adherence. In: Shumaker SA, Schron EB, Ockene JK, eds. *The Handbook of Health Behavior Change.* New York: Springer Publishing Company, Inc; 1990:5–43.

54. O'Brien MK, Petrie K, Raeburn J. Adherence to medication regimens: updating a complex medical issue. *Med Care Rev.* 1992;49: 435–453.

55. Haynes RB. Determinants of compliance: the disease and the mechanics of treatment. In: Haynes RB, Taylor DW, Sackett DL, eds. *Compliance in Health Care.* Baltimore: The Johns Hopkins University Press; 1979:49–61.

56. Meichenbaum D, Turk DC. *Facilitating Treatment Adherence: A Practitioner's Guidebook.* New York: Plenum Press; 1987.

57. Grueninger UJ. Arterial hypertension: lessons from patient education. *Patient Educ Couns.* 1995;26:37–55.

58. Sluijs EM, Kok GJ, van der Zee J. Correlates of exercise compliance in physical therapy. *Phys Ther.* 1993;73:771–782.

59. Donovan JL. Patient decision making: the missing ingredient in compliance research. *Int J Technol Assess Health Care.* 1995;11: 443–455.

60. Davey P, Parker S. Cost effectiveness of once-daily oral antimicrobial therapy. *J Clin Pharmacol.* 1992;32:706–710.

61. Dunbar-Jacob J, Erlen JA, Schlenk EA, Ryan CM, Sereika SM, Doswell WM. Adherence in chronic disease. *Annu Rev Nurs Res.* 2000;18:48–90.

62. Garcia Popa-Lisseanu MG, Greisinger A, Richardson M, O'Malley KJ, Janssen NM, Marcus DM, Tagore J, Suarez-Almazor ME. Determinants of treatment adherence in ethnically diverse, economically disadvantaged patients with rheumatic disease. *J Rheumatol.* 2005;32:913–919.

63. Smith BA, Shuchman M. Problem of nonadherence in chronically ill adolescents: strategies for assessment and intervention. *Curr Opin Pediatr.* 2005;17:613–618.

64. Klareskog L, Lindblad S. How is clinical progress achieved? *Best Pract Res Clin Rheumatol.* 2004;18:1–5.

65. Engstrom LO, Oberg B. Patient adherence in an individualized rehabilitation programme: a clinical follow-up. *Scand J Public Health.* 2005;33:11–18.

66. DiMatteo MR, Giordani PJ, Lepper HS, Croghan TW. Patient adherence and medical treatment outcomes: a meta-analysis. *Med Care.* 2002;40:794–811.

# Chapter 5

# Client Examination for Massage

This chapter reviews selected issues for therapists to consider when conducting a client examination prior to using massage techniques. These topics include the focus of an examination for the use of massage techniques, body structures and functions that are relevant to massage, client reports that arise during the course of history taking that can suggest soft tissue dysfunction, and the use of palpation and nonpalpatory examination techniques. Therapists can integrate this information into a client examination that is appropriate for their scope of practice and their clients' conditions. Numerous clinical texts document client examination techniques for musculoskeletal, neurological, cardiopulmonary, and psychological conditions for the various health care professions. Consequently, this chapter assumes that readers will consult those texts for details on the client examination approach and techniques that are within their scope of practice.

## Client Examination for Massage: Foundations

## FOCUS OF THE CLIENT EXAMINATION FOR MASSAGE

Chapter 3, Clinical Decision Making for Massage, outlined the purpose and steps in the Evaluative Phase of clinical decision making. Conducting a client examination for the use of massage techniques requires more than the addition of a few soft tissue examination techniques to one's customary approach to examination. To be effective, therapists need to expand the focus of their examinations to include the following objectives:

1. Treatment of Impairments Resulting from Medical Conditions
   - Identification of soft tissue dysfunction related to the client's clinical condition

■ Identification of other primary and secondary impairments that therapists can treat with massage techniques

■ Identification of the limitations in the client's level of activity that are associated with the impairments identified in the previous two bulleted items

2. Wellness Interventions

■ Identification of the body structures and functions in the client's wellness goals that therapists can treat with massage techniques

The assessment of soft tissue function and dysfunction can involve the use of tests and measures, such as palpation, that directly assess soft tissue.[1–38] In addition, therapists can extend their interpretation of the findings from standard musculoskeletal, neurological, cardiopulmonary, or psychological measures to include an analysis of how soft tissue dysfunction may be contributing to the client's symptoms. The extent to which therapists will have to modify their customary approach to the client examination will depend on how relevant soft tissue dysfunction is to the client's medical condition. For example, a strong focus on soft tissue dysfunction is less appropriate for the client with a longstanding below-knee amputation and a referral for gait training. By contrast, this focus would be more relevant if the client presents with chronic neck and shoulder pain. Nevertheless, therapists are wise to consider, even briefly, the role of soft tissue dysfunction and potential uses of massage techniques during their client examinations.

# RELEVANT CLINICAL OUTCOMES FOR MASSAGE

In the International Classification of Functioning, Disability and Health model (see Chapter 1), medical conditions result in impairments in body structures and functions.[1,2] These impairments are, in turn, associated with limitations in the client's ability to perform activities. During the client examination, therapists identify and measure the client's impairments. At this point, not all of the impairments will be amenable to treatment with massage techniques. In addition, failure to identify impairments may compromise the effectiveness of the treatment. The task of sorting impairments into those that are or are not amenable to treatment with massage techniques comes later in the treatment planning process. Nevertheless, it is useful to consider whether a reported or observed impairment may involve soft tissue dysfunction. Table 5-1 summarizes some of the impairments that are relevant to the use of massage techniques and gives examples of relevant examination techniques. This chapter discusses the assessment of impairments and functional limitations in preparation for using massage techniques.

| **Table 5-1** | Examples of Outcomes and Examination Techniques for Massage[1–376] | |
|---|---|---|
| **Impairment** | **Outcome** | **Tests and Measures** |
| **Musculoskeletal**<br>■ Adhesions/scarring | ■ Increased tissue mobility<br>■ Decreased scarring | ■ Visual inspection<br>■ Measurement of dimensions<br>■ Palpation<br>■ Ultrasonography<br>■ Magnetic resonance imaging<br>■ Arthroscopy |
| ■ Impaired connective tissue integrity:<br>　■ Fascial restrictions<br>　■ Abnormal connective tissue density<br>　■ Decreased mobility of skin, superficial and deep fascia | ■ Separation and lengthening of fascia<br>■ Promotion of dense connective tissue remodeling<br>■ Increased connective tissue mobility | ■ Visual inspection of static and dynamic postural alignment<br>■ Palpation<br>■ Skin mobility |

*(continued)*

**Table 5-1** continued

| Impairment | Outcome | Tests and Measures |
|---|---|---|
| ■ Impaired joint integrity:<br>　■ Inflammation of joint capsule or ligaments<br>　■ Restrictions of joint capsule and ligaments | ■ Decreased signs of inflammation of joint capsule, tendons, or ligaments<br>■ Decreased capsular and ligament restrictions<br>■ Increased joint mobility<br>■ Increased joint integrity | ■ Palpation<br>■ Selective tissue tension testing<br>■ Ligament stability tests<br>■ Magnetic resonance imaging<br>■ Arthroscopic examination<br>■ Arthrography<br>■ Stress radiography<br>■ Ultrasonography<br>(See measures of impaired joint mobility) |
| ■ Impaired joint mobility:<br>　■ Decreased voluntary range of motion | ■ Increased joint mobility<br>■ Increased voluntary range of motion | ■ Universal goniometer<br>■ Parallelogram goniometer<br>■ Visual estimation of range of motion<br>■ Fingers-to-floor distance<br>■ Schoeber (tape measure) method<br>■ Passive accessory motion testing<br>■ Palpation of end feel on overpressure<br>■ Two-dimensional and three-dimensional computer-aided motion analysis<br>■ Computerized six–degree of freedom electromagnetic tracker<br>■ Self-report range of motion measures<br>■ Cervical range of motion (CROM) instrument<br>■ Single and double inclinometer<br>■ Electrogoniometers<br>■ Pelvic Palpation Meter<br>■ Arthrometer |
| ■ Impaired muscle integrity:<br>　■ Decreased muscle extensibility<br>　■ Muscle strains and tears<br>　■ Tendinopathies<br>　■ Trigger points | ■ Increased muscle extensibility<br>■ Decreased signs of inflammation and promotion of healing of tendons<br>■ Decreased signs of inflammation and promotion of healing of muscle<br>■ Decreased trigger point activity<br>■ Increased joint mobility | ■ Muscle extensibility tests<br>■ Selective tissue tension testing<br>■ Palpation<br>■ Trigger point tests: twitch response, presence of taut bands, patterns of pain referral, electromyography<br>■ Pressure sensitivity testing (pressure algometer)<br>■ Universal goniometer<br>■ Isokinetic dynamometer<br>■ Dynamic ultrasonography |
| ■ Impaired muscle performance (strength, power, endurance) | ■ Enhanced muscle performance secondary to the enhancement of muscle extensibility, reduction of pain, reduction of muscle spasm, enhancement of joint mobility, normalization of joint integrity, reduction of trigger point activity, etc.<br>■ Balance of agonist/antagonist muscle function | ■ Manual muscle testing<br>■ Hand-held dynamometer<br>■ Repeated isotonic motion<br>■ 1-repetition maximum test<br>■ Single-leg hop test<br>■ Myotome testing<br>■ Modified sphygmomanometer<br>■ Pinch meter<br>■ Self-report measures of perceived exertion<br>■ Isokinetic dynamometer<br>■ Isoinertial devices<br>■ Pedaling devices<br>■ Electromyogram<br>■ Kinematic and kinetic gait analysis with two- or three-dimensional computer assisted motion analysis and force analysis |

(*continued*)

**Table 5-1** continued

| Impairment | Outcome | Tests and Measures |
|---|---|---|
| ■ Abnormal muscle resting tension<br>■ Muscle spasm | ■ Decreased muscle spasm<br>■ Normalized muscle resting tension<br>■ Increased joint mobility | ■ Palpation<br>■ Tissue compliance meter<br>■ Continuous electromyogram<br>■ Thermography |
| ■ Postural malalignment | ■ Normalized postural alignment<br>■ Increased postural awareness | ■ Visual inspection of static and dynamic posture<br>■ Postural grid<br>■ Posture Analysis forms<br>■ Universal goniometer<br>■ Plumb line<br>■ Inclinometer<br>■ Tape measure<br>■ Photography<br>■ Kyphometer<br>■ Flexible ruler<br>■ Video image and frame analysis<br>■ Two- or three-dimensional computer-assisted motion analysis<br>■ Three-dimensional electrogoniometers<br>■ X-ray line drawing analysis<br>■ Force platforms<br>■ Functional postural analysis measures |
| ■ Impaired sensation (secondary to entrapment neuropathy or nerve root compression) | ■ Normalized sensation (secondary to the reduction of nerve and nerve root compression due to fascial restrictions and trigger points) | ■ Sensory discrimination (kinesthesia, graphesthesia, stereognosis)<br>■ Vibrometer<br>■ Dermatome testing: light touch, pin prick, temperature<br>■ Filament testing (pressure)<br>■ Palpation of nerve<br>■ Neural tension testing<br>■ Myotome testing<br>■ Electrophysiological (nerve conduction) testing<br>■ Electroneurotomy<br>■ Single-frequency vibrometry tests<br>■ Magnetic resonance imaging |
| ■ Swelling: edema, joint effusion, lymphedema | ■ Increased lymphatic return<br>■ Increased venous return<br>■ Decreased joint effusion<br>■ Decreased edema<br>■ Increased joint integrity<br>■ Increased joint mobility | ■ Visual inspection<br>■ Volumetric analysis<br>■ Girth measurements: tape measure, wire, jeweler's ring<br>■ Palpation<br>■ Multiple-frequency bioelectrical impedance analysis<br>■ Magnetic resonance imaging<br>■ Laser-Doppler flowmetry |
| **Psychoneuroimmunological**<br>■ Stress | ■ Systemic sedation<br>■ Increased perceived relaxation<br>■ Decreased levels of cortisol, epinephrine, and norepinephrine | ■ Interview regarding perceived stress levels and symptoms of stress<br>■ Self-report stress measures<br>■ Galvanic skin response<br>■ Heart rate<br>■ Blood pressure<br>■ Finger pressure<br>■ Blood work: lipid peroxide, prolactin, cortisol, testosterone, glycated hemoglobin<br>■ Salivary cortisol levels |

*(continued)*

**Table 5-1** continued

| Impairment | Outcome | Tests and Measures |
|---|---|---|
| **Multisystem**<br>■ Pain | ■ Pain reduction through primary treatment of dysfunction, e.g., active trigger points<br>■ Counterirritant analgesia<br>■ Systemic sedation resulting in decreased perception of pain | **Pain Behavior**<br>■ Interview regarding location, quality, and behavior of pain<br>■ Pain diagram (used in conjunction with interview)<br>■ Self-report measures of pain intensity and affective component<br>■ Self-report measures of the impact of pain on function<br>■ Palpation<br>■ Pressure sensitivity testing (pressure algometer)<br>■ Selective tissue tension testing<br><br>**Tests and Measures of Pain Syndromes**<br>■ Neural tissue tension tests<br>■ Neural provocation tests<br>■ Trigger point tests: twitch response, presence of taut bands, patterns of pain referral, electromyography<br>■ Dynamic surface electromyography<br>■ Electrophysiological studies<br>■ Thermography |
| **Cardiopulmonary**<br>■ Impaired airway | ■ Increased respiration/gaseous exchange<br>■ Increased airway clearance/mobilization of secretions<br>■ Decreased dyspnea | ■ Interview regarding frequency and effectiveness of cough<br>■ Visual inspection of effectiveness of cough<br>■ Visual inspection of quality and quantity of sputum<br>■ Visual inspection and palpation of respiration rate and pattern<br>■ Auscultation of breath sounds<br>■ Pulse oximetry<br>■ Self-report dyspnea rating scales<br>■ Arterial blood gases<br>■ Pulmonary function tests<br>■ Self-report measures of quality of life<br>■ Standardized measures of self-care |
| ■ Dyspnea | ■ Decreased dyspnea due to increased airway clearance<br>■ Decreased dyspnea due to increased perceived relaxation | ■ Visual inspection of respiratory pattern and effort of breathing<br>■ Self-report perceived exertion and dyspnea rating scales<br>■ Self-report measures of outcome of dyspnea<br>■ 6-minute walk test of functional exercise capacity<br>■ Respiration rate<br>■ Oxygen saturation<br>■ Arterial blood gases<br>■ Capnography |
| ■ Impaired rib cage mobility (other than bony abnormality) | ■ Increased rib cage mobility<br>■ Increased muscle extensibility<br>■ Increased ventilation | ■ Visual inspection and palpation of lateral costal, sternal, and diaphragmatic motion during respiration<br>■ Palpation of rib cage motion during respiration<br>■ Changes in girth of rib cage during respiration |
| **Neurological**<br>■ Abnormal neuromuscular tone: spasticity, rigidity, clonus | ■ Normalized neuro-muscular tone<br>■ Alteration of movement responses through proprioceptive and exteroceptive stimulation techniques<br>■ Balance of agonist/antagonist muscle function | ■ Palpation<br>■ Graded passive range of motion tests, e.g., Ashworth scale<br>■ Quick stretch tests<br>■ Reflexes<br>■ Pendulum test<br>■ Isokinetic dynamometer<br>■ Hand-held dynamometer<br>■ Electromyogram with isokinetic dynamometer<br>■ Electrophysiological testing<br>■ Standardized measures of motor control<br>■ Standardized measures of self-care |

The Wellness Interactions Model guides therapists' examinations of clients who request wellness interventions (see Chapter 1). First, therapists will determine clients' perceived level of wellness and how this relates to their health status. Often, clients who have no medical condition and state that they seek only wellness or relaxation, will present with significant impairments such as anxiety, increased muscle resting tension, postural shortening, muscle weakness, limited range of motion, and pain. If this is the case, therapists may have to explain how these impairments can affect a client's well-being. In this situation, the assessment of impairments and limitations in activity performance may still be relevant. Technically, in a true wellness client, impairments are at a grade zero. When this occurs, therapists still assesses body structures and functions to determine which are amenable to optimized function or to determine when prevention of a potential impairment may be a desired outcome. Furthermore, this examination must also identify the client's current wellness behaviors and any barriers and facilitators to wellness such as social attitudes, available wellness services, education, and the individual's financial status.

## ISSUES IN THE CLIENT HISTORY FOR MASSAGE

Numerous clinical texts detail the nuances of history taking for the various health care professions. During the course of taking the standard client history, therapists can integrate questions to identify **soft tissue dysfunction**. Box 5-1 contains a brief list of issues that may prompt further exploration of a soft tissue lesion.

### ❓ Critical Thinking Question
What specific modifications do therapists need to make to their approach to client examination so that their examination findings will guide their use of massage techniques?

## USING PALPATION IN THE CLIENT EXAMINATION

Skilled **palpation** is an art, a required component of many client examination techniques, and a prerequisite skill for the effective execution of all massage techniques.[3-38] Therapists can use palpation to assess and reassess the client's impairments throughout the client examination and treat-

---

**Box 5-1** | **Issues in a Client History That Suggest Soft Tissue Dysfunction**

- Reports of any longstanding musculoskeletal condition because this may result in chronic soft tissue tightening[4,6,7,9,23-36]
- A history of prolonged infection
- Reports of a change in pain over time from an initially specific, localized pain to a more diffuse, generalized pain
- A history of chronic pain
- A history of pain combined with anxiety or stress
- Idiopathic pain with a complex history of multiple injuries or multiple surgeries because these events that would predispose the client to scarring
- A history of ambiguous symptoms, particularly when motion testing yields inconclusive results and subjective reports of symptoms are vague or ambiguous
- A history of multiple conflicting assessments or multiple ineffective treatments
- A history of a gradual onset of symptoms with a clearly perceived alteration of posture over approximately the same time period
- A history of having a relief of symptoms through massage or stretching
- The reported prior treatments do not include comprehensive treatment of soft tissue lesions; for example, treatment with ultrasound but not frictions for tendinitis
- During history taking, the client refers to the texture of her soft tissue as "tight," "hard," or "wired" and makes a connection between this texture and her symptoms
- A history of bony malalignment such as a leg length discrepancy, scoliosis, or dental malocclusion
- A history of emotional trauma

---

ment process. Furthermore, continuous palpation throughout the application of massage techniques allows therapists to use the client's response to the techniques to guide them in refining the intervention as it proceeds. This is one of the advantages of massage techniques over nonmanual treatment techniques.

There are many ways to perform palpation that are determined by the purpose of palpation, the object of palpation, the client's condition, and the therapist's abilities.[3-38] Regardless of how therapists are performing the palpation, all forms of palpation share common characteristics. During palpation, therapists attempt to identify subtle characteristics of the selected object of palpation and distinguish between normal and abnormal findings. Since palpation is comparative in nature, it involves movement of the contact surface or of therapists' attention. Although the emphasis of this chapter is on the client examination, the comments on palpation are also relevant to the treatment process.

## Basic Principles of Palpation

Palpation is moving inquiry that requires an unhurried, nonabrupt manner and a quiet, listening mind.[3–38] As therapists perform palpation, they seek answers to a variety of questions that inform effective palpation such as: What is this structure or quality? How does this finding differ from other structures or qualities that I have palpated? How does this finding relate to the client's history? How does this structure reflect the client's demonstrated and reported function? After extensive practice, therapists can move from the point at which conscious questioning guides their palpation to a point at which they are more adept at the practice of Intelligent Touch (see Chapter 1).

## Objects of Palpation

Therapists identify the client's impairments through the palpation of specific **objects of palpation**.[3–38] These objects of palpation are the focus of therapists' attention during palpation. They are not necessarily physical objects; instead, they may be a characteristic, such as temperature, or a phenomenon, such as resistance to movement. The nature of the object of palpation influences therapists' choice of method of palpation. For example, it is difficult to palpate skin temperature using deep thumb pressure. In the same way, it is less effective to palpate tissue resistance to barriers in the superficial fascia using a fast scanning palmar contact. Consequently, therapists should specify the object(s) of their inquiry prior to beginning palpation and select a palpation technique that is suited to the object of palpation.

## Contact Surfaces Used for Palpation

Therapists' hands must be supple and relaxed at all times during palpation.[3–38] Since therapists' dominant hands are generally more sensitive, they should use that hand for palpating very subtle objects. As they perform palpation, they may use their hands to do similar things such as comparing left and right sides. Conversely, their hands may perform different tasks, as is the case when one hand moves a body segment and the other evaluates the resulting motion.

Therapists can use virtually any surface to palpate: fingers and thumbs, the whole palmar surface, the thenar and

hypothenar eminences, or the back of their hands.[3–38] They should select a surface that relates to the particular aim of palpation. For example, the finger and thumb tips and pads have the greatest discriminatory ability and are best for palpating subtle objects. On the other hand, grasping forms of palpation may use the index and thumb together like a pincer or the whole hand.

## Force of Palpation

As with massage techniques, therapists should match the force they apply to the tissues during palpation to the task at hand.[3–38] This force can vary in rate, pressure, direction, and duration.

### Rate of Palpation

Therapists can use different rates of palpation to obtain different types of information.[3–38] A scanning or stroking type of palpation moves relatively quickly over a large area. Consequently, therapists use this when they want to collect information from a wide area. An example of this would be comparing bilateral tissue contours or assessing resting muscular tone of the client's entire back. A **scanning, or stroking, palpation** works best when static palpation would distort findings. By contrast, **static palpation** involves no movement of the palpating hand and is best suited for palpating moving phenomena such as pulse or respiratory rhythm.

### Pressure of Palpation

Lack of concentration, too much pressure, and too much movement are among the other common errors of palpation. Therapists should use the minimum pressure required to contact the chosen tissue or structure.[3–38] In doing so, they proceed from exerting a lighter force to a greater force, which results in the palpation of superficial tissue layers prior to deeper layers. Therapists do not need to apply pressure slowly. Nevertheless, therapists' touch should be firm, not tentative or abrupt, regardless of the rate at which they are applying pressure. There will be occasions when therapists need to apply a considerable amount of compression to the client's tissues. In these situations, therapists need to gauge how the clients' compressed tissues are deforming under the controlled application of their body weight. This type of palpation might be better termed "proprioceptive" palpation, as opposed to "manual" palpation, because therapists use their entire body to sense the movement of tissues.

## Direction of Palpation

Therapists can apply the **force of palpation** as a **shearing** force perpendicular to or parallel to the client's tissues.[3–38] Different directions of force will result in different responses of the client's tissues.

When the force of palpation is perpendicular to the client's tissues, it will produce a vertical compression. This form of palpation has several uses. For example, therapists can use perpendicular forces to palpate a pulse or pitting edema. They can also use them when measuring the sensitivity of a trigger point.

Tension along a tissue layer and **drag** occur when therapists apply the force of palpation in a direction that is parallel to the client's tissues (horizontal force).[3–38] Drag is a term used to describe both the therapist's palpation and the tissue layer's resistance to lengthening in response to that force. External and internal factors can result in an increase or decrease of the amount of drag that occurs during palpation. External factors include the presence of moisture on the skin, which can increase or decrease drag, and the presence of skin oil or lubricant, which can generally decrease it. Internal factors include tissue dystrophy. The assessment of drag is an integral part of therapists' examination of connective tissues such as skin and fascia.

Therapists can also use palpation to exert a shearing force on the client's tissues.[3–38] Shear involves adjacent, parallel tissue layers sliding over one another and displacing adjacent laminar elements. When drag is applied to a specific tissue layer, shear occurs between that layer and the layer that is adjacent and parallel to it. Therapists can use shearing forces, in combination with compression, when assessing muscle tone and bulk.

In practice, any palpation technique or massage technique combines elements of compression, drag, and shear.[3–38] In general, the direction of the force that therapists apply during the palpation of a particular tissue is often the same as the direction that they would use to treat that tissue.

## Duration of Palpation

Although therapists should not hurry palpation, their palpation of most objects need not take longer than a few seconds.[3–38] Indeed, the effects of prolonged palpation on tissues can confound the client examination. This occurs because maintaining a position or pressure can result in the adaptation of tissue receptors in the therapists' hands. In addition, it can also produce changes in the client's tissues. For example, when palpating a myofascial trigger point located in a deep layer, sustained pressure would have the same effect as the specific compression technique used for treatment of this condition. The palpation of barriers in connective tissue is an exception to this rule because it requires longer than a minute as a result of the biochemical nature of the tissue. In this situation, palpation will merge into treatment.

# Integration of Information from Other Senses

Effective palpation is the result of appropriate interplay of therapists' senses.[3–38] For example, therapists' vision may be useful in corroborating some of the findings of palpation such as posttraumatic swelling. Visual inspection may, however, interfere with therapists' ability to palpate more subtle objects such as the small intrinsic movements of connective tissue under traction.

# Assessing Objects of Palpation

Therapists need to match palpation techniques to the object of palpation. The following are examples of objects of palpation and appropriate palpation techniques.

## Temperature

The palpation of temperature can provide information about the status of inflammation, circulation, and organ function.[3–38] There are several approaches to palpating temperature. In one method, therapists place the back of their hands in direct contact with the client's skin. The pressure used for this method must be very light; otherwise, vasodilatation will occur and confound the findings. Another method is to use the palm of the dominant hand to scan approximately 4 inches (10 cm) off the surface of the client's body. In this technique, the motion of the therapist's hands must be continuous to avoid vasodilatation, insulation, and reradiation effects.

## Contour and Bulk

Contour and bulk refer to the gross shape and size of the client's body. Therapists can best examine these characteristics with a relatively fast-moving scanning palpation using a large contact surface such as the entire palmar surface of their hand.[3–38] Therapists should correlate the information they obtain from their palpation of contour and bulk with the findings from their visual inspection of the client's body.

## Texture and Consistency

Texture and consistency refer to variations in the density of tissues, regardless of the depth of the layer in which the tissues occur.[3-38] In other words, they describe the density of superficial tissues, such as the skin, or deeper tissues, such as the hamstring attachment to the ischial tuberosity.

There are two categories of tissue texture that are important because they reflect the presence of inflammation.[3-38] The first is acute inflammation, which generally produces different degrees of tissue softness that reflect the presence of extravasated fluid in the tissues. The terms "distended," "spongy," or "boggy" describe this texture. The second is chronic inflammation, which typically produces varying degrees of tissue "hardness" as a result of the deposit of collagen into the tissues. Some descriptors for the tissue "hardness" associated with chronic inflammation are "indurated," "ropy," and "stringy."

## Fluid Status

Therapists can use palpation to measure turgidity, which is fluid pressure or fluid tension.[3-38] Fluid tests, such as the ballottement test, involve the use of large contact surfaces to palpate excess fluid and push it from one place to another. These tests enable therapists to gauge the amount of excess fluid in an area and the pressure of the fluid. They can also assess whether the fluid is located in the intra- or extra-articular space, that is, whether it is an edema or an effusion. Finally, therapists can use sustained digital compression to determine whether "pitting" is present.

Viscosity refers to the "thickness" or "stickiness" of semi-liquid materials.[3-38] Therapists can assess viscosity using palpation. This is valuable because muscle and connective tissue commonly become less viscous in response to interventions such as the local application of neuro-muscular or connective tissue massage techniques or heat.

## Palpating Soft Tissue Layers ("Layer Palpation")

Traditionally, the term **soft tissue** describes any tissue that is not bone or articular surface.[9,16,25,26] More specifically, soft tissue includes the **epithelium**, the **connective tissues**, and the **contractile tissues**. Therapists frequently encounter a succession of layers of tissue that are oriented from surface to deep as they palpate clients' bodies. In doing so, they can use differences between the characteristics of these layers, such as hardness, density, texture, and mobility, to distinguish between tissue layers.

There are several distinct tissue layers.[9,16,25,26] The epithelium consists of closely packed columnar or squamous cells that have little intercellular material between them. Connective tissue consists of several different types of cells, such as fibroblasts and fat cells, and elastin and collagen fibers embedded in a matrix of gelatinous material, the consistency of which varies in response to many factors. Nerves, blood vessels, and lymph vessels lie in the connective tissue. Contractile tissue is comprised of muscle, its enveloping fascial layers, its associated tendon(s), and its periosteal attachments.

As Figure 5-1 shows, the skin consists of a layer of epithelium, the epidermis, and the dermis, which is the first layer of connective tissue.[9,16,25,26] Deep to the skin lies the **superficial fascia**, which houses fat and water, provides a path for nerves and vessels, and sometimes contains striated muscle that controls the movement of the skin. The investing layer of the **deep fascia** is dense connective tissue that lies between the superficial fascia and muscle. The investing layer of the deep fascia is continuous with the superficial fascia and the deep fascia that lie between muscle fibers. The primary functions of the deep fascia are to allow muscles to move freely, to carry nerve and blood vessels, to fill the space between muscles, and to provide an origin for muscles. For example, aponeuroses, retinacula, and interosseous membranes are all deep fascia. The deep fascia around muscle is continuous with the periosteum. In areas in which there is no muscle, the investing layer of the deep fascia is continuous with the periosteum. Finally, connective tissue exists in synovial joints; for example, the synovial membrane and the extrinsic ligaments are modified connective tissue.

## Skin

Therapists should use minimal force and note the following characteristics as they palpate clients' skin.[4,8,9,16,24-26] First, there are normal variations in skin thickness, for example, the thickness of the sole versus the dorsum of the foot. Second, skin has elastic rebound that varies with age. Third, there are variations in the tightness of the attachment of the skin, for example, the tightness of the attachment of the skin of the elbow versus the skin of the scalp. Therapists can also assess the level of moisture on the skin surface and the hydration of the skin itself because these may reflect a client's circulatory, trophic, or nutritional status. Finally, therapists may also be able to distinguish between the epidermis and the dermis by using gentle horizontal drag at the very surface of the skin.

Therapists can assess segmental or nerve root dysfunction and imbalance of visceral function by noting

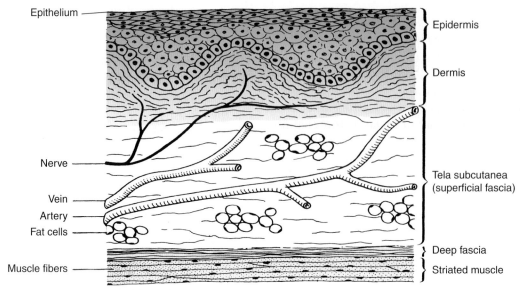

**Figure 5-1** Skin layers. (From Thomson JS. *Core Textbook of Anatomy.* Philadelphia: J. B. Lippincott Company; 1977:15. Used with permission of Lippincott Williams & Wilkins.)

whether there is tightness or resistance during the following sequence of movements[4,8,9,16,24–26]:

1. Stretch the skin horizontally in one direction at a time without gliding or engaging underlying issues.
2. Let the skin recoil.
3. Stretch the skin, and sustain this position at the barrier.
4. Note how soon the skin begins to elongate.

### Superficial Fascia

Therapists can engage the superficial fascia and the fat deposits it contains by increasing the compressive force they apply.[4,8,9,16,24–26] They can try to gauge the "turgor," or fluid pressure, of the tissues since edema often deposits into this tissue layer. They can also estimate the thickness of the superficial fascial layer by comparing different regions. The mobility tests outlined in Steps 1 to 4 above are also appropriate for assessing the superficial fascia. In addition, therapists can test the mobility of the superficial fascia by folding it or by lifting and rolling it over the surface of the underlying tissues. See Skin Rolling in Chapter 10, Connective Tissue Techniques. Therapists should compare the results they obtain for superficial fascia with those they obtained for the skin.

### The Investing Layer of the Deep Fascia

The investing layer of the deep fascia is smooth, firm, and continuous and lies between the superficial fascia and muscle.[4,8,9,16,24–26] Consequently, therapists may need practice to locate it precisely. The client examination procedure for connective tissue massage includes the assessment of the investing layer of the deep fascia. Therapists use techniques similar to those for the more superficial layers, described earlier, to assess the mobility of this connective tissue layer. The difference between these two approaches is that assessing the investing layer of the deep fascia requires more refined palpation skills because there is more intervening tissue. Tissue restrictions identified by therapists will often correlate with the restrictions that they find in the more superficial layers. These restrictions may indicate underlying muscle tension, segmental dysfunction, or visceral imbalance.

### Muscle

Therapists assess resting muscle tension during palpation by noting a muscle's response to the compressive and shearing forces that they deliver with their finger(s) or hands.[4,8,9,16,24–26] During palpation, their hand(s) may compress the whole muscle or bow it. They can also slowly enter the muscle tissue and tease its fibers apart using their fingers or thumbs. The higher the resting level of tone, the denser and harder the tissue will be on palpation. Increases and decreases in muscle resting tension are relative states because degrees of tone vary greatly from one person to another and between one segment of an individual's body and another. Spasm is more dramatic and, thus, more readily distinguished by therapists. Elevated resting tone can result from a wide variety of clinical conditions, including injury, degenerative diseases, and stress.

In addition to assessing muscle resting tension during the palpation of muscle, therapists can note whether high turgor (fluid distention) is present since this can indicate a postexercise condition or an inflammatory condition.[4,8,9,16,24–26]

### Periosteum

This tissue layer is only accessible to palpation in areas where there is no overlying muscle.[4,8,9,16,24–26] Therapists can use compressive fingertip force to palpate the thin, dense, spongy layer superimposed on the hardness of the underlying bone.

## Critical Thinking Question

What palpation techniques do therapists use to assess each of the soft tissue layers? Copy Figure 5-1, and label it with the relevant palpation techniques.

### *Tissue Mobility and Restrictive Barriers*

#### Normal Soft Tissue Range of Motion

Soft tissues have an available range of motion that is comparable to the range of motion available in joints.[4,8,9,16,24–26] Within this range of motion, normal soft tissue has three barriers, or resistances, that can limit movement (Figure 5-2). Therapists are "engaging" these tissue barriers at the point when they palpate a resistance to tissue motion. The physiological barrier (Ph) is the resistance that determines the range of motion that is available under normal conditions. In other word, the tissue's range of motion lies between the two physiological barriers, with the least amount of resistance being apparent at the midrange (M). The elastic barrier (E) is the resistance that therapists feel at the end of the passive range of motion when they have taken the "slack" out of or "engaging" the tissue. The anatomical barrier (A) is the final resistance to normal range of motion that the bone, ligament, or soft tissue can provide. Motion beyond the anatomical barrier results in tissue damage.

#### Restrictive Barriers

**Restrictive, or pathological, barriers in soft tissue** occur when soft tissue dysfunction is present.[4,8,9,16,24–26] Restrictive barriers may occur in skin, fascia, muscle, ligament, joint cap-

sule, or a combination of these tissues. They can be located anywhere between the normal physiological barriers, can limit the available range of motion within the tissues, and can alter the position of the midrange. Furthermore, the presence of a restrictive barrier will change the quality of the movement and the "feel" at the end of the tissue range of motion. This is similar to the abnormal end feels therapists observe in joints. An example of a restrictive barrier (R) and its impact on the position of the midrange (M2) appears in Figure 5-3.

#### Barrier-Release Phenomenon

Therapists engage the tissue barrier at the point at which therapists palpate a resistance to tissue motion.[4,8,9,16,24–26] If therapists sustain the pressure on the tissue barrier, a "release" may occur after a latency period that will vary with the nature of the tissue and its state of health. This release results in a reduction of the resistance that will enable therapists to move the tissue beyond the location of the original barrier without increasing the pressure of palpation. This phenomenon is called the **barrier-release phenomenon**.

Different types of tissue will respond differently to sustained pressure.[4,8,9,16,24–26] For example, connective tissue is most responsive to sustained pressure and will demonstrate a slow, palpable stretch of tissues called creep or viscoelastic creep. This stretch occurs beyond the elastic barrier (E) shown in Figure 5-3. In the case of pathological or restrictive barriers, this release can last for up to 30 seconds or longer and can result in normalized tissue mobility and pain reduction. Since connective tissue forms a portion of all soft tissues, some creep will be evident in all soft tissues in proportion to the amount of connective tissue that is present in that tissue.

Therapists can observe the barrier-release phenomenon during their application of horizontal drag, vertical compression, or shear forces to the tissues using either small or large contact surfaces.[4,8,9,16,24–26] Consequently, they can use palpation to identify the feel at the end of the available range of motion of tissue using a variety of palpation techniques including digital compression or a palmar drag on the superficial fascia. The barrier-release phenomenon is

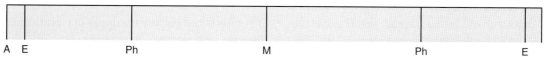

**Figure 5-2** Normal tissue barriers. A, anatomical barrier; E, elastic barrier; Ph, physiological barrier; M, midrange. (Reprinted with adaptations from Greenman PE. *Principles of Manual Medicine.* 2nd ed. Philadelphia: Lippincott Williams & Wilkins; 1996:43. Used with permission of Lippincott Williams & Wilkins.)

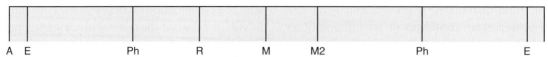

**Figure 5-3** Restrictive tissue barriers. A, anatomical barrier; E, elastic barrier; Ph, physiological barrier; R, restrictive barrier; M, midrange; M2, pathological midrange. (Reprinted with adaptations from Greenman PE. *Principles of Manual Medicine.* 2nd ed. Philadelphia: Lippincott Williams & Wilkins; 1996:43. Used with permission of Lippincott Williams & Wilkins.)

most useful when palpating connective tissue, but therapists can also apply it to any tissue or structure.

### Palpation of Tissue Mobility

Therapists can apply a compression or drag force, or a combination of the two, to a given tissue or structure within a client's body and observe the resulting movement.[4,8,9,16,24–26] In doing so, they can observe whether the normal range of motion is present in the tissues or whether restrictive barriers exist. If therapists palpate a restrictive barrier, they must note the available range of motion in the tissues, the quality of movement through the range of motion, and the feel of the point at which they engage the restrictive barrier.

### Critical Thinking Question

What are the similarities and differences between the range of motion available in joints and the range of motion of soft tissue?

### *Anatomical Structures*

The ability to palpate anatomical structures systematically is an absolute prerequisite for therapists who use massage.[3–38] This is the case because this ability has a direct impact on the accuracy of the therapists' examination using palpation, the effectiveness of the massage techniques they perform, and whether the client achieves treatment outcomes. The palpation of anatomical structures, detailed in comprehensive texts on this topic, involves the ability to discriminate between tissue types and to distinguish a structure from its surrounding structures with accuracy. Through palpation, therapists can identify bone, joint space (joint line), ligament, tendon (including junctions to both periosteum and to muscle), aponeurosis, fascia (septae, sheathes, retinacula), nerves, vessels, and viscera. Each anatomical structure has a characteristic "feel," which stems from its structure and histology. Therapists need to use compressive contact when they palpate anatomical structures. They also need to

select contact surfaces and levels of pressure for palpation based on the structure that they are palpating.

### *Body Rhythms*

Therapists assess **pulses** and **respiratory rhythms** using static palpation with minimal to moderate compression and a contact surface of appropriate size.[3–38] The amount of force they apply during the palpation of pulses is important because the use of excessive compression can result in inaccurate findings. Therapists assess pulses using a single hand. By contrast, they can use two hands, placed on opposite sides of the ribcage, to produce a three-dimensional test when they are palpating respiratory rhythms. Therapists can palpate both pulse and respiration at a distance to the site, although this technique sometimes confuses novices. Therapists with advanced skills or specialized training can palpate more subtle pulsations of inherent tissue motions using a broad-contact static palpation.

### *Tremors and Fasciculations*

**Fasciculations** are localized, subconscious muscle contractions.[3–38] They do not involve the entire muscle because they result from the contraction of the muscle cells innervated by a single motor axon. **Tremors**, by contrast, are rhythmic movements of a joint that result from involuntary contractions of antagonist and agonist muscle groups. Therapists can palpate both tremors and fasciculations statically with minimal to moderate compression and contact surfaces of varying sizes.

### *Vibration*

Therapists can palpate two types of vibration: **crepitus** and **fremitus**.[3–38] Crepitus is a vibration of variable fineness that is associated with a roughened gliding surface of a tendon, a tendon sheath, or the articulating surfaces of a joint. Therapists can sometimes hear crepitus, in addition to palpating it. Fremitus is another palpable vibration. Therapists can palpate this pulmonary vibration over the ribcage as the client speaks or vocalizes.

## Client's Response to Palpation

Therapists must observe and interpret the different verbal and physiological responses that palpation can evoke in a client.[3–38] **Local reflex signs** include discoloration of the skin (blanching or flushing) or more general autonomic responses such as sweating and nausea. Neuromuscular responses include twitching, spasm, or clonus. Clients may indicate that they are experiencing pain by grimacing, vocalizing, or making sudden involuntary movements.

Therapists must remember that pain is a common response to palpation, which they need to respect and observe carefully. Therapists can also quantify pain with, for example, a 4-point rating scale for grading tenderness or visual analog scales. The various types of pain responses differ in their significance and reliability. Tenderness to deep palpation, for example, is an unreliable finding since tenderness can be referred from other sites. Pain on percussion may have specific meaning for certain musculoskeletal conditions. Finally, during palpation, therapists need to be aware that palpation itself can sometimes produce negative or positive changes in the tissues they are palpating.

In summary, Box 5-2 outlines some of the body structures and functions that therapists assess using palpation.

---

| Box 5-2 | **Selected Impairments Evaluated through Palpation** |
|---|---|

- Abnormal connective tissue density[3–38]
- Abnormal levels of resting muscle tension
- Abnormal neuromuscular tone
- Adhesions
- Impaired extensibility of contractile and noncontractile tissues
- Impaired integrity of contractile and noncontractile tissues
- Decreased rib cage mobility
- Fascial restrictions
- Muscle spasm
- Pain
- Scarring
- Swelling: edema, effusion, lymphedema
- Trigger points

---

### Critical Thinking Question

What are the common "objects of palpation"? Which palpation techniques and types of force of palpation do therapists use to assess these objects of palpation?

# MUSCULOSKELETAL EXAMINATION

## Adhesions and Scarring

### *Definitions and Etiology*

#### Scar

A **scar** is the fibrous tissue that replaces normal tissues that a burn, wound, surgery, radiation, or disease has destroyed.[39]

#### Adhesions

Like scars, **adhesions** result from the replacement of normal tissue with connective tissue after a burn, wound, surgery, radiation, or disease destroys the original tissues.[3–39] Adhesions may be fibrous or fibrinous. Fibrinous adhesions have fine bands of fibrin that form as a result of an exudate of plasma or lymph or an extravasation of blood. Fibrous adhesions come from the organization of fibrinous adhesions into fibrous strands. Unlike scarring, adhesions are characterized by a loss of mobility of tissues that normally glide or move in relation to each other. Adhesions can contribute to impaired muscle, joint, and connective tissue integrity, which is described in detail in other sections of this chapter.

### *Overview of Examination Techniques*

Adhesions are of greater clinical significance than scars since they are associated with impaired tissue mobility.[3–38] The measurement of adhesions through observation and palpation is, unfortunately, less accurate than that of scars. Therapists can confirm the presence of scar through visual inspection, an important component to include in the measurement of scars since many clients forget scars. Ultrasonography, magnetic resonance imaging, and arthroscopy are more accurate, although clinically less practical, approaches. Therapists with training in visceral manipulation can perform more detailed examinations of visceral adhesions.

---

**Theory in Practice 5-1**

### Steps in Performing Palpation of Scarring

1. Position the patient so that the scar is not in a stretched position and is readily accessible to you.[3-38]

2. Prior to initiating palpation, explain the purpose and procedures of palpation to the patient. In particular, instruct the patient to tell you when she feels any discomfort. In doing so, inform her that you will cease applying pressure as soon as she indicates discomfort, so that she does not experience undue discomfort. This is especially important if the patient has reported that the scar is painful.

3. Begin palpation using a light pressure. Then, gradually increase the depth of palpation.

4. Assess whether the scar tissue moves as freely as the surrounding tissues. As you palpate the scar, identify differences in the mobility of different areas of the scar tissue. In addition, note areas in which the scar appears to be adherent to adjacent or deeper tissues. Document this information using the positions of a clock, for example, 3:00 (with 12:00 being in the cephalad direction).

5. During palpation, ask the patient to report when she experiences pain at the site of the scar or elsewhere during palpation. Movement of the scar should be pain free.

6. Identify areas of the scar that are puckered, and document this information.

7. Adjuncts to palpation used to assess changes in the dimensions of scars include the measurement of the depth of the scar using a ruler and photography. Follow your facility's guidelines for obtaining the patient's written permission for photographs.

---

## Connective Tissue Integrity

### Definitions and Etiology

#### Fascial Restrictions

**Fascial restrictions** are the adhesion of one fascial layer to another with the associated development of elasto-collagenous cross-links and loss of fluid consistency of fascial ground substance.[25,37-56] Fascial restrictions may be caused by trauma, adhesion, inflammatory or infectious processes, osseous restrictions, chronic fascial compartment syndromes, neurological or circulatory compression syndromes, or postural malalignment such as leg length discrepancy, pelvic malalignment, and dental malocclusion. Finally, fascial restrictions may cause pain, impaired motion, and general dysfunction throughout the body. These symptoms may occur at a distance from the restriction and may result in impaired cellular metabolism, nutrition, elimination, respiration, or lymphatic flow.

#### Abnormal Connective Tissue Density

**Abnormal connective tissue density** is irregular connective tissue remodeling that occurs during the consolidation and maturation stages of connective tissue healing.[25,37-56] This can be associated with chronic orthopedic injuries, including strains, fractures, and repetitive strain injuries, such as tendinitis, tenosynovitis, bursitis, and plantar fasciitis, in which there is ongoing microtrauma, low-grade inflammation, and tissue remodeling.

### Overview of Examination Techniques

Techniques for evaluating connective tissue impairments include visual inspection of the client's static and dynamic postural alignment; palpation of tissue, skin mobility, and vasomotor response; and assessment of craniosacral rhythm characteristics.[3-56] Therapists need to evaluate the client's entire body, regardless of the client's complaint, because imbalances in the fascial system can have significant effects at locations other than the site of the restriction.

## Posture

### Definitions and Etiology

#### Posture

**Posture** is the positioning and alignment of the skeleton and associated soft tissues in relation to gravity, the body's center of mass, and the body's base of support.[6,27-30,39,57-71]

#### Postural Malalignment

**Postural malalignment** is abnormal joint alignment or deformity within a bone.[6,27-30,39,57-71] Since all tissue growth and repair can be influenced by mechanical loading and body posture, postural malalignment can contribute to the development of neurovascular and musculoskeletal dysfunction. This contribution can be direct or as a result of the compensatory motions or postures that can accompany postural malalignment. For example, chronic placement of the head anterior to the body's center of gravity is a common postural malalignment that is associated with neurological and musculoskeletal dysfunction.

## Overview of Examination Techniques

Soft tissues exert a stress on bony structures; consequently, pathological changes in the tension of muscles and connective tissue can affect bony alignment.[6,27–30,39,57–71] The purpose of the postural analysis is, therefore, to document both soft tissue and bony structure and alignment. This information provides objective data that therapists can use to corroborate or refute findings from other examination techniques and the client's functional limitations. This will assist in the identification of appropriate outcomes (Box 5-3).

Visual inspection of the symmetry of bony landmarks, muscle contours, and other tissues with the client in static postures, such as sitting, standing, or lying, is the common clinical approach to assessing postural alignment.[6,27–30,39,57–71] Visual inspection of dynamic posture is of greater importance in the assessment of fascial restrictions. The technique of visual inspection can be refined through the use of postural grids, photography, and various posture analysis forms such as the Portland State University Posture Analysis Form. In addition, therapists can obtain information on the client's postural awareness during the client interview.

Goniometry, plumb lines, inclinometers, tape measures, and video image and frame analysis are among the tools that are available for quantifying postural malalignment.[6,27–30,39,57–71] For example, sagittal plane postural alignment of the head and shoulder in relationship to the lateral malleolus can be measured using a carpenter's tri-square with a line level attached to the horizontal arm and a goniometer with a line level attached to the horizontal arm.

More sophisticated measures of postural alignment include three-dimensional electrogoniometers, such as the Metrecom Skeletal Analysis System; a force platform; X-ray line drawing analysis for sagittal plane spinal displacement; and visual estimation of lumbar lordosis from radiographs (which can be inaccurate and unreliable).[6,27–30,39,57–71] Dynamic postural analysis can be performed using three-dimensional computer-assisted motion analysis, with or without electromyography. Finally, postural alignment during functional activity can be assessed using measures such as the Ovako Working Analysis System.

---

**Box 5-3** | **Incorporating Postural Data into Outcomes**

**Subjective Findings:** Client reports pain after performing keyboarding tasks for 5 minutes.

**Objective Findings:** Client has an anterior head posture; ear lobe is 2.5 cm anterior to the acromion.

**Analysis:** Client's anterior head position is biomechanically inefficient, decreases her endurance in performing keyboarding tasks, and contributes to her pain as a result of excessive loading of the posterior cervical and shoulder musculature. Correction of the soft tissue restrictions that contribute to this posture may reduce the client's complaints of pain and facilitate enhanced alignment of head and cervical spine, biomechanical efficiency, and work tolerance.

**Functional Outcome:** Client will be able to perform keyboarding tasks with the ear lobe in vertical alignment over the acromion for 30 continuous minutes without complaints of pain.

---

**Theory in Practice 5-2**

### Using Visual Postural Analysis

**Practitioner's Position for the Postural Analysis**

Anterior view: The practitioner stands directly in front of the patient at a distance of approximately 5–8 feet, with the patient in standing or sitting.[6,27–30,39,57–71] If the patient is in supine, the practitioner stands at the foot of the treatment table. Standing on a stool may offer a clearer view.

Posterior view: The practitioner stands directly behind the patient at a distance of approximately 5–8 feet, with the patient in standing or sitting. If the patient is prone, the practitioner stands at the foot of the treatment table (standing on a stool may offer a clearer view).

Lateral view: The practitioner positions himself to the side of the patient in alignment with the patient's external auditory meatus for the examination of the lateral view with the patient in standing or sitting. If the patient is in side lying, the practitioner is positioned at the side of the treatment table (standing on a stool may offer a clearer view). Standing at the side of the treatment table may provide a less obstructed view of the patient's upper body, compared with the anterior view, if the patient has a large abdomen or considerable amounts of pectoral or breast tissue.

**Patient's Position for the Postural Analysis**

Observation of the patient from different views and in different positions can provide the practitioner with a greater understanding of the patient's postural alignment. For example, a patient whose postural alignment differs in standing versus supine may have a pelvic malalignment, a leg length discrepancy, muscular weakness, or an impaired postural awareness. In addition, the practitioner can also identify whether the patient has a pelvic malalignment or a leg length discrepancy by comparing the patient's postural alignment in sitting and standing. If the patient is non-ambulatory, the practitioner may use sitting and supine for this purpose.

### Steps in Performing a Postural Analysis

1. Ask the patient to remove her shoes and don clothing or a gown that allows the therapist to view landmarks, while ensuring appropriate draping.
2. Select a view to assess, for example the anterior view, and identify the appropriate position for doing so.
3. Position the posture grid or plumb line.
4. Position the patient in relation to the posture grid or plumb line so that the selected view of the patient is unobstructed and the posture grid or plumb line provides an appropriate frame of reference.
5. Ask the patient to assume a relaxed posture, rather than what she thinks is "good" posture. Allow the patient to settle into that position for a minute to get a more accurate representation of her usual posture. If this is painful, then decrease the amount of time the patient spends in this position.
6. Assume the appropriate position from which to observe the landmarks for the selected view.
7. Perform the visual inspection of the selected view, identifying the positions of the landmarks listed in Landmarks for Visual Postural Analysis and noting the symmetry of body contours and muscle bulk throughout the patient's body. Ensure that you perform a bilateral comparison wherever this is appropriate.
8. Confirm or refute the findings of visual analysis with palpation.
9. Document the findings of visual analysis.
10. Note findings that will be an indication for further patient examination using other tests and measures.
11. Reposition the patient for the next view in the assessment.

### Landmarks for Visual Postural Analysis

#### Anterior View

Head and Neck
1. Orientation of the end of the nose with the manubrium, xiphoid process, and umbilicus (the umbilicus is often not in vertical alignment with these other landmarks)
2. Vertical alignment of the head, for example, excessive lateral flexion or rotation
3. Level of the eyes
4. Vertical alignment of the jaw
5. Contours of trapezius muscle

Upper Extremities
1. Carrying angle of elbows (5–15 degrees is the normal range of the carrying angle for an elbow)
2. Levels of hands (used in identifying asymmetrical shoulder levels)
3. Direction of palms (used in identifying asymmetrical shoulder rotation)

Trunk
1. Trunk in vertical alignment: note asymmetry of skin folds or the distances of the patient's arms to her trunk
2. Level of acromioclavicular joints
3. Level and length of clavicles
4. Sternum and costocartilage aligned: note superior, inferior, or lateral deviations of these landmarks
5. Ribs aligned and symmetrical bilaterally
6. Differences in weight bearing on the lower extremities as reflected by the position of the trunk over the extremities

Lower Extremities and Pelvis
1. Levels of the anterior superior iliac spines
2. Torsion of the tibia or femurs
3. Orientation of the knees, for example, varus or valgus
4. Orientation of the patellae
5. Levels of the fibular heads
6. Levels of lateral malleoli
7. Levels of the medial malleoli
8. Foot angle (10 degrees of external rotation or toeing out is normal)
9. Orientation of the arches of the feet, for example, neutral, pronated, supinated, pes cavus, or pes planus with the feet in their usual posture and then with the great toes aligned; if the patient wears orthotics, it may be appropriate to observe foot position with the patient's shoes on.

#### Lateral View

1. Deviation from an imaginary vertical line running through the following landmarks: ear lobe through the bodies of the cervical vertebrae, through the acromion process, through the lumbar vertebrae, through the highest point of the iliac crest, through the hip joint, anterior to the knee joint, and anterior to the ankle joint
2. Position of the glenohumeral joint
3. Position of the sternum: note if it is overly prominent or depressed
4. Tilt of the pelvis
5. Alignment of the knees: note recurvatum or excessive flexion

*Posterior View*

Head and Neck
1. Vertical alignment of the head

Upper Extremities
1. Level of the shoulders

Trunk
1. Levels and alignment of the spines and inferior angles of the scapulae (the scapulae should rest on the thorax between the levels of T2 and T8; note whether the scapulae are abducted, adducted, elevated, or depressed)
2. Position of the scapulae against the thorax: note if they are winging
3. Distance of the vertebral borders of scapulae from the thoracic vertebrae
4. Vertical alignment of the spine: note any lateral curvature
5. Distance between the twelfth rib and the iliac crest

Lower Extremities and Pelvis
1. Level of the iliac crests
2. Level of the posterior superior iliac spines
3. Levels of the gluteal folds
4. Levels of the knee joints
5. Angle of Achilles tendons (should be vertical)
6. Position of hindfoot with the feet in their usual posture and then with the great toes aligned. If the patient wears orthotics, it may be appropriate to observe foot position with the patient's shoes on. Note whether the hindfoot is in varus or valgus.

**Note**

Pelvic malalignment or a small hemipelvis can present as changes in thoracic alignment in sitting. In addition, consider a more detailed examination of pelvic misalignment if the patient's anterior superior iliac spines or posterior superior iliac spines are asymmetrical. Therapists can refer to other sources for detailed guidelines on the examination of pelvic alignment.

# PSYCHONEUROIMMUNO-LOGICAL EXAMINATION

## Stress

### *Definitions and Etiology*

#### Chronic Stress

**Chronic stress** is a prolonged and heightened state of arousal that has negative physiological and psychological consequences.[72–112] Chronic stress responses occur over the cog-

nitive, physiological, affective, or behavioral domains and may have consequences such as impaired cognitive function, depression, anxiety, muscle tension, and impaired social functioning.

#### Stress Response

**Stress response** is the individual's cognitive, physiological, affective, or behavioral response to the stressor or stress-provoking situation.[72–112]

#### Cognitive Transactional Model of Stress

The **Cognitive Transactional Model of Stress** views stress as the condition that results when a person's interactions with his environment leads him to perceive a discrepancy, whether real or not, between the demands of the situation and the resources of his biological, psychological, or social systems.[72–112]

#### Physiological Model of Stress

Hans Selye discovered that the adrenal cortex and neuroendocrine and immune systems interact during stress, a finding that current research supports.[72–112] He defined stress as the body's automatic response ("fight or flight") to a demand that is placed on it. Selye also made the distinction between negative and positive stress (distress and eustress, respectively).

#### Life Events Model of Stress

Holmes and Rahe defined a model of stress that examined the nature and consequences of negative life events and proposed that interpersonal stressors are predictive of increases in disease activity.[72–112]

Chronic psychosocial stress has numerous pathophysiological effects that may stem from excessive sympathetic nervous system activation.[72–112] In particular, adrenal glucocorticoid hormones may play a major role in the stress response because of their profound effects on mood, behavior, neurochemical transmission, and neuroendocrine control. The pathophysiological effects of chronic stress include insulin resistance, hyperinsulinemia, coronary heart disease risk, infertility in females, therapy-resistant periodontitis, and impaired hippocampus-mediated memory processes. In children, chronic stress may be associated with impaired mental and affective stability, integrity, and development.

Because of the subjective nature of stress, clients' perceptions of their symptoms and stress levels are a critical component of the client examination.[72–112] Client interviews can elicit clients' reports of physical, mental, emotional, and behavioral symptoms of stress and descriptions of the situations they perceive to be stress provoking. Therapists can use a visual analog scale to obtain a basic rating of the client's perceived stress level. There are also numerous standardized self-report stress-rating questionnaires that therapists can use to assess their clients' perceived level of stress and the factors contributing to the stress that their clients experience. These tests provide a well-defined set of information and are usually designed and validated for a specific population. Therapists who wish to use a standardized measure of stress should consult the manual for details of the professional training required prior to administering the measure. This will enable them to determine whether their training and scope of practice allow them to administer the measure. Some of these measures use dominant models of stress as their basis. For example, the Schedule of Recent Experience, Impact of Events Scale, and Social Readjustment Ratings Scale are classic measures based on Holmes and Rahe's Life Events Model of Stress. The Cognitive Transactional Model of Stress provides the basis for the Hassles and Uplifts and the Ways of Coping Questionnaire from Folkman and Lazarus.[95] In addition, there are health-related stress questionnaires such as the Cardiac Event Threat Questionnaire. Buros Mental Measurement Yearbook[96] is a useful source of information on standardized stress questionnaires that includes the test population, test purpose, test details, and reviews. Box 5-4 lists some of the many tests described in Buros.[96]

Therapists can also use any of the range of physiological measures of chronic stress that are available.[72–112] Clin-

ical measures include heart rate, systolic and diastolic blood pressure, finger pulse volume, skin conductance levels, and finger temperature. Electromyography, especially lateral frontalis electromyogram responses, is an indicator of stress. Laboratory measures of blood samples include levels of lipid peroxides in venous blood samples; levels of the stress-related hormones prolactin, cortisol, and testosterone; and glycated hemoglobin levels. Finally, analysis of saliva identifies salivary cortisol levels, a common physiological indicator of stress.

# MULTISYSTEM EXAMINATION

## Pain

### *Definitions and Etiology*

#### Pain

**Pain** is an unpleasant sensation associated with actual or potential tissue damage that is mediated by specific nerve fibers to the brain where its conscious appreciation may be modified by various factors.[27–30,39,40,113–155]

#### Acute Pain

**Acute pain** is pain provoked by noxious stimulation produced by injury and/or disease with unpleasant sensory and emotional experiences.[27–30,39,40,113–155]

#### Chronic Pain

**Chronic pain** is pain that persists beyond the usual course of healing of an acute disease or beyond the reasonable time in which therapists expect the injury to heal.[27–30,39,40,113–155] There is some ambiguity in the definition of chronic pain. Some authors define it in terms of duration of pain, with a lower limit of duration ranging from 6 weeks to 6 months. Conversely, others define chronic pain in terms of an increasing dissociation from the physical etiology and increasing affective and cognitive dimensions of pain (see the definition of Chronic Pain Syndrome).

#### Chronic Pain Syndrome

**Chronic pain syndrome** is a clinical syndrome in which clients present with high levels of pain that is chronic in duration, in conjunction with functional limitations and depression.[27–30,39,40,113–155] This clinical pattern is seen more often in younger and middle-aged clients than in geriatric clients.

---

| Box 5-4 | **Examples of Standardized Measures of Stress from the Buros Mental Measurement Yearbook**[96] |
| --- | --- |

- Adolescent Coping Scale
- Coping Inventory for Stressful Situations
- Coping with Stress
- Daily Stress Inventory
- Life Stressors and Social Resources Inventory–Youth Form
- Personal Stress Assessment Inventory
- Questionnaire on Resources and Stress
- Stokes-Gordon Stress Scale
- Stress Analysis System
- Stress Audit
- Stress Impact Scale
- Stress Indicator and Health Planner
- Stress Management Questionnaire
- Stress Resiliency Profile
- Stress Response Scale
- Understanding and Managing Stress

## Nociceptive Pain

**Nociceptive pain** is the sensitization of peripheral nociceptors as a result of injury to a muscle or a joint that causes an increased release of neurotransmitters in the dorsal horn of the spinal cord.[27–30,39,40,113–155] The sensitized dorsal horn neurons demonstrate an increased background activity, an increased receptive field size, and increased responses to peripherally applied stimuli. Nociceptive pain may be implicated in the majority of the clients seen in clinical practice.

## Neurogenic Pain

**Neurogenic pain** is pain that occurs as a result of noninflammatory dysfunction of the peripheral or central nervous system that does not involve nociceptor stimulation or trauma.[27–30,39,40,113–155]

## Referred Pain

**Referred pain** is pain that the client feels at another location of the body that is at a distance from the tissues that have caused it.[27–30,39,40,113–155] This occurs because the same or adjacent neural segments supply the referred site. Therapists can identify referred pain because clients report pain in a generalized area, which they feel deeply, that radiates segmentally without crossing the midline and that has indistinct boundaries.

## Radiculopathy

**Radiculopathy** is pain that the client feels in a dermatome, myotome, or sclerotome because of direct involvement of a spinal nerve or nerve root.[27–30,39,40,113–155] It is also known as radicular or nerve root pain.

- **Dermatomal pain**: A **dermatome** is an area of skin supplied by one dorsal nerve root.[27–30,39,40,113–155] Injury of a dorsal root can result in sensory loss in the skin or can be experienced by the client as a burning or electric pain. For example, irritation of the C7 nerve root can lead to sensory changes in the C7 dermatome: lateral arm and forearm to the index, long, and ring fingers on the palmar and dorsal aspect.
- **Sclerotomal pain**: Pain in a sclerotome, an area of bone or fascia innervated by one segmental nerve root.[27–30,39,40,113–155] For example, hip pain can be referred to the groin, sacroiliac joints, lumbar spine, knee, or ankle.
- **Myotomal pain**: Pain in a myotome, a group of muscles supplied by one nerve root.[27–30,39,40,113–155] For example, injury to the teres minor can result in referred pain near the insertion of the deltoid.

## Visceral Pain

**Visceral pain** is pain in areas of the viscera supplied by a nerve root.[27–30,39,40,113–155] For example, injury to the small intestine can refer pain to the same area supplied by the T9–10 dermatome: an area encircling the trunk reaching the level of the umbilicus.

## Trigger Point Pain

Referred **trigger point pain** arises in a trigger point, but the client feels it at a distance that is often entirely remote from its source.[23–28,113–155] The pattern of referred pain relates to its site of origin. The distribution of referred trigger point pain rarely coincides entirely with the distribution of a peripheral nerve or dermatomal segment. Untreated trigger points can be associated with pain syndromes that include, but are not limited to, radiculopathy, tennis elbow, tension headache, occipital headache, and frozen shoulder.

## *Overview of Examination Techniques*

Therapists have a variety of options for measuring the different aspects of a client's pain.[113–155] They can elicit the client's general experience of pain through pain interviews about the 24-hour pain behavior. They can augment this interview with the use of body diagrams that the client can use to map the locations and quality of pain. They can assess pain intensity using a visual analog scale, the Verbal Rating Scale, the Numerical Rating Scale, and the Descriptor Differential Scale. They can use the McGill Pain Questionnaire, the Verbal Rating Scale, the visual analog scale, the Pain Discomfort Scale, and the Descriptor Differential Scale to assess the affective component of pain (how the client behaves in response to pain). The impact of the client's pain on his or her level of function is often evaluated using standardized self-report measures such as the Oswestry Back Pain Questionnaire, the Sickness Impact Profile, the Dallas Pain Questionnaire, and the Millon Visual Analog Scale. Finally, pain that the client reports that remains constant, regardless of activity, rest, or sleep, may be from a nonmusculoskeletal cause, such as cancer, that warrants a referral to the client's physician for further assessment.

Physical tests that therapists use to identify pain syndromes include: neural tissue tension or provocation tests, active and passive moment analysis, and nerve or tissue palpation.[113–155] The client's sensitivity to the pressure of palpation can be quantified accurately and reliably (interrater reliability interclass correlation coefficients [ICCs] ranging from 0.75 to 0.84, intrarater reliability ICCs ranging from 0.64 and 0.96) using a pain threshold meter or pressure algometer. The combination of client history and palpation is the primary clinical means of identifying trigger points, although the palpation of latent trigger points may be less reliable than that of active trigger points. The electrophysiological studies (nerve conduction) of electromyography and thermography are among the laboratory or instrumented tests used in the diagnosis of pain syndromes.

# Swelling

## *Definitions and Etiology*

### Swelling

**Swelling** is an abnormal enlargement of a segment of the body.[27,39,156–166]

### Edema

**Edema** is an accumulation of fluid in cells, tissues, or serous cavities.[27,39,156–166] Edema has four main causes: increased permeability of capillaries, decreased plasma protein osmotic pressure, increased pressure in capillaries and venules, and lymphatic flow obstruction.

---

### Theory in Practice 5-3

#### Using a Visual Analog Scale

The visual analog scale (Figure 5-4) is a written rating scale of pain intensity that is widely used both clinically and in research because of the ease with which therapists can administer it.[113–155] The visual analog scale (VAS) consists of a straight line measuring 10 cm in length. "No pain" is at the left end of the line, and "the worst pain I have ever experienced" is at the right end. Test-retest reliability for the VAS has been reported as $r = 0.99$. Concurrent validity between the VAS and the Numeric Pain Rating Scale ranged between $r = 0.77$ to $r = 0.91$.

#### Steps in Administering the Visual Analog Scale

1. Explain the pain rating levels at both extremes of the scale to the patient.
2. Ask the patient to mark the line at the point that corresponds to the intensity of pain that she is experiencing at the time at which she is completing the VAS.
3. Measure the distance from the beginning of the line to the patient's mark; this is the value that represents the patient's intensity of pain.
4. On re-examination, present the patient with a new diagram rather than her previous pain rating.

---

### Effusion

**Effusion** is excessive fluid in the joint capsule, indicating irritation or inflammation of the synovium.[27,39,156–166]

### Lymphedema

**Lymphedema** is accumulation of abnormal amounts of lymph fluid and associated swelling of subcutaneous tissues that results from the obstruction, destruction, or hypoplasia of lymph vessels.[27,39,156–166]

### Dependent Edema

**Dependent edema** is an increase in extracellular fluid volume that is localized in a dependent area such as a limb.[27,39,156–166] Dependent edema can be associated with swelling or pitting.

### Pitting Edema

**Pitting edema** is edema that retains the indentation produced by the pressure of palpation.[27,39,156–166]

### Solid Edema

**Solid edema** is the infiltration of subcutaneous tissues by mucoid material.[27,39,156–166]

## *Overview of Examination Techniques*

Therapists can obtain the client's description of her swelling and related symptoms through the client interview, in conjunction with the use of a body diagram.[27,39,156–166] Visual inspection of swelling can assist therapists in determining how best to measure the client's swelling. Palpation of swelling provides data on the quality of the swelling and the degree of edema that is present. Grading scales for edema include a 4-point scale for the degree of pitting and a 3-point scale for stage of lymphedema. Therapists can measure the girth of swollen body segments using a flexible tape measure, jeweler's ring, or wire. Volumetric analysis, in which the amount of fluid displaced by the limb is measured, provides a simple means of quantifying the extent of swelling that is more appropriate for swelling of the extremities. Comparison of volumetric analysis and estimation of limb volume using measurements of the limb perimeter showed that there was no significant difference between the two measures of limb volume for the arm but that volumetric analysis was more reliable and accurate for the hand. Laboratory or instrumented measures of swelling include multiple frequency bioelectrical impedance analysis, magnetic resonance imaging, and laser-Doppler flowmetry.

No pain |⎯⎯⎯⎯⎯⎯⎯⎯⎯⎯⎯⎯⎯⎯⎯⎯⎯⎯⎯⎯⎯⎯⎯| The worst pain I have
ever experienced

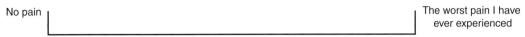

Figure 5-4  Visual analog scale for pain measurement.

## Theory in Practice 5-4

### Using a Pain Drawing

Practitioners often use the pain drawing to guide the patient systematically through a description of her pain and related symptoms.[113–155] The pain drawing that a patient produces on a body diagram can serve several purposes. First, practitioners can use it as an adjunct to the pain interview as a means of facilitating the patient's discussion of her symptoms. It is a simple and reliable method of identifying the location of a patient's pain and associated symptoms such as paresthesia and tightness. In addition, they can also use it to guide treatment planning and to document the patient's response to treatment.

#### Steps in Using the Pain Drawing

1. Provide the patient with a diagram of the human body (Figure 5-5) and colored pens.

2. Explain the purpose of the pain drawing and any pre-defined symbols, such as dotted lines, that represent pain and associated symptoms.

3. Inform the patient what time period the pain drawing is intended to represent. For example, this may be pain and symptoms experienced over the previous 24 hours. This time period will vary with the nature of the patient's clinical condition.

4. Ask the patient to indicate the location of any pain and associated symptoms that she has experienced during the specified time period on the diagram, using colors and predefined symbols. If the patient is unable to complete this task independently, the practitioner may provide the appropriate level of assistance.

5. When the patient has completed the pain drawing, discuss the drawing to clarify and expand on the information that the patient has provided. Practitioners can do this as part of the pain interview. Document this supplemental information on the pain drawing or elsewhere in

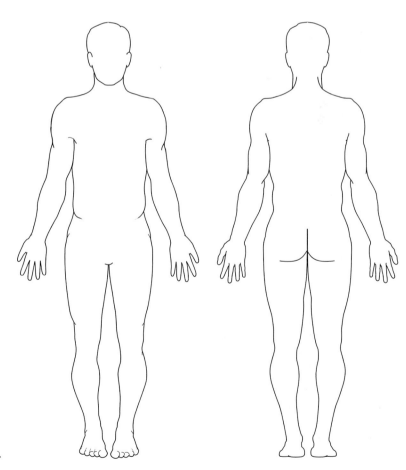

Figure 5-5  Body diagram for the pain drawing.

the patient's chart. The section on general pain behavior in the pain interview notes some issues that may be worthy of additional attention depending on the patient's clinical condition.

The practitioner may wish to identify asymptomatic areas that are immediately adjacent to the symptomatic area on the pain drawing.

12. In addition to palpating the locations of pain the patient has reported, you may also wish to palpate the following:
    (a) Trigger points that may refer to the painful areas
    (b) Related dermatomes
    (c) Related sclerotomes
13. Document all locations in which the palpation reproduces the patient's symptoms, and note the patterns of referred pain that result from palpation.

Note: Tenderness on palpation of a given area may be referred tenderness from another area and may not be a reliable finding. The practitioner needs to corroborate the findings of palpation for pain with other clinical tests and measures.

## Theory in Practice 5-5

### Using Palpation for Pain

Practitioners can use palpation to obtain further information on the location of the patient's pain and the sensitivity of the patient's tissues.[113–155]

#### Steps in Performing Palpation for Pain

1. Ensure that your hands are warm and dry.
2. Position the patient in a comfortable position in which the area to be palpated is readily accessible to you.
3. Drape the patient appropriately (see Chapter 6, Preparation and Positioning for Massage).
4. Explain the purpose of palpation and the procedures to be followed to the patient.
5. Ask the patient to inform you when she experiences tenderness, a referral of pain, or tingling or any other symptoms as a result of your palpation.
6. Select the location where you will begin palpation based on the patient's reports of the locations of pain, patterns of referred pain, or areas of tissue tightness that may be contributing to a postural dysfunction.
7. Begin palpation using a light pressure. Gradually increase the depth of palpation because a rapid change of depth may elicit a guarding response.
8. As you palpate each location, ask the patient if pressure on a given area causes any tenderness, localized pain, or referred pain. Move between locations slowly to avoid eliciting a painful spasm.
9. Observe the patient for twitching, vasomotor responses, and changes in breathing.
10. As you progress with palpation, identify and palpate areas in which the there are abnormalities of tissue texture such as bogginess or taut tissue bands.
11. Increase the depth of palpation and repeat the process if palpation with light pressure does not reproduce the patient's symptoms or the results of this palpation are inconclusive.

# CARDIOPULMONARY EXAMINATION

## Dyspnea

### *Definitions and Etiology*

#### Dyspnea

**Dyspnea** is shortness of breath, labored or difficult breathing, or an uncomfortable awareness of one's breathing.[39,167–187] Dyspnea is usually an indication of inadequate ventilation or insufficient amounts of oxygen in the circulating blood. Dyspnea is a complex sensation that involves: (a) the physiological and psychological events or stimuli preceding the development of dyspnea, (b) the characteristics of an individual or his or her environment that mediates his or her response to the dyspnea, and (c) the outcomes that result once the individual has reacted to the dyspnea.

### *Overview of Examination Techniques*

Clinical examination of a client with dyspnea can include visual inspection for posture used during respiration; quality, rate, and pattern of breathing; accessory muscle use; color; and affect.[39,167–187] Laboratory tests of decreased ventilation include arterial blood gases, which show oxygenation, acidosis, alkalosis, compensatory mechanisms, and buffer systems, and capnography, which determines levels of carbon dioxide.

There is only a fair association between perceived dyspnea and actual physiological lung function, possibly because of the different components that are the antecedents, mediators, and outcomes of dyspnea outlined earlier.[39,167–187] For this reason, self-report measures of dyspnea are important. Measures such as the British Medical Research Council Questionnaire, the American Thoracic Questionnaire, and the Dyspnea Interview Schedule can assess the events or stimuli that precede the dyspnea. The American Thoracic Questionnaire, the Chronic Respiratory Questionnaire, the Dyspnea Interview Schedule, the Pulmonary Functional Status Scale, and the Therapy Impact Questionnaire may measure characteristics that mediate the dyspnea. The Dyspnea Visual Analog Scale, the Therapy Impact Questionnaire, and the Borg Perceived Exertion Scale measure an individual's reactions to dyspnea. In addition, the Therapy Impact Questionnaire, the Baseline Dyspnea Index, the Transition Dyspnea Index, the Chronic Respiratory Questionnaire, the Oxygen Cost Diagram, the Dyspnea Interview Schedule, and the Modified Medical Research Council Dyspnea Scale measure the consequences of an episode of dyspnea. Finally, since decreased exercise capacity is one of the consequences of dyspnea, measures of functional exercise capacity, such as the 6-minute walk test, can be a valuable inclusion.

## Rib Cage Mobility

### Definitions and Etiology

#### Rib Cage Mobility

**Rib cage mobility** is the capacity of the ribcage to move within the available anatomical range of motion during respiration, based on the arthrokinematics of the joints of the ribcage and the thoracic spine, and the ability of the periarticular connective tissue to deform.[39,167–187]

### Overview of Examination Techniques

Examination of rib cage mobility involves both visual inspection and palpation.[39,167–187] The visual inspection performed by therapists should include general posture, breathing pattern, chest wall shape, symmetry of chest wall movement, accessory muscle use, and muscle contours. Palpation of chest wall excursion during respiration should address lateral costal and diaphragmatic excursion, thorough palpation of the intercostal spaces, sternal motion, and apical motion. Therapists can also use palpation to assess the mobility of the thoracic spine, the costovertebral joints, and the sternocostal joints. Palpation of muscle tension in the accessory muscles of breathing, such as the sternocleidomastoid and the intercostal muscles, will complete the palpation process. Finally, therapists can quantify rib cage mobility by measuring ribcage excursion during respiration with a tape measure using a consistent measurement site and position.

# FUNCTIONAL EXAMINATION

## Self-Care Activities

**Self-care activities** refer to those daily tasks that an individual needs to perform in order to be independent.[188–203] These tasks include dressing, feeding, grooming, hygiene, functional mobility, and functional communication. Therapists consider an inability to perform any of these tasks a functional limitation. Furthermore, they are more frequently using standardized measures of self-care to assess the clients' functional limitations and their progress on the identified functional outcomes. For example, the Barthel Index is a self-care measure that consists of the following 10 items that represent basic self-care activities: feeding, wheelchair transfer, grooming, bathing, walking on level surface, climbing stairs, dressing, bowel control, bladder control, and toilet use. Although it is one of the oldest self-care measures, ongoing studies are evaluating its validity and reliability. The Barthel Index is still widely used for the examination of clients with strokes, hip fractures, liver transplants, Parkinson's disease, amputations, and other clinical conditions. The relevant sections on impairments discuss other self-care measures.

## Health-Related Quality of Life

**Health-related quality of life** can be an issue to address in the client examination for massage since the impairments described earlier can have an impact on the client's level of activity and participation in society.[204–223] Measures of health-related quality of life have a broader focus than self-care measures and they typically cover the domains of physical, psychological, emotional, and social function. For example, the Medical Outcomes Survey–Short Form-36 (MOS SF-36) is a frequently used health-related quality of life measure that researchers have validated for several diseases and translated into other languages. Box 5-5 lists other health-related quality of life measures. In addition, therapists are using disease-specific quality of life measures, such as the Rheumatoid Arthritis Quality of Life Scale, more frequently in clinical examination and studies.

## REVIEWING THE BASICS

The client examination plays a critical role in Outcome-Based Massage by providing the clinical findings on which therapists can base their confirmation of their

These measures assess different components of quality of life.[204–223]
- Medical Outcomes Study Health Status Questionnaire
- Duke-UNC Health Profile
- The Sickness Impact Profile
- McMaster Health Index Questionnaire
- Functional Status Questionnaire
- Nottingham Health Profile

clinical hypothesis and their treatment planning. Consequently, therapists who are conducting client examinations with a view to using massage as a primary or complementary treatment modality need to expand the focus of their standard approach to examination to include the assessment of soft tissue dysfunction and the impairments that are relevant to the use of massage techniques.

Palpation provides an important means of assessing a variety of aspects of soft tissue function that can suggest the presence of impairments such as temperature, tissue mobility, fluid status, tissue texture, and tissue consistency. In addition, the client's response to palpation can give therapists other information about the client's presenting impairments. However, palpation is not the only means of assessing a client's impairments. Therapists can also extend their interpretation of the findings from standard musculoskeletal, neurologic, cardiopulmonary, and psychological tests and measures to include an analysis of the contribution of soft tissue dysfunction. Finally, the client examination conducted by therapists should also address the client's level of ability to perform functional activities and quality of life, so that therapists have data on which to base the identification of appropriate functional outcomes.

# Client Examination for Massage: Further Study and Practice

## UNDERSTANDING MUSCLE RESTING TENSION

### Definitions and Conceptual Framework

Traditionally, the literature describes muscle resting tension as the result of the biomechanical properties of muscle such as viscosity, elasticity, and plasticity. Furthermore, it notes that, in some situations, contractile activity can also contribute to resting tension. Clinicians know that the firmness and texture of skeletal muscle varies greatly from person to person.[23–28,34,39,98,332–340] Moreover, different muscles in the same client or the same muscle at different times can also vary in resting tension. Clinicians can observe the manner in which massage techniques can quickly produce dramatic changes in resting tension. These palpable changes in resting tension may relate to changes in a client's pain, other impairments, and level of activity.

One prevalent theory was that resting tension arises from a constant low-level contraction of skeletal muscle fibers, although recent research questions that theory.[23–28,34,39,98,332–340]

The emerging conceptual framework is that muscle resting tension results from a complex interaction among several components: myofibril contractile tissue, connectin and titin, giant structural proteins of striated muscle, connective tissue and its components, and nerve. The framework described in this section takes into account some observations about skeletal muscle that clinicians can notice during palpation (Box 5-6).

### Biomechanical Contributions to Resting Tension

This category refers to the contribution to resting tension made by the physical substances contained in muscle.[23–28,34,39,98,332–340] It has also been termed viscoelastic tone or passive tone. Muscle is a tissue composed of "subtissues": water, simple organic molecules, complex unchained organic molecules, and more complex biopolymers. Each of these has different physical or material properties such as density, stiffness, and deformability. The behavior of muscle during palpation reflects the properties of these components (Figure 5-6).

Box 5-6

### Observations about Skeletal Muscle That Can Be Noted during Palpation[23–28,34,39,98,332–340]

- Clinicians can change the shape of muscle by applying force.
- A deformed muscle reverts quickly to its former size and shape, although the muscle's shape and resting tension may change slightly.
- The texture of the same muscle can differ temporally. Sometimes, it feels softer, more flexible, and more liquid; at other times, it may feel harder, stiffer, and more solid. This texture is partly dependent on the muscle's position.
- The texture of a muscle can differ spatially. Relatively soft areas in a muscle may surround harder "knots."
- Clinicians can observe a wider range of textures across a selection of healthy clients. This range is along the same continuum from soft to hard.
- Fibers are commonly palpable in muscle at rest. These are similar to, but less pronounced than, those fibers clinicians feel when a working muscle contracts.
- Sometimes, a muscle that is "at rest" feels as though it is contracting.
- Palpation or massage can provoke a low-grade transient contraction. Therapists can sometimes observe a similar "twitching" when the muscle is at rest.
- After an injury, clinicians may find that the characteristic texture of muscle tissue is obscured. More specifically, it goes from feeling as though it contains fluid, in the period early after an injury, to feeling as though it contains something more like modeling clay, in the later period after injury.

### Water

Water associated with muscle tissue exists in several places[23,34,39,98,332–340]:

1. Contained in associated vessels such as arteries, veins, or lymphatics
2. In the interstitium, restrained in compartments formed by connective tissue
3. Freely in the interstitium
4. Loosely bonded to the hydrophilic molecules of the connective tissue matrix

Water normally flows relatively freely between these places.[23–28,34,39,98,332–340] Changing a muscle's position from fully shortened to fully lengthened results in increased fluid pressure within the muscle, which causes the muscle to feel harder during palpation. Pathology or injury may also shift water balance towards or away from one location, resulting in palpable changes in resting tension. For example, excess interstitial water may feel soft during the initial stages of edema and lymphedema, or it may feel harder in compartment syndromes when pressure builds as a result of the water restrained behind the thick fasciae. Some therapists believe that it is also possible to identify when the matrix is less hydrated through palpation.

### Connective Tissue

Fascia contributes to a varying proportion of the firmness of muscles at rest, as assessed by palpation.[23–28,34,39,98,332–340] This firmness is the result of two components: collagen fibers and the connective tissue matrix in which the collagen fibers are embedded. Poor modeling of the connective tissue within the muscle is one of several processes that

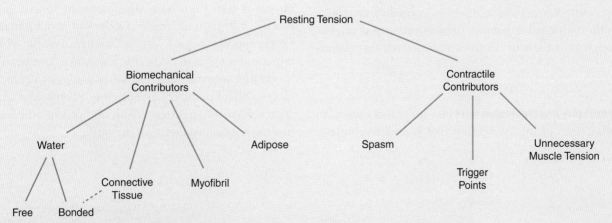

**Figure 5-6** Components of muscle resting tension. (Adapted from Mense S, Simon DG. *Muscle Pain: Understanding Its Nature, Diagnosis, and Treatment.* Philadelphia: Lippincott Williams & Wilkins; 2001.)

may contribute to the increased resting tension that clinicians palpate in the chronic stages of orthopedic injuries.

### Other Tissues

The contractile tissue—myofibrils composed of sarcomeres in series—affords little resistance to pressure when the muscle is not contracting.[23–28,34,39,98,155,332–340] A discussion of the contributions of active contraction to resting tension follows. Muscle also contains variable amounts of embedded fat (the marbling seen in meat), which gives little resistance to pressure during palpation under normal circumstances.

### Biomechanical Behavior of Muscle as a Whole

The mechanical behavior of noncontracting muscle is complex.[23–28,34,39,98,155,332–340] A force that clinicians apply quickly to muscle, such as a stretch or digital compression, will produce an initial deformation known as elastic deformation. When they apply the same force slowly, it produces further deformation, called viscous (or plastic) deformation. Furthermore, the amount of deformation of the tissues depends on the rate of application of the force. In addition, muscle tissue shows thixotropy, which means that it becomes more fluid and its stiffness decreases in response to movement. These behaviors depend on a complex interaction between the several components listed earlier that specialized texts discuss in detail.

## Myofibril Contraction Contributions to Resting Tension

The contractile activity of the sarcomeres that make up the myofibril contributes to resting tension.[23–28,34,39,98,155,332–340] Some authors define this as active tone or hypertonicity. This contractile activity is absent in normally innervated healthy muscle tissue. Figure 5-6 shows examples of ways in which contractile activity causes increased resting tension.

### Unnecessary Muscle Tension

**Unnecessary muscle tension** refers to "unwitting muscular contraction" or muscle tension that is under voluntary control.[23–28,34,39,98,332–340] Clinically, clinicians commonly see it in clients with muscle tension due to situational stress. Clinicians often observe unnecessary muscle tension in clients who request massage for wellness or to address the effects of stress.

### Trigger Points

**Trigger points** involve sarcomere shortening and myofibril activity, possibly as a result of calcium leakage at dysfunctional motor end plates.[23–28,34,39,98,155,332–340] In this situation, motor neuron and EMG activity are absent. The contraction knots and taut bands of trigger points frequently cause elevated resting tension.

### Spasm

**Spasm** involves involuntary contractile activity that is associated with motor neuron and EMG activity.[23–28,34,39,98,332–340] Spasm produces pain in one of three ways: by overloading parts of the muscle, by subjecting nociceptors between active and nonactive parts of the muscle to shearing forces, or through ischemia. Spasm is a common result of orthopedic injuries.

## A Vocabulary for Resting Tension

Poorly defined terminology and a lack of clarity on the source of muscle tension hamper the understanding of musculoskeletal pain and of muscle pain in particular.[23–28,34,39,98,155,332–340] Clinicians often develop an informal language for describing states of resting tension in otherwise healthy individuals. Some words such as "hard," "tight," "soft," "wiry," and "ropy" directly describe the texture of the muscle at rest. Expressions like "normally toned," "well-toned," or "hypertonic" make a judgment about function. Descriptors like "boggy," "dry," or "leathery" have unspoken implications about tissue health. Terms like "taut band" or "facilitated segment" link palpatory findings to complex theories about pathology of muscle or other tissue. Clinicians need to use these terms with caution since the literature has not defined them systematically.

## Client Examination for Massage: Advanced Examination Techniques

This section documents advanced examination techniques that are relevant to Outcome-Based Massage.

# MUSCULOSKELETAL EXAMINATION

## Joint Integrity

### Definitions and Etiology

#### Joint Integrity

**Joint integrity** is the extent to which a joint conforms to the expected anatomical and biomechanical norms.[39,141,56–58,224–245]

#### Capsular Restrictions

**Capsular restriction** is anatomical or pathological shortening of the joint capsule.[39,141,56–58,224–245] Capsular restrictions occur as a result of a variety of clinical conditions such as disuse, immobility, venous congestion, and diabetes. "Frozen shoulder" or adhesive capsulitis, for example, is a common capsular lesion seen in rehabilitation. This adherence of the shoulder capsule to the humeral head may be the consequence of altered supporting structures of and around the shoulder or autoimmune, endocrine, or other systemic diseases.

#### Capsular Laxity

**Capsular laxity** is anatomical or pathological lengthening of the joint capsule.[39,141,56–58,224–245] For example, global (anterior, inferior, and posterior) excessive laxity of the glenohumeral joint capsule leads to multidirectional instability of the shoulder.

#### Capsulitis and Synovitis

**Capsulitis and synovitis** describe inflammation of the synovium and the joint capsule and associated internal ligaments.[39,141,56–58,224–245] This can be associated with capsular distention secondary to increased levels of fluid in the joint, for example, as in rheumatoid arthritis.

#### Ligament Insufficiency

**Ligament insufficiency** is anatomical or pathological shortening of the capsular ligament.[39,141,56–58,224–245] For example, anterior capsular ligament length insufficiency in the gleno-

humeral joint can contribute to altered glenohumeral joint mechanics and shoulder pain.

#### Ligament Laxity

**Ligament laxity** is anatomical or pathological lengthening of the capsular ligament.[39,141,56–58,224–245] Anterior cruciate ligament laxity, for example, is a common cause of knee instability, pain, and functional limitations in athletes.

#### Nonmyofascial Trigger Points

**Nonmyofascial trigger point** is a hyperirritable spot in scars, fascia, periosteum, ligaments, and joint capsules that is associated with a hypersensitive palpable nodule in a taut band.[23,28,39,141,56–58,224–245]

### Overview of Examination Techniques

Cyriax[240] defined "capsular patterns," which are clinical signs of capsular lesions that are demonstrated during selective tissue tension testing that are supported by recent research.[23,28,39,141,56–58,224–245] Selective tissue tension testing involves the performance of a specific sequence of active range of motion, passive range of motion, and resisted isometric testing of the joint in question, during which clinicians observe sequences of pain and limitations of motion. Clinicians can identify clinical conditions with high levels of reliability (kappa = 0.875) using selective tissue tension testing.

The integrity of ligaments is best assessed clinically using a variety of static stability tests that demonstrate the stability of the ligaments of selected joints.[23,28,39,141,56–58,224–245] An example of these tests is the Lachman test of knee collateral ligament stability. Laboratory or instrumented tests of impaired joint integrity include magnetic resonance imaging, arthroscopic examination, arthrography, stress radiography, and ultrasonography.

## Joint Mobility

### Definitions and Etiology

#### Joint Range of Motion

**Joint range of motion** is the capacity of the joint to move within the anatomical or physiological range of motion that is available at that joint based on its arthrokinematics and the ability of the periarticular connective tissue to deform.[39,155,246–289] Range of motion reflects the function of the contractile, nervous, inert, and bony tissues and the client's willingness to perform a movement.

### Passive Range of Motion:

**Passive range of motion** is the amount of joint motion available when an examiner moves a joint through its anatomical or physiological range, without assistance from the client, while the client is relaxed.[39,155,246–289]

### Active Range of Motion

**Active range of motion** is the amount of joint motion that can be achieved by the client during the performance of unassisted voluntary joint motion.[39,155,246–289]

### Accessory Joint Motion

**Accessory joint motion** is the range of motion within synovial and secondary cartilaginous joints that is not under voluntary control. Consequently, clinicians can only obtain this measure passively.[39,155,246–289] These motions, also known as joint play movements, are essential for full and pain-free active range of motion.

### End Feel

**End feel** is the quality of motion or sensation that clinicians "feel" in the joint during overpressure at the end of passive range of motion.[39,155,246–289]

Impaired joint mobility can be the result of numerous primary impairments such as impaired muscle extensibility, altered muscle tone, capsular restriction or inflammation, tendinopathy, neurological deficit, pain, or bony deformity.[39,155,246–289] For the sake of clarity, this chapter defines relevant impairments in separate sections, although it outlines examination techniques for general range of motion testing here.

## Overview of Examination Techniques

Goniometry is the established approach to measuring joint range of motion for peripheral joints, and the universal goniometer is accurate and efficient.[155,246–289] Numerous studies have documented high degrees of intrarater reliability (ICCs of 0.88 to 0.93) and relatively lower levels of interrater reliability (ICCs of 0.80 to 0.85) for the universal goniometric measurements of a variety of upper and lower extremity joints by novice and experienced clinicians. Less sophisticated techniques for range of motion testing include visual estimation of range of motion. The findings from this technique may be more variable for many peripheral joints, regardless of therapists' level of experience, but more reliable in joints, such as the forefoot, that are more difficult to measure with goniometry. A parallelogram goniometer is under investigation and shows good reliability ($r = 0.85$ and $r = 0.87$) for the knee joint. Other techniques for assessing range of motion of peripheral joints include wire tracing for joints of the hand and a gravitational protractor. Two-dimensional and three-dimensional computer-aided motion analyses can provide information on the range of motion of multiple joints in static and dynamic postures, which can be more reliable than goniometry, particularly in complex joints. Although clinicians have traditionally measured joint range of motion with the client's joints uncovered, recent studies have explored measurement of clothed range of motion. In this situation, a computerized 6–degree of freedom electromagnetic tracker may be more accurate than goniometry. Finally, clinicians now use standardized measures of self-reported range of motion such as the Single Assessment Numeric Evaluation method, which asks clients to rate their range of motion as a percentage of normal.

Clinicians have used a variety of tools for the measurement of the range of motion of the spine and pelvis.[155,246–289] Measures of spinal range of motion include the Cervical Range of Motion (CROM) instrument, three-dimensional electromagnetic tracking systems, double inclinometers, electrogoniometers, computer-assisted motion analysis, and the combination of flexible rulers and trigonometric calculations. There are more simplistic measures of spinal range of motion that involve the measurement of various distances using a tape measure. The use of measured distances of the client's fingers to the floor in the testing of spinal range of motion may be the least reproducible approach and also reflects the range of motion of joints other than the spine. Another approach, the Schoeber method of using a tape measure placed on spinal landmarks to evaluate the motion of the spine, may be associated with considerable error. Pelvic range of motion can be difficult to measure. Consequently, clinicians can use devices such as the Palpation Meter, a caliper-inclinometer combination, or basic inclinometry to facilitate accurate measurement.

Clinicians measure accessory, or joint play, movements with the joint in the loose-packed position.[155,246–289] One technique described by Kaltenborn involves the palpation of glide and traction/compression ranges of motion during passive movements and the use of a 6-point grading system as follows: hypomobile (0–2), normal (3), or hypermobile (4–6). Accessory movement testing has shown poor to fair intrarater ($r = 0.75$) and interrater ($r = 0.45$) reliability. Laboratory or instrumented measures of accessory joint motion are now available. For example, clinicians use arthrometers to measure anterior-posterior translation (glide) in the knee joint.

The quality of movement is as important as the quantity of range that is available.[155,246–289] Therefore, clinicians should assess the quality of the movement throughout the range and at the end of the range as they perform passive range of motion. In doing so, they should apply overpressure at the end of the range and note whether the "end feel" is normal (bone-to-bone, soft tissue approximation, or tissue stretch) or abnormal (muscle spasm, hard capsular, soft capsular, bone-to-bone, empty, or springy block) for that joint.

# Muscle Integrity

## Definitions and Etiology

### Muscle Integrity

**Muscle integrity** is the extent to which a muscle conforms to the expected anatomical and biomechanical norms.[27–30,39,290–306]

### Muscle Extensibility

**Muscle extensibility** is the ability of the muscle and fascia to deform during the movement of a joint through its anatomical range.[27–30,39,290–306]

### Contracture

**Contracture** is a permanent muscular shortening due to a variety of physiological changes in muscle such as fibrosis or loss of muscular balance.[27–30,39,290–306] Physiological contractures are permanent muscular contractions or shortening that do not involve motor activity. The shortening of involved muscles in Volkman's ischemic contracture, for example, involves prolonged ischemia, myonecrosis, proliferation of fibroblasts, scar contraction, and formation of myotendinous adhesions. Muscle contractures may be associated with muscle imbalances that result from neurological disorders such as the presence of hypertonia in cerebellar lesions. They can also be associated with atrophy and fibrosis, as is the case in Duchenne's muscular dystrophy in which biopsies of contractures in selected muscles show a combination of muscle fiber atrophy with perimysial and endomysial fibrosis.

### Muscle Strain or Tear

**Muscle strain or tear** is a lesion or inflammation of muscle fibers that can occur in response to trauma.[27–30,39,290–306]

### Tendinitis

**Tendinitis** is inflammation of the peritendinous tissues that can occur in response to repetitive mechanical trauma.[27–30,39,290–306]

### Tendinosis

Unlike tendinitis, which is an inflammatory condition, **tendinosis** refers to common overuse tendon conditions with a histopathology that is consistent with a non-inflammatory, degenerative condition of unknown etiology.[27–30,39,290–306]

### Myofascial Trigger Point

**Myofascial trigger point** is a hyperirritable spot in skeletal muscle that is associated with a hypersensitive palpable nodule in a taut band.[23–28]

- Active trigger points are painful even when no one is palpating them.[23–28]
- Latent trigger points are not painful in and of themselves unless clinicians are palpating them.[23–28]

## Overview of Examination Techniques

Impaired muscle extensibility is measured clinically using stretch tests, defined as passive range of motion tests in which the muscle in question is placed in a stretched position, that have been defined for the given muscle group.[23–28,89–96] Extensibility of the hamstring muscles, for example, can be measured using goniometric measures of passive knee extension with the pelvis stabilized; this test can be reliable (r = 0.99) and performed with little associated pelvic motion. The Sit-and-Reach Test is another commonly used measure of hamstring extensibility. It is less accurate than the measurement of hip joint angle in this test position because the Sit-and-Reach Test also appears to reflect spinal mobility and anthropometric factors. Laboratory or instrumented measures of muscle extensibility include the use of force/angle data from isokinetic dynamometers, such as the KinCom to measure muscle extensibility with high levels of reliability (ICC = 0.81 to 0.95) for selected muscle groups, and dynamic ultrasonography.

Tendinopathies, muscle strains, and muscle tears are assessed using the methods of selective tissue tension testing outlined earlier in this chapter.[23–28,89–96] In this case, clinicians are looking for a relatively strong contraction of the muscle, with pain on contraction of the muscle (active movement in one direction), pain on stretch of the muscle (passive movement in the opposite direction), pain on isometric movement, and a possible decrease in range of motion if there is a gross hematoma. The distinction between tendinous and muscular lesions depends on the location of pain during testing and the results of palpation of tenderness. Clinicians can use magnetic resonance imaging when they require additional diagnostic information.

Impaired muscle integrity will also be associated with impaired muscle performance and pain that other sections describe in detail.[23–28,89–96]

---

### Theory in Practice 5-6

#### Using Palpation for Trigger Points

**Steps in Performing Palpation for Trigger Points**[23–28,89–96]

1.  Explain the purpose of palpation and the procedures to be followed to the patient.
2.  Ask the patient to inform you when she experiences tenderness, a referral of pain, or tingling or any other symptoms as a result of your palpation.
3.  Determine the muscle you will palpate for the presence of trigger points. This may include a review of the patient's reported pain behavior in the subjective examination for references to possible trigger point referral zones. Other potential locations of trigger points include muscles that showed limited range of motion on examination.
4.  Ensure that your hands are warm and dry.
5.  Position the patient with the muscle you will be examining in approximately two-thirds of its normal stretch position. Refer to *Travell and Simons' Myofascial Pain and Dysfunction: The Trigger Point Manual*[23,28] for the test positions for specific trigger points.
6.  Drape the patient appropriately (Chapter 6, Preparation and Positioning for Massage).
7.  Ensure that the patient is warm and the muscle you plan to palpate is relaxed.
8.  Identify the possible location of the trigger point.
9.  Palpate the location of the trigger point using one of the following approaches:
    (a) Flat palpation: Slide your finger or thumb along the taut band in the patient's muscle until the patient reports that you have reached the location of maximum tenderness, which represents the trigger point.
    (b) Pincer palpation: You can use this for muscles that you can lift easily. Grasp the belly of the muscle between your finger and thumb. Squeeze and roll the muscle tissue between your fingers to locate the taut band in the muscle. You can repeat this

maneuver along the muscle belly until you locate the trigger point.
    (c) Snapping palpation: Once you locate the taut band using pincer palpation, roll the taut band quickly under your fingers to produce a local twitch response.
10. During palpation determine whether the following are present:
    (a) Taut bands. The fiber direction and the pain referral pattern will enable you to identify the involved muscle.
    (b) Local hardness. The trigger point itself may present as a very small area of focal hardness (palpable nodule) in the taut band. Compress this area against the underlying tissues, and determine whether you reproduce the characteristic pain referral pattern for the trigger point in question.
    (c) Twitch responses. You can palpate twitch responses in superficial muscles.
    (d) Jump sign. A patient may produce a large involuntary contraction and other gross affective signs of pain if you palpate the trigger point too forcefully.
    (e) Generalized hardness. If there are adjacent trigger points in overlapping layers, the practitioner may find it difficult to palpate anything other than a generalized hardness. For example, this commonly occurs between the scapulae.
11. During palpation, have the patient compare the pain you produce by palpating the trigger point to her presenting symptoms. The patient should be able to recognize the pattern of pain referral if the trigger point is the contributing cause of her pain.

---

## Muscle Performance

### *Definitions and Etiology*

#### Muscle Performance
**Muscle performance** is the muscle's capacity to do work based on its length, tension, and velocity.[27–30,39,226–268,306–331] Neurological stimulus, fuel storage, fuel delivery, and balance, timing, and sequencing of muscle contraction all influence integrated muscle performance.

#### Muscle Strength
**Muscle strength** is the force or torque produced by a muscle or group of muscles to overcome a resistance during a maximum voluntary contraction.[27–30,39,226–268,306–331]

## Muscle Power

**Muscle power** is the work produced by a muscle per unit of time (strength × speed).[27-30,39,226-268,306-331]

## Muscle Endurance

**Muscle endurance** is the muscle's ability to contract, or maintain torque, over a number of contractions or a period of time.[27-30,39,226-268,306-331] Conversely, fatigue is a muscle's inability to maintain torque or the loss of power over time.

Because of the multiple inputs required for integrated muscle performance, impaired muscle performance can be the result of adhesions, impaired muscle integrity, abnormal neuromuscular tone, impaired joint mobility, impaired joint integrity, swelling, impaired connective tissue integrity, pain, and postural malalignment, which are described in detail in other sections of this chapter.[27-30,39,226-268,306-331] This chapter does not describe muscle weakness, a primary cause of impaired muscular performance, because massage techniques do not have a direct effect on increasing muscle strength.

## Overview of Examination Techniques

Muscle strength can be measured isometrically, isotonically, and isokinetically.[27-30,39,226-268,306-331] The graded manual muscle test is a longstanding clinical approach to isotonic strength testing that has questionable interrater reliability but good intrarater reliability (r = 0.88). Other options for isotonic testing include the one-repetition maximum test. Hand-held dynamometers are an accurate and reliable means of measuring isometric muscle strength and have become the mainstay of clinical practice. Clinicians typically perform hand strength testing with the grip strength dynamometer, the modified sphygmomanometer, and the pinch meter. They can measure isokinetic strength in a variety of ways using isokinetic dynamometers such as peak torque, mean peak torque, and force–frequency relationship. Muscle power is described in terms of peak power, mean power, instantaneous power, and torque–velocity relationships achieved through isokinetic testing. Isoinertial devices produce constant resistance to a movement that enables clinicians to measure isoinertial performance, particularly in trunk muscle testing.

Muscle endurance can be assessed using simple clinical measures, such as the number of repetitions performed, the single-leg hopping test, or more complex tests that include endurance time to limit of endurance and mean power frequency derived from an electromyogram.[27-30,39,226-268,306-331]

The client's perceived rate of exertion can be measured using rate of perceived effort tests, such as the Borg Perceived Effort Test, and correlated with objective measures of fatigue.

Clients with certain clinical conditions may require modifications to the usual muscle performance testing measures.[27-30,39,226-268,306-331] The modified sphygmomanometer is a reliable means (ICCs for interrater reliability of up to 0.85) of assessing isometric strength, particularly in geriatric clients and those with rheumatoid arthritis. Clinicians can also use pedaling activities to measure mechanical work and joint power generation patterns in clients who have had cerebrovascular accidents.

Clinicians can also assess the impact of an individual's muscle performance on his ability to perform functional tasks.[27-30,39,188,189,226-268,306-331] The Sit-to-Stand Test, for example, shows the impact of lower extremity strength on the client's ability to perform a functional transfer. The functional capacity evaluations used in occupational medicine measure a client's ability to perform work-related tasks such as pulling, lifting, carrying, and handling weights that reflect muscle performance. Kinematic and kinetic gait analysis using two- or three-dimensional computer-assisted motion analysis and force analysis show the impact of muscle performance on gait.

# Muscle Resting Tension
## Definitions and Etiology

### Muscle Resting Tension

**Muscle resting tension** is the firmness to palpation at rest observed in muscles with normal innervation or the perceived texture of muscle during palpation.[23-28,34,39,98,332-340]

### Muscle Spasm

**Muscle spasm** is involuntary contraction of a muscle that results in increased muscular tension and shortness that cannot be released voluntarily.[23-28,34,39,98,332-340] Research suggests that increased excitability of alpha-motor neuron pools contributes to the occurrence of muscle spasm.

## Overview of Examination Techniques

Clinicians can assess muscle resting tension and muscle spasm using a variety of tests. Nevertheless, research suggests that palpation is still the most important and exact method for measuring spasm.[23-28,34,39,98,332-340] The other tests for muscle spasm include the tissue compliance meter, which measures the consistency of soft tissue, badismography, continuous electromyogram, and thermography.

# MULTISYSTEM EXAMINATION

## Pain

### Definitions and Etiology

See Pain in the Client Examination for Massage: Foundations section of this chapter.

### Overview of Examination Techniques

#### The Pain Interview

Pain is a subjective experience. Consequently, the pain interview is an important means of eliciting information on the different components of the client's experience of pain, such as pain intensity, pain location, pain behavior, and the client's response to pain.[27-30,57-98] Through the pain interview, clinicians can determine the nature of the client's symptoms and the behavior of the client's symptoms over a 24-hour period. General guidelines for a pain interview appear in this chapter. Clinicians should modify the number of issues they cover in the pain interview based on the clinical setting and the client's clinical condition. For example, a more detailed pain interview may be appropriate for a client with chronic back pain in an occupational medicine clinic than it would be for a client with an acute episode of shoulder pain. Readers can refer to the texts on client examination for their health care profession to locate guidelines on issues related to pain assessment for specific clinical conditions. Clinicians can use the information from the pain interview during the Evaluative Phase of clinical decision making to confirm or refute their hypothesis about the client's clinical condition. They can also use the pain interview findings to clarify the impact of the client's pain on his or her functional level and to guide their identification of functional outcomes. The key areas in the pain interview appear in Theory in Practice 5-7: Using the Pain Interview.

#### Measuring Tissue Sensitivity Using a Pressure Algometer or Pain Threshold Meter

Clinicians can use a pain threshold meter or pressure algometer to measure tissue sensitivity to pressure.[23-28,85-96] There are a variety of types of pressure algometers available. Typically, these devices consist of a component for applying pressure, such as a hard rubber tip, attached to a

---

### Theory in Practice 5-7

#### Using the Pain Interview

**Location of Pain and 24-Hour Pain Behavior**

Discuss the following issues with the patient as a means of outlining the behavior of the patient's pain over a 24-hour period.[27-30,57-98] Bear in mind that the relevance of these issues will vary with the patient's clinical condition.

(a) Location of symptoms: The patient clarifies any locations marked on the pain drawing that are unclear.

(b) Priority of symptoms: The patient distinguishes between primary and secondary symptoms that she noted on the pain drawing.

(c) Nature of pain: The patient selects a pain identifier, such stabbing or burning, that best describes the pain in a particular location.

(d) Intensity of pain: The patient defines the intensity of pain that has occurred during a specified time period. The practitioner may use a numeric rating scale of 0 to 10, in which 0 represents the absence of pain and 10 represents the most pain the patient has ever experienced.

(e) Additional symptoms: The patient describes associated symptoms, such as paresthesia, that she has noted on the diagram.

(f) Frequency and duration of symptoms: The patient indicates whether pain is constant or intermittent. The patient also indicates how frequently and for how long the symptoms occur. A distinction between the duration of symptoms that occur during the day versus the night may be relevant to the patient's clinical condition. The frequency of the symptoms may be stated as a percentage, such as "50% of waking hours," or in relation to a time of day or an activity, such as "pain starts after 11:00 AM and persists until bedtime" or "burning sensation occurs after 30 minutes of keyboarding."

**Positions That Aggravate Pain**

1. Ask the patient to list the positions, such as sitting or standing, in which she notices an increase in her pain and associated symptoms.

2. For each position, elicit the following information:

   (a) How long can the patient maintain the position before noticing that the symptoms start or before they increase when there is a constant baseline level of pain?

   (b) How long can the patient maintain the position before the symptoms reach a level of intensity that causes her to move out of the position?

(c) When the symptoms change, as a result of being in the position, what is the change in level of intensity of the symptoms? Use the scale of 0 to 10 discussed earlier to show the difference.

(d) What does the patient do to ease her pain and other symptoms once the position aggravates them? For example, note the positions, modalities, exercises, and medications the patient uses to ease pain.

(e) Once the patient has moved out of the position and used some means of pain relief, how much time elapses before the patient notices that the symptoms have returned to the original level?

### Activities That Aggravate Pain

1. Ask the patient to list the activities during which she notices an increase in her pain and associated symptoms. These activities can include:
   (a) Self-care activities such as grooming, feeding, and functional mobility
   (b) Community management activities (instrumental activities of daily living) such as driving, taking the bus, and grocery shopping
   (c) Work-related activities such as lifting, keyboarding, and telephone use
   (d) Leisure activities such as sexual activity, walking, watching television, and playing sports
   (e) Sleeping. Since patients' symptoms are frequently aggravated during sleep, this activity usually warrants additional discussion of issues such as sleep position, bed type, and sleeping behavior.

2. For each activity, elicit the following information:
   (a) What is the time period for which the patient can perform the activity before noticing that the symptoms start (or increase if there is a constant baseline level of pain)?
   (b) What is the time period for which the patient can perform the activity before the symptoms reach a level of intensity that causes her to cease the activity?
   (c) When the symptoms change as a result of performing the activity, what is the change in level of intensity of the symptoms (use a scale of 0 to 10 to show the difference)?
   (d) What does the patient do to ease her pain and other symptoms once performing the activity aggravates then? For example, note the activities, modalities, exercises, and medications the patient uses to ease the pain.

(e) Once the patient has ceased the activity and used some means of pain relief, how much time elapses before the patient notices that the symptoms have returned to the original level?

### Self-Management

1. Ask the patient to describe the strategies she uses to manage her symptoms. Include details of the frequency, duration, and effects of these activities.
2. Ask the patient if she has received a self-care program in the past. Determine whether she is still performing it. If so, discuss the frequency, duration, and effects of this self-care program.

### Ergonomics

1. Ask the patient to describe and demonstrate the following:
   (a) Usual positions in which she performs her work
   (b) Any repetitive activities that are associated with performance of her job
   (c) Positions that she uses at work that she feels are safe and comfortable
   (d) Positions that she uses at work that she feels cause her pain
   (e) Positions that she uses at work that she feels are adaptations to her pain or that she uses to minimize her pain
2. Ask the patient whether the placement of the furniture and equipment in her work area appears to be contributing to her pain.
3. Ask whether the patient has had an ergonomic evaluation of her work place by a qualified professional. If so, what were the results?

pressure (force) gauge. The dial of the gauge shows pressure readings in $kg/cm^2$ or $lbs/cm^2$. Clinicians obtain pressure sensitivity readings by using the algometer to apply a gradually increasing force on the client's tissues and noting the pressure reading at the time at which the client reports experiencing pain or discomfort. Interrater reliability for pressure algometer scores varies (ICCs of greater than $r = 0.78$ and Pearson correlation coefficients of $r > 0.82$). The pressure algometer is valuable for documenting and reassessing the effects of trigger point therapy and other interventions that change tissue sensitivity because it provides a means of quantifying the client's subjective complaints.

## Using a Pressure Algometer to Test Tissue Sensitivity

1. Stand in a position that will enable you to apply an even pressure to the patient's tissues when the pressure algometer is positioned perpendicular to the patient's skin.[23–28,85–96]
2. Position the patient in a relaxed and well-supported position.
3. Explain the overall procedure to the patient, and demonstrate the application of the pressure algometer on an unaffected area of the patient's body. In particular, instruct the patient to say "Yes" when she first feels discomfort, and explain that you will cease the application of pressure as soon as she does so, so that she does not experience undue discomfort. Explain that rubor and capillary breakage can occur following tissue sensitivity testing with a pressure algometer, and provide basic instructions for the application of ice to the affected areas.
4. Identify the location where you want to test tissue sensitivity. For example, in the case of a trigger point, palpate for a taut band and an area of tenderness in the location specified for that trigger point. Once you have located the area to be tested, you may wish to mark it.
5. Ensure that the pressure gauge is at zero. Place the contact surface of the pressure algometer on the location you wish to test.
6. Hold the pressure algometer so that the shaft of the instrument is at a 90-degree angle to the surface of the patient's skin.
7. Using your free hand, gradually apply pressure on the patient's tissues with the pressure algometer. Continue to increase the pressure gradually until the patient reports feeling discomfort.
8. Cease applying pressure as soon as the patient reports discomfort, and note the pressure algometer reading at that point.
9. Reset the gauge to zero prior to the next episode of testing.

## Impaired Sensation Secondary to Entrapment Neuropathy

### Definitions and Etiology

#### Entrapment Neuropathy

**Entrapment neuropathy** is nerve compression that can result from muscle and connective tissue shortening and inflammation associated with trigger point activity, fascial re-strictions, overuse syndromes, and other clinical conditions.[27–30,39,70,341–350] The client with an entrapment neuropathy will present with pain, paresthesia, numbness, or loss of range of motion. Common peripheral entrapment neuropathies include carpal tunnel syndrome, cubital tunnel syndrome, and tarsal tunnel syndrome. Less common entrapment neuropathies include posterior interosseous nerve syndrome and anterior interosseous nerve syndrome.

### Overview of Examination Techniques

There are a several neurological and musculoskeletal examination techniques that are applicable to assessing entrapment neuropathies.[27–30,39,70,341–350] Dermatome testing includes light touch, hot/cold, pinprick, and filament testing. Myotome testing uses isometric movements and reflexes. In addition, therapists can use sensory discrimination testing (kinesthesia, graphesthesia, and stereognosis), palpation of the nerve in the area of possible compression, vibrometer testing, and neural tension testing.

Electrophysiological testing (nerve conduction studies) evaluates late responses (F waves and H reflexes) and long latency reflexes.[27–30,39,70,341–350] These studies enable clinicians to identify the location and severity of the neuropathy. Electroneurometry (skin surface electrical stimulation of the motor nerve), single-frequency (120-Hz) vibrometry tests, and magnetic resonance imaging are also of value in the diagnosis of entrapment neuropathies.

# NEUROLOGICAL EXAMINATION

## Neuromuscular Tone

### Definitions and Etiology

#### Muscle Tone

**Muscle tone** is resting tension and responsiveness of muscles to passive elongation or stretch.[39,332–340,351–376]

#### Postural Tone

**Postural tone** is the development of muscular tension in skeletal muscles that participate in maintaining the positions of different parts of the skeleton.[39,332–340,351–376] The cerebellum regulates postural tone. Unlike muscle resting tension, constant muscle activation is required for the maintenance of postural tone. Furthermore, the self-sustained firing of motor neurons may reduce the need for prolonged synaptic input.

## Hypertonia

**Hypertonia** is a general term used to refer to muscle tone that is above normal resting levels, regardless of the mechanism for the increase in tone.[39,332–340,351–376]

## Hypotonia or Flaccidity

**Hypotonia**, or flaccidity, is a general term used to refer to muscle tone that is below normal resting levels, regardless of the mechanism for the decrease in tone.[39,332–340,351–376]

## Spasticity

**Spasticity** is increased muscular tone that is a result of an upper motor neuron lesion that may or may not be associated with reflex hyperexcitability.[39,332–340,351–376] Spastic muscle exhibits a velocity-dependent increase in tonic stretch reflexes. The quicker the stretch is, the more pronounced the resistance of the spastic muscle.

## Rigidity

**Rigidity** is increased muscular tone that occurs as a result of brainstem or basal ganglia lesions.[39,332–340,351–376] Rigidity involves a uniformly increased resistance in both agonist and antagonist muscles, resulting in stiff, immovable body parts, independent of the velocity of the stretch stimulus. Patients exhibit two types of rigidity: (1) **cogwheel rigidity**, which is a ratchet-like response to passive movement, alternating between giving way and increased resistance, and (2) **lead pipe rigidity**, which is constant response to passive movement.

- **Decorticate rigidity** occurs as a result of brainstem lesions.[39,332–340,351–376] It presents clinically as sustained contraction and posturing of the trunk and lower limbs in extension and the upper limbs in flexion.
- **Decerebrate rigidity** occurs as a result of brainstem lesions.[39,332–340,351–376] It presents clinically as sustained contraction and posturing of the trunk and lower limbs in extension.
- **Parkinsonian rigidity** occurs as a result of basal ganglia lesions.[39,332–340,351–376] It presents clinically as a tight contraction of both agonist and antagonist muscles throughout the movement (lead pipe rigidity). Clients with Parkinson's disease will eventually present with rigidity.

## Clonus

**Clonus** is a cyclical, spasmodic hyperactivity of antagonistic muscles that occurs at a regular frequency in response to a quick stretch stimulus.[39,332–340,351–376]

## Overview of Examination Techniques

The measurement of abnormal muscular tone requires an understanding of neurological lesions.[39,332–340,351–376] Manual passive motion testing and the use of tone grading scales, such as the Ashworth scale, are central to the examination of abnormal tone. The client examination for spasticity can also use the pendulum test (using isokinetic dynamometers or a goniometer), torque/electromyogram curves for ramp and hold or sinusoidal oscillation, or the use of hand-held or isokinetic dynamometers to measure resistance to passive movement.

Some standardized assessments of motor control, such as the Fugl-Meyer assessment and the Montreal Evaluation, include sections on manual testing of muscle tone.[39,332–340,351–376] In addition to manual passive motion testing, spasticity can be evaluated using electrophysiological measures that measure the electrical and mechanical features of hypertonic muscle. These measures include electromyographical testing of reflexes such as the T reflexes, H reflexes, F responses, long-latency stretch reflexes, the tonic vibration reflex, and flexor reflexes. Research suggests, however, that there is a stronger correlation between Ashworth scale scores and spasticity than with laboratory or instrumented tests of reflex activity. Therapists can also test for exaggerated or clonic deep tendon reflexes in hypertonic individuals or absent or decreased reflexes for hypotonic states.

In light of the impact that neurological conditions can have on an individual's functional level, there are numerous functional measures that are used in the client examination.[39,332–340,351–376] These measures are similar in their emphasis on motor recovery and the functional tasks that are most often affected in individuals who have had strokes. They differ, however, in the philosophical principles on which they are based. For example, the measures that reflect neurodevelopmental therapy principles include the Rivermead Motor Assessment Protocol and the Montreal Assessment. The Fugl-Meyer assessment uses Brunnstrom's sequence of motor recovery. The Functional Test for the Hemiparetic Upper Extremity is based on both Brunnstrom and neurodevelopmental therapy principles. The structure of other measures, such as the Motor Assessment Scale, the Physical Assessment for

Stroke Patients, and the Arm Function Test, is not based on either philosophy.

# CARDIOPULMONARY EXAMINATION

## Airway Clearance

### Definitions and Etiology

#### Airway Clearance

**Airway clearance** is the ability to move pulmonary secretions effectively through the use of normal mechanisms of cough and the mucociliary escalator.[39,167-187]

#### Chronic Obstructive Pulmonary Disease

**Chronic obstructive pulmonary disease** is a pulmonary disorder characterized by the presence of increased airway resistance.[39,167-187] These disorders are associated with increased sputum production and cough that can predispose the individual to recurrent bronchial infection. Examples of chronic obstructive pulmonary disease include emphysema, chronic bronchitis, and asthma.

#### Chronic Restrictive Pulmonary Disease

**Chronic restrictive pulmonary disease** is a pulmonary disorder characterized by the restriction of lung expansion, such as interstitial fibrosis.[39,167-187]

### Overview of Examination Techniques

Clinicians base the clinical examination of impaired airway clearance on a number of clinical signs and symptoms.[39,167-187] The Respiratory Nursing Diagnosis Scale (RNDS), which defines major and minor characteristics of impaired airway clearance, summarizes many of these clinical signs and symptoms. According to this scale, the most important characteristic of impaired airway clear-

ance is an ineffective cough. The minor characteristics include tenacious sputum; subjective complaints of inability to cough up secretions; increased or copious sputum; absent, decreased, or abnormal breath sounds; air hunger; abnormal respiratory pattern; nasal flaring; anxiety; dyspnea at rest; cyanosis or other change in color; and restlessness. Characteristics deemed less relevant to impaired airway clearance include asymmetric chest excursion, abnormal inspiratory-to-expiratory ratio, dyspnea on exertion, diaphoresis, and pain.

A number of clinical tests collect the data on which to base the identification of impaired airway clearance.[39,167-187] Visual inspection of cough, visual inspection of the volume and quality of sputum, respiration rate and pattern, color, and accessory muscle use are essential starting points. Pulse oximeters measure oxygen saturation, which is the degree to which arterial blood is oxygenated. Unfortunately, the reliability of this measure decreases when clients' skin has a darker pigmentation. Breath sounds and heart rate are assessed using auscultation. Finally, clinicians can use self-report measures to elicit a client's perception of breathlessness (measured on a visual analog scale), rating of dyspnea on a Dyspnea Rating Scale, or perceived exertion on a Perceived Exertion Rating Scale.

There are several laboratory tests of symptoms associated with impaired airway clearance.[39,167-187] Arterial blood gases show oxygenation, acidosis, alkalosis, compensatory mechanisms, and buffer systems. Pulmonary function tests show inspired volume, respiratory exchange ratio, forced expiratory volumes, inspiratory capacity, and vital capacity. In addition, there are a variety of measures of oxygen consumption. Finally, laboratory measures of actual particle clearance rates are not yet appropriate for use with humans, although they are common in animal research.

A variety of self-report functional measures, such as the Nottingham Health Profile for quality of life and the Self-Efficacy for Functional Activities questionnaire, measure the client's perception of the impact of impaired airway clearance and chronic respiratory disease on his or her functional level and quality of life.[39,167-187]

## References

1. World Health Organization. Towards a common language for functioning, disability and health: ICF—the International Classification of Functioning, Disability and Health. Geneva, Switzerland: World Health Organization; 2002.
2. World Health Organization. ICF Checklist. Geneva, Switzerland: World Health Organization; 2003.
3. Childs JD, Whitman JM, Sizer PS, Pugia ML, Flynn TW, Delitto A. A description of physical therapists' knowledge in managing musculoskeletal conditions. *BMC Musculoskelet Disord.* 2005;6:32.
4. Chaitow L. *Palpation Skills: Assessment and Diagnosis Through Touch.* Philadelphia: WB Saunders; 1996.
5. Casterline MR. Trail guide to the body: how to locate muscles, bones and more. *J Athl Train.* 1998;33:284–285.

6. Protopapas MG, Cymet TC. Musculoskeletal examination: a complete review. *Compr Ther.* 2005;31:12–20.

7. Field D, Hutchinson JO. *Anatomy, Palpation, and Surface Markings.* 4th ed. Oxford, England: Butterworth-Heinemann; 2006.

8. Lewit K. Soft tissue and relaxation techniques in myofascial pain. In: Hammer WI, ed. *Functional Soft Tissue Examination and Treatment by Manual Methods: New Perspectives.* 2nd ed. Gaithersburg, MD: Aspen; 1999:479–532.

9. Greenman PE. *Principles of Manual Medicine.* 2nd ed. Baltimore: Williams and Wilkins; 1996.

10. Starkey C, Ryan J. *Evaluation of Orthopedic and Athletic Injuries.* 2nd ed. Philadelphia: F. A. Davis; 2001.

11. McKenzie AM, Taylor NF. Can physiotherapists locate lumbar spinal levels by palpation? *Physiotherapy.* 1997;83:235–239.

12. Najm WI, Seffinger MA, Mishra SI, Dickerson VM, Adams A, Reinsch S, Murphy LS, Goodman AF. Content validity of manual spinal palpatory exams: a systematic review. *BMC Complement Altern Med.* 2003;3:1.

13. Humphreys BK, Delahaye M, Peterson CK. An investigation into the validity of cervical spine motion palpation using subjects with congenital block vertebrae as a "gold standard." *BMC Musculoskelet Disord.* 2004;5:19.

14. Abbott JH, McCane B, Herbison P, Moginie G, Chapple C, Hogarty T. Lumbar segmental instability: a criterion-related validity study of manual therapy assessment. *BMC Musculoskelet Disord.* 2005;6:56.

15. Keating J, Matyas TA, Bach TM. The effect of training on physical therapists' ability to apply specified forces of palpation. *Phys Ther.* 1993;73:38–46.

16. Fritz S. *Fundamentals of Therapeutic Massage.* 2nd ed. St. Louis, MO: Mosby-Lifeline; 2000.

17. Downey BJ, Taylor NF, Niere KR. Manipulative physiotherapists can reliably palpate nominated lumbar spinal levels. *Manual Ther.* 1999;4:151–156.

18. Latimer J, Adams R, Lee M. Training with feedback improves judgments of non-biological linear elastic stiffness. *Manual Ther.* 1998;3:85–89.

19. American Physical Therapy Association. *Guide to Physical Therapist Practice.* 2nd ed. Alexandria, VA: American Physical Therapy Association; 1999.

20. Nicholson L, Adams R, Maher C. Reliability of a discrimination measure for judgments of non-biological stiffness. *Manual Ther.* 1997;2:150–156.

21. Inscoe EL, Witt PL, Gross MT, Mitchell RU. Reliability in evaluating passive intervertebral motion of the lumbar spine. *J Manual Manipulative Ther.* 1995;3:135–143.

22. Cox NH. Palpation of the skin: an important issue. *J R Soc Med.* 2006;99:598–600.

23. Simons DG, Travell JG, Simons LS. *Travell and Simons' Myofascial Pain and Dysfunction: the Trigger Point Manual. Volume 1: Upper Half of Body.* 2nd ed. Baltimore: Williams & Wilkins; 1999.

24. DiGiovanna EL, Schiowitz S. *An Osteopathic Approach to Diagnosis and Treatment.* 2nd ed. Philadelphia: Lippincott-Raven; 1997:18.

25. Cantu R, Grodin A. *Myofascial Manipulation: Theory and Clinical Application.* 2nd ed. Gaithersburg, MD: Aspen Publishers; 2000.

26. Thomson JS. *Core Textbook of Anatomy.* Philadelphia: Lippincott Williams & Wilkins; 1990.

27. Magee DJ. *Orthopedic Physical Assessment.* 4th ed. Philadelphia: WB Saunders; 2005.

28. Simons DG, Travell JG, Simons LS. *Travell and Simons' Myofascial Pain and Dysfunction: the Trigger Point Manual. Volume 2: Lower Half of Body.* 2nd ed. Baltimore: Williams & Wilkins; 1999.

29. Hoppenfeld S. *Physical Examination of the Spine and Extremities.* New York: Appleton-Century-Crofts; 1976.

30. Hertling D, Kessler RM. *Management of Common Musculoskeletal Disorders.* 4th ed. Philadelphia: Lippincott Williams & Wilkins; 2005.

31. Hoeksma AF, Faber WR. Assessment of skin temperature by palpation in leprosy patients: interobserver reliability and correlation with infrared thermometry. *Int J Lepr Other Mycobact Dis.* 2000;68:65–67.

32. Oerlemans HM, Perez RS, Oostendorp RA, Goris RJ. Objective and subjective assessments of temperature differences between the hands in reflex sympathetic dystrophy. *Clin Rehabil.* 1999;13:430–438.

33. Murff RT, Armstrong DG, Lanctot D, Lavery LA, Athanasiou KA. How effective is manual palpation in detecting subtle temperature differences? *Clin Podiatr Med Surg.* 1998;15:151–154.

34. Lederman E. *The Science and Practice of Manual Therapy.* 2nd ed. Edinburgh: Elsevier Churchill Livingstone; 2005.

35. Kisner C, Colby LA. *Therapeutic Exercise: Foundations and Techniques.* 5th ed. Philadelphia: FA Davis; 2007.

36. de Domenico G, Wood EC. *Beard's Massage.* 4th ed. Philadelphia: WB Saunders; 1997.

37. Rolf IP. *Rolfing: The Integration of Human Structure.* New York: Harper and Row; 1977.

38. Chaitow L. *Modern Neuromuscular Techniques.* 2nd ed. New York: Churchill-Livingston; 2003.

39. Stedman TL. *Stedman's Medical Dictionary.* 28th ed. Baltimore: Lippincott Williams & Wilkins; 2005.

40. Mannheim CJ. *The Myofascial Release Manual.* 3rd ed. Hightstown, NJ: McGraw Hill; 2001.

41. Sucher BM. Thoracic outlet syndrome: a myofascial variant: Part 1. Pathology and diagnosis. *J Am Osteopath Assoc.* 1990; 90:686–696,703–704.

42. Sucher BM, Heath DM. Thoracic outlet syndrome: a myofascial variant: Part 3. Structural and postural considerations. *J Am Osteopath Assoc.* 1993;93:334,340–345.

43. Boyling J, Jull G, eds. *Grieve's Modern Manual Therapy: The Vertebral Column.* 3rd ed. New York: Churchill-Livingston; 2005.

44. Cisler TA. Whiplash as a total-body injury. *J Am Osteopath Assoc.* 1994;94:145–148.

45. Hanten WP, Chandler SD. Effects of myofascial release leg pull and sagittal plane isometric contract-relax techniques on passive straight-leg raise angle. *J Orthop Sports Phys Ther.* 1994; 20:138–144.

46. Drape JL, Silbermann Hoffman O, Houvet P, Dubert T, Thivet A, Benmelha Z, Frot B, Alnot JY, Benacerraf R. Complications of flexor tendon repair in the hand: MR imaging assessment. *Radiology.* 1996;198:219–224.

47. Tillman LJ, Chasan N. Properties of dense connective tissue. In: Hertling D, Kessler RM, eds. *Management of Common*

*Musculoskeletal Conditions.* 4th ed. Philadelphia: Lippincott Williams & Wilkins; 2006:3–13.

48. Tillman LJ, Cummings GS. Biologic mechanisms of connective tissue mutability. In: Currier DP, Nelson RM, eds. *Dynamics of Human Biologic Tissues.* Philadelphia: FA Davis; 1992:1–44.

49. Kessler RM, Hertling D. Friction massage. In: Hertling D, Kessler RM, eds. *Management of Common Musculoskeletal Conditions.* 3rd ed. Philadelphia: Lippincott-Raven; 1996: 133–139.

50. Hammer WI. Friction massage. In: Hammer WI, ed. *Functional Soft Tissue Examination and Treatment by Manual Methods.* 2nd ed. Gaithersburg, MD: Aspen; 1999:463–478.

51. Palastanga N. The use of transverse frictions for soft tissue lesions. In: Grieve GP, ed. *Modern Manual Therapy for the Vertebral Column.* New York: Churchill-Livingston; 1986:819–825.

52. Brosseau L, Casimiro L, Milne S, Robinson V, Shea B, Tugwell P, Wells G. Deep transverse friction massage for treating tendinitis. *Cochrane Database Syst Rev.* 2002;4:CD003528.

53. Cyriax J, Cyriax PJ. *Cyriax's Illustrated Manual of Orthopaedic Medicine.* 2nd ed. Stoneham, MA: Butterworth-Heinemann; 1993.

54. Cyriax J. Deep massage. *Physiotherapy.* 1977;63:60–61.

55. Fernandez-de-las-Penas C, Alonso-Blanco C, Fernandez-Carnero J, Carlos Miangolarra-Page J. The immediate effect of ischemic compression technique and transverse friction massage on tenderness of active and latent myofascial trigger points: a pilot study. *J Bodywork Move Ther.* 2006;10:3–9

56. Hammer WI. The use of friction massage in the management of chronic bursitis of the hip or shoulder. *J Manipulative Physiol Ther.* 1993;16:107–111.

57. Grindel S. Evidence based medicine in the musculoskeletal examination. *Br J Sports Med.* 1998;32:278–279.

58. Riegger Krugh C, Keysor JJ. Skeletal malalignments of the lower quarter: correlated and compensatory motions and postures. *J Orthop Sports Phys Ther.* 1996;23:164–170.

59. Dunk NM, Lalonde J, Callaghan JP. Implications for the use of postural analysis as a clinical diagnostic tool: reliability of quantifying upright standing spinal postures from photographic images. *J Manipulative Physiol Ther.* 2005;28:386–392.

60. Champain N, Dupuis R, Pomero V, Mouilleseaux B, Dubousset J, Skalli W. Geometric and postural analysis of mild idiopathic scoliotic patients. *Stud Health Technol Inform.* 2002;91:267–271.

61. Dunk NM, Chung YY, Compton DS, Callaghan JP. The reliability of quantifying upright standing postures as a baseline diagnostic clinical tool. *J Manipulative Physiol Ther.* 2004;27:91–96.

62. Seegert EM, Shapiro R. From the field. Effects of alternative exercise on posture. *Clin Kinesiol.* 1999;53:41–47.

63. Grimmer K. An investigation of poor cervical resting posture. *Aust J Physiother.* 1997;43:7–16.

64. Villanueva MB, Jonai H, Sotoyama M, Hisanaga N, Takeuchi Y, Saito S. Sitting posture and neck and shoulder muscle activities at different screen height settings of the visual display terminal. *Ind Health.* 1997;35:330–336.

65. Harrison AL, Barry Greb T, Wojtowicz G. Clinical measurement of head and shoulder posture variables. *J Orthop Sports Phys Ther.* 1996;23:353–361.

66. Franklin ME, Chenier TC, Brauninger L, Cook H, Harris S. Effect of positive heel inclination on posture. *J Orthop Sports Phys Ther.* 1995;21:94–99.

67. Harrison DE, Harrison DD, Troyanovich SJ. Reliability of spinal displacement analysis on plain X-rays: a review of commonly accepted facts and fallacies with implications for chiropractic education and technique. *J Manipulative Physiol Ther.* 1998;21:252–266.

68. Tuck AM, Peterson CK. Accuracy and reliability of chiropractors and Anglo-European College of Chiropractic students at visually estimating the lumbar lordosis from radiographs. *Chiropract Techniq.* 1998;10:19–26.

69. Capodaglio EM, Capodaglio P, Panigazzi M, Bazzini G. An ergonomic study of postures of toll collectors. *G Ital Med Lav Ergon.* 1998;20:24–30 (Abstract).

70. Novak CB, Mackinnon SE. Repetitive use and static postures: a source of nerve compression and pain. *J Hand Ther.* 1997; 10:151–159.

71. Christensen HW. Precision and accuracy of an electrogoniometer. *J Manipulative Physiol Ther.* 1999;22:10–14.

72. Lazarus RS. Toward better research on stress and coping. *Am Psychol.* 2000;55:665–673.

73. Lutgendorf SK, Costanzo ES. Psychoneuroimmunology and health psychology: an integrative model. *Brain Behav Immun.* 2003;17:225–232.

74. Berczi I. The stress concept and neuroimmunoregulation in modern biology. *Ann N Y Acad Sci.* 1998;851:3–12.

75. Szabo-S. Hans Selye and the development of the stress concept. Special reference to gastroduodenal ulcerogenesis. *Ann N Y Acad Sci.* 1998;851:19–27.

76. Sarafino E. *Health Psychology: Biopsychosocial Interactions.* New York: Wiley; 1990.

77. Rozanski A, Blumenthal JA, Kaplan J. Impact of psychological factors on the pathogenesis of cardiovascular disease and implications for therapy. *Circulation.* 1999;99:2192.

78. Fuchs E, Flugge G. Stress, glucocorticoids and structural plasticity of the hippocampus. *Neurosci Biobehav Rev.* 1998;23: 295–300.

79. Wilbert-Lampen U, Trapp A, Modrzik M, Fiedler B, Straube F, Plasse A. Effects of corticotropin-releasing hormone (CRH) on endothelin-1 and NO release, mediated by CRH receptor subtype R2: a potential link between stress and endothelial dysfunction? *J Psychosom Res.* 2006;61:453–460.

80. Oei NY, Everaerd WT, Elzinga BM, van Well S, Bermond B. Psychosocial stress impairs working memory at high loads: an association with cortisol levels and memory retrieval. *Stress.* 2006;9:133–141.

81. Steptoe A, Donald AE, O'Donnell K, Marmot M, Deanfield JE. Delayed blood pressure recovery after psychological stress is associated with carotid intima-media thickness: Whitehall psychobiology study. *Arterioscler Thromb Vasc Biol.* 2006;26: 2547–2551.

82. Jansen LM, Gispen-de Wied CC, Wiegant VM, Westenberg HG, Lahuis BE, van Engeland H. Autonomic and neuroendocrine responses to a psychosocial stressor in adults with autistic spectrum disorder. *J Autism Dev Disord.* 2006;36:891–899.

83. Elsenbruch S, Lucas A, Holtmann G, Haag S, Gerken G, Riemenschneider N, Langhorst J, Kavelaars A, Heijnen CJ, Schedlowski M. Public speaking stress-induced neuroendocrine responses and circulating immune cell redistribution in irritable bowel syndrome. *Am J Gastroenterol.* 2006;101: 2300–2307.

84. Duncko R, Makatsori A, Fickova E, Selko D, Jezova D. Altered coordination of the neuroendocrine response during psychosocial stress in subjects with high trait anxiety. *Prog Neuropsychopharmacol Biol Psychiatry.* 2006;30:1058–1066.

85. Keltikangas Jarvinen L, Ravaja N, Raikkonen K, Hautanen A, Adlercreutz H. Relationships between the pituitary-adrenal hormones, insulin, and glucose in middle-aged men: moderating influence of psychosocial stress. *Metabolism.* 1998;47:1440–1449.

86. Sanders KA, Bruce NW. A prospective study of psychosocial stress and fertility in women. *Hum Reprod.* 1997;12:2324–2329.

87. Axtelius B, Soderfeldt B, Edwardsson S, Attstrom R. Therapy-resistant periodontitis (I). Clinical and treatment characteristics. *J Clin Periodontol.* 1997;24:640–645.

88. Ohl F, Fuchs E. Differential effects of chronic stress on memory processes in the tree shrew. *Brain Res Cogn Brain Res.* 1999;7:379–387.

89. Rothenberger A, Huther G. The role of psychosocial stress in childhood for structural and functional brain development: neurobiological basis of developmental psychopathology. *Prax Kinderpsychol Kinderpsychiatr.* 1997;46:623–644 (Abstract).

90. Diniz DH, Schor N, Blay SL. Stressful life events and painful recurrent colic of renal lithiasis. *J Urol.* 2006;176:2483–2487.

91. Savoia MG, Bernik M. Adverse life events and coping skills in panic disorder. *Rev Hosp Clin Fac Med Sao Paulo.* 2004;59:337–340.

92. Clarke D, Singh R. Life events, stress appraisals, and hospital doctors' mental health. *N Z Med J.* 2004;117:U1121.

93. Holmes TH, Rahe RH. The Social Readjustment Rating Scale. *J Psychosom Res.* 1967;11:213–218.

94. Lazarus RS, Folkman S. *Hassles and Uplifts Scales Research Edition.* Palo Alto, CA: Consulting Psychologists Press Inc; 1989.

95. Folkman S, Lazarus RS. *Ways of Coping Questionnaire Research Edition.* Palo Alto, CA: Consulting Psychologists Press Inc; 1988.

96. Plake B, Spies R, eds. *The Sixteenth Mental Measurements Yearbook.* Lincoln, NE: Buros Institute of Mental Measurements; 2005.

97. Bennett SJ, Puntenney PJ, Walker NL, Ashley ND. Development of an instrument to measure threat related to cardiac events. *Nurs Res.* 1996;45:266–270.

98. Shalev AY, Bloch M, Peri T, Bonne O. Alprazolam reduces response to loud tones in panic disorder but not in posttraumatic stress disorder. *Biol Psychiatry.* 1998;44:64–68.

99. Rief W, Shaw R, Fichter MM. Elevated levels of psychophysiological arousal and cortisol in patients with somatization syndrome. *Psychosom Med.* 1998;60:198–203.

100. Stones A, Groome D, Perry D, Hucklebridge F, Evans P. The effect of stress on salivary cortisol in panic disorder patients. *J Affect Disord.* 1999;52:197–201.

101. Eller NH, Netterstrom B, Hansen AM. Psychosocial factors at home and at work and levels of salivary cortisol. *Biol Psychol.* 2006;73:280–287.

102. Rohleder N, Wolf JM, Herpfer I, Fiebich BL, Kirschbaum C, Lieb K. No response of plasma substance P, but delayed increase of interleukin-1 receptor antagonist to acute psychosocial stress. *Life Sci.* 2006;78:3082–3089.

103. Koo-Loeb JH, Pedersen C, Girdler SS. Blunted cardiovascular and catecholamine stress reactivity in women with bulimia nervosa. *Psychiatry Res.* 1998;80:13–27.

104. Demaree HA, Harrison DW. Physiological and neuropsychological correlates of hostility. *Neuropsychologia.* 1997;35:1405–1411.

105. Dahlgren A, Kecklund G, Akerstedt T. Overtime work and its effects on sleep, sleepiness, cortisol and blood pressure in an experimental field study. *Scand J Work Environ Health.* 2006;32:318–327.

106. Davis PA, Holm JE, Myers TC, Suda KT. Stress, headache, and physiological dysregulation: a time-series analysis of stress in the laboratory. *Headache.* 1998;38:116–121.

107. Artinian NT, Washington OG, Flack JM, Hockman EM, Jen KL. Depression, stress, and blood pressure in urban African-American women. *Prog Cardiovasc Nurs.* 2006;21:68–75.

108. Podbevsek D. Hyperlipidemia with disseminated eruptive xanthomas and hyperglycemia caused by mental stress: a case report. *Lijec Vjesn.* 2005;127:220–223.

109. Wilhelm FH, Roth W. Acute and delayed effects of alprazolam on flight phobics during exposure. *Behav Res Ther.* 1997;35:831–841.

110. Schneider RH, Nidich SI, Salerno JW, Sharma HM, Robinson CE, Nidich RJ, Alexander CN. Lower lipid peroxide levels in practitioners of the Transcendental Meditation program. *Psychosom Med.* 1998;60:38–41.

111. Anderzen I, Arnetz BB. Psychophysiological reactions to international adjustment. Results from a controlled, longitudinal study. *Psychother Psychosom.* 1999;68:67–75.

112. Schuck P. Glycated hemoglobin as a physiological measure of stress and its relations to some psychological stress indicators. *Behav Med.* 1998;24:89–94.

113. Heitz NA, Eisenman PA, Beck CL, Walker JA. Hormonal changes throughout the menstrual cycle and increased anterior cruciate ligament laxity in females. *J Athl Train.* 1999;34:144–149.

114. von Baeyer CL. Children's self-reports of pain intensity: scale selection, limitations and interpretation. *Pain Res Manag.* 2006;11:157–162.

115. Heck JF, Sparano JM. A classification system for the assessment of lumbar pain in athletes. *J Athl Train.* 2000; 35(2):204–211.

116. Main CJ, Williams AC. Musculoskeletal pain. *BMJ.* 2002;325:534–537.

117. Goddard G, Karibe H, McNeill C. Reproducibility of Visual Analog Scale (VAS) pain scores to mechanical pressure. *J Craniomandibular Pract.* 2004;22:250–256.

118. Main CJ, Watson PJ. Psychological aspects of pain. *Man Ther.* 1999;4:203–215.

119. Puttick MP. Rheumatology: 11. Evaluation of the patient with pain all over. *CMAJ.* 2001;164:223–227.

120. Laslett M, McDonald B, Tropp H, Aprill CN, Öberg B. Agreement between diagnoses reached by clinical examination and available reference standards: a prospective study of 216 patients with lumbopelvic pain. *BMC Musculoskelet Disord.* 2005;6:28.

121. Koes BW, van Tulder MW, Thomas S. Diagnosis and treatment of low back pain. *BMJ.* 2006;332:1430–1434.

122. Chaplin ER: Chronic pain and the injured worker: a sociobiological problem. In: Kasdan ML, ed. *Occupational Hand and Upper Extremity Injuries and Diseases.* Philadelphia: Hanley and Belfus, Inc.; 1991:13–45.

123. Simon JM. Chronic pain syndrome: nursing assessment and intervention. *Rehabil Nurs.* 1996;21:13–19.

124. van Herk R, van Dijk M, Baar FP, Tibboel D, de Wit R. Observation scales for pain assessment in older adults with cognitive impairments or communication difficulties. *Nurs Res.* 2007;56:34–43.

125. Carr JL, Moffett JA, Sharp DM, Haines DR. Is the Pain Stages of Change Questionnaire (PSOCQ) a useful tool for predicting participation in a self-management programme? Further evidence of validity, on a sample of UK pain clinic patients. *BMC Musculoskelet Disord.* 2006;7:101.

126. Fink R. Pain assessment: the cornerstone to optimal pain management. *Proc (Bayl Univ Med Cent).* 2000;13:236–239.

127. Corran TM, Farrell MJ, Helme RD, Gibson SJ. The classification of patients with chronic pain: age as a contributing factor. *Clin J Pain.* 1997;13:207–214.

128. Sluka KA. Pain mechanisms involved in musculoskeletal disorders. *J Orthop Sports Phys Ther.* 1996;24:240–254.

129. Katavich L. Pain mechanisms underlying peripheral nerve injury: implications for mobilisation of the nervous system. *N Z J Physiother.* 1999;27:24–27.

130. Khalsa PS. Muscle pain due to mechanical stimuli. *J Neuromusculoskeletal Syst.* 1999;7:1–8.

131. Seaman DR, Cleveland C III. Spinal pain syndromes: nociceptive, neuropathic, and psychologic mechanisms. *J Manipulative Physiol Ther.* 1999;22:458–472.

132. Hall TM, Elvey RL. Nerve trunk pain: physical diagnosis and treatment. *Man Ther.* 1999;4:63–73.

133. Ross RG, LaStayo PC. Clinical assessment of pain. In: Van Deusen J, Brunt D, eds. *Assessment in Occupational Therapy and Physical Therapy.* Philadelphia: WB Saunders; 1997.

134. Downie W, Leatham P, Rhind V, Wright V, Branco J, Anderson J. Studies with pain rating scales. *Ann Rheum Dis.* 1978;37:378–381.

135. McDougall JJ. Arthritis and pain. Neurogenic origin of joint pain. *Arthritis Res Ther.* 2006;8:220.

136. Weinstein SM. Cancer pain. *Phys Med Rehabil State Art Rev.* 1994;8:279–296.

137. Elvey RL. Physical evaluation of the peripheral nervous system in disorders of pain and dysfunction. *J Hand Ther.* 1997;10:122–129.

138. Lewis J, Ramot R, Green A. Changes in mechanical tension in the median nerve: possible implications for the upper limb tension test. *Physiotherapy.* 1998;84:254–261.

139. Song KM, Morton AA, Koch KD, Herring JA, Browne RH, Hanway JP. Chronic musculoskeletal pain in childhood. *J Pediatr Orthop.* 1998;18:576–581.

140. Marovino T, Blackmon CB, Sherman M, Carzon M, Tworek R. Pain assessment. The accuracy and test-retest reliability of dolorimetry measurements in a healthy and chronic pain population. *Am J Pain Manage.* 1995;5:94–97.

141. Antonaci F, Sand T, Lucas GA. Pressure algometry in healthy subjects: inter-examiner variability. *Scand J Rehabil Med.* 1998;30:3–8.

142. Hong C. Algometry in evaluation of trigger points and referred pain. *J Musculoskeletal Pain.* 1998;6:47–59.

143. Scott J, Huskisson E. Vertical or horizontal visual analogue scales. *Ann Rheum Dis.* 1979;38:560.

144. Nussbaum EL, Downes L. Reliability of clinical pressure-pain algometric measurements obtained on consecutive days. *Phys Ther.* 1998;78:160–169.

145. Swift T, Brescia N. Intra and inter-rater reliability of pressure algometer measurements taken by student physical therapists. Unpublished Masters Research Paper. Oakland, CA: Samuel Merritt College; 1997.

146. Brown FF, Robinson ME, Riley JL 3rd, Gremillion HA, McSolay J, Meyers G. Better palpation of pain: reliability and validity of a new pressure pain protocol in TMD. *Cranio.* 2000;18: 58–65.

147. Lew PC, Lewis J, Story I. Inter-therapist reliability in locating latent myofascial trigger points using palpation. *Man Ther.* 1997;2:87–90.

148. Hsieh CY, Hong CZ, Adams AH, Platt KJ, Danielson CD, Hoehler FK, Tobis JS. Interexaminer reliability of the palpation of trigger points in the trunk and lower limb muscles. *Arch Phys Med Rehabil.* 2000;81:258–264.

149. Cohen H, Pertes R. Diagnosis and management of fascial pain. In: Rachlin ES, ed. *Myofascial Pain and Fibromyalgia: Trigger Point Management.* St. Louis, MO: Mosby Year Book Inc; 1994:361–382.

150. Delaney G, McKee A. Inter- and intra-rater reliability of the pressure threshold meter in measurement of myofascial trigger point sensitivity. *Am J Phys Med Rehabil.* 1993;72:136–139.

151. Alvarez DJ, Rockwell PG. Trigger points: diagnosis and management. *Am Fam Physician.* 2002;65:653–660.

152. Rivner MH. The neurophysiology of myofascial pain syndrome. *Curr Pain Headache Rep.* 2001;5:432–440.

153. Ingber RS. Myofascial pain in lumbar dysfunction. *Phys Med Rehabil State Art Rev.* 1999;13:473–498.

154. Hammond E. Electrodiagnosis of the neuromuscular system. In: Van Deusen J, Brunt D, eds. *Assessment in Occupational Therapy and Physical Therapy.* Philadelphia: WB Saunders; 1997.

155. Mense S, Simons DG. *Muscle Pain: Understanding Its Nature, Diagnosis, and Treatment.* Baltimore: Lippincott Williams & Wilkins; 2001.

156. Knight CA. Peripheral vascular disease. In: O'Sullivan SB, Schmitz TJ, eds. *Physical Rehabilitation.* 6th ed. Philadelphia: FA Davis Company; 2006:583–619.

157. Johansson K, Albertsson M, Ingvar C, Ekdahl C. Effects of compression bandaging with or without manual lymph drainage treatment in patients with postoperative arm lymphedema. *Lymphology.* 1999;32:103–110.

158. Moholkar K, Fenelon G. Diurnal variations in volume of the foot and ankle. *J Foot Ankle Surg.* 2001;40:302–304.

159. Todd JE. Symptom management. Lymphedema: a challenge for all healthcare professionals. *Int J Palliat Nurs.* 1998;4: 230–239.

160. Ramadan A. Hand analysis. In Van Deusen J, Brunt D, eds. *Assessment in Occupational Therapy and Physical Therapy.* Philadelphia: WB Saunders; 1997.

161. Palmada M, Shah S, O'Hare K. Issues in the measurement of hand edema. *Physiother Theory Pract.* 1998;14:139–148.

162. Acebes O, Renau E, Sansegundo R, Santos FJ, Aguilar JJ. Evaluation of post-mastectomy lymphedema. Comparative study of two measurement methods. *Rehabilitacion.* 1999;33:190–194 (Abstract).

163. Klauser A, Frauscher F, Halpern EJ, Mur E, Springer P, Judmaier W, Schirmer M. Remitting seronegative symmetrical synovitis with pitting edema of the hands: ultrasound, color Doppler ultrasound, and magnetic resonance imaging findings. *Arthritis Rheum.* 2005;53:226–233.

164. del Olmo J, Espana A, Richter J. The usefulness of isotopic lymphoscintigraphy in the study of lymphedemas. *Actas Dermosifiliogr.* 2005;96:419–423.

165. Khan O, Maharaj P, Rampaul R, Archibald A, Naipaul R, Loutan N. Lymphoscintigraphic evaluation of chronic lower limb edema. *West Indian Med J.* 2003;52:136–139.

166. Cornish BH, Bunce IH, Ward LC, Jones LC, Thomas BJ. Bioelectrical impedance for monitoring the efficacy of lymphoedema treatment programmes. *Breast Cancer Res Treat.* 1996; 38:169–176.

167. Frownfelter DL, Dean E. *Cardiovascular and Pulmonary Physical Therapy: Evidence and Practice.* 4th ed. St. Louis, MO: Mosby; 2005.

168. Ries AL. Minimally clinically important difference for the UCSD Shortness of Breath Questionnaire, Borg Scale, and Visual Analog Scale. *COPD.* 2005;2:105–110.

169. Gunen H, Hacievliyagil SS, Kosar F, Gulbas G, Kizkin O, Sahin I. The role of arterial blood gases, exercise testing, and cardiac examination in asthma. *Allergy Asthma Proc.* 2006;27:45–52.

170. Hutter BO, Wurtemberger G. Functional capacity (dyspnea) and quality of life in patients with chronic obstructive lung disease (COPD): instruments of assessment and methodological aspects. *Pneumologie.* 1999;53:133–142 (Abstract).

171. Geiger R, Strasak A, Treml B, Gasser K, Kleinsasser A, Fischer V, Geiger H, Loeckinger A, Stein JI. Six-minute walk test in children and adolescents. *J Pediatr.* 2007;150:395–399.

172. Carlson Catalano J, Lunney M, Paradiso C, Bruno J, Luise BK, Martin T, Massoni M, Pachter S. Clinical validation of ineffective breathing pattern, ineffective airway clearance, and impaired gas exchange. *Image J Nurs Sch.* 1998;30:243–248.

173. Dallimore K, Jenkins S, Tucker B. Respiratory and cardiovascular responses to manual chest percussion in normal subjects. *Aust J Physiother.* 1998;44:267–274.

174. McChesney JA, McChesney JW. Auscultation of the chest and abdomen by athletic trainers. *J Athl Train.* 2001;36:190–196.

175. Protas E. Cardiovascular and pulmonary function. In: Van Deusen J, Brunt D, eds. *Assessment in Occupational Therapy and Physical Therapy.* Philadelphia: WB Saunders; 1997.

176. Basoglu OK, Atasever A, Bacakoglu F. The efficacy of incentive spirometry in patients with COPD. *Respirology.* 2005;10: 349–353.

177. Thomas JR, von Gunten CF. Management of dyspnea. *J Support Oncol.* 2003;1:23–32.

178. de Torres JP, Pinto-Plata V, Ingenito E, Bagley P, Gray A, Berger R, Celli B. Power of outcome measurements to detect clinically significant changes in pulmonary rehabilitation of patients with COPD. *Chest.* 2002;121:1092–1098.

179. Aaron SD, Vandemheen KL, Clinch JJ, Ahuja J, Brison RJ, Dickinson G, Hebert PC. Measurement of short-term changes in dyspnea and disease-specific quality of life following an acute COPD exacerbation. *Chest.* 2002;121:688–696.

180. Fujimoto K, Kubo K, Miyahara T, Matsuzawa Y, Kobayashi T, Ono C, Ito N. Effects of muscle relaxation therapy using specially designed plates in patients with pulmonary emphysema. *Intern Med.* 1996;35:756–763.

181. Oberdorster G, Cox C, Gelein R. Intratracheal instillation versus intratracheal inhalation of tracer particles for measuring lung clearance function. *Exp Lung Res.* 1997;23:17–34.

182. Fuchs Climent D, Le Gallais D, Varray A, Desplan J, Cadopi M, Prefaut C. Quality of life and exercise tolerance in chronic obstructive pulmonary disease: effects of a short and intensive inpatient rehabilitation program. *Am J Phys Med Rehabil.* 1999;78:330–335.

183. Resnick B. Reliability and validity testing of the Self-Efficacy for Functional Activities scale: three studies. *J Nurs Meas.* 1999;7:5–20.

184. Springhouse. *Professional Guide to Diseases.* 8th ed. Springhouse, PA: Springhouse Corporation; 2005.

185. Mancini I, Body JJ. Assessment of dyspnea in advanced cancer patients. *Support Care Cancer.* 1999;7:229–232.

186. Hill J, Johansen J, Pedersen S, LaPier TK. Site of measurement and subject position affect chest excursion measurements. *Cardiopulmonary Phys Ther J.* 1997;8:12–17.

187. Fruth SJ. Differential diagnosis and treatment in a patient with posterior upper thoracic pain. *Phys Ther.* 2006;86:254–268.

188. Mueller BA, Adams ED. Work activities. In: Van Deusen J, Brunt D, eds. *Assessment in Occupational Therapy and Physical Therapy.* Philadelphia: WB Saunders; 1997.

189. King PM, Tuckwell N, Barrett TE. A critical review of functional capacity evaluations. *Phys Ther.* 1998;78:852–866.

190. Law M. Self care. In: Van Deusen J, Brunt D, eds. *Assessment in Occupational Therapy and Physical Therapy.* Philadelphia: WB Saunders; 1997.

191. Finch E, Brooks D, Stratford P, Mayo N. *Physical Rehabilitation Outcome Measures.* Philadelphia: Lippincott Williams & Wilkins; 2002.

192. Mahoney F, Barthel D. Functional evaluation: The Barthel Index. *MD State Med J.* 1965:61–65.

193. De Groot IJ, Post MW, Van Heuveln T, Van Den Berg LH, Lindeman E. Measurement of decline of functioning in persons with amyotrophic lateral sclerosis: responsiveness and possible applications of the Functional Independence Measure, Barthel Index, Rehabilitation Activities Profile and Frenchay Activities Index. *Amyotroph Lateral Scler.* 2006;7:167–172.

194. Langhammer B, Stanghelle JK. Co-variation of tests commonly used in stroke rehabilitation. *Physiother Res Int.* 2006; 11:228–234.

195. Bennett M, Ryall N. Using the modified Barthel index to estimate survival in cancer patients in hospice: observational study. *BMJ.* 2000;321:1381–1382.

196. Ceran F, Ozcan A. The relationship of the Functional Rating Index with disability, pain, and quality of life in patients with low back pain. *Med Sci Monit.* 2006;12:435–439.

197. Engberg A, Bentzen L, Garde B. Rehabilitation after stroke: predictive power of Barthel Index versus a cognitive and a motor index. *Acta Neurol Scand.* 1995;91:28–36.

198. Levi SJ. Posthospital setting, resource utilization, and self-care outcome in older women with hip fracture. *Arch Phys Med Rehabil.* 1997;78:973–979.

199. Kakurai S, Akai M. Clinical experiences with a convertible thermoplastic knee-ankle-foot orthosis for post-stroke hemiplegic patients. *Prosthet Orthot Int.* 1996;20:191–194.

200. Hui E, Lum CM, Woo J, Or KH, Kay RL. Outcomes of elderly stroke patients. Day hospital versus conventional medical management. *Stroke.* 1995;26:1616–1619.

201. Jonsson B, Overend T, Kramer J. Functional measures following liver transplantation. *Physiother Can.* 1998;50:141–146.

202. Patti F, Reggio A, Nicoletti F, Sellaroli T, Deinite G, Nicoletti F. Effects of rehabilitation therapy on Parkinson's disability and functional independence. *J Neurol Rehabil.* 1996;10:223–231.

203. Condie E, Treweek S, Jones D, Scott H. A one-year national survey of patients having a lower limb amputation. *Physiotherapy.* 1996;82:14–20.

204. Jette AM. Using health-related quality of life measures in physical therapy outcomes research. *Phys Ther.* 1993;73:528–537.

205. Mielenz T, Jackson E, Currey S, DeVellis R, Callahan LF. Psychometric properties of the Centers for Disease Control and Prevention Health-Related Quality of Life (CDC HRQOL) items in adults with arthritis. *Health Qual Life Outcomes.* 2006;4:66.

206. Whitfield K, Buchbinder R, Segal L, Osborne RH. Parsimonious and efficient assessment of health-related quality of life in osteoarthritis research: validation of the Assessment of Quality of Life (AQoL) instrument. *Health Qual Life Outcomes.* 2006;4:19.

207. Ware J, Sherbourne C. The MOS 36-item Short Form Health Survey (SF-36). *Med Care.* 1992;30:473–483.

208. McHorney CA, Haley SM, Ware JE Jr. Evaluation of the MOS SF-36 Physical Functioning Scale (PF-10): II. Comparison of relative precision using Likert and Rasch scoring methods. *J Clin Epidemiol.* 1997;50:451–461.

209. Thumboo J, Fong KY, Ng TP, Leong KH, Feng PH, Thio ST, Boey ML. Validation of the MOS SF-36 for quality of life assessment of patients with systemic lupus erythematosus in Singapore. *J Rheumatol.* 1999;26:97–102.

210. Daeppen JB, Krieg MA, Burnand B, Yersin B. MOS-SF-36 in evaluating health-related quality of life in alcohol-dependent patients. *Am J Drug Alcohol Abuse.* 1998;24:685–694.

211. Lam CL, Gandek B, Ren XS, Chan MS. Tests of scaling assumptions and construct validity of the Chinese (HK) version of the SF-36 Health Survey. *J Clin Epidemiol.* 1998;51:1139–1147.

212. Duncan PW, Samsa GP, Weinberger M, Goldstein LB, Bonito A, Witter DM, Enarson C, Matchar D. Health status of individuals with mild stroke. *Stroke.* 1997;28:740–745.

213. Russo J, Trujillo CA, Wingerson D, Decker K, Ries R, Wetzler H, Roy-Byrne P. The MOS 36-Item Short Form Health Survey: reliability, validity, and preliminary findings in schizophrenic outpatients. *Med Care.* 1998;36:752–756.

214. Schlenk EA, Erlen JA, Dunbar Jacob J, McDowell J, Engberg S, Sereika SM, Rohay JM, Bernier MJ. Health-related quality of life in chronic disorders: a comparison across studies using the MOS SF-36. *Qual Life Res.* 1998;7:57–65.

215. Wu AW, Hays RD, Kelly S, Malitz F, Bozzette SA. Applications of the Medical Outcomes Study health-related quality of life measures in HIV/AIDS. *Qual Life Res.* 1997;6:531–554.

216. de Jong Z, van der Heijde D, McKenna SP, Whalley D. The reliability and construct validity of the RAQoL: a rheumatoid arthritis-specific quality of life instrument. *Br J Rheumatol.* 1997;36:878–883.

217. Vo TX, Guillemin F, Deschamps JP. Psychometric properties of the DUKE Health Profile-adolescent version (DHP-A): a generic instrument for adolescents. *Qual Life Res.* 2005;14:2229–2234.

218. Guillemin F, Paul-Dauphin A, Virion JM, Bouchet C, Briancon S. The DUKE health profile: a generic instrument to measure the quality of life tied to health. *Sante Publique.* 1997;9:35–44.

219. Nanda U, McLendon PM, Andresen EM, Armbrecht E. The SIP68: an abbreviated sickness impact profile for disability outcomes research. *Qual Life Res.* 2003;12:583–595.

220. Lipsett PA, Swoboda SM, Campbell KA, Cornwell E 3rd, Dorman T, Pronovost PJ. Sickness Impact Profile Score versus a Modified Short-Form survey for functional outcome assessment: acceptability, reliability, and validity in critically ill patients with prolonged intensive care unit stays. *J Trauma.* 2000;49:737–743.

221. Kim KU, Yoon SJ, Lee JL, Ahn HS, Park HJ, Lee SI, Jo MW. Validation of the Korean version of the McMaster Quality of Life Scale in terminal cancer patients. *J Palliat Care.* 2006;22:40–45.

222. Reardon JZ, Lareau SC, ZuWallack R. Functional status and quality of life in chronic obstructive pulmonary disease. *Am J Med.* 2006;119(Suppl 1):32.

223. Rubenstein LM, Voelker MD, Chrischilles EA, Glenn DC, Wallace RB, Rodnitzky RL. The usefulness of the Functional Status Questionnaire and Medical Outcomes Study Short Form in Parkinson's disease research. *Qual Life Res.* 1998;7:279–290.

224. Tillman LJ, Hanks JE. Wound healing: injury and repair of dense connective tissues. In: Hertling D, Kessler RM, eds. *Management of Common Musculoskeletal Conditions.* 4th ed. Philadelphia: Lippincott Williams & Wilkins; 2006:15–26.

225. Junger M, Steins A, Zuder D, Klyscz T. Physical therapy of venous diseases. *Vasa.* 1998;27:73–79 (Abstract).

226. Ogilvie Harris DJ, Myerthall S. The diabetic frozen shoulder: arthroscopic release. *Arthroscopy.* 1997;13:1–8.

227. Siegel LB, Cohen NJ, Gall EP. Adhesive capsulitis: a sticky issue. *Am Fam Physician.* 1999;59:1843–1852.

228. Gam AN, Schydlowsky P, Rossel I, Remvig L, Jensen EM. Treatment of "frozen shoulder" with distension and glucocorticoid compared with glucorticoid alone. A randomised controlled trial. Scand J Rheumatol. 1998;27:425–430.

229. Schenk TJ, Brems JJ. Multidirectional instability of the shoulder: pathophysiology, diagnosis, and management. *J Am Acad Orthop Surg.* 1998;6:65–72.

230. Dias R, Cutts S, Massoud S. Frozen shoulder. *BMJ.* 2005;331:1453–1456.

231. Baker CL Jr, Merkley MS. Clinical evaluation of the athlete's shoulder. *J Athl Train.* 2000;35:256–260.

232. Cornelissen BP, Rijkenhuizen AB, van den Hoogen BM, Rutten VP, Barneveld A. Experimental model of synovitis/capsulitis in the equine metacarpophalangeal joint. *Am J Vet Res.* 1998;59:978–985.

233. Sevier TL, Wilson JK. Treating lateral epicondylitis. *Sports Med.* 1999;28:375–380.

234. Barozzi L, Olivieri I, De Matteis M, Padula A, Pavlica P. Seronegative spondylarthropathies: imaging of spondylitis, enthesitis and dactylitis. *Eur J Radiol.* 1998;27(Suppl 1):S12–S17.

235. Coari G, Paoletti F, Iagnocco A. Shoulder involvement in rheumatic diseases. Sonographic findings. *J Rheumatol.* 1999;26:668–673.

236. Hjelm R, Draper C, Spencer S. Anterior-inferior capsular length insufficiency in the painful shoulder. *J Orthop Sports Phys Ther.* 1996;23:216–222.

237. Rozzi SL, Lephart SM, Gear WS, Fu FH. Knee joint laxity and neuromuscular characteristics of male and female soccer and basketball players. *Am J Sports Med.* 1999;27:312–319.

238. Messina DF, Farney WC, DeLee JC. The incidence of injury in Texas high school basketball: a prospective study among male and female athletes. *Am J Sports Med.* 1999;27:294–299.

239. Harris NL. Physical diagnosis of collateral ligament and combined ligament injuries. *Oper Techniq Sports Med.* 1996;4:148–157.

240. Cyriax J. *Textbook of Orthopedic Medicine. Vol 1. Diagnosis of Soft Tissue Lesions.* 7th ed. London: Bailliere Tindall; 1978.

241. Fritz JM, Delitto A, Erhard RE, Roman M. An examination of the selective tissue tension scheme, with evidence for the concept of a capsular pattern of the knee. *Phys Ther.* 1998;78:1046–1056.

242. Pellecchia GL, Paolino J, Connell J. Intertester reliability of the cyriax evaluation in assessing patients with shoulder pain. *J Orthop Sports Phys Ther.* 1996;23:34–38.

243. Wilk KE, Andrews JR, Arrigo CA. The physical examination of the glenohumeral joint: emphasis on the stabilizing structures. *J Orthop Sports Phys Ther.* 1997;25:380–389.

244. Blevins FT. Rotator cuff pathology in athletes. *Sports Med.* 1997;24:205–220.

245. van Dijk CN, Mol BW, Lim LS, Marti RK, Bossuyt PM. Diagnosis of ligament rupture of the ankle joint. Physical examination, arthrography, stress radiography and sonography compared in 160 patients after inversion trauma. *Acta Orthop Scand.* 1996;67:566–570.

246. White DJ. Musculoskeletal assessment. In: O'Sullivan SB, Schmitz TJ, eds. *Physical Rehabilitation.* 6th ed. Philadelphia: FA Davis Company; 2006:101–133.

247. Norkin CC, White JD. *Measurement of Joint Motion: A Guide to Goniometry.* 3rd ed. Philadelphia: FA Davis Company; 2003.

248. Gilliam J, Barstow IK. Joint range of motion. In: Van Deusen J, Brunt D, eds. *Assessment in Occupational Therapy and Physical Therapy.* Philadelphia: WB Saunders; 1997.

249. MacDermid JC, Chesworth BM, Patterson S, Roth JH. Intratester and intertester reliability of goniometric measurement of passive lateral shoulder rotation. *J Hand Ther.* 1999;12:187–192.

250. Thoms V, Rome K. Effect of subject position on the reliability of measurement of active ankle joint dorsiflexion. *Int J Clin Foot Sci.* 1997;7:153–158.

251. Bruton A, Ellis B, Goddard J. Comparison of visual estimation and goniometry for assessment of metacarpophalangeal joint angle. *Physiotherapy.* 1999;85:201–208.

252. Somers DL, Hanson JA, Kedzierski CM, Nestor KL, Quinlivan KY. The influence of experience on the reliability of goniometric and visual measurement of forefoot position. *J Orthop Sports Phys Ther.* 1997;25:192–202.

253. Meyer DC, Werner CM, Wyss T, Vienne P. A mechanical equinometer to measure the range of motion of the ankle joint: interobserver and intraobserver reliability. *Foot Ankle Int.* 2006;27:202–205.

254. Ellis B, Bruton A, Goddard JR. Joint angle measurement: a comparative study of the reliability of goniometry and wire tracing for the hand. *Clin Rehabil.* 1997;11:314–320.

255. Neumann D. *Kinesiology of the Musculoskeletal System.* St. Louis, MO: Mosby; 2002.

256. O'Sullivan SB, Schmitz TJ, eds. *Physical Rehabilitation.* 6th ed. Philadelphia: FA Davis Company; 2006.

257. Gajdosik RL. Comparison and reliability of three goniometric methods for measuring forearm supination and pronation. *Percept Mot Skills.* 2001;93:353–355.

258. Flowers KR, Stephens-Chisar J, LaStayo P, Galante BL. Intrarater reliability of a new method and instrumentation for measuring passive supination and pronation: a preliminary study. *J Hand Ther.* 2001;14:30–35.

259. Brosseau L, Balmer S, Tousignant M, O'Sullivan JP, Goudreault C, Goudreault M, Gringras S. Intra- and intertester reliability and criterion validity of the parallelogram and universal goniometers for measuring maximum active knee flexion and extension of patients with knee restrictions. *Arch Phys Med Rehabil.* 2001;82:396–402.

260. Ellis B, Bruton A. A study to compare the reliability of composite finger flexion with goniometry for measurement of range of motion in the hand. *Clin Rehabil.* 2002;16:562–570.

261. Menadue C, Raymond J, Kilbreath SL, Refshauge KM, Adams R. Reliability of two goniometric methods of measuring active inversion and eversion range of motion at the ankle. *BMC Musculoskelet Disord.* 2006;7:60.

262. Stam HJ, Ardon MS, den Ouden AC, Schreuders TA, Roebroeck ME. The compangle: a new goniometer for joint angle measurements of the hand. A technical note. *Eura Medicophys.* 2006;42:37–40.

263. Brosseau L, Tousignant M, Budd J, Chartier N, Duciaume L, Plamondon S, O'Sullivan JP, O'Donoghue S, Balmer S. Intratester and intertester reliability and criterion validity of the parallelogram and universal goniometers for active knee flexion in healthy subjects. *Physiother Res Int.* 1997;2:150–166.

264. Ellis B, Bruton A, Goddard JR. Joint angle measurement: a comparative study of the reliability of goniometry and wire tracing for the hand. *Clin Rehabil.* 1997;11:314–320.

265. Holm I, Bolstad B, Lutken T, Ervik A, Rokkum M, Steen H. Reliability of goniometric measurements and visual estimates of hip ROM in patients with osteoarthrosis. *Physiother Res Int.* 2000;5:241–248.

266. Chiu HY, Su FC. The motion analysis system and the maximal area of fingertip motion. A preliminary report. *J Hand Surg Br.* 1996;21:604–608.

267. Klein PJ, DeHaven JJ. Accuracy of three-dimensional linear and angular estimates obtained with the Ariel Performance Analysis System. *Arch Phys Med Rehabil.* 1995;76:183–189.

268. Friedrichsen K. The validity and reliability of a two-dimensional computer-assisted video gait analysis system. *Diss Abstr Int.* 1995;33-06:1863.

269. Mueller MJ, Norton BJ. Reliability of kinematic measurements of rear-foot motion. *Phys Ther.* 1992;72:731–737.

270. Maulucci RA, Eckhouse RH. A technique for measuring clothed range of joint motion. *J Appl Biomech.* 1997;13:316–333.

271. Williams GN, Gangel TJ, Arciero RA, Uhorchak JM, Taylor DC. Comparison of the Single Assessment Numeric Evaluation method and two shoulder rating scales: outcomes measures after shoulder surgery. *Am J Sports Med.* 1999;27:214–221.

272. Love S, Gringmuth RH, Kazemi M, Cornacchia P, Schmolke M. Interexaminer and intraexaminer reliability of cervical

passive range of motion using the CROM and Cybex 320 EDI. *J Can Chiropract Assoc.* 1998;42:222–228.

273. Barrett CJ, Singer KP, Day R. Assessment of combined movements of the lumbar spine in asymptomatic and low back pain subjects using a three-dimensional electromagnetic tracking system. *Manual Ther.* 1999;4:94–99.

274. Nitschke JE, Nattrass CL, Disler PB, Chou MJ, Ooi KT. Reliability of the American Medical Association guides model for measuring spinal range of motion. Its implication for whole-person impairment rating. *Spine.* 1999;24:262–268.

275. Evans K, Refshauge KM, Adams R. Measurement of active rotation in standing: reliability of a simple test protocol. *Percept Mot Skills.* 2006;103:619–628.

276. Ng JK, Kippers V, Richardson CA, Parnianpour M. Range of motion and lordosis of the lumbar spine: reliability of measurement and normative values. *Spine.* 2001;26:53–60.

277. Troke M, Moore AP, Cheek E. Reliability of the OSI CA 6000 Spine Motion Analyzer with a new skin fixation system when used on the thoracic spine. *Manual Ther.* 1998;3:27–33.

278. Harrison DE, Haas JW, Cailliet R, Harrison DD, Holland B, Janik TJ. Concurrent validity of flexicurve instrument measurements: sagittal skin contour of the cervical spine compared with lateral cervical radiographic measurements. *J Manipulative Physiol Ther.* 2005;28:597–603.

279. Piva SR, Erhard RE, Childs JD, Hicks G, Al-Abdulmohsin H. Reliability of measuring iliac crest level in the standing and sitting position using a new measurement device. *J Manipulative Physiol Ther.* 2003;26:437–441.

280. Viitanen JV, Kokko ML, Heikkila S, Kautiainen H. Assessment of thoracolumbar rotation in ankylosing spondylitis: a simple tape method. *Clin Rheumatol.* 1999;18:152–157.

281. Hresko MT, Mesiha M, Richards K, Zurakowski D. A comparison of methods for measuring spinal motion in female patients with adolescent idiopathic scoliosis. *J Pediatr Orthop.* 2006;26:758–763.

282. Morphett AL, Crawford CM, Lee D. The use of electromagnetic tracking technology for measurement of passive cervical range of motion: a pilot study. *J Manipulative Physiol Ther.* 2003;26:152–159.

283. Hagins M, Brown M, Cook C, Gstalder K, Kam M, Kominer G, Strimbeck K. Intratester and intertester reliability of the Palpation Meter (PALM) in measuring pelvic position. *J Manual Manipulative Ther.* 1998;6:130–136.

284. Katenborn F. Manual Mobilization of the Joints: The Extremities. Minneapolis: Orthopedic Physical Therapy Products, 2002.

285. Fjellner A, Bexander C, Feleij R, Strender L. Interexaminer reliability in physical examination of the cervical spine. *J Manipulative Physiol Ther.* 1999;22:511–516.

286. Ellem D. Assessment of the wrist, hand and finger complex. *J Manual Manipulative Ther.* 1995;3:9–14.

287. Olson KA, Paris SV, Spohr C, Gorniak G. Radiographic assessment and reliability study of the craniovertebral sidebending test. *J Manual Manipulative Ther.* 1998;6:87–96.

288. Huber FE, Irrgang JJ, Harner C, Lephart S. Intratester and intertester reliability of the KT-1000 arthrometer in the assessment of posterior laxity of the knee. *Am J Sports Med.* 1997;25:479–485.

289. Malanga GA, Andrus S, Nadler SF, McLean J. Physical examination of the knee: a review of the original test description and

scientific validity of common orthopedic tests. *Arch Phys Med Rehabil.* 2003;84:592–603.

290. Zchezewski JE. Improving flexibility. In: Scully RM, Barnes MR, eds. *Physical Therapy.* Philadelphia: J. B. Lippincott Company; 1989.

291. Simons DG, Mense S. Understanding and measurement of muscle tone as related to clinical muscle pain. *Pain.* 1998; 75:1–17.

292. Santi MD, Botte MJ. Volkmann's ischemic contracture of the foot and ankle: evaluation and treatment of established deformity. *Foot Ankle Int.* 1995;16:368–377.

293. O'Dwyer NJ, Ada L, Neilson PD. Spasticity and muscle contracture following stroke. *Brain.* 1996;119:1737–1749.

294. Niamane R, Birouk N, Benomar A, Benabdejlil M, Amarti A, Yahyaoui M, Chkili T, Hajjaj Hassouni N. Rigid spine syndrome. Two case-reports. *Rev Rhum Engl Ed.* 1999;66:347–350.

295. Noonan TJ, Garrett WE Jr. Muscle strain injury: diagnosis and treatment. *J Am Acad Orthop Surg.* 1999;7:262–269.

296. Almekinders LC. Tendinitis and other chronic tendinopathies. *J Am Acad Orthop Surg.* 1998;6:157–164.

297. Khan KM, Cook JL, Bonar F, Harcourt P, Astrom M. Histopathology of common tendinopathies. Update and implications for clinical management. *Sports Med.* 1999;27:393–408.

298. Fredriksen H, Dagfinrud H, Jacobsen V, Maehlum S. Passive knee extension test to measure hamstring muscle tightness. *Scand J Med Sci Sports.* 1997;7:279–282.

299. Jones CJ, Rikli RE, Max J, Noffal G. The reliability and validity of a chair sit-and-reach test as a measure of hamstring flexibility in older adults. *Res Q Exerc Sport.* 1998;69:338–343.

300. Tyler TF, Roy T, Nicholas SJ, Gleim GW. Reliability and validity of a new method of measuring posterior shoulder tightness. *J Orthop Sports Phys Ther.* 1999;29:262–269.

301. Scully RM, Barnes MR, eds. *Physical Therapy.* Philadelphia: J. B. Lippincott Company; 1989.

302. Reese NB, Bandy WD. Use of an inclinometer to measure flexibility of the iliotibial band using the Ober test and the modified Ober test: differences in magnitude and reliability of measurements. *J Orthop Sports Phys Ther.* 2003;33:326–330.

303. Reid DA, McNair PJ. Passive force, angle, and stiffness changes after stretching of hamstring muscles. *Med Sci Sports Exerc.* 2004;36:1944–1948.

304. Cornbleet SL, Woolsey NB. Assessment of hamstring muscle length in school-aged children using the sit-and-reach test and the inclinometer measure of hip joint angle. *Phys Ther.* 1996;76:850–855.

305. Allison GT, Weston R, Shaw R, Longhurst J, James L, Kyle K, Nehyba K, Low SM, May M. The reliability of quadriceps muscle stiffness in individuals with Osgood-Schlatter disease. *J Sport Rehabil.* 1998;7:258–266.

306. Siems JJ, Breur GJ, Blevins WE, Cornell KK. Use of two-dimensional real-time ultrasonography for diagnosing contracture and strain of the infraspinatus muscle in a dog. *J Am Vet Med Assoc.* 1998;212:77–80.

307. Kendall E, Provance P, Rodgers M, Romani W. *Muscles: Testing and Function, with Posture and Pain.* Philadelphia: Lippincott Williams & Wilkins; 2005.

308. Knepler C, Bohannon RW. Subjectivity of forces associated with manual-muscle test grades of 3+, 4−, and 4. *Percept Mot Skills.* 1998;87:1123–1128.

309. Jain M, Smith M, Cintas H, Koziol D, Wesley R, Harris-Love M, Lovell D, Rider LG, Hicks J. Intra-rater and inter-rater reliability of the 10-point Manual Muscle Test (MMT) of strength in children with juvenile idiopathic inflammatory myopathies (JIIM). *Phys Occup Ther Pediatr.* 2006;26:5–17.

310. Fournier K, Bourbonnais D, Bravo G, Arsenault J, Harris P, Gravel D. Reliability and validity of pinch and thumb strength measurements in de Quervain's disease. *J Hand Ther.* 2006;19:2–10.

311. Li RC, Jasiewicz JM, Middleton J, Condie P, Barriskill A, Hebnes H, Purcell B. The development, validity, and reliability of a manual muscle testing device with integrated limb position sensors. *Arch Phys Med Rehabil.* 2006;87:411.

312. Hogrel JY, Ollivier G, Desnuelle C. Manual and quantitative muscle testing in neuromuscular disorders. How to assess the consistency of strength measurements in clinical trials? *Rev Neurol (Paris).* 2006;162:427–436.

313. Krause DA, Schlagel SJ, Stember BM, Zoetewey JE, Hollman JH. Influence of lever arm and stabilization on measures of hip abduction and adduction torque obtained by hand-held dynamometry. *Arch Phys Med Rehabil.* 2007;88:37–42.

314. Ladeira CE, Hess LW, Galin BM, Fradera S, Harkness MA. Validation of an abdominal muscle strength test with dynamometry. *J Strength Cond Res.* 2005;19:925–930.

315. Burns SP, Spanier DE. Break-technique handheld dynamometry: relation between angular velocity and strength measurements. *Arch Phys Med Rehabil.* 2005;86:1420–1426.

316. Bohannon RW. Internal consistency of manual muscle testing scores. *Percept Mot Skills.* 1997;85:736–768.

317. Bohannon RW. Manual muscle testing: does it meet the standards of an adequate screening test? *Clin Rehabil.* 2005;19:662–667.

318. Bohannon RW. Research incorporating hand-held dynamometry: publication trends since 1948. *Percept Mot Skills.* 1998;86:1177–1178.

319. Reinking MF, Bockrath Pugliese K, Worrell T, Kegerreis RL, Miller-Sayers K, Farr J. Assessment of quadriceps muscle performance by hand-held, isometric, and isokinetic dynamometry in patients with knee dysfunction. *J Orthop Sports Phys Ther.* 1996;24:154–159.

320. Risberg MA, Holm I, Tjomsland O, Ljunggren E, Ekeland A. Prospective study of changes in impairments and disabilities after anterior cruciate ligament reconstruction. *J Orthop Sports Phys Ther.* 1999;29:400–412.

321. Binder Macleod SA, Lee SCK, Fritz AD, Kucharski LJ. New look at force-frequency relationship of human skeletal muscle: effects of fatigue. *J Neurophysiol.* 1998;79:1858–1868.

322. Wilkerson GB, Pinerola JJ, Caturano RW. Invertor vs. evertor peak torque and power deficiencies associated with lateral ankle ligament injury. *J Orthop Sports Phys Ther.* 1997;26:78–86.

323. Whitcomb LJ, Kelley MJ, Leiper CI. A comparison of torque production during dynamic strength testing of shoulder abduction in the coronal plane and the plane of the scapula. *J Orthop Sports Phys Ther.* 1995;21:227–232.

324. Bridgewater KJ, Sharpe MH. Trunk muscle performance in early Parkinson's disease. *Phys Ther.* 1998;78:566–576.

325. Fleming SL, Jansen CW, Hasson SM. Effect of work glove and type of muscle action on grip fatigue. *Ergonomics.* 1997;40:601–612.

326. Moller M, Lind K, Styf J, Karlsson J. The reliability of isokinetic testing of the ankle joint and a heel-raise test for endurance. *Knee Surg Sports Traumatol Arthrosc.* 2005;13:60–71.

327. Wang SS, Normile SO, Lawshe BT. Reliability and smallest detectable change determination for serratus anterior muscle strength and endurance tests. *Physiother Theory Pract.* 2006;22:33–42.

328. Kaegi C, Thibault M, Giroux F, Bourbonnais D. The interrater reliability of force measurements using a modified sphygmomanometer in elderly subjects. *Phys Ther.* 1998;78:1095–1203.

329. Sherrington C, Lord SR. Reliability of simple portable tests of physical performance in older people after hip fracture. *Clin Rehabil.* 2005;19:496–504.

330. Perell KL, Gregor RJ, Scremin AME. Lower limb cycling mechanics in subjects with unilateral cerebrovascular accidents. *J Appl Biomech.* 1998;14:158–179.

331. Bohannon RW. Alternatives for measuring knee extension strength of the elderly at home. *Clin Rehabil.* 1998;12:434–440.

332. Smith LK, Weiss EL, Lehmkuhl LD. *Brunnstrom's Clinical Kinesiology.* 5th ed. Philadelphia: FA Davis Company; 1996.

333. Maruyama K. Connectin, an elastic protein of striated muscle. *Biophys Chem.* 1994;50:73–85.

334. Prado LG, Markarenko I, Andresen C, Kruger M, Opitz CA, Linke WA. Isoform diversity of giant proteins in relation to passive and active contractile properties of rabbit skeletal muscles. *J Gen Physiol.* 2005;126:461–480.

335. Campbell KS, Lakie M. A cross-bridge mechanism can explain the thixotropic short-range elastic component of relaxed frog skeletal muscle. *J Physiol Lond.* 1998;510:941–962.

336. O'Sullivan SB. Strategies to improve motor learning and motor control. In: O'Sullivan SB, Schmitz TJ, eds. *Physical Rehabilitation.* 6th ed. Philadelphia: FA Davis Company; 2006:363–411.

337. Katavich L. Neural mechanisms underlying manual cervical traction. *J Manual Manipulative Ther.* 1999;7:20–25.

338. Katavich L. Differential effects of spinal manipulative therapy on acute and chronic muscle spasm: a proposal for mechanisms and efficacy. *Manual Ther.* 1998;3:132–139.

339. Kovac C, Krapf M, Ettlin T, Mennet P, Stratz T, Muller W. Methods for detection of changes in muscle tonus. *Z Rheumatol.* 1994;53:26–36 (Abstract).

340. Dvorak J. Epidemiology, physical examination, and neurodiagnostics. *Spine.* 1998;23:2663–2673.

341. Maigne JY, Doursounian L. Entrapment neuropathy of the medial superior cluneal nerve: nineteen cases surgically treated, with a minimum of 2 years' follow-up. *Spine.* 1997;22:1156–1159.

342. van Deursen RW, Sanchez MM, Derr JA, Becker MB, Ulbrecht JS, Cavanagh PR. Vibration perception threshold testing in patients with diabetic neuropathy: ceiling effects and reliability. *Diabet Med.* 2001;18:469–475.

343. Billi A, Catalucci A, Barile A, Masciocchi C. Joint impingement syndrome: clinical features. *Eur J Radiol.* 1998;27(Suppl 1)S39–S41.

344. Idler RS. General principles of patient evaluation and nonoperative management of cubital syndrome. *Hand Clin.* 1996;12:397–403.

345. Nakano KK. Nerve entrapment syndromes. *Curr Opin Rheumatol.* 1997;9:165–173.

346. Huang KC, Chen YJ, Hsu RW. Anterior tarsal tunnel syndrome: case report. *Chang Keng I Hsueh Tsa Chih.* 1999;22: 503–507.

347. Preston DC. Distal median neuropathies. *Neurol Clin.* 1999; 17:407–424.

348. Lee CY. Lower limb entrapment neuropathies. *Phys Med Rehabil State Art Rev.* 1999;13:231–249.

349. Cherniack MG, Moalli D, Viscolli C. A comparison of traditional electrodiagnostic studies, electroneurometry, and vibrometry in the diagnosis of carpal tunnel syndrome. *J Hand Surg Am.* 1996;21:122–131.

350. Kleindienst A, Hamm B, Hildebrandt G, Klug N. Diagnosis and staging of carpal tunnel syndrome: comparison of magnetic resonance imaging and intra-operative findings. *Acta Neurochir Wien.* 1996;138:228–233.

351. Manni E, Petrosini L. Luciani's work on the cerebellum a century later. *Trends Neurosci.* 1997;20:112–116.

352. Gorassini MA, Bennett DJ, Yang JF. Self-sustained firing of human motor units. *Neurosci Lett.* 1998;247:13–16.

353. O'Dwyer NJ, Ada L. Reflex hyperexcitability and muscle contracture in relation to spastic hypertonia. *Curr Opin Neurol.* 1996;9:451–455.

354. Jepsen JR, Laursen LH, Hagert CG, Kreiner S, Larsen AI. Diagnostic accuracy of the neurological upper limb examination II: relation to symptoms of patterns of findings. *BMC Neurol.* 2006;6:10.

355. Agostinucci J. Upper motor neuron syndrome. In: Van Deusen J, Brunt D, eds. *Assessment in Occupational Therapy and Physical Therapy.* Philadelphia: WB Saunders; 1997.

356. Clarkson HM, Gilewich BG. *Musculoskeletal Assessment: Joint Range of Motion and Manual Muscle Strength.* Baltimore: Williams and Wilkins; 1989.

357. Shaw J, Bially J, Deurvorst N, Macfie C, Brouwer B. Clinical and physiological measures of tone in chronic stroke. *Neurol Rep.* 1999;23:19–24.

358. Yam WK, Leung MS. Interrater reliability of Modified Ashworth Scale and Modified Tardieu Scale in children with spastic cerebral palsy. *J Child Neurol.* 2006;21:1031–1035.

359. Mehrholz J, Wagner K, Meissner D, Grundmann K, Zange C, Koch R, Pohl M. Reliability of the Modified Tardieu Scale and the Modified Ashworth Scale in adult patients with severe brain injury: a comparison study. *Clin Rehabil.* 2005;19:751–759.

360. Smith AW, Jamshidi M, Lo SK. Clinical measurement of muscle tone using a velocity-corrected modified Ashworth scale. *Am J Phys Med Rehabil.* 2002;81:202–206.

361. Singer BJ, Dunne JW, Singer KP, Allison GT. Velocity dependent passive plantar flexor resistive torque in patients with acquired brain injury. *Clin Biomech.* 2003;18:157–165.

362. Smith AW, Kirtley C, Jamshidi M. Fleuren JF, Nederhand MJ, Hermens HJ. Intrarater reliability of manual passive move-

363. Fleuren JF, Nederhand MJ, Hermens HJ. Influence of posture and muscle length on stretch reflex activity in poststroke patients with spasticity. *Arch Phys Med Rehabil.* 2006;87: 981–988.

364. Kakebeeke TH, Lechner H, Baumberger M, Denoth J, Michel D, Knecht H. The importance of posture on the isokinetic assessment of spasticity. *Spinal Cord.* 2002;40:236–243.

365. Lin CC, Ju MS, Huang HW. Muscle tone in diabetic polyneuropathy evaluated by the quantitative pendulum test. *Arch Phys Med Rehabil.* 2007;88:368–373.

366. Lechner HE, Frotzler A, Eser P. Relationship between self- and clinically rated spasticity in spinal cord injury. *Arch Phys Med Rehabil.* 2006;87:15–19.

367. McDonald MF, Kevin Garrison M, Schmit BD. Length-tension properties of ankle muscles in chronic human spinal cord injury. *J Biomech.* 2005;38:2344–2353.

368. Rabita G, Dupont L, Thevenon A, Lensel-Corbeil G, Perot C, Vanvelcenaher J. Quantitative assessment of the velocity-dependent increase in resistance to passive stretch in spastic plantar flexors. *Clin Biomech.* 2005;20:745–753.

369. Peng Q, Shah P, Selles R, Gaebler-Spira D, Zhang LQ. Measurement of ankle spasticity in children with cerebral palsy using a manual spasticity evaluator. *Conf Proc IEEE Eng Med Biol Soc.* 2004;7:4896–4899.

370. Sabari J. Motor control. In: Van Deusen J, Brunt D, eds. *Assessment in Occupational Therapy and Physical Therapy.* Philadelphia: WB Saunders; 1997.

371. Vattanasilp W, Ada L. The relationship between clinical and laboratory measures of spasticity. *Aust J Physiother.* 1999;45: 135–139.

372. Rabadi MH, Rabadi FM. Comparison of the action research arm test and the Fugl-Meyer assessment as measures of upper-extremity motor weakness after stroke. *Arch Phys Med Rehabil.* 2006;87:962–966.

373. Hsueh IP, Hsieh CL. Responsiveness of two upper extremity function instruments for stroke inpatients receiving rehabilitation. *Clin Rehabil.* 2002;16:617–624.

374. Shelton FD, Volpe BT, Reding M. Motor impairment as a predictor of functional recovery and guide to rehabilitation treatment after stroke. *Neurorehabil Neural Repair.* 2001;15: 229–237.

375. Chae J, Labatia I, Yang G. Upper limb motor function in hemiparesis: concurrent validity of the Arm Motor Ability test. *Am J Phys Med Rehabil.* 2003;82:1–8.

376. Kelly PJ, Furie KL, Shafqat S, Rallis N, Chang Y, Stein J. Functional recovery following rehabilitation after hemorrhagic and ischemic stroke. *Arch Phys Med Rehabil.* 2003;84:968–972.

# Part II  Treatment and Discharge

The chapters in Part II cover the later phases of the clinical decision-making process: the Treatment Phase and the Discharge Phase. Chapter 6, Preparation and Positioning for Massage, describes how the therapist prepares for treatment, as well as the techniques for positioning and draping the client for treatment. Chapters 7 through 12 introduce categories of related massage techniques, describe in detail how to apply each technique, and describe common uses of these techniques in interventions. These chapters also include discussions of the descriptive components (see Box 1), outcomes of care, research evidence, indications, contraindications, and cautions associated with each technique. Chapter 13, Sequencing Massage Techniques, describes the principles and processes that therapists can use to design regional and general sequences of massage techniques. Finally, Chapter 14, Using Massage to Achieve Clinical Outcomes, demonstrates how to use massage techniques to achieve clinical outcomes within interventions for wellness and the treatment of impairments related to common medical conditions. This chapter also describes how to craft comprehensive interventions and progress them from the initial intervention to discharge.

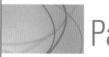 Part II Objectives

After studying Part II, the reader will have the information required to:

1. Outline the materials used to perform massage and how to prepare them.
2. Outline and demonstrate how to position a client for massage of different regions of the body.

---

**Box 1** | **Descriptive Components of Massage Techniques**

**Contact Surface:** The portion of the therapist's hand or arm that is used to execute the stroke.

**Pressure:** The amount of force per unit area of contact surface that the therapist applies. We define categories of pressure as: minimal, engages skin; light, engages subcutaneous fascia and fat; moderate, engages superficial muscle layers; and heavy, engages deeper muscle layers.

**Tissues Engaged:** The target tissues or layers of tissue to which the therapist directs the pressure of the stroke and that are mechanically deformed by the application of the technique.

**Direction:** The direction of the applied force. The direction given in the description of techniques is the direction in which the greatest force is applied during the pressure phase of the stroke. Directions that are commonly specified include: centripetal (towards the heart), centrifugal (away from the heart), and transverse or parallel to the fibers of a reference structure.

**Amplitude:** An indication of the size of the area that is covered by a technique.

**Rate:** An indication of how fast the force is applied. This is a critical component because many desired effects occur only at certain rates of application. The rate may describe the speed of the movement of the therapist's hand over the client's skin (distance per second), the frequency of repetitions of a described technique (repetitions per second), or both.

**Duration:** An estimate of a reasonable length of time for which a single technique may have to be applied by a competent therapist in order to achieve the specified impairment-level outcomes of care. This text provides a minimum duration that can be exceeded at the discretion of the therapist, for example, "10 minutes or greater." If a longer duration of application of a technique can result in side effects or risks, this text provides a suggested upper limit, for example "1 to 10 minutes," and discusses how to determine an appropriate duration of treatment in the accompanying text.

**Variations:** Two common variations are presented in this text: "intergrades with" and "combines with." When one technique is said to "intergrade" with another, the two techniques can be performed consecutively and will merge gradually one into another since there are intermediate hybrid forms of the technique that lie between and resemble both techniques. When one technique is said to "combine" with another, it means that the two techniques may be executed simultaneously.

**Context:** A brief description of how the technique is conventionally sequenced in relation to other techniques.

---

3. Describe and demonstrate how to perform appropriate draping techniques for different regions of the body.

4. Identify six basic categories of massage techniques and describe how each category affects different types of tissues.

5. Describe each massage technique in terms of the contact surface, pressure, tissues engaged, amplitude, direction, and rate.

6. Demonstrate how to perform each massage technique and how to apply it in the context of a practice sequence.

7. Speculate about the mechanisms by which massage techniques achieve their effects.

8. Describe the outcomes of care, indications, contraindications, and common uses associated with each massage technique.

9. Describe evidence-based massage interventions to address specific impairments and wellness goals.

10. Create and progress plans of care for clients with multiple impairments and wellness goals.

# INTELLIGENT PRACTICE OF MASSAGE TECHNIQUES

We advise novice therapists to consider the following guidelines when practicing the application of the massage techniques outlined in Part II.

- Locate the tissues selected for treatment through palpation and be specific in your contact of these tissues.
- Palpate continuously for the response of the client's tissues to your application of the technique.
- Frequently observe and elicit feedback on the client's response to your application of techniques.
- First attempt to achieve penetration to deeper tissue layers through repetition of the technique rather than by increasing the pressure of application.
- Decrease the rate of application when you are treating deeper tissue layers in order to provide a sufficient amount of time for the displacement of fluid and the intervening tissues.
- Obtain feedback on the client's level of comfort after changes of position to eliminate positioning as a source of discomfort during the application of techniques.

- Minimize client discomfort during treatment by modifying your application of techniques to ensure the client's comfort.
- Adapt your application of each technique to the region of the body to which you are applying it.
- Practice each technique individually to achieve competence in the execution of that technique before attempting to combine techniques into massage sequences. Unthinking repetition of any sort of routine may result in an inflexibility of treatment approach that may later impede your appropriate use of techniques in clinical situations.

# Chapter 6
## Preparation and Positioning for Massage

Using massage techniques in treatment requires more than a laying-on of hands during a treatment session. Several other important activities are involved. First, you need to prepare yourself physically and mentally before you begin to interact with the client. Second, you must also select and prepare a variety of treatment materials such as tables, lubricants, and linen. Third, during the intervention, you need to ensure that you have positioned the client appropriately and draped the client both prior to and during the massage. Finally, you need to ensure that you have positioned yourself well and use correct body mechanics during the intervention.

## Preparation and Positioning for Massage: Foundations

### THERAPISTS' PHYSICAL PREPARATION FOR TREATMENT (SELF-CARE)

The practice of massage places considerable strain on your body. In particular, the soft tissues of the back and the upper limb are prone to muscular fatigue, tightness, **trigger point syndromes**, and **repetitive strain injury**. Anyone who uses massage techniques extensively in treatment must develop a comprehensive exercise program that includes aerobic, flexibility, resistance, and balance training in order to maintain a trouble-free level of function and to prevent ongoing damage. Failure to pursue an exercise program can place you at greater risk of injury and increases the likelihood that you will experience burnout. Comprehensive programs are beyond the scope of this book and are detailed elsewhere.[1–3] The following is a selection of exercises that are of particular relevance for therapists who use massage techniques in treatment.

## Movement

Therapists can use different types of **active exercises** for different purposes. Brisk active exercise increases heart rate, local blood flow, tissue temperature, and tissue **extensibility**. You can use active exercise prior to stretching exercises to warm up at the beginning of the workday and after breaks. Figures 6-1 to 6-4 show several shaking and "swinging" exercises for the whole body, which you can use to loosen the muscles of the shoulder girdle, back, and hips in preparation for performing massage.

Very slow, active movements are excellent for tension release and relaxation (Figures 6-5 and 6-6). When performing these exercises, sit or recline comfortably to promote relaxation throughout your body. Then choose a single isolated motion, such as shoulder abduction, and perform it very slowly and at a consistent rate. The rate of movement should be sufficiently slow that it takes 30 to 60 seconds to complete movement through the available range. At the end of the movement, relax completely and rest for several seconds. You may then either repeat that movement or perform a movement for another joint. This procedure is most effective when you use it on several joints.

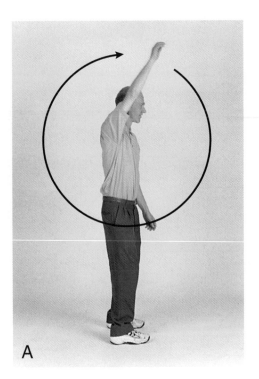

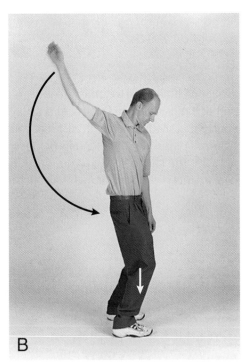

**Figure 6-2** A. Circumduct each arm vigorously 10 to 20 times. This movement opens the shoulder girdle and pushes blood in a centrifugal direction to the hand. B. Perform the movement in both directions. Coordinate bending your knees as your arm descends and straightening your knees as your arm ascends.

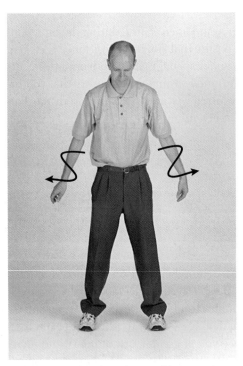

**Figure 6-1** Shaking the hands, wrists, and forearms is a good way to relieve local neuromuscular tension immediately before or after massage. You can do this slowly and in a relaxed fashion or more briskly.

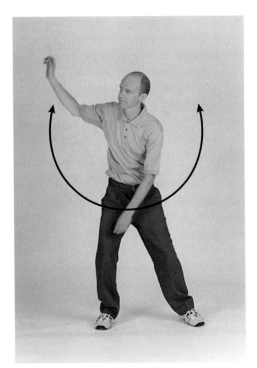

**Figure 6-3** Swing the arms from side to side in the frontal plane; lift both arms up to one side, then relax and allow them to drop passively back down and in front of the body. Then swing them up to the other side, and then relax down again to the center. Produce a continuous movement back and forth like a pendulum.

## Stretching

Stretching techniques are an excellent way to maintain and improve soft tissue **flexibility**, relieve neuromuscular tension, improve capacity for activity, and relieve pain and soreness related to activity.[4-7] There are many different stretching techniques. The following are the basic guidelines for effective static stretching.[5,6]

1. Warm up first with slow active movement.
2. Move to the end of range to the point at which a comfortable stretch is experienced.
3. Breathe deeply throughout the stretch.
4. Hold the stretch position for 15 to 30 seconds.
5. Gently move farther into the range without bouncing.
6. Hold the stretch position for an additional 30 seconds.
7. Stretch both sides equally.
8. Never stretch to the point of experiencing pain.

These stretches target areas that are frequently of concern to therapists who use massage in treatment. You can assemble these into short routines to use at the beginning or end

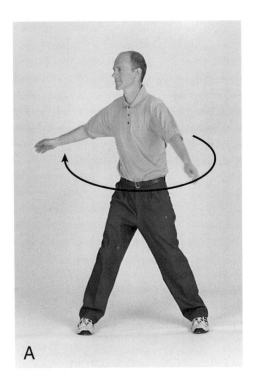

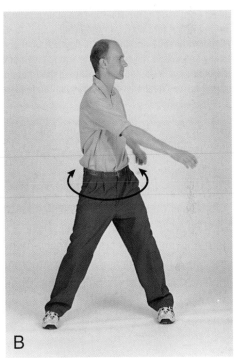

**Figure 6-4** A. Swing the arms in the horizontal plane around the body in one direction and then back again. Allow the movement of the arms to be as loose as possible, so that the hands swing round to tap the opposite shoulder and hip at the end of each movement. B. You can power the movement of the arms by generating a forceful rotation of the trunk and pelvis in one direction and then back again (like a washing machine); the arms follow this movement.

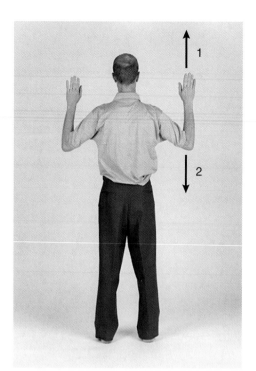

Figure 6-5  Lie supine on the floor in this position. Keep hands, arms, and shoulders as relaxed as possible and maintain maximum contact with the floor without forcing. Slide the arm(s) very slowly up as if reaching "over the head" and then back down. Pause occasionally to relax totally and take a full breath. Allow at least 2 minutes to go through the entire cycle up and down. Repeat the entire movement or concentrate on less fluid portions of the joint range of motion.

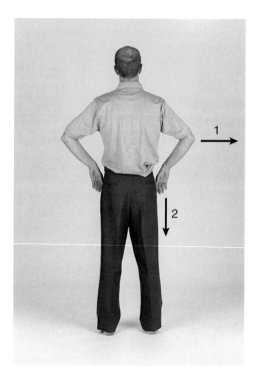

Figure 6-6  Lie supine on the floor in this position. Keep hands, arms, and shoulders as relaxed as possible, and maintain maximum contact with the floor without forcing. Slide the hands very slowly beside the body up toward the armpits (the elbows move out to the side) and then back down. Pause occasionally to relax totally and take a full breath. Allow at least 2 minutes to go through the entire cycle up and down. Repeat the entire movement, or concentrate on less fluid portions of the joint range of motion.

of the work day or even in the brief intervals that arise between clients (Figures 6-7 to 6-25).

## ❓ Critical Thinking Question

Some systems of exercise such as **Hatha Yoga** teach physical conditioning and physical awareness together. Which other systems teach both physical conditioning and physical awareness together? Choose one system and describe how the conditioning and awareness involved in that system will help you to perform massage.

## Self-Massage

Once you acquire some expertise with performing the different massage techniques described later in this text, you can perform them on yourself. Self-massage is particularly useful for relieving the tension that accumulates in your forearms and hands during treatment. You can also incorporate these techniques into your warm-up and cool-down routines (Figures 6-26 to 6-33).

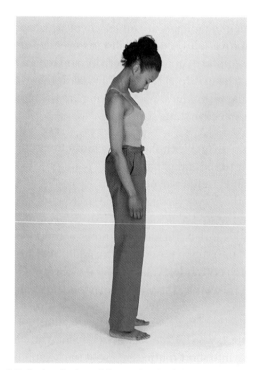

Figure 6-7  Active flexion of the neck—"chin to chest."

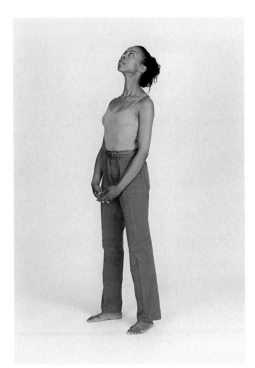

**Figure 6-8** Active extension of the neck. Attempt to elongate the entire neck as cervical extension occurs, rather than just moving the occiput toward the first thoracic vertebra.

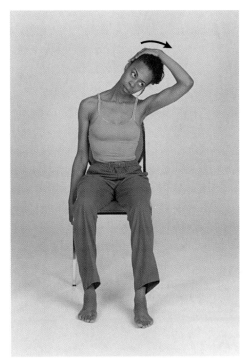

**Figure 6-10** Cervical side-bending with gentle overpressure. You can stabilize the shoulder girdle by holding under the edge of the chair.

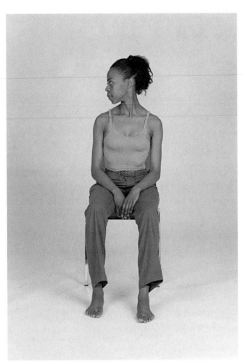

**Figure 6-9** Active cervical rotation.

## Receipt of Skilled Massage

In recent years, as various forms of massage have received growing attention in scientific and public forums, there has been a trend toward allowing students to perform massage with little or no personal experience with skilled massage or related forms of structured touch. This lack of on-the-table experience can make it difficult for students to acquire more than the most basic proficiency in massage. Students cannot rely on each other to demonstrate refined touch in classroom exchanges. In addition, the brief exposure to the touch of qualified teachers in the classroom does not demonstrate overall flow, pacing, and rhythm to the students. Furthermore, although watching experienced therapists work is extremely useful, it fails to convey the subtleties of touch. In addition, the authors have observed that students who have received touch from competent professionals prior to studying massage techniques often demonstrate much more rapid improvement in their manual skills. On this basis, the authors propose that few preparations will facilitate students' achievement of mastery of the craft of massage as much as the repeated receipt of massage or other manual techniques from competent, experienced professionals. This repeated exposure to "Intelligent Touch" can impart certain kinesthetic essentials that cannot be conveyed in words, ideas, or images.

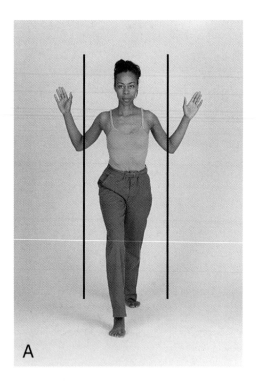

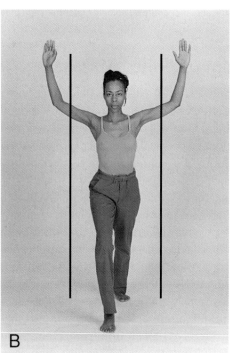

Figure 6-11 A. The "in doorway" stretch for pectoral muscles (the sides of the door frame are represented by the bars). The therapist pushes gently through the door frame toward the viewer, without arching the lower back. This position stretches the clavicular fibers of the pectoralis major. B. The "in doorway" stretch with the arms in the upper position stretches the sternal fibers of the pectoralis major.

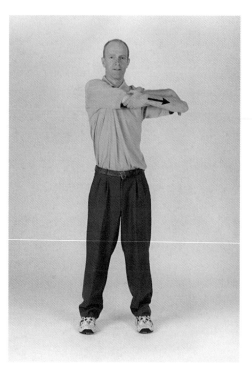

Figure 6-12 To stretch the posterior deltoid, draw the arm across the front of the body toward the opposite shoulder.

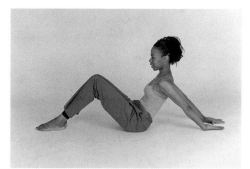

Figure 6-13 You can stretch the biceps brachii in several positions as long as you extend your shoulder and elbow and pronate your forearm. In this position, extending the thoracic spine will intensify the stretch.

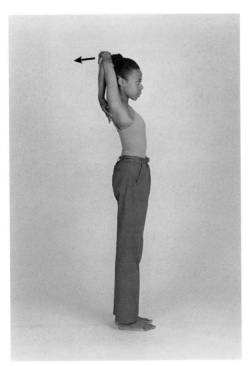

Figure 6-14 To stretch all of the triceps brachii you need to flex your shoulder and your elbow.

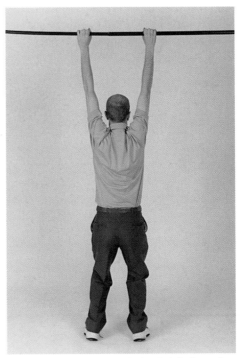

Figure 6-16 Hang from a bar of suitable height (or a door or door frame) to lengthen the entire torso. Maintain contact with ground. Perform a posterior pelvic tilt (tuck the pelvis) to stretch the latissimus dorsi.

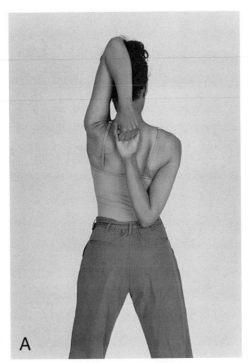
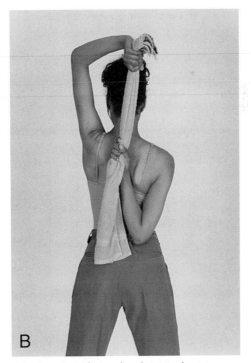

Figure 6-15 A. This behind-the-back clasped-hand position lengthens internal and external rotators of the shoulder on opposite sides. B. A towel can help a less flexible person attain the position. The hands can pull up or down to stretch the opposite shoulder.

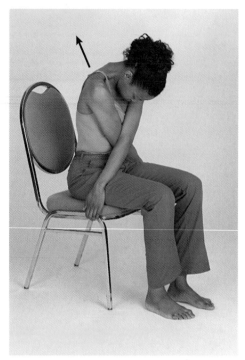

**Figure 6-17** To stretch the interscapular area, assume this position, round the thoracic spine, and push through the sixth thoracic vertebra toward the ceiling.

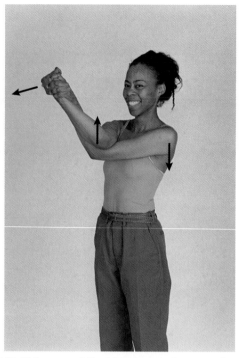

**Figure 6-18** If done carefully, this yoga pose is an excellent stretch for the mid-trapezius. Wrap your arms around each other and simultaneously depress the shoulder girdle, raise your elbows, and push your hands away from your face.

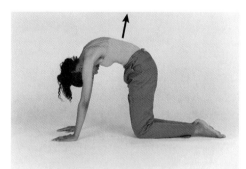

**Figure 6-19** Arch upward to stretch the extensors of your spine. You can shift your weight forward over your arms or back over your knees to focus the stretch more toward the thoracic or the lumbar extensors, respectively.

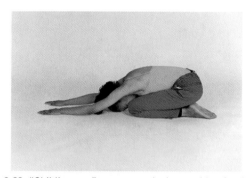

**Figure 6-20** "Child's pose"—a most relaxing position for the back. The buttocks rest on the heels. A less flexible person can place one or two pillows over the posterior calves or the thighs for support.

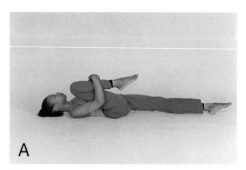

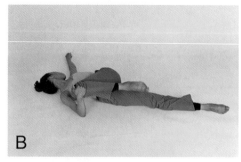

**Figure 6-21** A. "Knee to chest" provides a unilateral stretch of the gluteus maximus in supine. B. "Knee to opposite chest" also stretches the gluteus maximus. To stretch the piriformis, bring the hip down from this position to exactly 90 degrees of flexion.

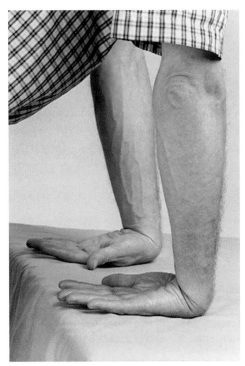

**Figure 6-22** To stretch the wrist extensors, extend the elbows and use a gentle pressure of the dorsum of the hands against a vertical or horizontal surface to move the wrist into flexion. Do not lean on the wrists in this position.

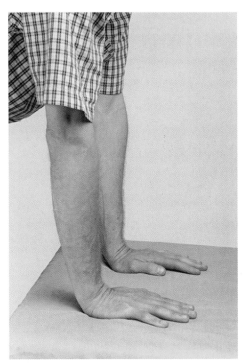

**Figure 6-23** To stretch the wrist flexors, extend the elbows and use a gentle pressure of the palms against a vertical or horizontal surface to take the wrists into extension.

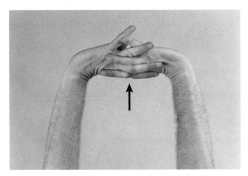

**Figure 6-24** Another flexor stretch. Interlock the fingers and push the hands as far away as possible.

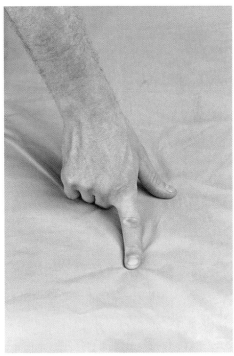

**Figure 6-25** "Finger-splits" stretch the intrinsic muscles of the hand. You can perform a maneuver between each pair of adjacent digits.

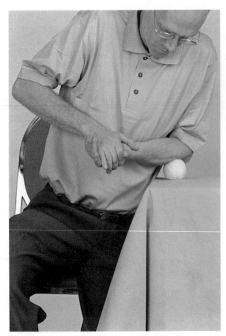

Figure 6-26 Compression administered to the extensors of the forearm with a tennis ball and body weight. See Chapter 9, Neuromuscular Techniques.

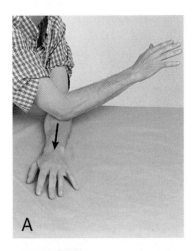

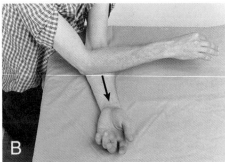

Figure 6-27 A. Self-administered direct fascial technique applied to the extensor surface of the forearm. See Chapter 10, Connective Tissue Techniques. B. Self-administered direct fascial technique applied to the flexor surface of the forearm. See Chapter 10, Connective Tissue Techniques.

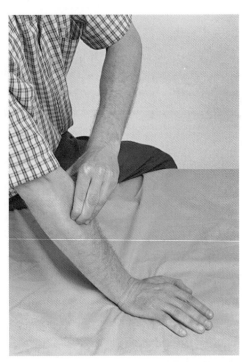

Figure 6-28 Near the common extensor origin is a frequent trouble spot for repetitive strain injuries. From this position, the therapist can apply stripping, direct fascial technique, or friction. See Chapter 9, Neuromuscular Techniques, and Chapter 10, Connective Tissue Techniques.

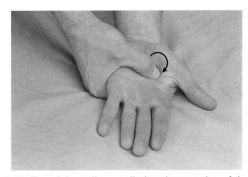

Figure 6-29 Thumb kneading applied to the muscles of the thenar eminence. You can continue this with good effects for 5 to 10 minutes or more per hand. See Chapter 9, Neuromuscular Techniques.

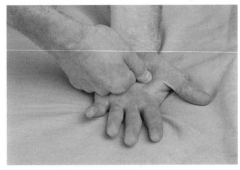

Figure 6-30 Specific digital compression applied with a reinforced thumb to the muscles of the thenar eminence. See Chapter 9, Neuromuscular Techniques.

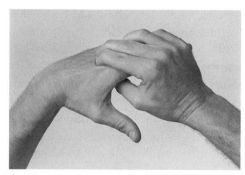

**Figure 6-31** The index finger and the thumb (hidden) work on opposite sides of the intermetacarpal space to free the intrinsic muscles of the hand. Techniques that you can apply in this position include specific compression, stripping, and direct fascial technique. See Chapter 9, Neuromuscular Techniques, and Chapter 10, Connective Tissue Techniques.

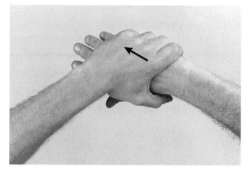

**Figure 6-32** Performing massage exerts considerable compressive force on joints of the wrist and hand that you can counter with the use of self-mobilization. Here, distraction of the wrist includes both proximal and distal carpal joints.

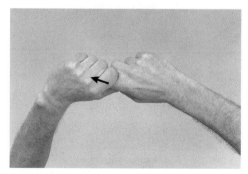

**Figure 6-33** You can perform distraction at the metacarpophalangeal joints and all other joints of the hand.

# THERAPISTS' PSYCHOLOGICAL PREPARATION FOR TREATMENT

You must ensure that you allot adequate time to perform the types of treatment you have scheduled, to review clients' files, to check reference material, and to think about each client. Ideally, you should be able to manage your own treatment schedule. This will enable you to consider and address clients' needs, the facility's policies, charting requirements, reimbursement issues, and your own capacity for performing treatments as you schedule clients. If another individual is responsible for booking, you will need to state your guidelines for booking clearly to that person so that they do not impose an unreasonable and rushed schedule on you.

Once you ensure that you have adequate time for treatment and other supporting activities, you can use some of the physical modalities previously described, such as gentle stretching, to assist your psychological preparation. In the same manner, conscious diaphragmatic breathing, correct body mechanics, and the use of controlled repetitive movement during the performance of massage techniques can deepen your level of relaxation.

Professions that use massage are usually service-oriented professions. You may draw upon a number of different resources for informing and deepening your ethical commitment to others and cultivating an attitude of peaceful, fulfilling service to others. These include a variety of forms of nonsectarian and sectarian spiritual practice such as the use of autogenic or visualization exercises for relaxation or drawing upon an established faith. It is invaluable for you to practice some routine of calming the mind throughout the workday, especially in the few minutes preceding sessions. Since isolation contributes to the experience of "**burnout**" that is so common in service-oriented professions, it is also wise to include in your clinical practice opportunities for interactions with colleagues, such as continuing education courses, review of clients, and professional meetings. Finally, service to others should not be at the expense of taking care of yourself.

# THERAPISTS' PREPARATION OF MATERIALS FOR TREATMENT

## Tables

The treatment table or massage table is an essential tool in the practice of massage. Since treatment tables come in a variety of makes and styles, you should consider your anticipated needs carefully prior to purchasing a table. Any table that you use for massage techniques must be solid, stable, easy to clean, at least 28 by 72 inches, and adjustable for height to accommodate different clients and types of work.

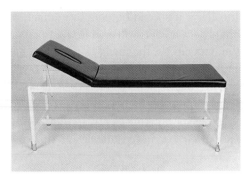

**Figure 6-34** A metal-frame stationary table with face hole and adjustable legs that you can tilt partially.

Ideally, the table will have high-density foam padding on both the top and sides of the tabletop because you may frequently lean or brace yourself against the sides of the table. A well-designed, adjustable face cradle or head support is a desirable addition to the basic treatment table. This is an appropriate alternative to the use of face holes, since the latter rarely fit all clients equally well.

Stationary tables are preferable for the clinic or office setting, since they are extremely strong and stable, although heavy and not easily moved (Figure 6-34). A hydraulic or electric height-adjustable table provides quick adjustment to the different heights that are required for the most efficient application of different techniques.

If you travel frequently to provide care, there are many styles of well-built portable tables from which to choose (Figure 6-35). These tables weigh between 10 and 20 kg, are strong and attractive, are equipped with face cradles and arm shelves, and only lack quick height adjustments. As a result, you may choose to use a portable table for your primary place of practice.

If you select a table that lacks a mechanism for quickly adjusting height, set the table up at a lower height. The use of a lower table height requires you to have training and practice in the correct use of your legs. Novice therapists frequently set their tables too high, which predisposes them to make many errors in body mechanics. When you are performing work that requires use of a substantial amount of body weight, such as **neuromuscular** and **connective tissue techniques**, you may set the height of the table to the level of your extended fingertips or even lower (Figure 6-36). For lighter work, such as superficial reflex and passive movement techniques, you may set the table height to the level of your wrist or even higher.

Portable massage chairs are specifically designed for "on-site" or "mobile" practices of massage (Figure 6-37A). These chairs offer comfort and ease of access to common problem areas for the office worker. They are not, however, very versatile, and some clients may find the half-kneeling position difficult to assume (Figure 6-37B).

Before and between clients, therapists should clean the table, bed, or chair surfaces that come in contact with clients with commercially available disinfectants, and draping should be washed with soap and hot water and rinsed with a 10% bleach solution.[8]

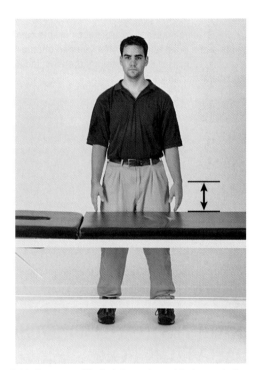

**Figure 6-36** Correct table height varies with the technique that is being performed and the size of the client. Usually, the working height of the table lies between the height of the therapist's wrist and the tips of the extended fingers. Occasionally, the optimal height may be as low as the therapist's knees or as high as the waist.

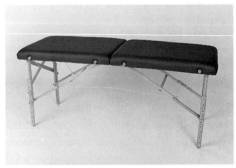

**Figure 6-35** A portable table.

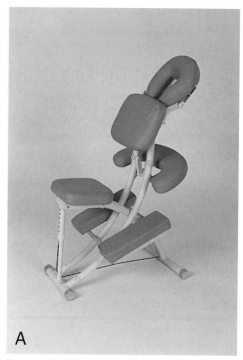
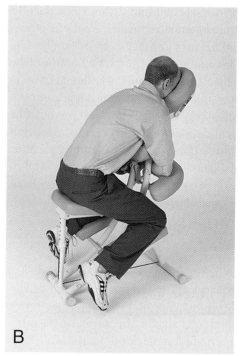

**Figure 6-37** A. Portable massage chair with a strong, light, upholstered frame that folds into an easily carried unit. B. It offers good access to the back and neck.

## Supports

You can use either a commercially designed set of bolsters or a set of pillows when positioning clients on a bed or the floor. In addition, you need a large selection of pillows and bolsters of various sizes and shapes, including at least six standard-sized pillows (Figure 6-38). If necessary, you can place foam- or kapok-filled mats on the floor. The physical demands of working on the floor are extreme, however, and the repertoire of techniques that can be adapted for floor work is limited. Before and between clients, thera-

pists should clean mat surfaces that come into contact with clients with commercially available disinfectants, and draping should be washed with soap and hot water and rinsed with a 10% bleach solution.[8]

## Linen

Sturdy, bleachable, opaque, cotton sheeting in white or pastels are common for clinical use. Although single (twin) flat sheets ensure ample coverage, a slightly narrower width of 50 to 54 inches is easier to handle and can reduce bunching of excess draping. Pillow cases, small and large towels, and blankets are among the basic linen supplies. You must launder any linen that comes into contact with clients after each use with detergent and hot water. Some facilities also use bleach and commercial degreaser. Whenever possible, use professional laundering.

## Lubricants

Therapists use lubricants to control the amount of **glide**, **friction**, and **drag** that occurs between their moving hands and their clients' skin. Although you may apply lubricants to the client's skin, they affect your ability to palpate and produce

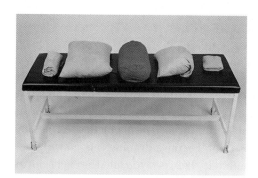

**Figure 6-38** The therapist will require supports in a variety of shapes and sizes.

changes in the client's subcutaneous tissues. Consequently, you require lubricant for some techniques, avoid it for others, and obtain potential benefit for other techniques only when you carefully choose and apply the lubricant. Because of the different requirements for lubricants, you should have on hand a selection of lubricants to facilitate application of a range of techniques. Any lubricant that you use must be hypoallergenic and dispensed in a hygienic manner that does not contaminate the supply such as a squeeze bottle, pump, or shaker. Clients must **consent** to the choice of lubricant and must consent before you add scent to the lubricant as, for example, in **aromatherapy**.

### Oils

Oils continue to be the lubricant of choice for classical **neuromuscular techniques**. You can use virtually any high-quality vegetable oil, including olive, sunflower, safflower, almond, jojoba, and coconut oils. Mineral oil, on the other hand, is considered to be less nutritious for the skin.[9] Each oil has a slightly different density, stickiness, and rate of absorption. Oil has two drawbacks: it goes rancid, and it stains. In addition, you must remove unabsorbed oil from the client's skin with disposable towels, which you can moisten with alcohol.

### Lotions

Lotions are opaque, liquid suspensions of particles in either oil or water. Since lotions are readily absorbed into the client's skin, their lubricating qualities decline quickly with time. This rapid absorption can be an advantage when you are preparing the client's tissues for deeper neuromuscular or **connective tissue techniques**.

### Creams

Creams are thicker suspensions, often oil based, that fall midway between oils and lotions in terms of their rate of absorption. Creams can be quite oily and promote glide. Alternatively, they may contain sticky ingredients, such as lanolin and beeswax, which reduce glide and increase your tendency to drag the client's skin. The ability of some creams to reduce glide may be useful for connective tissue techniques.

### Powders

Use fine powder in the form of French chalk, cornstarch, or unscented baby powder for techniques that require glide and when clients refuse oil. Furthermore, powder is the preferred lubricant for most **lymph-drainage techniques**.

 **Critical Thinking Question**

Assemble a group of different lubricants. Spread them on a variety of body parts in differing amounts. What do you perceive to be the advantages and disadvantages of each type of lubricant?

## POSITIONING AND DRAPING THE CLIENT DURING TREATMENT

### Positioning

In selecting the position for massage, consider the aims of treatment, the areas you wish to access, and your client's preferences and comfort. Prone, supine, side-lying, seated, seated inclined, and long-sitting are common options, each of which has its own specific requirements for pillow placement and support. Box 6-1 summarizes which muscles, tissues, and regions are readily accessible in the common positions used for treatment.

Once you have positioned the client correctly on the treatment table, adjust, add, or remove the pillows, bolsters, or rolled towels used for support to ensure that the client is comfortable. Figures 6-39 to 6-45 illustrate some common positions and how you can support them with pillows. In practice, place pillows beneath the bottom sheet so that you can reuse them without having to recover them. Many other configurations are possible and will be required if you work in a hospital, rehabilitation, sports, or office setting.

### Draping

Draping does more than place the client in a safe, warm, modest, and comfortable position in which to receive the intended massage. Appropriate draping can also serve to achieve and maintain appropriate client–therapist boundaries that therapists need in all practice settings, including the classroom. Because draping sets a symbolic and an actual boundary between you and the client during treatment, you must make draping comfortable yet precise and secured when exposing the client's body for treatment purposes.

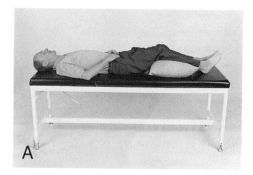

## Box 6-1 — Treatment Positions for Various Muscles

**Prone is an excellent treatment position for:**
Posterior cervical muscles
Latissimus dorsi
Rhomboids
Mid and lower trapezius
Spinal extensors
Gluteus maximus
Hamstrings
Triceps surae
Intrinsic foot muscles

**Supine is an excellent treatment position for:**
All muscles of the head and neck
Pectorals
All muscles of the arm
Abdominals
Quadriceps
Muscles of the anterior compartment

**Side-lying is an excellent treatment position for:**
*On uppermost side of the client's body*
Scalenes
Rotator cuff
Pectoralis minor
Serratus anterior
Abdominals
Quadratus lumborum
Iliocostalis
Gluteus medius and minimus
Iliotibial tract
Peronei

*On lower side of the client's body*
Adductors of the hip
Triceps surae

**Seated upright position is an excellent treatment position for:**
Upper trapezius

**Seated inclined position is an excellent treatment position for:**
All muscles of the posterior aspect of the head and neck
All muscles of the upper back
All muscles of the posterior aspect of the upper arms

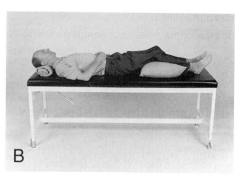

**Figure 6-39** A. Typically therapists use one or two pillows under the knees when a client is in supine to reduce the strain on the lower back. B. You may need an additional pillow or towel roll under the cervical spine for the comfort of clients who have an anterior-head posture.

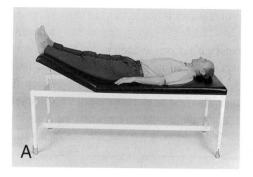

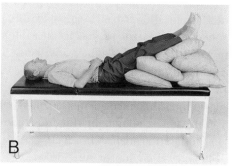

**Figure 6-40** Legs can be elevated for drainage with (A) a tilted treatment table or (B) a mound of pillows.

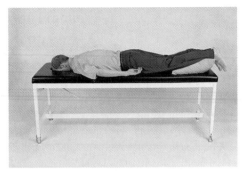

**Figure 6-41** In prone, a single pillow under the ankles takes pressure off the knees.

Your scope of practice, the professional code of conduct, and local laws will dictate what is permissible in terms of exposing the client's body during treatment. When undraping the client, adhere to these rules:

1. Only undrape one body segment at a time.
2. Only undrape areas that are to be treated.
3. Do not undrape the gluteal cleft, perineum, genitals, and female breast.

There are three possible legitimate exceptions to these rules.[10,11] In each case, you must know whether your local laws supersede the exception.

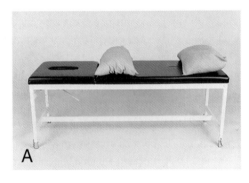

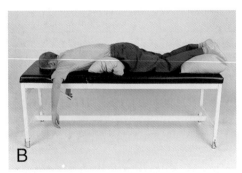

**Figure 6-42** A, B. In prone, an additional small pillow placed under the abdomen can raise the lumbar spine into a less lordotic position. This may reduce the back pain of some clients with low back pain such as those with acute facet derangement.

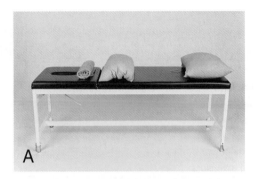

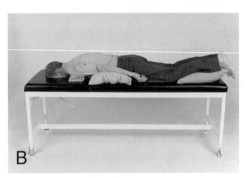

**Figure 6-43** A, B. Add another towel roll under the upper chest to improve comfort for large-breasted women or to take the pressure off the thyroid cartilage.

1. You may expose the female breasts if breast massage is clinically indicated and the client has provided voluntary **informed consent** to this exposure prior to treatment.
2. You may undrape the pelvis if the client has provided voluntary informed consent to massage for the purposes of labor support and/or delivery. Therapists who have the treatment of pelvic floor dysfunction in their professional scope of practice should consult their professional organization for guidelines on draping.
3. You may treat infants undraped with parental consent.

Use the following steps for carrying out draping when massage is a primary modality and you are in a clinical setting with individual treatment rooms and tables. You may modify these procedures if you use massage techniques as an adjunct to other manual or exercise techniques or if you practice in a hospital, rehabilitation, sports, or other setting. Once you have negotiated the plan of care with the client, identify the articles of clothing and jewelry that she will need to remove and explain the rationale for doing so. If the client chooses to remain clothed or partially clothed, you must explain the technical consequences of this choice to the client. Then give the client clear instructions on how to position herself on the table and how to arrange the draping and supports that you have provided. Once you are sure that you have answered the client's questions, leave the room so that the client can

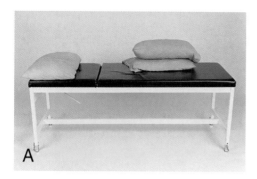

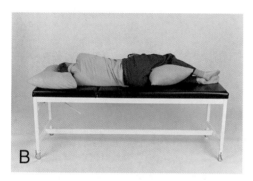

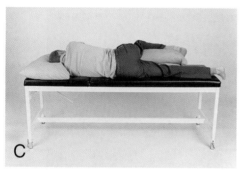

Figure 6-44 A. In side-lying, use pillows for the head and legs. B. Place one or two pillows between the client's knees to enhance comfort. C. To access the medial tissues of the thigh and leg nearest the table, flex the hip and knee of the upper leg to 90 degrees, and use pillows to support the upper leg so that the pelvis does not rotate.

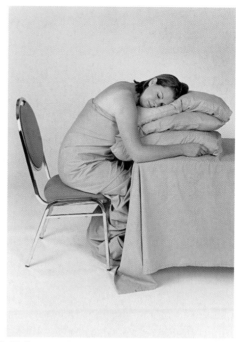

Figure 6-45 Several pillows support a relaxed seated position that offers good access to the upper back, shoulders, and posterior neck.

undress in privacy.[10] If the client requires assistance undressing or getting onto the table, you must clearly explain which items of the client's clothing—if any—you will be removing and where you will be touching or moving her; you also need to obtain and record consent for this assistance before assisting the client. Clean your hands and other contact surfaces thoroughly with soap and hot water or alcohol-based hand sanitizer for at least 10 seconds prior to beginning draping procedures and subsequent massage.[8,10]

Students must practice the process of appropriate draping repeatedly and extend appropriate respect to each other during classroom practice. In addition, it is useful for students to perform initial classroom practice with the practice partners clothed until they develop a reasonable level of skill in draping.

The draping sequences in Figures 6-46 to 6-59 all use two single (twin) flat sheets and a few towels. Therapists can also perform the sequences with sheets as narrow as 4 feet wide. When therapists perform these draping sequences as described, the draping will be comfortable and secure and will ensure privacy for unclothed clients. You can easily modify the sequences for the legs should the client choose to wear her underwear. In addition, you will need to modify the draping if you are using massage as an adjunct to other modalities and if the clinical setting or client preference requires the use of a gown.

Following a clinical session, if there is sufficient time, invite the client to rest before rising. Then instruct the client on how to get off the table safely, using statements such as "roll onto your side, let your legs drop off the table, and slowly come to a sitting position, using your arms to push up." If the client has physical limitations, you may also be required to give the client discreet assistance to sit up, stand, or dress after the session.

## Critical Thinking Question

How would you adapt the positioning and draping procedures illustrated in this chapter for use at the following locations: a public hospital ward, a private home, an office, and a sports competition in an arena?

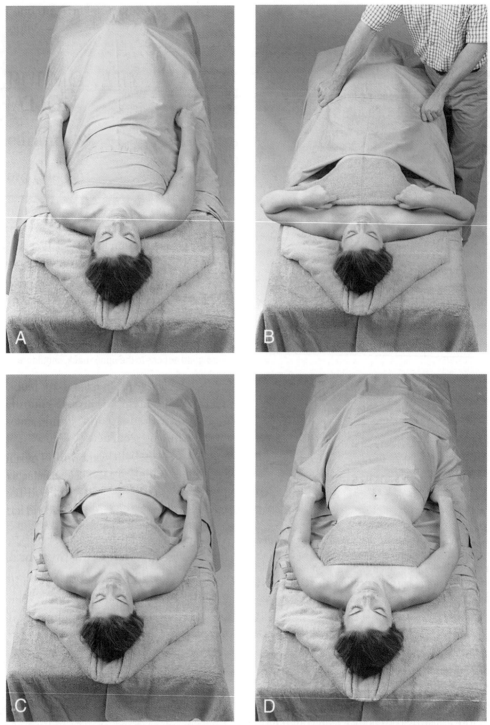

**Figure 6-46** A. Starting position for undraping the female torso in supine. B. Place a folded towel on top of the sheet over the breasts. The client holds the top edge of the towel while the therapist withdraws the sheet from under the towel. C. Tuck the towel under the torso or arms, and then expose the abdomen. D. In the final position, the drape is securely tucked, and the client's abdomen is exposed from the xiphoid process to the anterior superior iliac spine.

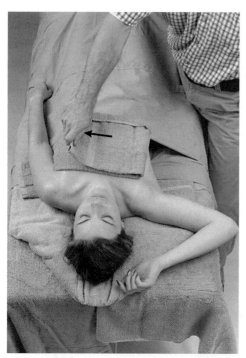

Figure 6-47  For women, the chest towel can be folded back to undrape one or both breasts if informed consent has been obtained and massage of breast tissue or the pectoral muscles is clinically indicated.

# THERAPISTS' POSTURE, ALIGNMENT, AND BODY MECHANICS DURING TREATMENT

Efficient posture and movement constitute the physical foundation of effective execution of massage techniques. The outcomes and characteristic "feel" of well-performed massage techniques depend as much on correct use of your feet, legs, pelvis, and respiratory apparatus as they do on the motion of your upper limbs. Students and therapists who aspire to achieve expertise in performing massage strokes may have postural habits that they must systematically retrain. Furthermore, this retraining must start before instruction in manual technique begins, since attention to your posture will decrease once you begin to learn manual technique. If you have habitually poor body mechanics that are not corrected, then you will experience fatigue and pain when performing massage strokes. For many, this unpleasant result can occur in as little as a few hours or weeks.

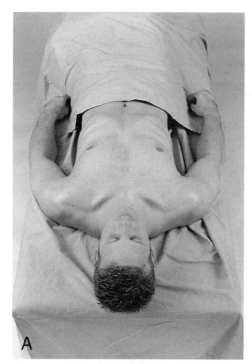

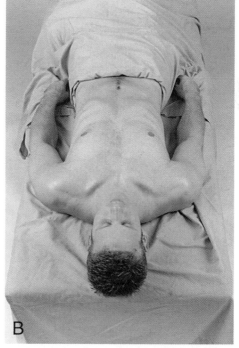

Figure 6-48  A. For men, the issue of consent to treat the anterior torso is less delicate. If you are to perform extensive work on a male client's torso, he can be undraped to the waist. If you only plan for abdominal massage, you should offer him a chest towel for warmth. B. The final drape tucked at the level of the anterior superior iliac spine.

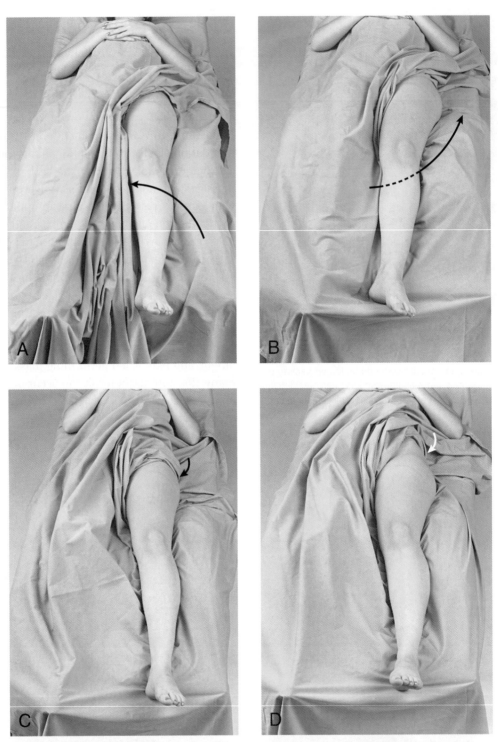

**Figure 6-49** A. Undraping the anterior leg. You expose the client's leg and gather the extra sheet between her legs. B. You then pull the extra sheet underneath the exposed leg back toward the side of the table. Here, the weight of the leg securely anchors the sheet. C. You can tuck the top edge of the drape under the gluteal at the level of the greater trochanter. D. Or you can roll the edge of the sheet higher to expose the anterior superior iliac spine and tuck it under the client's lower back.

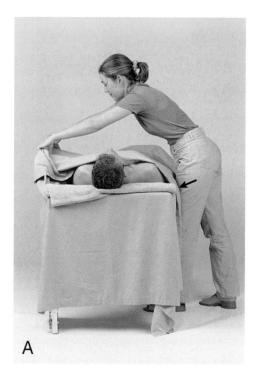
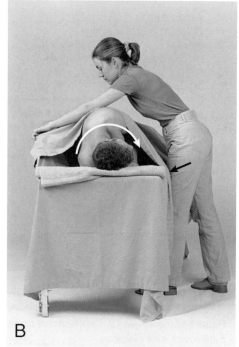

A B

Figure 6-50 A. Turning to prone. The basic procedure is similar for turning from supine to prone, from prone to supine, or from either position to or from side-lying. Use the front of your thigh to pin the sheets against the near edge of the table while your hands secure both sheets across the table. Instruct the client to turn. B. Throughout the turn, maintain control of both sheets at both sides of the table. Failure to do this will result in exposure of the client or a migrating bottom sheet that bunches uncomfortably under the client. Take care to minimize inadvertent touching of the client during the turn.

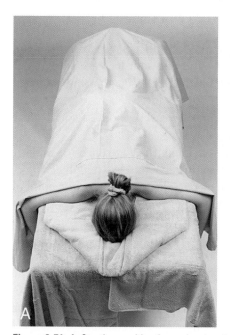
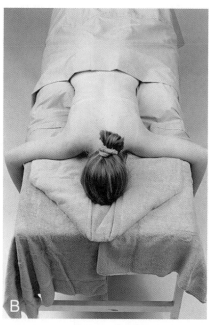
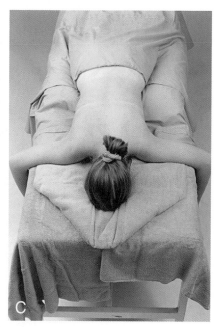

Figure 6-51 A. Starting position for undraping the torso in prone. B. For general back massage, the back is exposed to just below the level of the posterior superior iliac spine. C. The drape is securely tucked.

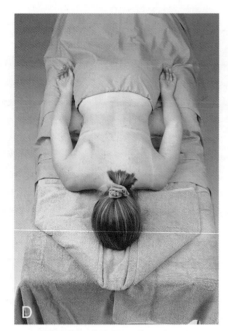 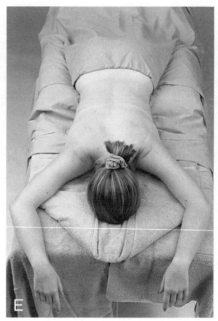

**Figure 6-51** *(Continued)* D. The client may choose to position her arms at her sides. E. Or the client may position her arms overhead.

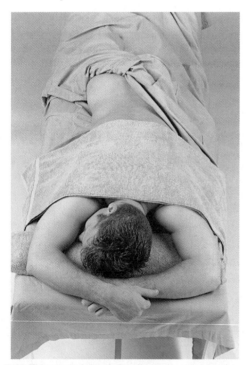

**Figure 6-52** This angled draping unilaterally exposes the superior gluteal insertions. Clinicians must work on these extensively when treating many lumbar conditions.

The following general principles of body mechanics apply during massage.

1. Keep your posture aligned and as upright as possible, except during controlled transfer of body weight.
2. Keep both feet in contact with the floor.
3. Reduce the vertical distance between yourself and the client by bending your knees, rather than by bending at the waist.
4. Reduce the horizontal distance between yourself and the client by repositioning your legs or shifting your weight onto your forward leg, rather than by bending at the waist or reaching excessively.
5. Point your navel area toward the body segment of the client that you are treating.
6. Increase pressure through the controlled use of body weight, rather than through muscle strength.
7. You may lean in a controlled way toward the point of contact with the client. When doing so, control the amount of your body weight that you are transferring to the client precisely and continuously.
8. Position your joints as close to neutral as possible and do not load them when they are in a close-packed position.
9. Change position (e.g., from sitting to kneeling) frequently to vary the mechanical stress that is being placed on your body.

The chapters on techniques use the postures and movements described in this chapter[8,9,12,13] during the application

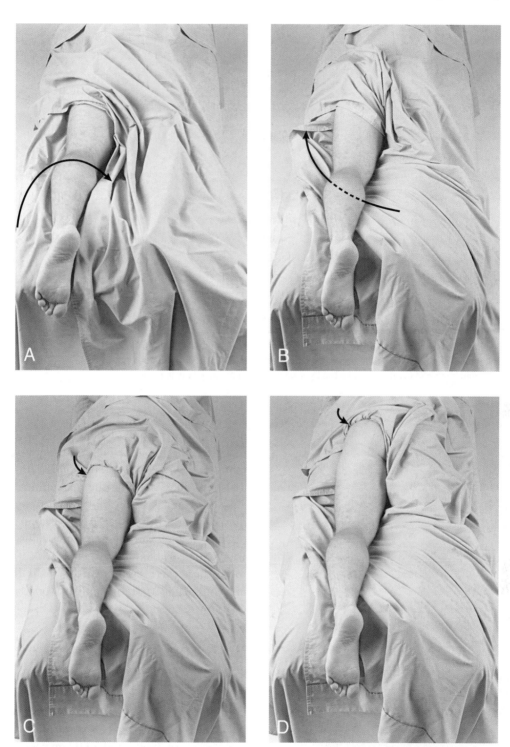

**Figure 6-53** A. The procedure for undraping the posterior leg is similar to that for the anterior leg. Expose the client's limb and gather the extra sheet between his legs. B. Pull the extra sheet underneath the exposed thigh back toward the side of the table. Here, the weight of the leg securely anchors the sheet. C. For a low drape, tuck the upper edge of the sheet under the anterior thigh at the level of the greater trochanter. D. A more common and much more useful technique is to roll the edge of the sheet toward the gluteal cleft and securely tuck it above the anterior superior iliac spine, thus exposing the bulk of the gluteals.

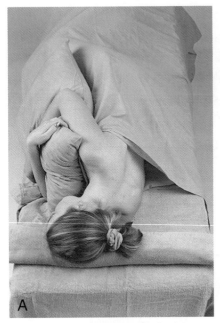
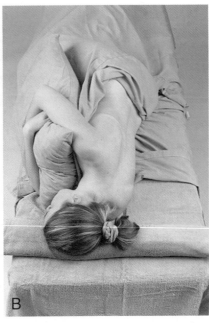
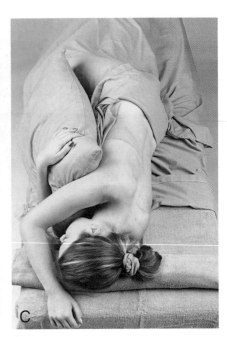

**Figure 6-54** A. To expose the back and the flank of a side-lying female, first instruct the client to clasp a standard-sized pillow in front. B. Undrape the back to the desired level. C. Then securely tuck the drape. The upper arm can be raised overhead, while the lower arm maintains the pillow in position.

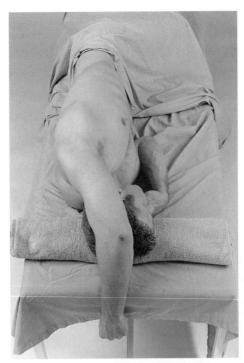

**Figure 6-55** The side-lying position potentially offers unparalleled access to the uppermost rotator cuff, serratus anterior, quadratus lumborum, and portions of the pectorals and spinal extensors.

of massage techniques. Ideally, practice them until they have become habitual before attempting to learn the manual parts of massage techniques. These exercises will assist you in developing the relaxation, awareness, balance, coordination, flexibility, and strength that are required to perform massage. A lack of familiarity with these or comparable exercises can compromise the quality of your manual technique and increase risk of injury. Furthermore, these exercises are worthwhile in their own right, and you can incorporate them into your daily warm-up or cool-down.

## Standing Aligned Posture

This deceptively simple posture can actually be quite difficult to maintain because it often reveals and accentuates chronic patterns of tension in the body when you first begin to use it. The steps for performing this posture follow (see figures 6-60A and 6-60B on page 179).

1. Stand with your feet positioned shoulder-width apart. Use the glenoid fossa as a landmark, rather than the lateral surface of the deltoid.
2. Breathe deeply and relax.
3. Let the weight settle down through your legs and into your feet.

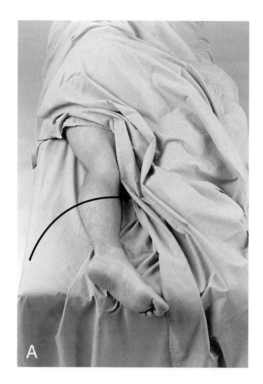

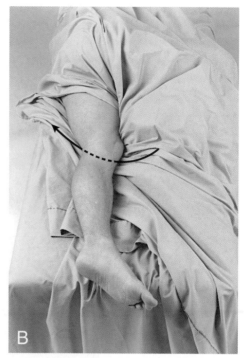

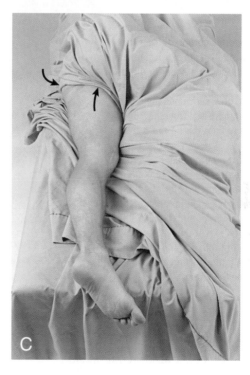

**Figure 6-56** A. To undrape the bottom leg in side-lying (for work on the adductors, triceps surae, and tibialis posterior), first flex the knee and hip of the top leg to 90 degrees and use pillows to keep it forward and out of the way (see Figure 6-44C). Then expose the bottom leg from behind and gather the extra sheet between the legs. B. Then pull the extra sheet underneath the exposed leg back toward the posterior side of the table at the level of mid-thigh or slightly higher. Here, the weight of the leg securely anchors the sheet. At this point, instruct a male client to move his genitals in a superior direction (e.g., "Adjust yourself."). C. The top edge of the drape is then rolled and pushed as close to the ischiopubic ramus as possible, and the posterior edge is tucked under the greater trochanter. You may best perform techniques on the adductor attachments onto the ramus through the sheet, for reasons of discretion.

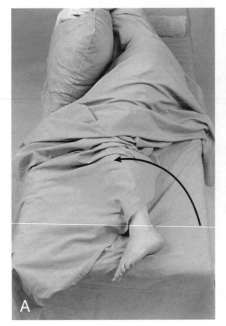
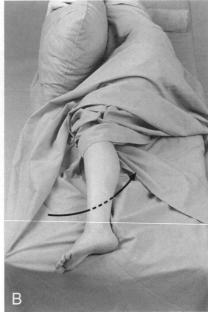
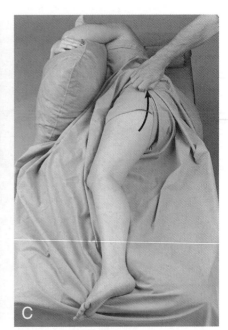
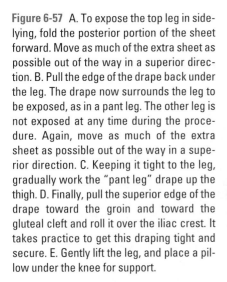
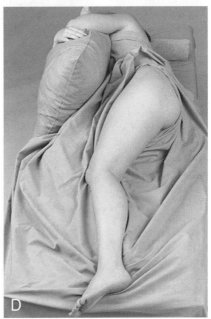
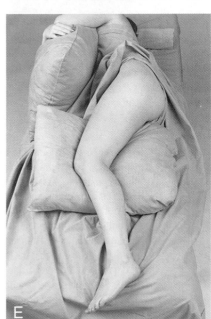

**Figure 6-57** A. To expose the top leg in side-lying, fold the posterior portion of the sheet forward. Move as much of the extra sheet as possible out of the way in a superior direction. B. Pull the edge of the drape back under the leg. The drape now surrounds the leg to be exposed, as in a pant leg. The other leg is not exposed at any time during the procedure. Again, move as much of the extra sheet as possible out of the way in a superior direction. C. Keeping it tight to the leg, gradually work the "pant leg" drape up the thigh. D. Finally, pull the superior edge of the drape toward the groin and toward the gluteal cleft and roll it over the iliac crest. It takes practice to get this draping tight and secure. E. Gently lift the leg, and place a pillow under the knee for support.

4. Explore the manner in which your feet contact the ground by rocking from front to back, shifting from left to right, and shifting the inside to the outside.

5. Attempt to find the foot position in which you distribute the weight of your body evenly through your feet.

6. Let the top of your head rise up gently. You may want to have someone check whether you are incorrectly positioning your head by flexing or extending your neck.

7. Try to hold a standing aligned posture for 10 minutes, progressively refining both your foot contact with the ground and your sense of vertical alignment.

## Standing Aligned Posture with Diaphragmatic Breathing

The following are the steps for performing this posture (Figure 6-60C).

1. Assume a standing aligned posture until you feel very stable and relaxed.

2. Focus your attention on your breathing.

3. Let your upper chest remain still, and breathe using your diaphragm so that your abdomen passively moves

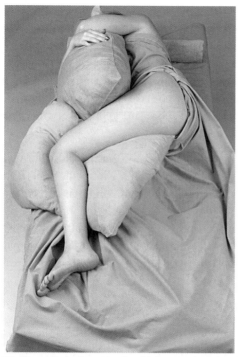

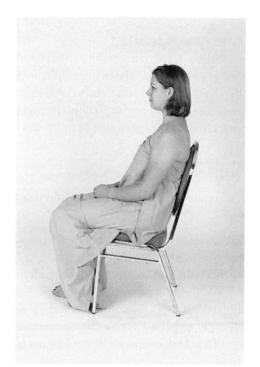

**Figure 6-58** The preferred position in which to work on the piriformis is with the knee and hip both flexed to 90 degrees. If you have applied the drape correctly, it will be possible for you to move the leg without the drape loosening.

**Figure 6-59** Wrap-around draping is useful for seated massage of the head, neck, and shoulders in a seated inclined position.

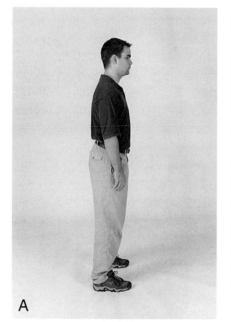

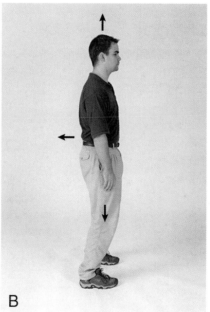

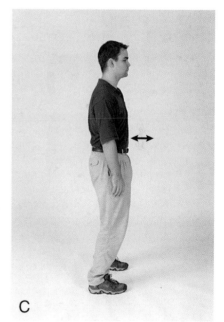

**Figure 6-60** A. Lateral view of standing posture shows a forward lean; a shortening in this therapist's lumbar muscles, with an accompanying anterior pelvic tilt; and an anterior-head posture. These may be due to postural habit or chronic fascial shortening. B. The therapist's lumbar spine is in a more neutral position, and the whole posture is better aligned after he balanced the weight on his feet, softened his knees, let his sacrum drop, and let his head rise. Here, the therapist has overcompensated by bending his knees more than necessary. C. Using the diaphragm to breathe produces a passive rise of the abdomen on inhalation. Use standing aligned posture when you perform superficial reflex techniques that do not require application of pressure and that you need to sustain for some time.

out during the inhalation and passively moves back during the exhalation.

4. Remain in this position and continue to focus on the passive movements of your abdomen. Gradually increase both the duration and depth of the inhalation.

5. Sustain focused breathing for 10 minutes, and periodically check the alignment of your body.

## Standing Pelvic Tilt

The following are the steps for performing this posture (Figure 6-61).

1. Assume a **standing aligned posture** until you feel very stable and relaxed.
2. Ensure that your knees are not hyperextended.
3. Focus your attention on your pelvis.
4. Keeping the legs and upper body motionless, perform a posterior pelvic tilt by letting your sacrum drop and rolling your anterior superior iliac spine in a posterior direction.
5. Place a hand on your lumbar spine and note whether you feel it flatten slightly; this indicates that the posterior pelvic tilt has occurred.

6. Hold the pelvic tilt and breathe deeply using your diaphragm in the manner outlined in the previous section.
7. Relax.
8. Perform this tilt and relax movement 10 to 20 times.
9. Vary your practice of this posture by making the movement larger or more subtle or by varying the amount you bend your knees.

Proper performance of a posterior pelvic tilt in standing requires some flexibility. If it is difficult to perform, practice this posture lying supine on a flat surface with your knees and hips flexed, progress to lying supine with your knees and hips extended, and then attempt to perform it standing with your back against a wall before reattempting the posture in unsupported standing.

## Seated Aligned Posture

The following are the steps for performing this posture (Figure 6-62).

1. Sit upright on a level, firm, well-padded chair that allows your knees and hips to rest at 90 degrees of flexion. Place your feet on the floor, shoulder-width apart or slightly wider.

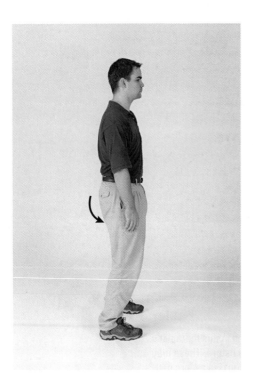

**Figure 6-61** During a standing slow pelvic tilt, the pelvis is tucked under, while the thorax remains in the same position. This results in a lengthening of the lumbar region and a reduction of the normal lordosis. This movement is a prerequisite for later movements that involve bending the knees.

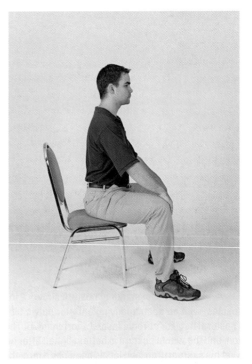

**Figure 6-62** Use seated aligned posture when applying many different techniques. Note the feet flat on the floor and the erect upper body supported by the ischiopubic rami.

2. First touch and then focus your attention on your ischial tuberosities.

3. Allow your spine to flex until you feel the weight of your upper body resting on your ischial tuberosities.

4. While maintaining your upper body in an upright position, slowly roll the contact point of your pelvis with the chair forward so that it shifts from being on the ischial tuberosities to being along the ischial rami in the direction of the symphysis pubis.

5. Since that movement should extend your lumbar spine, place your hand in the small of your back and note whether you feel the erector spinae muscles tighten in your lumbar region.

6. Very slowly rock back and forward several times and locate the point on your pelvis, between your ischial tuberosities and symphysis pubis, at which your upper body feels upright and most comfortably balanced over the pelvis (somewhere around the perineum). The erector spinae muscles in your lumbar region should not be engaged in that position.

7. Breathe deeply using your diaphragm.

8. Let the top of your head rise up gently. You may want to have someone check whether you are incorrectly positioning your head by flexing or extending your neck.

9. Sit for 10 minutes, progressively refining both the contact of your pelvis with the chair and your sense of vertical alignment.

## Lunge

This position is also known as walk-standing, bow stance, or archer stance. The following are the steps for performing this posture (Figures 6-63A and 6-63B).

1. Stand with your feet together.

2. Externally rotate your left hip to 20 to 45 degrees so that your left foot is turned out.

3. With your right foot, step forward and to the right of the left foot a comfortable distance.

4. Maintaining an upright torso, slowly straighten your left (back) leg without hyperextending your knee, and bend your right (forward) leg as you move your body over your forward foot.

5. Straighten your right (forward) leg and bend your left (back) knee as you shift your weight onto your back leg. Slowly shift your weight back and forth from your left to right foot, while keeping your torso perfectly poised and upright. Your head should remain equidistant from the floor throughout the movement.

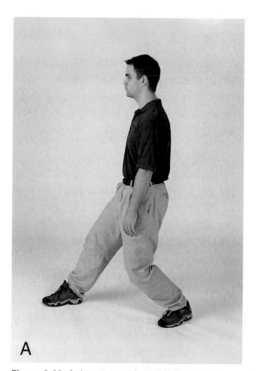
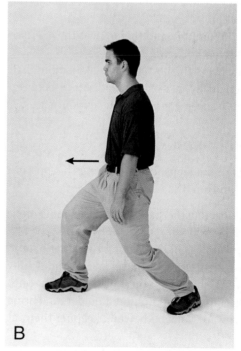

**Figure 6-63** A. Lunge position with the weight over the back leg. B. Lunge position, shifting the weight toward the front leg (the rear leg can still be straightened some more). As you shift your weight back and forth, your torso remains balanced and motionless in relation to the moving legs. This basic leg movement, used for many techniques, requires some quadriceps strength.

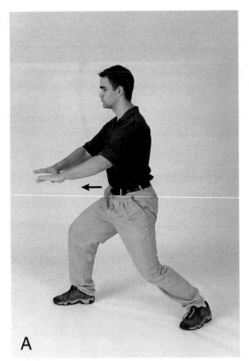 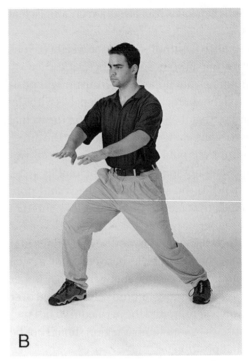

**Figure 6-64**  A, B. Lunge and reach. Arms extend from an upright torso as you shift your weight to the forward leg. This exact movement is used for superficial effleurage.

6. You may also synchronize your breathing with the movement by inhaling as you shift your weight in the posterior direction and exhaling as you shift your weight in the anterior direction.
7. Continue for 5 minutes, and then repeat the exercise with the other foot forward.
8. Vary your practice of this posture and make it more challenging by gradually increasing the distance between your feet and the degree to which you flex your knees.

## Lunge and Reach

The following are the steps for performing this posture (Figures 6-64A and 6-64B).

1. Begin by performing the steps in the **lunge** movement previously described.
2. As you shift your weight onto your forward leg, extend both arms straight ahead at navel level without fully extending your elbows. As you shift your weight onto your back leg, flex your elbows and shoulders and bring your arms toward your body while keeping them at waist level.
3. Vary your practice of this posture by increasing the distance between your feet, by changing the degree to which you flex your knees, by varying the level of your arms, and by using different breathing patterns.

**Theory in Practice 6-1**

### Preparation and Positioning for Massage

Practitioner Profile:
A healthy 30-year-old practitioner in good physical condition began to experience frequent tightness and aching in his lower back after doubling his weekly workload of massage. His pain level has been increasing each week and is now affecting his ability to work.

Subjective Findings:
The practitioner reports that his symptoms appear after a couple of hours of work, get progressively worse until the end of the work day, and then disappear after an hour of rest. Stretching, especially stretching his spinal extensors, relieves his symptoms. He cannot identify which actions are contributing to his symptoms while he works and reports that both standing and seated positions seem to be at fault.

Objective Findings:
The practitioner is right-hand dominant. His posture shows a minor **upper-cross** pattern. Active lumbar range of motion is within normal limits. Abdominal strength is grade 5/5. He has hamstring tightness based on the sit-and-reach test. On palpation, there is **elevated resting tension** in the thoracic and lumbar erector spinae and related **latent trigger points** that reproduce his pain.

Treatment Approach:

The practitioner's profile and findings suggest that his back pain is biomechanical. A likely mechanism is that he is overusing his spinal extensors—a common result of trying too hard to maintain an upright posture.

He has several options:

■ He can have a colleague monitor his posture during work to look for signs of lumbar hyperextension. He can then correct this with feedback.

■ While working, he can periodically place a hand in the small of his back to monitor his lumbar extensors for signs of excessive contraction or tightness.

■ In order to refine his awareness of pelvic position and related extensor contraction, he can practice pelvic tilt daily in lying, seated, and standing aligned positions.

■ He can follow a daily program of lumbar stretching.

■ When working, he can train himself to stop at the first sign of tightness or pain, stand back briefly, relax, take a breath, and adjust his posture before continuing.

■ He can adjust the **ergonomic** load while he is working by modifying his posture during treatments.

■ He can decide whether these symptoms stem from general fatigue secondary to overworking and reduce his workload.

# Preparation and Positioning for Massage: Further Study and Practice

## THERAPISTS' POSTURE, ALIGNMENT, AND BODY MECHANICS DURING TREATMENT

### Lunge and Lean

The following are the steps for performing this posture (Figure 6-65).

1. Begin by performing the steps in the **lunge** movement previously described.
2. Rather than keeping your torso upright throughout the movement, incline it forward (lean) as you shift your weight onto the forward leg. At the forward portion of the motion, there should be a straight line from the top of your head, through your torso, to the heel of your back leg. The movement of this posture is from upright with your weight on your back leg, to leaning with the weight on your front leg, and back again.
3. Once you have mastered the performance of the lean during the weight shift, add the arm movement previously described in the lunge and reach posture.

### Wide-Stance Knee Bend

This position is also known as the horse or warrior stance. The following are the steps for performing this posture (Figures 6-66, 6-67A, and 6-67B).

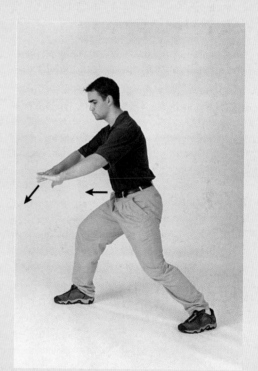

**Figure 6-65** Lunge and lean. The therapist is shifting his weight over the front leg as he leans forward; extending his back knee slightly will complete the forward movement. Using exactly this movement, the therapist transfers pressure to the client during various neuromuscular and connective tissue techniques.

1. Stand with your feet placed more than shoulder-width apart and your feet pointed straight forward or in a small degree of external rotation.

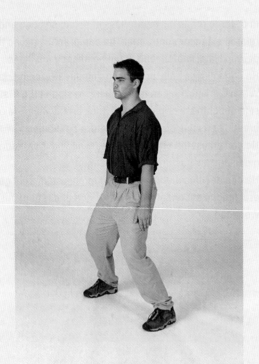

**Figure 6-66** First, practice the wide stance (horse stance) without movement (the "upper bent-knee position").

2. While keeping your upper body upright, flex your hips and knees a few degrees. Hold this position. This is the "upper bent-knee position."
3. Adjust the distance (width) between your feet until you are in a position that you can comfortably hold for 2 to 3 minutes.
4. Slowly increase the degree of knee flexion so that you lower your body 6 to 8 inches. This is the "lower bent-knee position."
5. While keeping your torso upright, perform a posterior pelvic tilt (using the steps previously described) so that your lower spine lengthens as you lower your body. Place a hand on your lumbar spine to monitor its position during this movement.
6. Slowly extend your knees and return to the upper bent-knee position without hyperextending your lumbar spine or your knees.
7. Repeat.
8. Gradually work up to 100 repetitions of this sequence of movements from neutral to the upper and lower bent-knee positions.

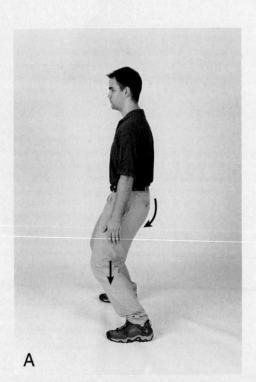

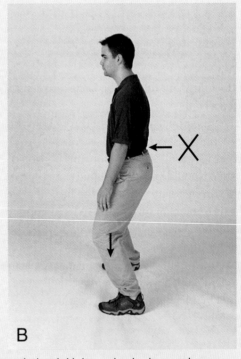

A                                                    B

**Figure 6-67**  A. Knee bend in the wide stance. As the therapist bends his knees, he simultaneously executes a posterior pelvic tilt so that the lumbar region lengthens. Use this type of leg movement for some neuromuscular techniques like wringing. B. A common error of movement is to increase the lumbar lordosis as the knees are bending.

9. Vary your practice of this posture in one of several ways:
   - Change the distance (width) between your feet.
   - Flex your knees more.
   - Rotate your upright torso in one direction as you go down and rotate to the original position as you come up.
   - Perform the knee bend beside a massage table while transferring a portion of your upper body weight to the table through your bent arms.

## Standing Controlled Lean

The following are the steps for performing this posture (Figure 6-68).

1. You need a massage table or other stable object against which you can lean to perform this posture. The table should be within reach of your partially extended arms.
2. Begin by performing the steps of the **lunge and lean** posture previously described.
3. As you shift weight onto your forward leg, lean forward and extend your arms. Allow your hands to contact the table and slowly transfer some of your weight to the table. As you do this, you should feel a shift of weight onto your extended back leg.
4. Slowly return your arms to their original position and shift your upper body back over your back leg.
5. Repeat this back-and-forth movement and transfer some of your body weight to the table at the appropriate point in each movement. The compression and release should be slow and controlled.

## Seated Controlled Lean

The following are the steps for performing this posture (Figures 6-69 and 6-70).

1. Begin in the **seated aligned posture** facing a massage table or other stable object against which you can lean.

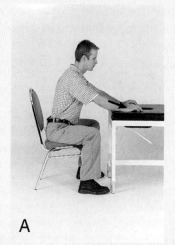

A

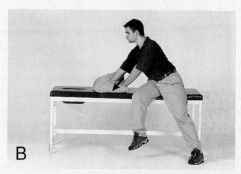

B

Figure 6-69  A. A seated controlled lean using a chair. This is often used when treating the client's shoulders. B. A seated controlled lean sitting on the edge of the table. When treating clients, it is acceptable to sit on the edge of the table as long as the therapist only contacts the client with his hands or forearms, not his thigh or pelvis.

2. Place your hands on the supporting surface.
3. Gradually lean forward from your waist and apply pressure to the supporting surface so that you feel balanced as you do so.
4. Alternatively, sit upright on the edge of a firm bed or massage table and face one end of it. If you are on a

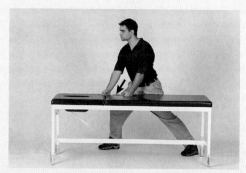

Figure 6-68  Use a standing controlled lean to apply pressure during many neuromuscular and connective tissue techniques.

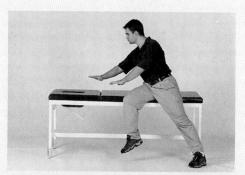

Figure 6-70  The therapist is obviously not using the client to support his body. He demonstrates flawless control of the amount of body weight that he could transfer to a client in this position.

massage table, the leg closest to the table will be off the ground and the other foot will have a secure contact with the floor.

5. Slowly lean forward to transfer your body weight in the manner described above.

6. Vary your practice of this posture by changing the amount of weight you transfer to the supporting surface, the height of contact, and the compression

time (without losing continuous control and relaxed shoulders).

## Critical Thinking Question
Which of the described postures do you find hardest to perform? Why? Use your understanding of your body structures to explain this difficulty.

## References

1. Sharkey B. *Fitness and Health.* 4th ed. Champaign, IL: Human Kinetics; 1997.
2. Anderson B, Pearl B, Burke E. *Getting in Shape.* Bolinas, CA: Shelter Publications; 2002.
3. Moffat M, Vickery S. *The American Physical Therapy Association Book of Body Maintenance and Repair.* New York: Henry Holt & Co.; 1999.
4. Alter MJ. *Science of Stretching.* 3rd ed. Champaign, IL: Human Kinetics; 2004.
5. Oswald C, Basco S. *Stretching for Fitness, Health and Performance: The Complete Handbook for All Ages and Fitness Levels.* New York: Sterling Publishing; 1998.
6. Anderson B. *Stretching.* Revised edition. Bolinas, CA: Shelter Publications; 2000.
7. Loving J. *Massage Therapy.* Stamford, CT: Appleton & Lange; 1999.
8. Fritz S. *Mosby's Fundamentals of Therapeutic Massage.* 3rd ed. St. Louis: Mosby; 2004.
9. Salvo SG. *Massage Therapy: Principles and Practice.* 2nd ed. Philadelphia: WB Saunders; 2003.
10. Quality Assurance Committee of the College of Massage Therapists of Ontario. *Code of Ethics and Standards of Practice.* Toronto: College of Massage Therapists of Ontario; 2006.
11. Curties D. *Breast Massage.* New Brunswick, Canada: Curties-Overzet Publications; 1999.
12. Beck MJ. Milady's *Theory and Practice of Therapeutic Massage.* 3rd ed. Albany, NY: Milady; 1999.
13. Hollis M. *Massage for Therapists.* 2nd ed. Oxford, England: Blackwell Science; 1998.

# Chapter 7
## Superficial Reflex Techniques

Superficial reflex techniques are those massage techniques that engage only the skin and primarily affect level of arousal, autonomic balance, and the perception of pain. These techniques include static contact, superficial stroking, and fine vibration. This chapter describes these techniques, how to perform them, and how to apply them in a practice sequence. A section on further study for each technique discusses relevant outcomes and evidence, cautions and contraindications, and how to use the technique in treatment.

**Table 7-1** Summary of Outcomes for Body Structures and Functions for Superficial Reflex Techniques

| Impairment-Level Outcome of Care | Technique | | |
|---|---|---|---|
| | Static Contact | Superficial Stroking | Fine Vibration |
| Increased sedation | ✓ | ✓ | ✓ |
| Decreased anxiety | ✓ | ✓ | P |
| Increased arousal | ? | ✓ | ? |
| Counterirritant analgesia | P | P | ✓ |
| Increased local resting muscle tension or neuromuscular tone | ? | ? | ✓ |
| Decreased local resting muscle tension or neuromuscular tone | > | ✓ | ? |
| Stimulated peristalsis | P | P | P |

✓: the outcome is supported by research summarized in this chapter. P: the outcome is possible. ?: the outcome is debatable (research results are absent or inconsistent).

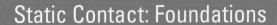

# Static Contact: Foundations

## DEFINITION

**Static contact**: Motionless contact of the therapist's hands with the client's body performed with minimal force.[1-7]

## USES

Therapists use static contact to establish rapport, to promote **relaxation**, and to assist with client education. They often use it when they must avoid more forceful techniques.

## PALPATION PRACTICE

The following palpation exercises will help you develop the manual skill and focus you need to perform static contact well.

1. Mold the entire palmar surface of your hand to household objects of varying sizes and shapes. The aim is to maximize hand contact without tensing your hand or compressing the object.
2. Chaitow[8] suggests palpating household objects made of different materials (e.g., metal, glass, plastic) that you perceive to be warm or cold when they are at normal room temperature. What would explain the perceived differences in temperature? Are different parts of your hand more sensitive to temperature?
3. With your eyes closed and hands placed lightly on a practice partner's ribcage, monitor the breathing rhythm. Try this with your hands more distant from the ribcage. Can you detect the breathing rhythm when contacting the pelvis, the knees, or the feet?
4. With your forearms supported on the table, cradle the client's occiput in both hands for 10 minutes. What rhythmical movements can you detect?

---

### Theory in Practice

### Superficial Reflex Techniques

**Patient Profile**

Your patient is a 35-year-old recently separated mother of two adolescents. The psychologist who is treating her for issues related to self-esteem, **body image**, and a history of physical abuse has referred her for treatment.

**Clinical Findings**

Subjective:
Her medical history is unremarkable, other than having had one Caesarean delivery. She requests help to cope with **stress**, learn how stress affects her body, and alleviate occasional neck pain and stiffness.

Objective:
- Observation: Postural analysis shows a moderate kyphosis.
- Range of motion: She has mildly limited range of motion in her cervical spine secondary to elevated resting tension and muscle tightness.

**Treatment Approach**

- Initial outcomes include: developing good rapport (trust), fostering relaxation, and improving body awareness.
- The patient's history of physical abuse necessitates that you pay special attention to the process of obtaining informed consent. As you obtain **informed consent**, com-

municate clearly and carefully and explain the intervention protocol fully. Offer her the option of doing the work fully clothed. In addition, ask her which areas of her body she does not want you to touch, or about which she has concerns. Finally, discuss the possibility of **touch-triggered memory** and **somato-emotional release** with her.

- Once the patient is on the table, remind her where you will be beginning. Gently apply static contact, and sustain it for a couple of minutes or until the patient indicates that you can proceed to an adjacent area. (The Practice Sequence later in this section gives one example of how you can proceed from place to place.) Communicate with the patient to encourage breathing and general relaxation, or guide her awareness of the areas of her body that you are treating. Allow the patient the freedom to talk about her experiences as the need arises. Once you have covered one region with static contact, apply superficial stroking to it for a minute or so. Remind her which region you will be treating next. Proceed through the regions of the body using the allotted treatment time.

- As this patient's episode of care proceeds, you will likely introduce other techniques, presented in later chapters, in order to address the kyphosis and muscle tension. At that time, continue to begin each subsequent **intervention** with several minutes of static contact and superficial stroking to establish safety and relaxation. End each session with static contact and superficial stroking to allow the patient time to reflect and to obtain closure.

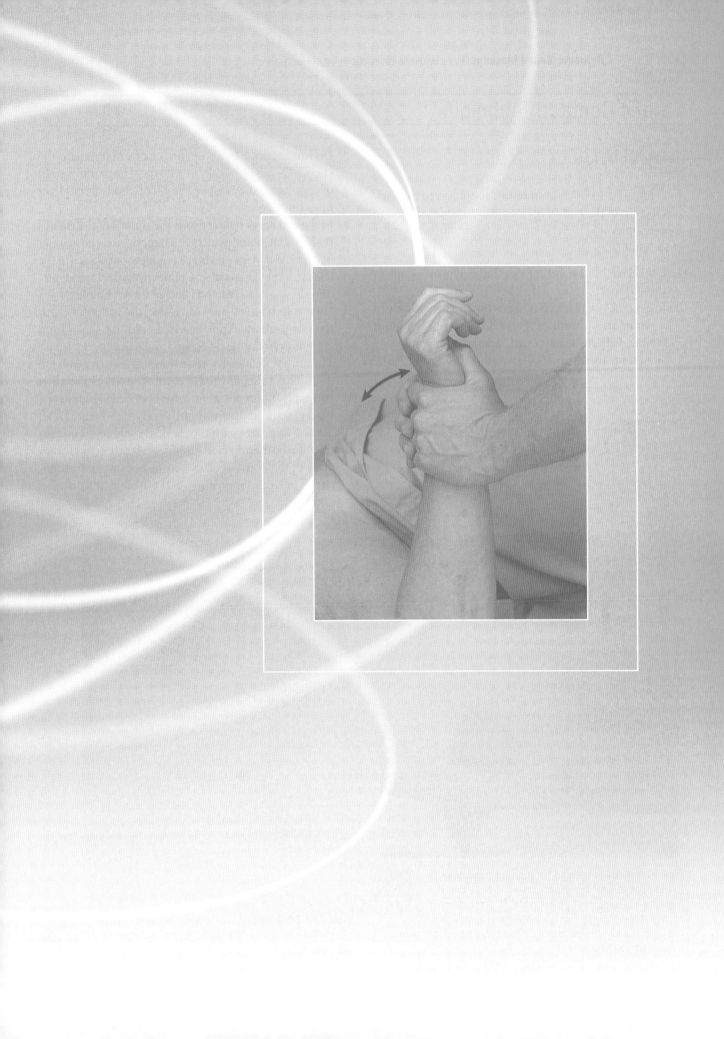

## Static Contact: Technique

# MANUAL TECHNIQUE

In Figures 7-1 to 7-7, static contact is applied to the various regions of the body. Figures are ordered from head to foot in supine and then prone. Each figure illustrates most of the guidelines for manual technique.

1. Use relaxed, full-hand contact that conforms evenly to the surface contours of the client's body.
2. In general, you place your hands on the client's body in a symmetrical position. This allows you to maintain contact with the left and right sides of the client's body simultaneously (Figures 7-1A and 7-1B, 7-3, and 7-6).

3. Do not attempt to apply force or to manipulate the client's tissues physically in any way. The partial weight of your hands may rest on the client's body if the client finds this tolerable.
4. Make and break contact with the surface of the client's body gradually and gently. To a large degree, the manner in which you make and break contact contributes to the client's level of **relaxation**. Changing contact frequently may decrease the **sedative** effect of this technique.
5. Hold your hands steady when they are in contact with the client's body. Your hands should not shake from fatigue, even during prolonged application.
6. The author's clinical observation suggests that you are more likely to achieve the effect of deep relaxation when you apply static contact for longer periods (5 minutes or longer) at the midsacrum and/or occiput[3] (Figures 7-1B and 7-7). Contact with the client's hands, feet, and face may also be more likely to produce relaxation than other areas of the body.[3,9,10] This may be because of the density of nervous innervation in these areas (Figures 7-5 and 7-6).

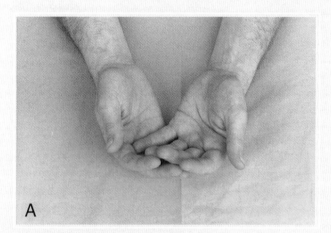

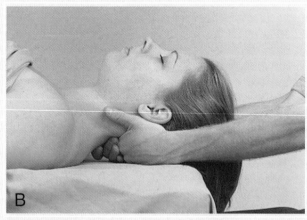

**Figure 7-1** A. Hand position for applying static contact to the occiput with the client in supine. Note that the forearms are supported on the table. B. Static contact applied to the occiput. This nonthreatening approach to reducing spasm or hypertonicity in the client's neck can also produce sedative effects.[3]

ON-LINE VIDEO

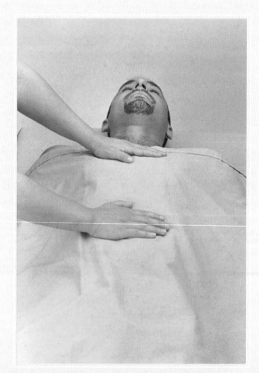

**Figure 7-2** Static contact used to draw the client's awareness to the movement of the upper ribs and abdomen during breathing.

ON-LINE VIDEO

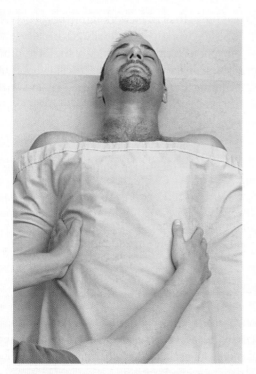

**Figure 7-3** Static contact used to facilitate instruction of the client in lateral costal breathing.

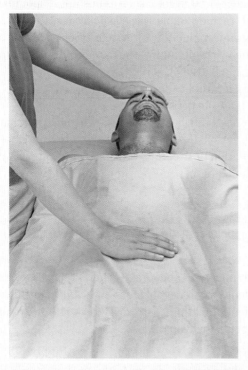

**Figure 7-4** Simultaneous contact to the forehead and abdomen.

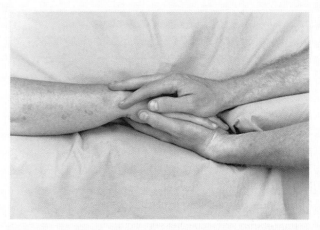

**Figure 7-5** Appropriate contact to the hand(s) can be both intimate and comforting.[10]

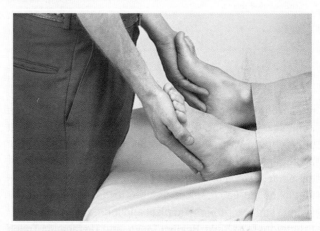

**Figure 7-6** Bilateral static contact to the soles of the feet.

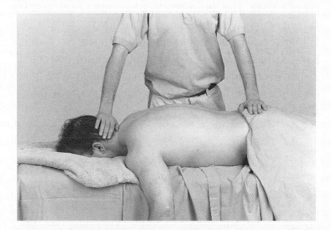

**Figure 7-7** Prolonged simultaneous contact at occiput and sacrum can produce relaxation in the client.[3]

---

**Box 7-1** | **Components of Static Contact**

**Contact:** Whole hand, fingertip(s), thumb

**Pressure:** Minimal

**Engages:** Skin

**Direction:** N/A

**Amplitude/length:** N/A

**Rate:** N/A

**Duration:** 60 seconds to 15 minutes or more

**Intergrades with:** Compression, vibration

**Context:** May be used alone. It is often used as a "framing technique," performed at the beginning and end of regional or full-body sequences that use other techniques to engage deeper tissues

---

## How static contact might work

Researchers are uncertain how this very simple technique achieves its therapeutic effects. In other words: How do cutaneous nerves generate a relaxation effect? It is possible that gentle stimulation of the skin boosts the activity of the **parasympathetic** nervous system.[11–14] This parasympathetic activity may result in changes in the neuroendocrine system such as reduced **cortisol** and increased **serotonin**.[15] Practitioners of **Reiki**, **Healing Touch**, and **Therapeutic Touch** propose that it is possible to use the simplest form of touch to manipulate the energy field or magnetic field of the client's body. The questions this position raises are: Do humans actually have a biomagnetic field? Can a skilled therapist project a magnetic field from his or her hands? Can this in turn affect the magnetic field of the client? James Oschman reviews the scientific evidence for these ideas at length in the book *Energy Medicine: The Scientific Basis* and related articles.[16–24]

## THERAPIST'S POSITION AND MOVEMENT

1. Use the basic positions described in Chapter 6, Preparation and Positioning for Massage, in the sections on **standing aligned**, seated aligned, **lunge**, and **lunge and reach** postures.
2. Select a posture that is comfortable and stable to minimize inadvertent shaking of your hands when you must sustain contact for longer periods.

3. You may prefer to sit when working on the client's feet and head or when working unilaterally. Sitting allows you to support your forearms on the edge of the table, providing increased stability and reducing the likelihood of arm fatigue during the technique (Figures 7-1A and 7-1B).

## PALPATE

As you perform the technique, palpate the client's skin for the following:

1. Skin texture
2. Skin temperature
3. Presence of perspiration and moisture

## OBSERVE

As you perform the technique, observe the client for changes in the **level of arousal** and **autonomic balance** that reflect increasing relaxation. The signs listed below may indicate increased relaxation:

1. Decrease in rate and depth of breathing
2. Deeper voice tone
3. Changes in skin color such as flushing. Pallor may indicate an undesirable **sympathetic response**.
4. Systemic reduction of **muscle resting tension**, as evidenced by softening of the tissue contours or broadening and flattening of body segments
5. Muscle twitches and jerks
6. Increases in peristaltic noises
7. Decreases in heart rate, as evidenced by change in pulses that are visible at the neck, wrist, and foot
8. Agitation or sweating, which may indicate an undesirable sympathetic response

## COMMUNICATION WITH THE CLIENT

Communicate to encourage general relaxation, to guide the client's awareness of areas of the body, or to facilitate the client's breathing pattern. Here are some examples of statements that you can use.

1. "Let your . . . relax, as much as you're able."
2. "Feel the weight of your body" or "Let your body sink into the table."
3. "Notice what's occurring in your body. It's not unusual to experience sensations some distance from the location of my hands."
4. "Let your awareness move to . . ."

5. "It's not unusual to have emotions or feelings arise in response to touch. Just observe them and express them if you need to."
6. "Deepen your breathing without forcing it in any way."
7. "Notice how your ribs move here when you inhale."
8. "What is happening with your pain?" You can use this statement when you are applying the technique to reduce pain. It allows you to check how the client perceives that the intervention is affecting her pain at intervals during the application of the technique.

 **A Practice Sequence for Static Contact**

Practice time: 30 or 60 minutes per person.
Hold each position bilaterally for about 1 minute for a 30-minute session or 2 minutes for a 1-hour session. Therapists who use static contact extensively often recommend a sequence that proceeds in a direction from head to toe, as is described here. We suggest that students try different orders and draw their own conclusions.

| SUPINE | PRONE |
| --- | --- |
| Vertex | Vertex |
| Occiput | Parietal bone |
| Eyes/frontal bone | Temporal bone |
| Cheeks/jaw | Occiput |
| Anterior neck | Posterior neck |
| Anterior shoulders | Upper trapezius |
| Upper ribs | Mid and upper thorax |
| Lower ribs | Lower thorax |
| Elbows | Elbows |
| Dorsum of hands | Palms |
| Upper abdomen | Lumbar area |
| Lower abdomen | Sacrum |
| Hips | Gluteal area |
| Knees | Knees |
| Ankles | Ankles |
| Dorsum of feet | Plantar surface of feet |

Home study: Devise comparable sequences that:

1. Move in a toe-to-head direction
2. Incorporate more contact between joints
3. Spend half of the allotted time on a specified region such as the legs

## Static Contact: Further Study and Practice

### NAMES AND ORIGINS

Static contact is probably the simplest, oldest, and most universal of massage techniques. In other texts or massage-related systems, the technique that we call static contact is also known as "resting position," "passive touch," "superficial touch," "light touch," "static touch," "maintained touch," or "stationary holding."[1,3-7] It is used extensively in **energetic approaches**, such as Therapeutic Touch, Reiki, and Polarity Therapy, that attempt to regulate the magnetic or energy field of the body.

### OUTCOMES AND EVIDENCE

Static contact is the least mechanically stimulating of the massage techniques. Therapists can use it to enhance the flow of interventions, to achieve **outcomes** related to clients' psychological and physiological impairments, and to clarify client education. Clinicians can use static contact to facilitate the flow and **coherence** of interventions in two ways: to establish a **therapeutic rapport** with the client[9,25,26] and to reduce **anxiety** and induce sedation[11-14] at the beginning and end of massage interventions that incorporate other techniques.[1,3,4] Static contact has many psychological effects. Clinicians can use it by itself to decrease anxiety and the perception of pain in conditions in which the use of movement or force is contraindicated or poorly tolerated. For example, it can be used in situations of trauma, acute conditions, extreme or **intractable** pain, illness, dying, postsurgery, systemic weakness, convalescence, emotional distress, hypersensitivity, and posttraumatic stress and when there is a history of violence, sexual abuse, or poor physical self-image.[27-34] Static contact is also indispensable when teaching a client breathing techniques (see Figures 7-2 and 7-3) or when cueing a client to become aware of any body segment.[35] Furthermore, clinicians can use it to facilitate movement. Finally, static contact is integrated into therapeutic approaches such as Therapeutic Touch, Reiki, and Polarity, which conceptualize the philosophy of treatment in terms of energy or life force.[13-14,31-33,36-44] Table 7-1 summarizes the main outcomes for body structures and functions for static contact.

The Center for Complementary Care in the United Kingdom performed an uncontrolled, preliminary evaluation of "healing by gentle touch" in 35 clients with cancer.[34] Clinicians used "a simple repeating pattern" of "non-invasive touch on the head, chest, arms, legs and feet for approximately 40 minutes" that would be difficult to replicate without reviewing the references cited in the study. Outcome measures included reasonable pre- and posttreatment measures of physical and psychological function. The most pronounced improvements were seen in the clients' subjective ratings of perceived stress and relaxation, severe pain/discomfort, and depression/anxiety. This was particularly evident in those clients who had the most severe symptoms on entry. This research study was conceptually clear, relevant, and well-reported. The study's primary drawback was its lack of a control group for its pretest, posttest design. The authors concluded that a more rigorous evaluation using a randomized pretest, posttest design with a control group was warranted.

Weze C, Leathard HL, Grange J, Tiplady P, Stevens G. Evaluation of healing by gentle touch in 35 clients with cancer. *Eur J Oncol Nurs.* 2004;8:40–49.

### Critical Thinking Question

What characteristics of static contact make it well suited to the treatment of seriously ill people?

## CAUTIONS AND CONTRAINDICATIONS

Clinicians need clinical training and supervised practice when learning static contact. Advanced training may be advisable when dealing with pathological conditions. Static contact is a **reflex technique**; consequently, the contraindications for the use of **mechanical techniques** do not generally apply (see Chapter 3, Clinical Decision Making for Massage).[1] The primary exception to this rule is that the use of static contact may be contraindicated locally in areas of acute inflammation because of pain. Furthermore, clients who are experiencing considerable pain or distress or who are dying may not tolerate touch at all.

There are several cautions for the use of static contact.[1] Because clinicians can use it with frail clients, high-risk infants, or terminally ill clients, they need to be sensitive to the emotional and physical needs of these clients. Static contact looks deceptively simple and causes minimal mechanical effects. Nevertheless, like all massage techniques, it can give rise to very complex physical and emotional responses, including **touch-triggered memory**.[45] As with all massage techniques, clinicians must obtain **informed consent** from the client prior to using this technique. When the client's condition results in an impairment of the client's cognitive function or level of consciousness, the clinician may have difficulty obtaining informed consent to treat. In addition, the clinician must maintain clear and consistent communication with the client throughout the intervention when she is applying the technique for long periods or over large areas of the client's body.

## USING STATIC CONTACT IN TREATMENT

Before considering the use of static contact for treatment, you should be able to perform **diaphragmatic breathing** while standing and sitting. You should also know how to assess and track autonomic function in a client.

### Relaxation

There are several modalities that you can use in a complementary manner with static contact to promote relaxation.

1. You can use **progressive relaxation or diaphragmatic breathing**[35] prior to, or simultaneously with, static contact to enhance sedative effects. For example, you can combine prolonged contact with the client's occiput, ribcage, or abdomen with instruction on diaphragmatic breathing.
2. Moist **hot packs** can enhance sedation and analgesia, if the use of heat is appropriate for the client's condition.[46]
3. Some **craniosacral** therapy techniques may have a calming effect on the client.[47]
4. Instruct the client to rest from 10 to 30 minutes and to resume activity slowly if experiencing the sedative effects of static contact.

## Superficial Stroking: Foundations

### DEFINITION

Superficial stroking: Gliding over the client's skin with minimal **deformation** of subcutaneous tissues. Therapists usually apply this stroke unidirectionally over large areas of the client's body.

### USES

Therapists can use superficial stroking to reduce pain and to relax or stimulate clients depending on the contact, direction, and rate of application. It may also have effects on resting muscle tension and neuromuscular tone.

### PALPATION PRACTICE

The following palpation exercises will help you develop the manual skill and focus you need to perform superficial stroking well.

1. Stroke a carpet or broadloom and determine the direction of the nap. Stroke textured woven fabrics and attempt to describe the pattern of the weave by palpation alone.
2. With closed eyes and constantly moving palmar contact, run your hand over large objects maintaining constant light pressure: car bodies, furniture, and wood and metal sculptures. Form a mental image of the shape. How much detail can you discern about the surface finish without using your eyes?
3. Stroke the bare limb of a practice partner in one direction. Try to perceive variations in temperature and texture between areas. Do you come to the same judgments if the stroke goes in the opposite direction?

## Superficial Stroking: Technique

### MANUAL TECHNIQUE

In Figures 7-8 to 7-15, superficial stroking is applied to the various regions of the body. The order of figures is from head to foot in supine and then in prone. Each figure illustrates most of the guidelines for manual technique outlined below.

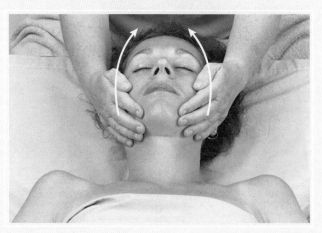

**Figure 7-8** Slow, bilateral superficial stroking of the face with palmar contact can produce sedative effects.[1,3,5]

1. Lubricant is not usually required to achieve glide without binding.
2. Relax your hands when you use the full palmar surface to perform the stroke. Use only enough hand weight to ensure good contact with the client's skin.
3. Perform superficial stroking in one direction, unless the desired outcome of the intervention is stimulation, since the reflex effects of superficial stroking are dependent on direction.
4. Return your hands to the starting position in the air for the **return stroke**. Use the same speed for the return stroke as for the stroke itself because this encourages a stable rhythm, which is necessary to achieve systemic sedation.
5. Although responses vary from person to person and with the context of treatment, you can achieve different effects by adjusting the type of contact, rate, and direction of the stroke.[1,3-7,48] Palmar contact, slow steady rate, **centrifugal** direction on the limbs, and caudal direction

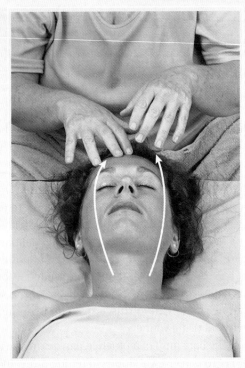

Figure 7-9 Fingertip superficial stroking of the face and scalp can provide a refreshing end to a massage sequence.

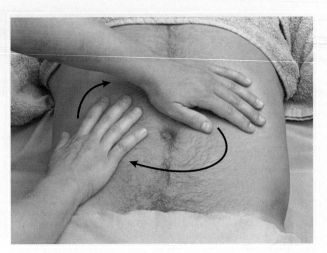

Figure 7-11 Continuous hand-over-hand palmar superficial stroking of the abdomen in the direction of colonic flow.

nique of breaking up a long stroke into overlapping shorter ones is called "layering," "shingling,"[3] or "thousand hands."[7,48] This technique enables you to cover a large area with less reaching for each stroke, and it creates a sensory experience that may help some clients to relax.

7. On the abdomen, you may perform the stroke across the abdomen or in the direction of colonic flow (Figures 7-10 and 7-11).[48]

on the back tend to produce sedation (Figure 7-13A). Conversely, fingertip contact, fast or irregular rate, **centripetal** direction on the limbs, and cephalad direction on the back tend to produce arousal (Figure 7-14). Fingertip stroking is usually stimulating and may sometimes be irritating (Figures 7-9, 7-13B, and 7-14).

6. You can substitute a succession of overlapping short strokes for a single long stroke (Figure 7-15). The tech-

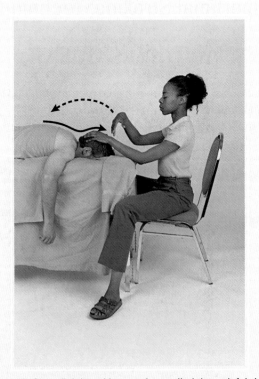

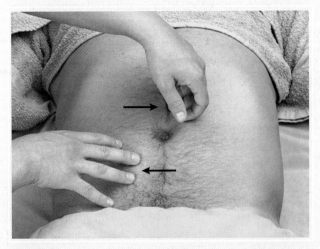

Figure 7-10 Dorsal and palmar contact surfaces alternate during transverse, bidirectional superficial stroking of the abdomen.

Figure 7-12 Superficial stroking can be applied through fabric, and the practitioner may choose a seated aligned posture.

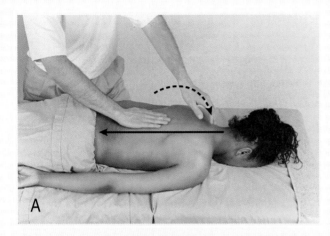

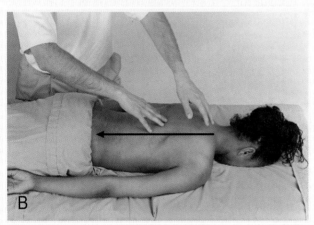

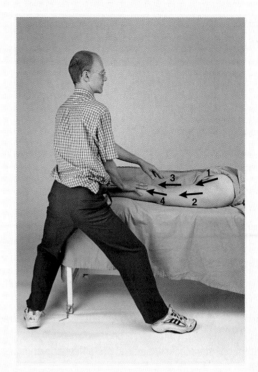

Figure 7-15 For long regions such as the posterior leg, the therapist may use overlapping short strokes instead of one long stroke.

Figure 7-13 A. Slow, regular palmar stroking down the spine produces sedative effects.[3] The return stroke in the air (dotted line) is made at the same rate as the stroke. B. Fingertip contact can yield a more stimulating effect than palmar contact, with other components being the same.[1,3,5]

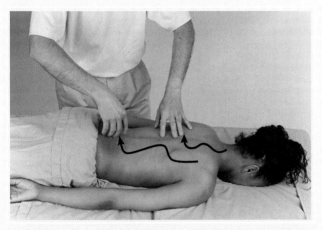

Figure 7-14 Fast, multidirectional, superficial fingertip stroking can be very stimulating and may be used judiciously to produce increased arousal in sedated clients.

8. Contact with the spinal column from occiput to sacrum, hands, feet, and face may produce stronger clinical effects than that with other areas of the body, possibly because of the density of nervous innervation in these areas (Figures 7-8, 7-9, and 7-13A).

9. You should use superficial stroking with caution on the plantar surface of the feet.

10. You can apply superficial stroking effectively through the client's clothes or a sheet (Figure 7-12). In this situation, take steps to prevent bunching of the fabric over the skin, since this will detract from the regularity of the sensory input that the client receives during the stroke. You may tuck the drape securely or use one hand to tighten the intervening fabric while your other hand performs the technique.

## How superficial stroking might work

The **"gate theory of pain"** first proposed by Melzack and Wall provides an explanation for the use of superficial stroking to reduce pain. Superficial stroking supplies a barrage of sensory information carried on large-fiber

| Box 7-2 | Components of Superficial Stroking |

**Contact:** Palmar surface of your hand, or fingertips

**Pressure:** Minimal

**Engages:** Skin only

**Direction:** Usually parallel to the long axis of the body segment being stroked

**Amplitude:** The full length of the body segment

**Rate:** 5 to 100 cm/second

**Duration:** 10 seconds to 10 minutes or more, depending on the therapist's intention

**Intergrades with:** Superficial effleurage

**Combines with:** May be combined with fine vibration or shaking

**Context:** May be used alone. Therapists often use it as a "framing technique," performed at the beginning and end of regional or full-body sequences that incorporate deeper techniques

cutaneous afferents that may reduce the transmission of pain impulses through the same level of the spinal chord to the higher centers of the central nervous system. Researchers have recently questioned whether the gate theory is the mechanism for massage's analgesic effects.[15] Nonetheless, stroking may reduce pain[49–53] by boosting levels of **oxytocin**.[49–52]

Superficial stroking adds components of rate and rhythm to the light touch of static contact. Could the element of periodicity cause a relaxing effect beyond that of the touch itself? Consider the idea of **entrainment**—the alteration of a biological rhythm in response to an external stimulus.[54–57] Research suggests that listening closely to music or sounds of specific frequencies can alter biological rhythms of the body such as breathing and heart rate.[1,56,57] Perhaps a rhythmical kinesthetic stimulus such as superficial stroking induces effects comparable to a rhythmical auditory stimulus, entraining the autonomic system towards a state of relaxation.

### Critical Thinking Question

Why is stroking usually performed *down* the limbs?

# THERAPIST'S POSITION AND MOVEMENT

1. Use the basic positions described in Chapter 6, Preparation and Positioning for Massage, in the sections on standing **aligned**, seated aligned, **lunge**, and lunge and reach positions.
2. Keep your shoulders and arms relaxed during the stroke, without straining to reach at the end; never fully extend your elbows.
3. It is easier to perform long strokes by using a relatively wide foot placement and shifting the weight of your upright torso from one leg to the other as the stroke proceeds.

# PALPATE

As you perform the technique, palpate the client's skin for the following:

1. Skin texture
2. Skin temperature
3. Presence of perspiration and moisture
4. Slight horizontal stretch of the skin that occurs in the direction of movement. Because of the light pressure and relatively fast rate, this stretch does not approach the **elastic barrier** of the skin.

# OBSERVE

As you perform the technique, observe the client for increases or decreases in the client's level of arousal and autonomic balance. The following signs may indicate increased relaxation:

1. Change of rate and depth of breathing
2. Changes in voice tone
3. Changes in skin color such as flushing or pallor
4. Systemic reduction of **muscle resting tension**, as evidenced by softening of the tissue contours or settling of body segments
5. Muscle twitches and jerks
6. Peristaltic noises
7. Change in heart rate as evidenced by change in pulses that are visible at the neck, wrist, and foot
8. Agitation or sweating may indicate an undesirable sympathetic response

# COMMUNICATION WITH THE CLIENT

Communicate to encourage general relaxation or guide the client's awareness of areas of the body. Here are some examples of statements that you can use.

1. "Let your . . . relax, as much as you're able."
2. "Feel the weight of your body" or "Let your body sink into the table."
3. "Notice what's occurring in your body. It's not unusual to experience sensations some distance from the location of my hands."
4. "Let your awareness move to . . ."
5. "It's not unusual to have emotions or feelings arise in response to touch. Just observe them and express them if you need to."
6. "What is happening with your pain?" You can use this statement when you are applying the technique to reduce pain. It allows you to check how the client perceives that the intervention is affecting her pain at intervals during the application of the technique.

## A Practice Sequence for Superficial Stroking

Practice time: 30 to 45 minutes per person.

Begin with palmar stroking down the spine from the crown to the sacrum. Begin at a fast rate (100 cm/second) and decrease the rate gradually over a period of 10 minutes until it is very slow (5–10 cm/second). Follow with 5 minutes of static contact at both the sacrum and occiput.

After communicating changes in your intentions to your client, experiment with a variety of combinations of contact, rate, and direction that include different regions of the body in any orderly sequence. Examples of these combinations are:

Moderate rate, palmar, layered from occiput to sacrum
Fast, palmar, across the back
Fast and irregular, fingertip, on the back
Slow, fingertip, down one limb
Fast, palmar, up the opposite limb
Moderate rate, palmar, across the abdomen
Slow, palmar or fingertip, up the face and scalp

Finish with palmar stroking down the spine and static contact at the sacrum and occiput. Ask the client for feedback.

Note: It takes time and repetition to produce sedative effects; it takes neither to achieve increased arousal.

# Superficial Stroking: Further Study and Practice

## NAMES AND ORIGINS

In other texts or massage-related systems, the technique that we call superficial effleurage is known as "light stroking," "feather stroking," "nerve stroking," or "reflex stroking."[7,48] Some authors do not distinguish between stroking and **effleurage**[1,6] or consider stroking to be similar to effleurage without the restriction of the direction of the stroke.[7,48] This is discussed further in Chapter 8, Superficial Fluid Techniques. This book uses **Mennell's**[58] definition, which considers superficial stroking to be a distinct reflex technique that is performed with a lighter pressure than that used with effleurage.

## OUTCOMES AND EVIDENCE

Clinicians can use superficial stroking to change the client's level of arousal, for pain reduction, and to facilitate changes in muscle resting tension and **neuromuscular tone**. Since superficial stroking can result in sedation or stimulation, depending on the contact, direction, and rate of application,[7,48] clinicians often use it at the beginning or end of an intervention session to adjust the client's **level of arousal**. Like static contact, this technique is well suited to difficult situations in which the use of pressure is contraindicated. Frequently, superficial stroking has been incorporated into interventions, such as the "**slow-stroke** back rub" described in the nursing literature,[59-67] that are used to improve mood and relieve anxiety in the critically ill.[60-63] Superficial stroking that can stimulate the client's level of arousal,[7,48] when judiciously applied, may temporarily ameliorate some symptoms of debility, convalescence, lethargy, and depression. Superficial stroking may have a role in treating pain when **mechanical techniques** are contraindicated. In this case, pain relief may occur because light touch and vibration increase large-diameter afferent nerve input and may reduce the transmission of "slow" pain impulses through the spinal gate of the segment being touched.[5,7] It may also occur because stroking boosts levels of oxytocin.[49-52] Superficial stroking may minimally facilitate or inhibit local muscle tone via musculocutaneous reflexes and may reduce **spasm**. Finally, clinicians can use it locally and over the posterior primary rami to decrease limb **spasticity**.[3,68]

Research also suggests that superficial stroking and gentle passive movement (infant massage) can have a positive effect on the physiological and psychological development of premature infants,[69-85] ill infants,[86,87] and full-term infants,[88-95] while enhancing maternal health and mother–child interaction.[96-101] Leading researchers[93] suggest that "light" (superficial) pressure is less effective in promoting weight gain than "moderate" pressure for normal infants.

Table 7-1 summarizes the main outcomes for body structures and functions for superficial stroking.

## EXAMINING THE EVIDENCE

In a recent randomized controlled trial, researchers at the University of Georgia and the University of Miami's **Touch Research Institute** examined the effects of 5 days of massage therapy on stable preterm infants who averaged 30 weeks at delivery.[70] The 15-minute intervention consisted of 5 minutes of "moderate pressure stroking with the flats of the fingers of both hands" that covered the whole body, 5 minutes of passive flexion/extension movements of the limbs, and 5 more minutes of stroking. The intervention was performed three times a day. The 16 massaged infants gained 53% more weight and slept less than 16 infants in the control group. No placebo treatment is described for the control; presumably, the researchers had a "no massage" control group. The small sample size was nonetheless large enough to show statistical significance in daily weight gain between the massage and nonmassage groups. Overall, this study is succinct, complete, and rigorous.

Dieter JN, Field T, Hernandez-Reif M, Emory EK, Redzepi M. Stable preterm infants gain more weight and sleep less after five days of massage therapy. *J Pediatr Psychol.* 2003;28:403–411.

# CAUTIONS AND CONTRAINDICATIONS

Clinicians need clinical training and supervised practice when learning superficial stroking. Advanced training may be advisable when dealing with pathological conditions. Superficial stroking is a reflex technique; consequently, the contraindications for the use of mechanical techniques do not generally apply (see Chapter 3, Clinical Decision Making for Massage).[1] The primary exception to this rule is that the use of superficial stroking may be contraindicated locally in areas of acute inflammation because of pain. In this situation, treat the client's pain by performing the technique on adjacent areas as tolerated by the client. Furthermore, clients who are experiencing considerable pain or distress or who are dying may not tolerate touch at all.

There are several cautions for the use of superficial stroking.[1] When the client's condition results in an impairment of the client's cognitive function or level of consciousness, the clinician may have difficulty obtaining informed consent to treat. Because clinicians can use superficial stroking with frail clients, high-risk infants, or terminally ill clients, they need to be sensitive to the emotional and physical needs of these clients. Although recent myocardial infarction was once considered to be a contraindication for massage, light massage is now considered to be permissible. A further cardiac-related caution is that a 48-hour wait is advisable after coronary artery bypass surgery.[102] Finally, if superficial stroking is being used for reflex stimulation, the clinician needs to ensure that the application of the technique does not become irritating. Ticklishness frequently occurs in areas where there is underlying muscular tension. If the application of superficial stroking tickles the client, the clinician should try the following strategies: switch to a broader contact, add lubricant, check that the stroke direction does not run against the grain of the client's body hair, or change to a technique that uses more pressure.

# USING SUPERFICIAL STROKING IN TREATMENT

Before considering the use of superficial stroking for treatment, you should be able to perform diaphragmatic breathing while standing and sitting, and you should know how to assess and track autonomic function in a client.

## Relaxation

There are several modalities that you can use in a complementary manner with superficial stroking to promote relaxation.

1. You can use progressive relaxation or diaphragmatic breathing[35] prior to, or simultaneously with, superficial stroking to enhance sedative effects.
2. Moist hot packs can enhance sedation and analgesia, if the use of heat is appropriate for the client's condition.[46]
3. Some craniosacral techniques may have a calming effect on the client.[47]
4. Instruct your client to rest from 10 to 30 minutes and to resume activity slowly if experiencing the sedative effects of superficial stroking.

---

## Fine Vibration: Foundations

### DEFINITION

Fine vibration: A fast, oscillating or trembling movement that is produced on the client's skin and that results in minimal deformation of subcutaneous tissues.[103–128]

### USES

Therapists can use fine vibration to achieve pain relief and produce changes in neuromuscular tone.

---

## Fine Vibration: Technique

### MANUAL TECHNIQUE

In Figures 7-16 to 7-21, fine vibration is applied to the various regions of the body. The order of figures is from head to foot in supine and then in prone. Each figure illustrates most of the guidelines for manual technique outlined here.

1. The amplitude of fine vibration is scarcely visible and is generally less than 1 to 5 mm. Fine vibration exerts minimal mechanical effects beyond the surface of the client's skin.
2. Use your forearm and wrist to produce the motion, with as little recruitment of your shoulder muscles as possible. One efficient method of generating fine vibration is to use a rapid, low-amplitude, alternating pronation and supination of the forearm—a "flutter" (Figures 7-16A and 7-16B). Do not attempt to compress and release the client's tissues with the whole contact surface during the application of fine vibration. This action will usually recruit your shoulder muscles and result in a more vigorous and fatiguing manipulation that has mechanical effects on the client's subcutaneous tissues.
3. Your two hands are rarely even in ability. You can improve the ability of the less competent hand by practicing the application of fine vibration with both hands together in mirror image. Some therapists choose to use only their dominant hand for fine vibration.
4. If you cannot produce an even vibration, try reducing the speed of the oscillation. It is preferable to produce a slow, controlled vibration than a fast, uncontrolled one. Control and speed of application come with practice.
5. You can combine fine vibration with superficial stroking to yield a "running" vibration whose reflex effects will also depend on the contact, rate, and direction of the stroking (Figure 7-18).

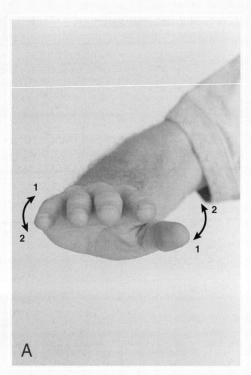

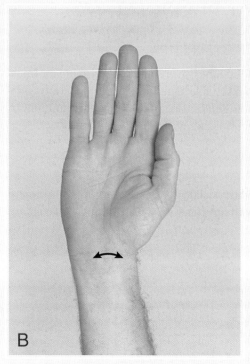

**Figure 7-16** A. To create a fine vibration, the practitioner may use low-amplitude alternating pronation and supination of the forearm. B. Or the practitioner may use alternating radial and ulnar deviation of the wrist or forearm.

## *How fine vibration might work*

The **gate theory of pain** first proposed by Melzack and Wall provides an explanation for the use of machine-produced fine vibration to reduce pain. Fine vibration supplies a barrage of sensory information that is carried on large-fiber cutaneous afferents and reduces the transmission of pain impulses through the same level of the spinal cord to the higher centers of the central ner-

vous system. Researchers have recently questioned whether the gate theory is the mechanism of massage's analgesic effects.[15] However, one recent study found that ipsilateral and contralateral applications of 100-Hz vibration produced equally significant changes in pain associated with temperomandibular joint dysfunction. This finding suggests that some type of central nervous system mechanism is at work[129] other than **endorphins** or another endogenous opioid.[114,119–122]

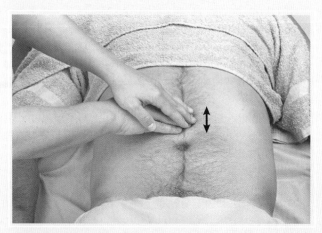

**Figure 7-17** Fine vibration with stabilized fingertip contact applied to the abdomen.

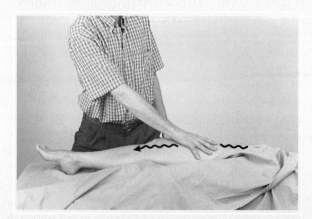

**Figure 7-18** Fine vibration may be combined with stroking to produce a "running vibration," here shown on the quadriceps and anterior leg.

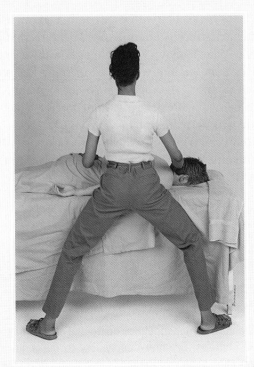

**Figure 7-19** Whatever the manual method, posture must be aligned (standing or seated), and particular care must be taken to let the shoulders relax.

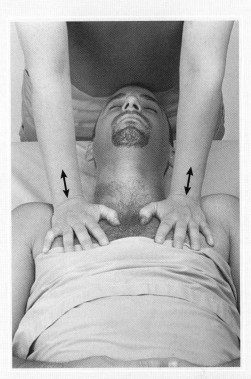

**Figure 7-21** Coarser types of vibration that move subcutaneous tissue—such as the repeated rapid pumping of the ribcage shown here—have significant mechanical and proprioceptive effects and are discussed in later chapters.

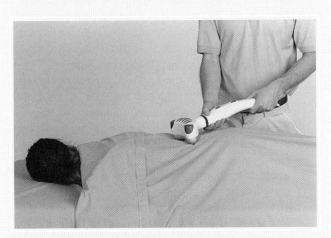

**Figure 7-20** A handheld device for producing fine vibration.

# THERAPIST'S POSITION AND MOVEMENT

1. Use the basic positions described in Chapter 6, Preparation and Positioning for Massage, in the sections on basic standing aligned and seated aligned postures. See also Figure 7-19.
2. Relax your shoulders (down) and flex your elbows. You will experience less fatigue if you engage your shoulder muscles as little as possible.

---

**Box 7-3**    **Components of Fine Vibration**

**Contact:** Palmar surface or fingertips are most common

**Pressure:** Minimal

**Engages:** Skin

**Direction:** N/A

**Amplitude/length:** Less than 1 to 5 mm

**Rate:** 4 to 10 Hz or more for manual vibration; 100 Hz is common for machine-produced vibration

**Duration:** 5 to 40 minutes for analgesia

**Intergrades with:** Shaking

**Combines with:** Can be combined with superficial stroking or compression

**Context:** Machine-produced vibration can be used alone. Manual fine vibration is often alternated with superficial stroking and/or static contact in situations in which the indications for treatment are similar

3. You may find it helpful to sit with your elbow or part of your forearm resting on the edge of the table.
4. Your body position must be stable, since inadvertent postural shifts will detract from the intended effects of fine vibration.

## PALPATE

As you perform the technique, palpate the client's skin for the following:

1. Skin texture
2. Skin temperature
3. Presence of perspiration and moisture

## OBSERVE

As you perform the technique, observe the client for decreases in level of pain or general signs of relaxation. The following signs may signal this.

1. Decrease in rate and depth of breathing
2. Deeper voice tone
3. Changes in skin color such as flushing. Pallor may indicate an undesirable sympathetic response.
4. Systemic reduction of muscle resting tension (see Observe sections in previous parts of this chapter), as evidenced by softening of the tissue contours or broadening and flattening of body segments
5. Muscle twitches and jerks
6. Increases in peristaltic noises
7. Decreases in heart rate as evidenced by change in pulses that are visible at the neck, wrist, and foot
8. Agitation or sweating, which may indicate an undesirable sympathetic response

## COMMUNICATION WITH THE CLIENT

Communicate to monitor the client's pain and to encourage general relaxation. Here are some examples of statements that you can use.

1. "What is happening with your pain?" You can use this statement when you are applying the technique to reduce pain. It allows you to check how the client perceives that the intervention is affecting her pain at intervals during the application of the technique.
2. "Deepen your breathing without forcing," "Let your body sink into the table," "Let yourself relax completely" can be used to facilitate relaxation. Altered autonomic functioning may, in turn, affect the perception of pain.

### A Practice Sequence for Manual Fine Vibration

Practice time: 15 minutes per day for several days.

1. Stand with your shoulders down and elbows flexed to 90 degrees. Breathe deeply. Try to make an even vibration of only your hand of less than 1 cm in the air. The wrist and forearm will move slightly, too. Continue for 1 minute, and then rest for a minute.
2. Begin again. Try to generate an equal movement of the two hands. Continue for a minute and then rest again.
3. Begin again. Slightly flex and extend your shoulders, then your elbows, and then your wrists. Move through various combinations of shoulder, elbow, and wrist flexion while continuing the vibration. Rest.
4. Place one hand on the opposite posterior deltoid. While vibrating with the free hand, can you tell if you are recruiting any shoulder girdle muscles to produce the vibration? Gradually increase the amplitude of the vibration to discover when your shoulder muscles begin to tense. Decrease the amplitude of the vibration and find the position and manual technique that recruits your shoulder muscles the least. Switch arms. Practice this sequence once a day, gradually extending the time for which you can perform the fine vibration continuously without fatigue until you have reached 5 minutes. Then begin practice on clients, alternating periods of fine vibrations with superficial stroking.

Note: Remember to relax, breathe, and let your shoulders drop.

## Fine Vibration: Further Study and Practice

## NAMES AND ORIGINS

In other texts or massage-related systems, the technique that we call fine vibration is known as "vibration," "mechanical vibration," "cutaneous vibration," "transcutaneous vibration," or "vibratory stimulation."[103-130] The term "vibration" has been used by some authors[3,5] to denote markedly differing techniques that involve shaking, compressing, or percussing the client's subcutaneous tissues with considerable force, as illustrated in Figure 7-21. This text distinguishes between fine vibration and the more vigorous forms of vibration, which have mechanical effects and are described in Chapter 9, Neuromuscular Techniques, Chapter 11, Passive Movement Techniques, and Chapter 12, Percussive Techniques. Recent research addresses fine vibration produced by small portable devices operating at frequencies varying from 20 to 200 Hz, with 100 Hz being the most commonly used.[103-129] The documented effects of machine-produced vibration, often referred to as mechanical vibration, cannot be extrapolated to manually produced fine vibration except with caution.

## OUTCOMES AND EVIDENCE

Clinicians can use machine-produced vibration to achieve pain relief and changes in neuromuscular tone. Machine-produced vibration can be an effective analgesic for acute and **chronic pain** of various causes such as dental pain, phantom limb pain, **myofascial pain**, tendinous pain, neurogenic pain, and idiopathic pain.[103-123,129] Although the mechanism of **analgesia** is not well understood, researchers have noted that the reduction of pain and accompanying elevation of the pain threshold can persist for some time after the intervention.[114,121,122] Analgesic effects are increased with sustained application of machine-produced vibration for 15 to 30 minutes or longer.[109,112] In addition, clinicians can obtain analgesic effects when they apply machine-produced vibration to different regions of the client's body in relation to the site of pain, including direct application to the site of pain over a large area, distal to the site of pain, to the antagonist muscle group, to adjacent **dermatomes**, or even contralateral to the site of pain.[107,113,114,116,123,129] Combining the vibration with moderate pressure, if the client's condition permits, may enhance the analgesic effects of the vibration.[106,109,112,113]

Machine-produced vibration can result in an elevation of resting tone of the muscles under the site of application.[124-126] This effect may be used, when treating clients with neurological conditions, to promote more balanced movement and to prepare the client to perform functional activity.[125,126] Other effects ascribed to fine vibration are reflex relaxation, especially when it is applied to the feet,[127] healing of chronic peripheral nerve lesions,[128] and reduction in frequency of postsurgical complications.[130] Table 7-1 summarizes the main outcomes for body structures and functions for fine vibration.

Effective application of manual fine vibration, using the technique described earlier, takes much practice. In addition, it requires considerable skill on the part of the clinician to perform sustained application of manual fine vibration for more than a few minutes, hence the frequent use of machine vibration. The light touch of superficial stroking is a less taxing manual alternative to manual fine vibration that also produces large-fiber afferent input.[131] Consequently, clinicians may alternate superficial stroking with, or substitute it for, fine vibration. In this situation, they may obtain similar analgesic effects if the duration of application is comparable.

### ? Critical Thinking Question
How could you use a fine vibration device during an intervention without reducing the time you have available to perform other hands-on techniques?

### EXAMINING THE EVIDENCE

A recent small (n = 17) uncontrolled study compared the ability of machine-produced 20-Hz vibration, 100-Hz vibration, and control treatment to reduce pain (both "magnitude" and "unpleasantness") in subjects with temporomandibular disorders (TMD).[129] **Visual analog scale** ratings and drawings both showed that pain was reduced by 100-Hz vibration but not by 20-Hz vibration. The results and analysis of spatial and temporal patterns of analgesia hint at the complexity of both the phenomena of pain and of its measurement. Spatial analysis showed that ipsilateral and contralateral effects of vibration were statistically equivalent for subjects with chronic temporomandibular joint pain. This suggests that vibratory analgesia for chronic pain relies, in part, on central nervous system mechanisms. Analgesic effects were statistically significant but judged to be too modest to be of clinical significance. However, this study used 10-minute applications of vibration, a much shorter time than previous researchers have recommended for maximizing analgesia using this technique.[109,112] It would be worthwhile to repeat this study using longer vibration times and including a separate control group.

Roy EA, Hollins M, Maixner W. Reduction of TMD pain by high-frequency vibration: a spatial and temporal analysis. *Pain.* 2003;101:267–274. Erratum in: *Pain.* 2003;104:717.

## CAUTIONS AND CONTRAINDICATIONS

Clinicians need clinical training and supervised practice when learning fine vibration. Advanced training may be advisable when dealing with pathological conditions. Fine vibration is a reflex technique; consequently, the contraindications for the use of mechanical techniques do not generally apply (see Chapter 3, Clinical Decision Making for Massage). If, however, the clinician is using fine vibration to treat pain in a client with an acute condition, the client may find the weight of the clinician's hand or a mechanical device intolerable. In this situation, the clinician should administer fine vibration in adjacent areas as tolerated by the client.

## USING FINE VIBRATION IN TREATMENT

### Analgesia

Before considering the use of fine vibration for treatment of pain you must perform a basic pain assessment and attempt to discover the cause of the client's pain. It is important to distinguish between acute nociceptive pain, chronic pain, and chronic pain syndrome. There are several modalities that you can use in a complementary manner to enhance pain relief while using fine vibration.

1. Application of transcutaneous electrical nerve stimulation (**TENS**) increases the analgesic effect of fine vibration.[119,120]
2. A variety of applications of heat, such as moist hot pack, **fluidotherapy**, and whirlpool, can enhance sedation and analgesia in the client.[47,132] Applications of cold, including cold packs, **ice massage**, and cold baths can enhance analgesia in the client.[47,132] You must ensure that the selected modality is appropriate for the client's condition.
3. You can instruct the client in the home use of a vibrating massage device and in appropriate hydrotherapy for analgesia.

## Clinical Case

### History of Present Illness

A 44-year-old male with late-stage **AIDS** who has been admitted to hospice from home for **palliative care**.

## Subjective

- General complaints of pain and stiffness at rest and with activity
- Complaints of pain during examinations of range of motion and functional activity
- Complaints of anxiety and depression regarding terminal condition
- Complaints of difficulty sleeping because of pain and anxiety

# Objective

## Impairments

▪ Marked wasting of upper and lower extremity muscles
▪ Range of motion—active and passive within normal limits in upper and lower extremities (pain throughout range)
▪ Mild muscle tightness in upper and lower extremities
▪ Generalized weakness of upper and lower extremities; strength is grade 2–3/5
▪ Exercise tolerance: General debility, complains of fatigue and pain with less than 5 minutes of activity

## Functional Limitations

▪ Bed mobility: Requires moderate assistance of one person
▪ Activities of daily living: Requires moderate assistance of one person for dressing and feeding
▪ Requires maximal assistance of one person for lying to/from sitting and sitting to/from standing and side of bed
▪ Mood: Appears anxious and depressed
▪ Limited social interaction

# Analysis

## Treatment Rationale

To provide relief of pain, stiffness, anxiety, and depression as the client's functional level declines

| Impairment | Outcomes and Role of Massage |
|---|---|
| Pain | Decreased complaints of pain<br>Primary treatment; analgesia is a direct effect |
| Decreased muscle **extensibility** | Increased muscle extensibility<br>Primary treatment; increased muscle extensibility is a direct effect |
| Muscle wasting | Decreased muscle wasting<br>Improbable effect; wasting is due to disuse |
| Muscle weakness | Increased muscle strength<br>Possible secondary effect; weakness is primarily due to disuse; pain reduction may facilitate willingness to perform movement through range |
| Poor **exercise tolerance** | Improved exercise tolerance<br>Possible secondary effect; poor exercise tolerance is a result of debility; pain reduction may facilitate willingness to perform activities |
| Anxiety | Decreased anxiety<br>Primary treatment; anxiety relief and systemic sedation are direct effects |
| Depression | Improved mood<br>Secondary effect; sensory arousal may ease some symptoms of depression and lethargy |

| *Activity Limitation* | *Functional Outcomes* |
|---|---|
| ▦ Decreased ability to perform self-care activities | ▦ Patient will be able to perform feeding and dressing with assistance as required with decreased complaints of pain and stiffness |
| ▦ Decreased ability to perform transfers | ▦ Patient will be able to perform bed mobility and transfers with assistance as required with decreased complaints of pain and stiffness |
| ▦ Decreased social interaction | ▦ Patient will demonstrate increased social interaction with decreased complaints of depression |
| ▦ Impaired sleep | ▦ Patient will demonstrate increased duration of sleep with decreased complaints of pain and anxiety interfering with sleep |

## *Plan*

| | |
|---|---|
| Massage Techniques | Static contact, soothing superficial stroking, and manually produced fine vibration will almost certainly be tolerated and will all reduce pain and anxiety; machine-produced fine vibration, superficial effleurage, and gentle petrissage (see later chapters) may be tolerated depending on the patient's sensitivity, level of debility, and previous familiarity with massage. |
| Other Appropriate Techniques and Interventions | Medical management, passive and active assisted range of motion, assisted activities of daily living, assisted bed mobility and transfers, counseling or pastoral care. |

## *References*

1. Fritz S. *Mosby's Fundamentals of Therapeutic Massage.* St Louis: Mosby-Lifeline; 2004.
2. American Physical Therapy Association. *Guide to Physical Therapist Practice.* 2nd ed. Alexandria, VA: American Physical Therapy Association; 1999.
3. Benjamin PJ, Tappan FM. *Tappan's Handbook of Healing Massage Techniques.* 4th ed. Upper Saddle River, NJ: Pearson Prentice Hall; 2005.
4. Loving J. *Massage Therapy.* Stamford, CT: Appleton & Lange; 1999.
5. de Domenico G, Wood EC. *Beard's Massage.* 4th ed. Philadelphia: WB Saunders; 1997.
6. Salvo SG. *Massage Therapy: Principles and Practice.* 2nd ed. Philadelphia: WB Saunders; 2003.
7. Holey E, Cook E. *Evidence-Based Therapeutic Massage.* 2nd ed. Edinburgh: Churchill Livingstone; 2003.
8. Chaitow L. *Palpation and Assessment Skills.* Edinburgh: Churchill-Livingston; 2003.
9. McKorkle R. Effects of touch on seriously ill patients. *Nurs Res.* 1974;3:125–132.
10. Weiss SJ. Psychological effects of caregiver touch on incidence of cardiac dysrhythmia. *Heart Lung.* 1986;15:496–503.
11. Anonymous. Research: Reiki induces relaxation, liminal state of awareness. *Massage Magazine.* 2002;129.
12. Oh HJ, Park JS. Effects of hand massage and hand holding on the anxiety in patients with local infiltration anesthesia. *Taehan Kanho Hakhoe Chi.* 2004;34:924–933.
13. Post-White J, Kinney ME, Savik K, Gau JB, Wilcox C, Lerner I. Therapeutic massage and healing touch improve symptoms in cancer. *Integr Cancer Ther.* 2003;2:332–344.
14. Wardell DW, Engebretson J. Biological correlates of Reiki touch healing. *J Adv Nurs.* 2001;33:439.
15. Moyer CA, Rounds J, Hannum JW. A meta-analysis of massage therapy research. *Psychol Bull.* 2004;130:3–18.
16. Oschman JL. *Energy Medicine: The Scientific Basis.* Edinburgh: Churchill Livingston, 2000.
17. Oschman JL. Energy and the healing response. *J Bodywork Movement Ther.* 2005;9:3–15.
18. Oschman JL. Clinical aspects of biological fields: an introduction for health care professionals. *J Bodywork Movement Ther.* 2002;6:117–125.
19. Oschman JL. The electromagnetic environment: implications for bodywork. Part 1: environmental energies. *J Bodywork Movement Ther.* 2000;4:56–67.
20. Oschman JL. Energy circles: energy review part 6B. *J Bodywork Movement Ther.* 1998;2:59–61.
21. Oschman JL. What is healing energy? Part 6: conclusions: is energy medicine the medicine of the future? Energy review part 6A. *J Bodywork Movement Ther.* 1998;2:46–59.
22. Oschman JL. What is healing energy? Part 2: measuring the fields of life. Energy review part 2A. *J Bodywork Movement Ther.* 1997;1:117–121.
23. Oschman JL. Polarity, therapeutic touch, magnet therapy and related methods. Energy review part 2B. *J Bodywork Movement Ther.* 1997;1:123–128.

24. Oschman JL. What is healing energy? Part 4: vibrational medicines. Energy review part 4A. *J Bodywork Movement Ther.* 1997;1:239–247.

25. Knable J. Handholding: one means of transcending barriers of communication. *Heart Lung.* 1981;10:1106.

26. Linn LS, Kahn KL. Physician attitudes toward the "laying on of hands" during the AIDS epidemic. *Acad Med.* 1989;64:408–409.

27. Lynch JJ, Thomas SA, Mills ME, et al. The effects of human contact on cardiac arrhythmia in coronary care patients. *J Nerv Mental Dis.* 1974;158:88–89.

28. Lynch JJ, Flaherty L, Emrich C, et al. Effects of human contact on the heart activity of curarized patients in a shock-trauma unit. *Am Heart J.* 1974;88:160–169.

29. McCaffery M, Wolff M. Pain relief using cutaneous modalities, positioning, and movement. *Hospice J.* 1992;8:121–153.

30. Werner R. A Massage Therapist's Guide to Pathology. 2nd ed. Philadelphia: Lippincott Williams & Wilkins; 2002.

31. Apostle-Mitchell M, MacDonald G. An innovative approach to pain management in critical care: therapeutic touch. *Off J Can Assoc Crit Care Nurs.* 1997;8:19–22.

32. Bracciante LE. Scientific validation for healing touch. *Massage Bodywork.* 2004;19:12.

33. Cook CAL, Guerrerio JK, Slater VE. Healing touch and quality of life in women receiving radiation treatment for cancer; a randomized controlled trial. *Altern Ther Health Med.* 2004;10:34–41.

34. Weze C, Leathard HL, Grange J, Tiplady P, Stevens G. Evaluation of healing by gentle touch in 35 clients with cancer. *Eur J Oncol Nurs.* 2004;8:40–49.

35. Kisner C, Colby LA. Therapeutic Exercise: Foundations and Techniques. 4th ed. Philadelphia: FA Davis; 2002.

36. Krieger D. The response of in-vivo human haemoglobin to an active healing therapy by direct laying on of hands. *Hum Dimens.* 1972;1:12–15.

37. Krieger D. Healing by the laying on of hands as a facilitator of bioenergetic change: the response of in-vivo human haemoglobin. *Psychoenerg Syst.* 1974;1:121–129.

38. Krieger D. Therapeutic touch: the imprimatur of nursing. *Am J Nurs.* 1975;75:784–787.

39. Krieger D, Peper E, Ancoli S. Physiologic indices of therapeutic touch. *Am J Nurs.* 1979;14:660–662.

40. Krieger D. The Therapeutic Touch. New York: Prentice-Hall; 1979.

41. Siedman M. Like a Hollow Flute: A Guide to Polarity Therapy. Santa Cruz, CA: Elan Press; 1982.

42. Gordon R. Your Healing Hands: The Polarity Experience. Santa Cruz, CA: Unity Press; 1979.

43. Stein D. Essential Reiki: A Complete Guide to an Ancient Healing Art. Freedom, CA: Crossing Press; 1995.

44. Richards K, Nagel C, Markie M, Elwell J, Barone C. Use of complementary and alternative therapies to promote sleep in critically ill patients. *Crit Care Nurs Clin North Am.* 2003;15:329–340.

45. Nathan B. Touch and Emotion in Manual Therapy. Edinburgh: Churchill Livingstone; 1999.

46. Fowlie L. Heat and Cold as Therapy. Toronto: Curties-Overzet Publications; 2006.

47. Upledger J, Vredevoogd JD. Craniosacral Therapy. Seattle, WA: Eastland Press; 1983.

48. Hollis M. Massage for Therapists. 2nd ed. Oxford, England: Blackwell Science; 1998.

49. Lund I, Lundeberg T, Kurosawa M, Uvnas-Moberg K. Sensory stimulation (massage) reduces blood pressure in unanaesthetized rats. *J Auton Nerv Syst.* 1999;78:30–37.

50. Lund I, Yu LC, Uvnas-Moberg K, et al. Repeated massage-like stimulation induces long-term effects on nociception: contribution of oxytocinergic mechanisms. *Eur J Neurosci.* 2002;16:330–338.

51. Kurosawa M, Lundeberg T, Agren G, Lund I, Uvnas-Moberg K. Massage-like stroking of the abdomen lowers blood pressure in anesthetized rats: influence of oxytocin. *J Auton Nerv Syst.* 1995;56:26–30.

52. Agren G, Lundeberg T, Uvnas-Moberg K, Sato A. The oxytocin antagonist 1-deamino-2-D-tyr-(oet)-4-thr-8-orn-oxytocin reverses the increase in the withdrawal response latency to thermal, but not mechanical, nociceptive stimuli following oxytocin administration or massage-like stroking in rats. *Neurosci Lett.* 1995;187:49–52.

53. Brooks WW, Conrad CH, Nedder AP, Bing OH, Slawsky MT. Thoracic massage permits use of echocardiography in unanesthetized rats. *Comp Med.* 2003;53:288–292.

54. Oschman JL. Therapeutic entrainment. Energy review part 3B. *J Bodywork Movement Ther.* 1997;1:189–194.

55. Oschman JL. What is healing energy? Part 3: silent pulses. Energy review part 3A. *J Bodywork Movement Ther.* 1997;1: 179–189.

56. Rider MS, Floyd JW, Kirkpatrick J. The effect of music, therapy, and relaxation on adrenal corticosteroids and the re-entrainment of circadian rhythms. *J Music Ther.* 1985;22:46–58.

57. McCaffrey R. Music listening as a nursing intervention: a symphony of practice. *Holist Nurs Pract.* 2002;16:70–77.

58. Mennell JB. Physical Treatment by Movement, Manipulation and Massage. 5th ed. Philadelphia: Blakiston; 1945.

59. Longworth JCD. Psychophysiological effects of slow stroke back massage in normotensive females. *Adv Nurs Sci.* 1982;6:44–61.

60. Sims S. Slow stroke back massage for cancer patients. *Nurs Times.* 1986;82:47–50.

61. Fakouri C, Jones P. Relaxation treatment: slow stroke back rub. *J Gerontol Nurs.* 1987;13:32–35.

62. Meek SS. Effects of slow stroke back massage on relaxation in hospice clients. *Image J Nurs Scholar.* 1993;25:17–21.

63. Lewis P, Nichols E, Mackey G, et al. The effect of turning and backrub on mixed venous oxygen saturation in critically ill patients. *Am J Crit Care.* 1997;6:132–140.

64. Mok E, Woo CP. The effects of slow-stroke back massage on anxiety and shoulder pain in elderly stroke patients. *Complement Ther Nurs Midwifery.* 2004;10:209–216.

65. Muller-Oerlinghausen B, Berg C, Scherer P, Mackert A, Moestl HP, Wolf J. Effects of slow-stroke massage as complementary treatment of depressed hospitalized patients. *Dtsch Med Wochenschr.* 2004;129:1363–1368.

66. Rowe M, Alfred D. The effectiveness of slow-stroke massage in diffusing agitated behaviors in individuals with Alzheimer's disease. *J Gerontol Nurs.* 1999;25:22–34.

67. Holland B, Pokorny ME. Slow stroke back massage: its effect on patients in a rehabilitation setting. *Rehabil Nurs.* 2001;26: 182–186.

68. Brouwer B, Sousa de Andrade V. The effects of slow stroking on spasticity in patients with multiple sclerosis: a pilot study. *Physiother Theory Pract.* 1995;11:13–21.

69. Aly H, Moustafa MF, Hassanein SM, Massaro AN, Amer HA, Patel K. Physical activity combined with massage improves

bone mineralization in premature infants: a randomized trial. *J Perinatol.* 2004;24:305–309.

70. Dieter JN, Field T, Hernandez-Reif M, Emory EK, Redzepi M. Stable preterm infants gain more weight and sleep less after five days of massage therapy. *J Pediatr Psychol.* 2003;28:403–411.

71. Ferber SG, Kuint J, Weller A, et al. Massage therapy by mothers and trained professionals enhances weight gain in preterm infants. *Early Hum Dev.* 2002;67:37–45.

72. Field T. Preterm infant massage therapy studies: an American approach. *Semin Neonatol.* 2002;7:487–494.

73. Field T. Massage therapy facilitates weight gain in preterm infants. *Current Dir Psychol Sci.* 2001;10:51–54.

74. Field TM. Massage therapy effects. *Am Psychol.* 1998;53: 1270–1281.

75. Hayes JA, Adamson-Macedo EN, Perera S. The mediating role of cutaneous sensitivity within neonatal psychoneuroimmunology. *Neuroendocrinol Lett.* 2000;21:187–193.

76. Hayes JA. TAC-TIC therapy: a non-pharmacological stroking intervention for premature infants. *Complement Ther Nurs Midwifery.* 1998;4:25–27.

77. Mathai S, Fernandez A, Mondkar J, Kanbur W. Effects of tactile-kinesthetic stimulation in preterms: a controlled trial. *Indian Pediatr.* 2001;38:1091–1098.

78. Vickers A, Ohlsson A, Lacy JB, Horsley A. Massage for promoting growth and development of preterm and/or low birthweight infants. *Cochrane Database Syst Rev.* 2004;2:CD000390.

79. Field T, Schanberg SM, Scafidi F, et al. Tactile/kinesthetic stimulation effect on preterm neonates. *Pediatrics.* 1986;77:654–658.

80. Schanberg SM, Evoniuk G, Kuhn CM. Tactile and nutritional aspects of maternal care: specific regulators of neuroendocrine function and cellular development. *Proc Soc Exp Biol Med.* 1984;175:135–146.

81. Jay SS. The effect of gentle human touch on mechanically ventilated very short-term gestation infants. *Matern Child Nurs J.* 1982;11:199–259.

82. White JL, Labarda RC. The effects of tactile and kinesthetic stimulation on neonatal development in the premature infant. *Dev Psychol.* 1976;9:569–577.

83. Kramer M, Chamorro I, Green D, Knudtson F. Extra tactile stimulation of the premature infant. *Nurs Res.* 1975;24:324–334.

84. Kattwinkel J, Nearman HS, Fanaroff AA, et al. Apnea of prematurity: comparative therapeutic effects of cutaneous stimulation and nasal continuous positive airway pressure. *J Pediatr.* 1975;86:588–592.

85. Solkoff N, Matuszak D. Tactile stimulation and behavioral development among low-birthweight infants. *Child Psychiatry Hum Dev.* 1975;6:33–37.

86. Lewis S. Utilising paediatric massage in an intensive care unit (PICU) in Saudi Arabia. *Aust J Holist Nurs.* 2000;7:29–33.

87. Onozawa K, Glover V, Adams D, Modi N, Kumar RC. Infant massage improves mother-infant interaction for mothers with postnatal depression. *J Affect Disord.* 2001;63:201–207.

88. Kim TI, Shin YH, White-Traut RC. Multisensory intervention improves physical growth and illness rates in Korean orphaned newborn infants. *Res Nurs Health.* 2003;26:424–433.

89. Agarwal KN, Gupta A, Pushkarna R, Bhargava SK, Faridi MM, Prabhu MK. Effects of massage and use of oil on growth, blood flow and sleep pattern in infants. *Indian J Med Res.* 2000; 112:212–217.

90. Kuhn CM, Schanberg SM. Responses to maternal separation: mechanisms and mediators. *Int J Dev Neurosci.* 1998;16: 261–270.

91. Bellieni CV, Bagnoli F, Perrone S, et al. Effect of multisensory stimulation on analgesia in term neonates: a randomized controlled trial. *Pediatr Res.* 2002;51:460–463.

92. Davanzo R. Newborns in adverse conditions: issues, challenges, and interventions. *J Midwifery Womens Health.* 2004; 49:29–35.

93. Field T, Hernandez-Reif M, Diego M, Feijo L, Vera Y, Gil K. Massage therapy by parents improves early growth and development. *Infant Behav Dev.* 2004;27:435–442.

94. Elias PM. Impact of topical oils on the skin barrier: possible implications for neonatal health in developing countries. *Acta Paediatr.* 2002;91:546.

95. Ferber SG, Laudon M, Kuint J, Weller A, Zisapel N. Massage therapy by mothers enhances the adjustment of circadian rhythms to the nocturnal period in full-term infants. *J Dev Behav Pediatr.* 2002;23:410–415.

96. Dennis CL. Treatment of postpartum depression. Part 2: a critical review of nonbiological interventions. *J Clin Psychiatry.* 2004;65:1252–1265.

97. Field T. Early interventions for infants of depressed mothers. *Pediatrics.* 1998;102:1305–1310.

98. Field T. Maternal depression effects on infants and early interventions. *Prev Med.* 1998;27:200–203.

99. Glover V, Onozawa K, Hodgkinson A. Benefits of infant massage for mothers with postnatal depression. *Semin Neonatol.* 2002;7:495–500.

100. Onozawa K, Glover V, Adams D, Modi N, Kumar RC. Infant massage improves mother-infant interaction for mothers with postnatal depression. *J Affect Disord.* 2001;63:201–207.

101. Porter LS, Porter BO. A blended infant massage–parenting enhancement program for recovering substance-abusing mothers. *Pediatr Nurs.* 2004;30:363–372,401.

102. Labyak SE, Metzger BL. The effects of effleurage backrub on the physiological components of relaxation: a meta-analysis. *Nurs Res.* 1997;46:59–62.

103. Hansson P, Ekblom A. Acute pain relieved by vibratory stimulus. *Br Dent J.* 1981;6:213.

104. Ottoson D, Ekblom A, Hansson P. Vibratory stimulation for the relief of pain of dental origin. *Pain.* 1981;10:37–45.

105. Lundeberg T, Ottoson D, Hakansson S, Meyerson BA. Vibratory stimulation for the control of intractable chronic orofacial pain. *Adv Pain Res Ther.* 1983;5:555–561.

106. Lundeberg TCM. Vibratory stimulation for the alleviation of chronic pain. *Acta Physiol Scand Suppl.* 1983;523:1–51.

107. Bini G, Cruccu G. Hagbarth KE, et al. Analgesic effect of vibration and cooling on pain induced by intraneural electrical stimulation. *Pain.* 1984;18:239–248.

108. Lundeberg T. The pain suppressive effect of vibratory stimulation and transcutaneous electrical nerve stimulation (TENS) as compared to aspirin. *Brain Res.* 1984;294:201–209.

109. Lundeberg T. Vibratory stimulation for the alleviation of pain. *Am J Chinese Med.* 1984;12:60–70.

110. Lundeberg T. A comparative study of the pain alleviating effect of vibratory stimulation, transcutaneous electrical nerve stimulation, electroacupuncture and placebo. *Am J Chinese Med.* 1984;12:72–79.

111. Lundeberg T. Long-term results of vibratory stimulation as a pain relieving measure for chronic pain. *Pain.* 1984;20:13–23.

112. Lundeberg T, Nordemar R, Ottoson D. Pain alleviation by vibratory stimulation. *Pain.* 1984;20:25–44.

113. Ekblom A, Hannson P. Extrasegmental transcutaneous electrical nerve stimulation and mechanical vibratory stimulation as compared to placebo for the relief of acute oro-facial pain. *Pain.* 1985;23:223–229.

114. Lundeberg T. Naloxone does not reverse the pain-reducing effect of vibratory stimulation. *Acta Anaesthesiol Scand.* 1985; 29:212–216.

115. Lundeberg T. Relief of pain from a phantom limb by peripheral stimulation. *J Neurol.* 1985;232:79–82.

116. Sherer CL, Clelland JA, O'Sullivan P, et al. The effect of two sites of high frequency vibration on cutaneous pain threshold. *Pain.* 1986;25:133–138.

117. Lundberg T, Abrahamsson P, Bondesson L, Haber E. Effect of vibratory stimulation on experimental and clinical pain. *Scand J Rehabil Med.* 1988;20:149–159.

118. Palmesamo TJ, Clelland JA, Sherer C, et al. Effect of high-frequency vibration on experimental pain threshold in young women when applied to areas of different size. *Clin J Pain.* 1989;5:337–342.

119. Guieu R, Tardy-Gervet MF, Blin O, Pouget J. Pain relief achieved by transcutaneous electrical nerve stimulation and/or vibratory stimulation in a case of painful legs and moving toes. *Pain.* 1990;42:43–48.

120. Guieu R, Tardy-Gervet MF, Roll JP. Analgesic effects of vibration and transcutaneous electrical nerve stimulation applied separately and simultaneously to patients with chronic pain. *Can J Neurol Sci.* 1991;18:113–119.

121. Guieu R, Tardy-Gervet MF, Giraud P. Metenkephalin and beta-endorphin are not involved in the analgesic action of transcutaneous vibratory stimulation. *Pain.* 1992;48:83–86.

122. Tardy-Gervet MF, Guieu R, Ribot-Ciscar E, Roll JP. Transcutaneous mechanical vibrations: analgesic effect and antinociceptive mechanisms. *Rev Neurol (Paris).* 1993;149:177–185 (Abstract).

123. Yarnitsky D, Kunin M, Brik R, Sprecher E. Vibration reduces thermal pain in adjacent dermatomes. *Pain.* 1997;69:75–77.

124. Cody FWJ, MacDermott N, Ferguson IT. Stretch and vibration reflexes of wrist flexor muscles in spasticity. *Brain.* 1987;110: 433–450.

125. Schmitt T, O'Sullivan S. *Physical Rehabilitation, Assessment and Treatment.* 2nd ed. Philadelphia: FA Davis; 1988.

126. Hagbarth KE, Eklund G. The muscle vibrator: a useful tool in neurological therapeutic work. *Scand J Rehabil Med.* 1969;1: 26–34.

127. Matheson DW, Edelson R, Hiatrides D, et al. Relaxation measured by EMG as a function of vibrotactile stimulation. *Biofeedback Self Regul.* 1976;1:285–292.

128. Spicher C, Kohut G. A significant increase in superficial sensation, a number of years after a peripheral neurologic lesion, using transcutaneous vibratory stimulation. *Ann Chir Main Memb Super (French).* 1997;16:124–129 (Abstract).

129. Roy EA, Hollins M, Maixner W. Reduction of TMD pain by high-frequency vibration: a spatial and temporal analysis. *Pain.* 2003;101:267–274. Erratum in *Pain.* 2003;104:717.

130. Strelis AA, Strelis AK, Roskoshnykh VK. Vibration massage in the prevention of postresection complications and in the clinical rehabilitation of patients with pulmonary tuberculosis after surgical interventions. *Probl Tuberk Bolezn Legk.* 2004;11: 29–34.

131. Hertling D, Kessler RM. *Management of Common Musculoskeletal Conditions.* 4th ed. Philadelphia: Lippincott Williams and Wilkins; 2006.

132. Michlovitz S. *Thermal Agents in Rehabilitation.* 3rd ed. Philadelphia: FA Davis; 1996.

*Further Reading*

Anonymous. Craniosacral therapy receives nod of approval from Blue Cross/Blue Shield of Michigan. *Connections (Connections Magazine).* 1999;3.

Benjamin PJ. A look back: massage in the nursery 100 years ago. *Massage Ther J.* 2004;43:144,146–148.

Bond C. Positive touch and massage in the neonatal unit: a British approach. *Semin Neonatol.* 2002;7:477–486.

Burke D, Hagbarth KE, Lofstedt L, Wallin BG. The responses of human muscle spindle endings to vibration of non-contracting muscles. *J Physiol.* 1976;261:673–693.

Carter A. The use of touch in nursing practice. *Nurs Stand.* 1995;9:31–35.

Cashar L, Dixon BK. The therapeutic use of touch. *J Psychiatr Nurs.* 1967;5:442–451.

Ching M. The use of touch in nursing practice. *Aust J Adv Nurs.* 1993;10:4–9.

Cochran-Fritz S. Physiological effects of massage on the nervous system. *Int J Altern Complementary Med.* 1993;September:21–25.

Cody FWJ, Plant T. Vibration-evoked reciprocal inhibition between human wrist muscles. *Brain Res.* 1989;78:613–623.

Darmstadt GL, Saha SK. Neonatal oil massage. *Indian Pediatr.* 2003; 40:1098–1099.

Darmstadt GL, Saha SK. Traditional practice of oil massage of neonates in bangladesh. *J Health Popul Nutr.* 2002;20:184–188.

Doering TJ, Fieguth HG, Steuernagel B, Brix J, Konitzer M, Schneider B, Fischer GC. External stimuli in the form of vibratory massage after heart or lung transplantation. *Am J Phys Med Rehabil.* 1999;78:108–110.

Doraisamy P. The management of spasticity—a review of options available in rehabilitation. *Ann Acad Med Singapore.* 1992;21:807–812.

Engle VF, Graney MJ. Biobehavioral effects of therapeutic touch. *J Nurs Scholarsh.* 2000;32:287–293.

Feldman R, Eidelman AI. Intervention programs for premature infants: how and do they affect development? *Clin Perinatol.* 1998;25:613–626.

Geis F, Viksne V. Touching: physical contact and level of arousal. *Proc Ann Convent Am Psychol Assoc.* 1972;7:179–180.

Gharavi B, Schott C, Linderkamp O. Value of kangaroo care, basal stimulation, kinesthesis awareness and baby massage in development promoting nursing of premature infants. *Kinderkrankenschwester.* 2004;23:368–372.

Helmig O. Vibrator therapy. History repeats itself. *Ugeskr Laeger.* 2001;163:7286–7288.

Hernandez Reif M, Field T, Diego M, Beutler J. Evidence-based medicine and massage. *Pediatrics.* 2001;108:1053.

Hernandez-Reif M, Oschman J. Energy medicine: correspondence: Oschman J 2002 Clinical aspects of biological fields: an introduction for health care professionals. *J Bodywork Movement Ther.* 6:117–125. *J Bodywork Movement Ther.* 2003;7:62–65.

Huhtala V, Lehtonen L, Heinonen R, Korvenranta H. Infant massage compared with crib vibrator in the treatment of colicky infants. *Pediatrics.* 2000;105:E84.

Issurin VB, Tenenbaum G. Acute and residual effects of vibratory stimulation on explosive strength in elite and amateur athletes. *J Sports Sci.* 1999;17:177–182.

Jones JE, Kassity N. Varieties of alternative experience: complementary care in the neonatal intensive care unit. *Clin Obstet Gynecol.* 2001;44:750–768.

Kubsch SM, Neveau T, Vandertie K. Effect of cutaneous stimulation on pain reduction in emergency department patients. *Accid Emerg Nurs.* 2001;9:143–151.

Kubsch SM, Neveau T, Vandertie K. Effect of cutaneous stimulation on pain reduction in emergency department patients. *Complement Ther Nurs Midwifery.* 2000;6:25–32.

Kuntz A. Anatomic and physiologic properties of cutaneo-visceral vasomotor reflex arc. *J Neurophysiol.* 1945;8:421–430.

Lewis N. Using the whole brain: integrating the right and left brain with hemi-sync sound patterns. *Noetic Sci Rev.* 1994:43.

MacManaway B, Turcan J. *Healing.* Wellingborough, England: Thorsons; 1983.

Malaquin-Pavan E. Therapeutic benefit of touch-massage in the overall management of demented elderly. *Rech Soins Infirm.* 1997;49:11–66 (Abstract).

Mansour AA, Beuche M, Laing G, Leis A, Nurse J. A study to test the effectiveness of placebo Reiki standardization procedures developed for a planned Reiki efficacy study. *J Altern Complement Med.* 1999;5:153–164.

Matthew PBC. The reflex excitation of the soleus muscle of a decerebrated cat caused by vibration applied to its tendon. *J Physiol.* 1966;184:450–472.

Megharfi W, Bughin V. Physical therapy-massage of children in a sterile isolator. *Rev Infirm.* 2002;86:33.

Miriutova NF, Levitskii EF, Abdulkina NG. Electromagnetic and mechanical vibrations in the therapy of myofascial pains. *Vopr Kurortol Fizioter Lech Fiz Kult.* 2000;1:14–16.

Modrcin-Talbott MA, Harrison LL, Groer MW, Younger MS. The biobehavioral effects of gentle human touch on preterm infants. *Nurs Sci Q.* 2003;16:60.

Mullany LC, Darmstadt GL, Khatry SK, Tielsch JM. Traditional massage of newborns in Nepal: implications for trials of improved practice. *J Trop Pediatr.* 2005;51:82–86.

Naliboff BD, Tachhiki KH. Autonomic and skeletal muscle responses to non-electrical cutaneous stimulation. *Percept Motor Skills.* 1991;72:575–584.

Oschman JL. Healing energy. Part 1: historical background. Energy review part 1A. *J Bodywork Movement Ther.* 1996;1:34–39.

Porter LS, Porter BO. A blended infant massage–parenting enhancement program for recovering substance-abusing mothers. *Pediatr Nurs.* 2004;30:363–372,401.

Sansone P, Schmitt L. Providing tender touch massage to elderly nursing home residents: a demonstration project. *Geriatr Nurs.* 2000;21:303–308.

Savage L. Preterm touch and massage. *Massage Australia.* 2003:12.

Schneider EF. The benefits of infant massage. *Massage Magazine.* 1997:41.

Seraia EV, Lapshin VP, Loginov LP, Artemova VV. Comparative efficacy of various massage techniques in the rehabilitation treatment of patients with inhalation trauma early after admission to the hospital. *Vopr Kurortol Fizioter Lech Fiz Kult.* 2002;5:32–33.

Spencer KM. The primal touch of birth: midwives, mothers and massage. *Midwifery Today Int Midwife.* 2004;70:11–13,67.

Stiles KG. A new look at energy work. *Massage Ther J.* 2005;44:88–99.

Stiles KG. An introduction to bowtech. *Massage Ther J.* 2003;42:92–104.

Tovar MK, Cassmeyer VL. Touch: the beneficial effects for the surgical patient. *AORN J.* 1989;49:1356–1361.

Tyler DO, Winslow EH, Clark AP, White KM. Effects of a one minute back rub on mixed venous saturation and heart rate in critically ill patients. *Heart Lung.* 1990;19:562–565.

Ulm G. The current significance of physiotherapeutic measures in the treatment of Parkinson's disease. *J Neural Transm Suppl.* 1995;46:455–460.

Wang R. Treatment of 40 cases of hydroceles with massage at qichong (st 30). *J Tradit Chin Med.* 1998;18:218–219.

White-Traut R. Providing a nurturing environment for infants in adverse situations: Multisensory strategies for newborn care. *J Midwifery Womens Health.* 2004;49:36–41.

# Chapter 8
## Superficial Fluid Techniques

**Superficial fluid techniques** are massage techniques that therapists apply to tissues superficial to muscle to increase the return flow of blood or lymph. These techniques include superficial effleurage and superficial lymph drainage technique. This chapter describes these techniques, how to perform them, and how to apply them in a practice sequence. A section on further study for each technique discusses relevant outcomes and evidence, cautions and contraindications, and how to use the technique in treatment.

| | Technique | |
|---|---|---|
| **Table 8-1** Summary of Outcomes for Superficial Fluid Techniques | | |
| **Outcome of Care** | **Superficial Effleurage** | **Superficial Lymph Drainage Technique** |
| Systemic sedation | ✓ | ✓ |
| Decreased anxiety | ✓ | ✓ |
| Counterirritant analgesia | P | P |
| Increased venous return | ? | ✓ |
| Decreased edema | P | ✓ |
| Increased lymphatic return | P | ✓ |

✓: the outcome is supported by research summarized in this chapter.
P: the outcome is possible. ?: the outcome is debatable (research results are absent or inconsistent).

## Superficial Effleurage: Foundations

# DEFINITION

**Superficial effleurage:** a gliding technique performed with light pressure in the direction of venous and lymphatic flow that deforms tissue down to the investing layer of the deep fascia.[1-8]

# USES

Therapists use superficial effleurage to increase **venous return** and **lymphatic return**, to spread oil at the start of regional massage, and to relax clients. They often use it at intervals during **classical massage** to give clients a "break" from deeper or more aggressive techniques.

# PALPATION PRACTICE

The following palpation exercises will help you develop the manual skill and focus you need to perform superficial effleurage well.

1. On a practice partner, estimate the thickness of the layer of fat (and associated **superficial fascia**) that lies on top of the most superficial muscle layer. Be sure to do this in several regions since fat is not evenly distributed. Compare several people. Compare men and women.
2. Palpate the superficial veins and arteries embedded in the superficial fat and fascia.
3. Try to locate and palpate the **investing layer of deep fascia.** This layer is harder than the fat above it and is often harder than the muscle beneath it. If you are palpating muscle fibers then you are too deep. Be sure to explore the following areas where this layer is thicker and easier to find: over the scapula, in the lumbar area, lateral to the shin, and on the palms of the hand and soles of the feet. It will be helpful to have a photographic atlas of anatomy at hand that shows this layer.

### Theory in Practice

## Superficial Fluid Techniques

### Patient Profile

Your patient is a recreational runner who rolled over on his right ankle 2 days ago during a cross-country run. His pain increased slowly after the injury. Twelve hours later, he went to the emergency department, where a doctor diagnosed a "grade 2 sprain" after taking X-rays. This injury is a repeat of a similar one that he had about 10 years ago.

### Clinical Findings

Subjective:
He complains of constant ankle pain, swelling, and reduced ability to bear weight on the affected ankle. He walks with a limp and cannot run.

Objective:
- Observation: He presents with an **antalgic** gait and an inability to bear weight on the right foot in standing. **Edema** on his right foot extends from the metatarsal heads to several inches above the malleoli. The skin is discolored in the region of the edema. He is using crutches.
- Palpation: There is exquisite point tenderness in the location of the anterior talofibular ligament.
- Range of motion: Right active and passive inversion and plantarflexion are limited by 50%, with pain at the end of range.
- Special tests: Anterior drawer and varus stress tests reproduce his pain.

### Treatment Approach

- Initial outcomes include edema reduction and pain relief.
- Explain that the course of recovery will be several weeks and that forcing himself to bear weight on his ankle when it is not ready will only compound problems.
- Place the patient on the table in supine, elevate the leg to 30° with several pillows, and apply ice to the ankle for 10 minutes. Instruct the patient on how to perform **diaphragmatic breathing**. Apply superficial effleurage to the proximal portion of the affected leg and then to the distal portion, only working as far distally as the proximal margin of swelling in the lower leg. Alternate back and forth from proximal to distal portions of the leg. Use contact that encircles the leg as much as possible and be sure to include the medial surface. Continue to apply superficial effleurage in this manner for as long as the treatment time allows. You can also apply **reflex** techniques, such as static contact and superficial stroking,

on the site of injury as the patient tolerates. Instruct the patient on how to use elevation and ice at home, to move the toes and ankle regularly without increasing pain, and to limit weight-bearing for several days.

■ As the patient's **episode of care** proceeds, you will introduce other massage techniques, presented in later chapters, to facilitate tendon healing and treat muscle tension in both legs. You can read about the progression of an episode of care for acute inflammation in Chapter 14, Using Massage to Achieve Clinical Outcomes.

■ Other treatment components would address strengthening, balance, proprioception, and gait training and any other **impairments** or **functional limitations** that are present.

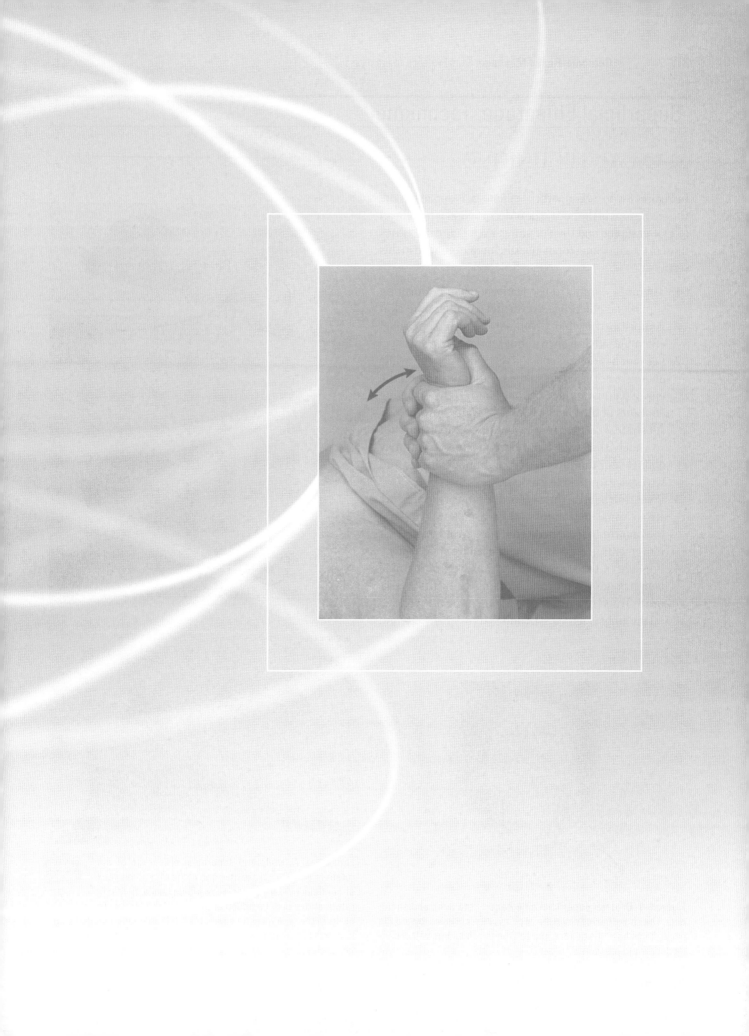

## Superficial Effleurage: Technique

# MANUAL TECHNIQUE

In Figures 8-1 to 8-9, superficial effleurage is applied to the various regions of the body. The order of figures is from head to foot in supine and then in prone. Each figure illustrates most of the guidelines for manual technique outlined in this section.

1. Therapists prefer to use **lubricant** when performing superficial effleurage. Nevertheless, unless the skin is moist or very hairy, you can perform superficial effleurage effectively without lubricant.
2. Let your hands be as soft and relaxed as possible while gliding over the client's skin. Continuously mold the entire palmar surface of your hand to the changing contours of the client's body, like water flowing over substrate. You may spread your fingers apart, but not so widely that your hand becomes tense. You may abduct your thumb and use your thumb, fingers, and web space to encircle a limb.
3. Point your hand in the general direction of the pressure stroke. Small deviations of the wrist allow your hand to conform to local body contours. Avoid large wrist movements in order to prevent **repetitive strain injury**.
4. Pressure of the stroke is toward axillary or inguinal lymph nodes when you are working on the trunk (Figure 8-3) and towards the heart when you are working on the limbs (Figures 8-4A and 8-4B, 8-5, 8-7, 8-10, and

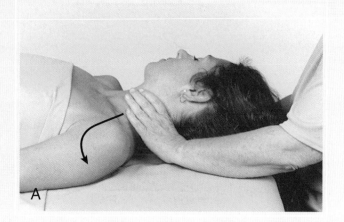

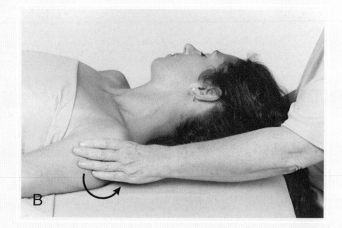

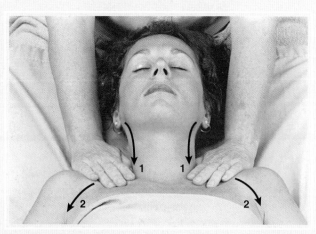

**Figure 8-1** Bilateral superficial effleurage of the neck and shoulders. The stroke moves down the neck, over the clavicles toward the axilla, finishing at the deltoid, and settling the shoulders with a gentle downward pressure.

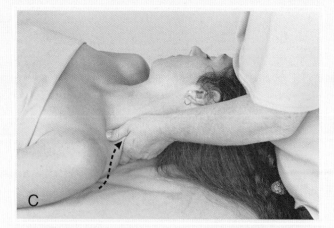

**Figure 8-2** A. Unilateral superficial effleurage of the rotated neck. The stroke may end at the root of the neck or continue over the clavicle toward the axilla. B. A light return stroke may be added at the end of the stroke. To perform this, the forearm supinates while the hand maintains contact with the client's skin. C. And the hand draws lightly back toward the occiput.

ON-LINE VIDEO

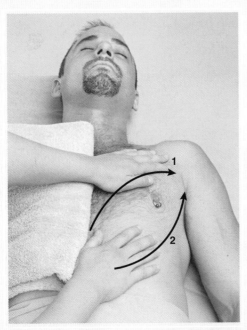

Figure 8-3 On the chest, for both men and women, strokes are directed toward the axilla while avoiding the region of the client's nipple. (For concepts related to the ethics of touching the breast, see Chapter 3, Clinical Decision Making for Massage, and Chapter 6, Preparation and Positioning for Massage.)

8-11). When you apply this technique to the client's back, the stroke typically begins at the sacrum and moves toward the axilla (Figure 8-6), although it can also be applied from the head down.

5. Engage progressively deeper layers of tissue with each repetition of the **centripetal** pressure stroke, advancing as deep as the investing layer of the deep fascia. Repeat strokes 5 to 10 times or more to overcome the **inertial**

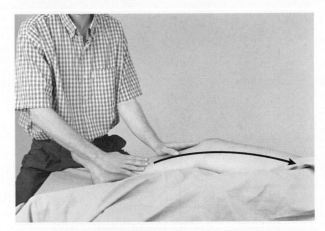

Figure 8-5 Medial and lateral surfaces of the client's leg can often be included in the same stroke. Note the therapist's upright posture.

**resistance** of fluid. Using the same pattern of movement, you can gradually increase the amount of pressure you apply and engage underlying muscle, if this is indicated (see Chapter 9, Neuromuscular Techniques).

6. Some authors suggest that the pressure of each stroke can be increased with increasing proximity of the hand(s) to the heart.[6,8] You can also use a distinct pause with slight **overpressure** at the proximal end of the stroke, preferably over a set of lymph nodes.

7. The rate of the stroke can vary from 5 to 50 cm/second. One author specifies a rate of 15 cm/second or 6 to 7 inches/second.[6]

8. There are varying opinions on the use of the **return stroke**. You may omit the return stroke, since the production of even a slight centrifugal pressure conflicts with the aim of assisting fluid return (Figures 8-1 and 8-2A). Alternatively, you may allow your hand(s) to

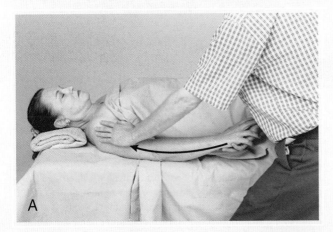

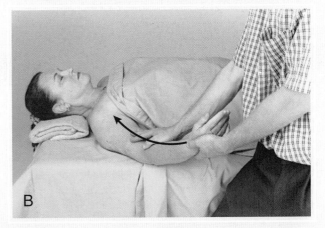

Figure 8-4 During superficial effleurage of the arm, the practitioner alternates application of the stroke to the lateral and medial surfaces of the client's arm. A. The lateral surface. B. The medial surface. Note the change in the practitioner's stance.

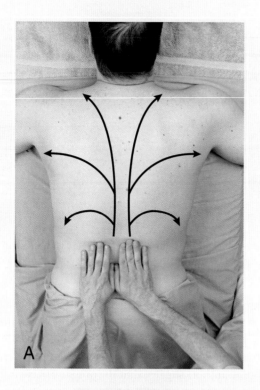

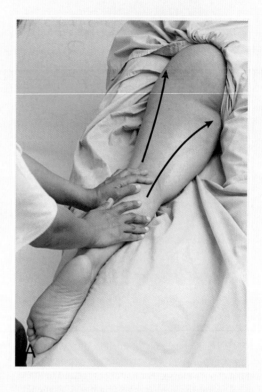

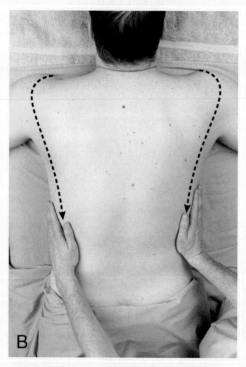

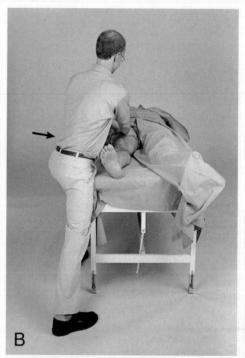

**Figure 8-6** A, B. Bilateral superficial effleurage of the back begins at the sacrum and can follow different paths. The practitioner may alternate these different paths on consecutive strokes.

**Figure 8-7** A. Superficial effleurage of the posterior leg, including the gluteals. B. For this technique, which requires light pressure, the therapist should achieve the stroke length primarily through leg movement while maintaining an upright torso. Here, on the other hand, the therapist is reaching and leaning; if repeated, this action will place unnecessary strain on the lower back.

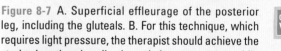

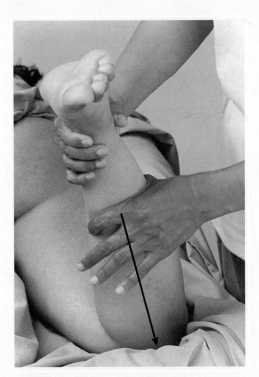

**Figure 8-8** Superficial effleurage applied to the ankle with an encircling "bracelet" contact.

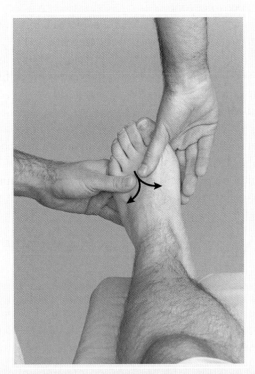

**Figure 8-9** Superficial effleurage with short thumb strokes will increase lymphatic return from the foot. Similar short strokes can be used to drain posttraumatic edema in a centrifugal direction, away from the periphery of swelling.

| Box 8-1 | Components of Superficial Effleurage |
|---|---|

**Contact:** Whole relaxed palmar surface of hand

**Pressure:** Light

**Engages:** Skin, superficial fascia, and fat

**Direction:** On limbs, **centripetal**; on torso, toward axillary or inguinal lymph nodes

**Amplitude:** Length of the region

**Rate:** 5 to 50 cm/second

**Duration:** 2 minutes or longer

**Intergrades with:** Petrissage and superficial stroking

**Context:** Used for extended periods alone or alternating with superficial lymph drainage technique to facilitate return of lymph and possibly blood. Often used as a prelude and follow-up to extended application of neuromuscular techniques.

remain in contact with the client's body for the return stroke but use minimal pressure while performing dragless superficial stroking with either palmar or fingertip contact (Figures 8-2B and 8-2C). If you choose to use a return stroke, you must make the transition from one direction to the other smooth.

9. Alternating, two-handed superficial effleurage, with the return strokes performed in the air, is a useful variation.

10. Use thumb or finger contact on smaller parts or around the periphery of swelling with the same general intention (Figures 8-8 and 8-9). Encircle forelimbs and digits with a "bracelet" or "ring" contact.

11. When you use superficial effleurage to treat localized swelling, it is preferable to treat proximal regions first. When you work near swelling, ensure that the individual strokes begin at the proximal margin or the periphery of the swelling so that you make no attempt to push fluid into or through an area of congestion. Later chapters discuss the design of massage sequences to increase lymphatic and venous return.

## How superficial effleurage might work

Superficial effleurage compresses veins and lymph vessels, mechanically pushing blood and lymph forward through these vessels, which contain valves to prevent backflow.[1-9]

Once a section of a vessel has emptied, a suction effect also draws distal fluid proximally.[7] The resulting increase in venous return may increase cardiac stroke volume,[9] although not overall systemic flow,[9-11] in healthy subjects.[9] In addition, light pressure on terminal lymphatics may stimulate the smooth muscle of these vessels to contract, pushing lymph forward.[12] Finally, repetitive rhythmic pressure may entrain a relaxation response. (See the discussion of entrainment in the section titled How Superficial Stroking Might Work in Chapter 7, Superficial Reflex Techniques.)

## THERAPIST'S POSITION AND MOVEMENT

1. Use the basic positions described in Chapter 6, Preparation and Positioning for Massage, in the sections on **standing aligned, lunge,** and **lunge and reach** postures.
2. When applying superficial effleurage to a large region such as the back or the legs, you achieve the full length of the strokes through correct movement of your legs, rather than through overreaching with your arms. Throughout the stroke, keep your torso upright to reduce repetitive flexion and extension of your lumbar spine (Figures 8-5 and 8-7B).

## PALPATE

As you perform the technique, palpate the client for the following:

1. Skin texture
2. Skin temperature
3. Presence of perspiration and moisture
4. Horizontal stretch of the skin and subcutaneous **superficial fascia**, which occurs in the direction of movement. Because lubricant reduces drag, these superficial tissues are not stretched to their elastic limit.
5. Subcutaneous fatty lipomas, which are common on the back,[13] and floating, hard fibrositic nodules, which are common around the iliac crest and occiput. Both of these can be tender on palpation.
6. Surface contours
7. Pliability of superficial subcutaneous tissues. This normally increases as these tissues become less viscous with continued application.
8. Inertial resistance of the subcutaneous tissue, which reflects its fluid content (i.e., interstitial fluid pressure)

9. Resorption of fluid from edematous tissue, which is accompanied by changes in surface contours and the **viscosity** and inertial resistance of the subcutaneous tissues

## OBSERVE

As you perform the technique, observe the client for signs of reduction of swelling or of relaxation. These signs are listed in the following sections.

### Reduction of Swelling

1. Normalization of skin color and texture
2. Change of surface contours
3. Visible reduction of swelling, which may often occur within 15 to 45 minutes. Cumulative reduction of swelling will occur during the course of the intervention, with resolution of an inflammatory process, or with resolution of circulatory and lymphatic dysfunction.

### Relaxation

1. Decrease in rate and depth of breathing
2. Deeper voice tone
3. Changes in skin color such as flushing. Pallor may indicate an undesirable **sympathetic response**.
4. Systemic reduction of **muscle resting tension**, as evidenced by softening of the tissue contours or broadening and flattening of body segments
5. Muscle twitches and jerks
6. Increases in peristaltic noises
7. Decreases in heart rate, as evidenced by change in pulses that are visible at the neck, wrist, and foot
8. Agitation or sweating, which may indicate an undesirable sympathetic response

## COMMUNICATION WITH THE CLIENT

Get feedback on the client's level of comfort during the technique. Here are some examples of statements that you can use.

1. "Let me know if this pressure becomes uncomfortable." When you are treating close to areas of acute or subacute inflammation, ensure that the pressure of the technique does not increase the client's level of pain.

2. "What is happening with your pain?" You can use this statement when you are applying the technique to reduce pain. It allows you to check how the client perceives that the intervention is affecting her pain at intervals during the application of the technique.
3. Encourage the client to perform deep diaphragmatic breathing during the intervention to assist lymphatic drainage and relaxation.

 ## Critical Thinking Question

Why is superficial effleurage performed with centripetal pressure? Why not with centrifugal pressure?

---

 ### A Practice Sequence for Superficial Effleurage

---

The following sequence of body regions, which you can complete in 30 minutes, proceeds from proximal to distal. Apply superficial effleurage to each region in succession.

Begin the strokes distally within each region, and cover the entire region with centripetal strokes that run the full length of the region. Repeat strokes several times.

> Supine: Neck, face, chest, arm, abdomen, anterior legs
> Prone: Back, gluteals, posterior legs

Try variations that:

- Use only the centripetal pressure stroke
- Use superficial stroking to return to the starting position
- Use constant pressure
- Increase pressure slightly as the strokes move proximally
- Pause over lymph nodes at the proximal end of the stroke
- Use different rates (5–50 cm/second)

How you would apply the technique using only side-lying positions while working from proximal to distal regions?

---

## Superficial Effleurage: Further Study and Practice

## NAMES AND ORIGINS

In other texts and massage-related systems, the technique that we call superficial effleurage is known as "effleurage," "gliding," "stroking," and "deep stroking."[1-8] The use of the word "effleurage" in current texts is (alas) highly variable with respect to the type and depth of tissues engaged by the stroke being described. Some authors use the terms "effleurage" and "stroking" interchangeably.[1-5] This book follows the convention used in many texts, including *Beard's Massage,*[6] which distinguishes between effleurage and stroking on the basis of the pressure, direction, tissues engaged, and clinical effects of the strokes.[6-8] Although superficial effleurage may be used to produce similar **reflex effects** to those produced with superficial stroking (discussed in Chapter 7, Superficial Reflex Techniques), it has additional effects on fluid dynamics. Additionally, this book makes a further distinction between superficial effleurage and the similarly patterned deep effleurage, which uses sufficient pressure to engage and **deform** muscle (see Chap-

ter 9, Neuromuscular Techniques). The precedent and clinical rationale for making this distinction is that clinicians must learn to discriminate clearly among the various tissue layers—skin, subcutaneous fascia and fat, and muscle.[1,3,5,7] This ability will enable the clinician to selectively direct the force of a massage stroke toward each tissue layer, as required to achieve the desired treatment **outcomes**.

## OUTCOMES AND EVIDENCE

Clinicians can use this light, flowing technique to improve the flow of interventions and to achieve circulatory effects, psychological effects, and a variety of physiological effects. Superficial effleurage is ideal for spreading lubricant, and clinicians often use it as an introductory stroke in regional massage and **general massage**. They can also use it as a transitional stroke and between deeper techniques that engage the client's muscles (see Chapter 9, Neuromuscular Techniques).

Superficial effleurage is best known for its circulatory effects. Numerous sources state that effleurage (in some form) increases **lymphatic and venous return** from the region to which it is applied.[1-8] One possible mechanism for this effect on lymphatic flow is that the gentle mechanical stresses of the technique cause a contraction of small lymphatic vessels, thereby increasing the formation and return of lymph.[10] Furthermore, superficial effleurage may produce direct movement of lymph when the pressure of the stroke is light and the rate of glide is slow. Notwithstanding its **mechanical effect** on lymphatic vessels, superficial effleurage does not appear to affect local arterial or venous flow, at least in healthy tissues.[11-13] Effects on lymphatic flow make superficial effleurage an indicated treatment for conditions of lymphatic congestion, including dependent **edema**; edema or effusion associated with the acute and subacute phases of common musculoskeletal injuries such as bursitis, sprains, strains, contusions, dislocations, separations, and fractures; **reflex sympathetic dystrophy**; and congestion of the breast associated with menses or lactation. It may also be of use when treating venous stasis[13] and related conditions such as varicosities and venous ulcers. Finally, superficial effleurage is useful in the treatment of **lymphedema** following surgical excision of lymphatics.[14] Because its range of effects on lymphatic flow, superficial effleurage is a component of some systems of **manual lymph drainage**.

Superficial effleurage also has a variety of other psychological and physiological effects. As with superficial stroking, superficial effleurage can be used to decrease anxiety, induce relaxation[15,16] (with one dissent[17]), temporarily decrease lower motor neuron excitability,[18,19] and stimulate peristalsis.[20,21] Because of its mild mechanical effects, clinicians can use superficial effleurage with superficial reflex techniques to induce **sedation**, increase general comfort, and reduce the perception of pain in postoperative situations. Finally, it is also indicated for infant colic.[21] Table 8-1 summarizes the main outcomes for superficial effleurage.

### EXAMINING THE EVIDENCE

Meta-analyses are uncommon in the massage literature, and those that examine the effects of a single massage technique are rare. In 1997, nursing researchers Labyak and Metzger[16] conducted a **meta-analysis** of nine studies that applied from 3 to 10 minutes of effleurage (**"slow-stroke backrub"**) to

those studies. Some of the studies were pretest, posttest designs but lacked control groups. Furthermore, treatment lengths in the studies were varied and brief. Finally, potentially confounding variables included: the presence of cardiovascular disease in clients, clients' age, and the gender of the therapist.

Labyak SE, Metzger BL. The effects of effleurage backrub on the physiological components of relaxation: a meta-analysis. *Nurs Res.* 1997;46:59–62.

## CAUTIONS AND CONTRAINDICATIONS

Clinicians need clinical training and supervised practice to master the proper application of superficial effleurage. Advanced training may be advisable in certain situations, particularly when dealing with pathological conditions. Although superficial effleurage only uses enough pressure to deform superficial fat and fascia, with their associated vessels, the clinician should consider all contraindications and cautions to massage (see Chapter 3, Clinical Decision Making for Massage).[1] There are several contraindications for clients with cardiac, orthopedic, and metabolic conditions. Critically ill clients typically tolerate superficial effleurage well.[16,22,23] Acute cardiac conditions are the exception to this rule. Although light massage is beneficial after myocardial infarction, there is a caution to allow a 48-hour wait after coronary artery bypass surgery before using massage.[22] Furthermore, the clinician must exercise caution when the client presents with cardiac insufficiency or congestive heart failure because an increase in venous return can compromise cardiac or pulmonary function.

Clients with acute orthopedic injuries or reflex sympathetic dystrophy may not tolerate local application of superficial effleurage. It may also be a contraindication for clients with these conditions. In these situations, the clinician should apply the technique proximal to the site of the injury to enhance drainage. In general, the clinician should not apply superficial effleurage over newly forming scars,[24] areas of confirmed or suspected infection, cellulitis, and thrombus. The use of superficial effleurage may increase the rate of kidney filtration in clients with serious kidney pathology or nutritional deficiency and lead to complications. Finally, even the use of light massage may reduce the duration of effectiveness of epidural anesthesia.[25]

# USING SUPERFICIAL EFFLEURAGE IN TREATMENT

Before you consider using superficial effleurage for treatment, you should be able to recognize the signs and symptoms of major vascular disease and major lymphatic dysfunction and understand their implications.

## Orthopedic Injuries

To treat **edema** secondary to trauma, apply extended, repetitive superficial effleurage proximal to the site of trauma. Combine this with ice or the application of cold, elevation of the limbs to 30 or 45 degrees, and passive movements and gentle joint mobilization techniques to reduce pain. Encourage the client to perform deep diaphragmatic breathing to assist lymphatic return. The postintervention self-care intervention for orthopedic injuries (RICE) includes: rest, ice or the application of cold, compression, and elevation of the limbs to 30 or 45 degrees.

## Lymphedema

The comprehensive treatment of **lymphedema** requires detailed, expert instruction on hygiene and skin care, regular use of compression bandages and garments, and specialized active exercises. Depending on the nature and extent of lymphedema, any of the following direct interventions may be indicated: gait, locomotion, balance, and **postural awareness** training; **strengthening**; and functional training in self-care and home management, including the use of assistive and adaptive devices.[2] Neuromuscular and connective tissue massage techniques may be useful for fibrosed edema.

## Venous Stasis

To treat edema associated with venous stasis, ensure that thrombus or thrombophlebitis are absent and then apply the technique proximal to the site of stasis, avoiding the immediate area of ulcers or varicosities. Elevation of a limb during the intervention and raised leg exercises for home-care may be helpful.[26]

# Superficial Lymph Drainage Technique: Foundations

## DEFINITION

**Superficial lymph drainage technique:** a nongliding technique performed in the direction of lymphatic flow, using short, rhythmical strokes with minimal to light pressure, that deforms subcutaneous tissue without engaging muscle.[27–37]

## USES

Therapists use superficial lymph drainage technique to increase lymphatic return. When they perform it correctly, this technique also has a secondary sedative effect.

## PALPATION PRACTICE

The following palpation exercises will help you develop the manual skill you need to perform superficial lymph drainage technique well.

1. Estimate the thickness of the layer of fat (and associated superficial fascia) that lies on top of the most superficial muscle layer. Be sure to do this in several regions because fat is not evenly distributed. Compare several people. Compare men and women.
2. Try to palpate the actual investing layer of deep fascia. This layer is harder than the fat above it and is often harder than the muscle beneath it. If you are palpating muscle fibers, then you are too deep. Be sure to explore the areas over the scapula, the lumbar area, the area lateral to the shin, the palms of the hand, and the soles of the feet.
3. Find the **elastic barrier** of the skin and superficial fat and fascia. How far can you stretch this tissue layer before your hand begins to slide over the skin? How far can you stretch this tissue layer without putting any pressure on the investing layer of deep fascia? Try this exercise in several regions, including those listed in the previous exercise.

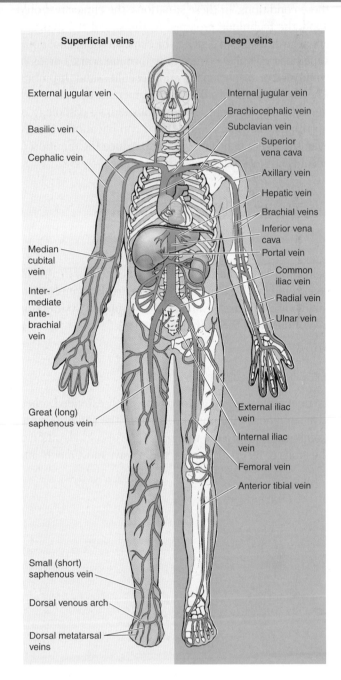

**Principal veins**

**Figure 8-10** Venous return to the heart. Reprinted with permission from Moore K. *Clinically Oriented Anatomy.* 4th ed. Philadelphia: Lippincott Williams & Wilkins; 1999:33).

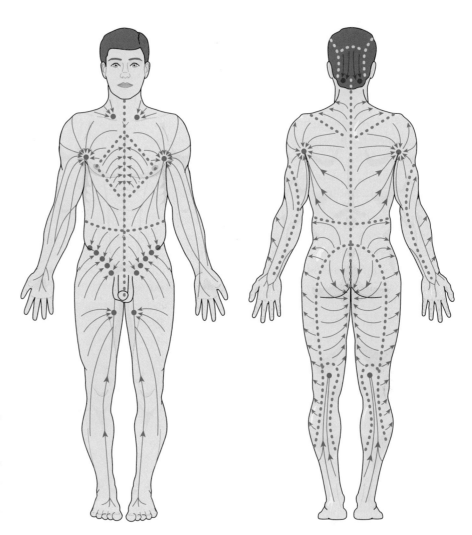

**Figure 8-11** Lymphatic watersheds with indication of the direction of flow of lymph. (Redrawn from Tappan FM, Benjamin PJ. *Tappan's Handbook of Healing Massage Techniques.* 3rd ed. Upper Saddle River, NJ: Prentice-Hall, Inc.; 1998:227. Copyright 1998. Adapted with permission from Prentice-Hall, Inc., Upper Saddle River, NJ.)

## Superficial Lymph Drainage: Technique

## MANUAL TECHNIQUE

In Figures 8-12 to 8-20, superficial lymph drainage technique is applied to the various regions of the body. The order of figures is from head to foot in supine and then in prone. Each figure illustrates most of the guidelines for manual technique outlined in this section.

1. Do not use oil. If either your skin or your client's skin is moist, you may apply enough unscented fine talc, cornstarch, or chalk to your hands to prevent sticking.

2. This technique demands supreme relaxation of your hands, which only comes from extensive practice. You can use any part of your hand, as long as the manual contact is soft and evenly distributed (Figures 8-15, 8-16, and 8-19). You may abduct your thumb so that the web space becomes a part of the contact surface (Figure 8-15). Fingerpad or thumb contact is useful when you are treating smaller parts of the body (Figures 8-12, 8-13, and 8-20).

3. Placing two hands side by side can create a larger contact, which is more suitable for broad areas such as the torso or thigh (Figure 8-16).

4. Use minimal pressure to engage the skin and sink slightly into the subcutaneous fat; little or no indentation should be visible. Then gently stretch the skin and

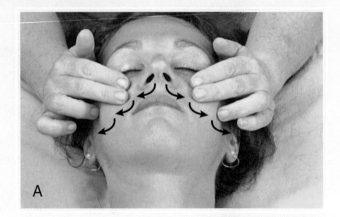

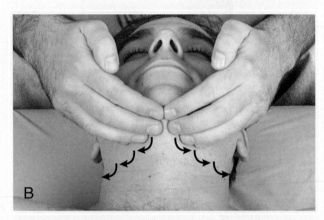

**Figure 8-13** A. Fingerpad contact can be used for superficial lymph drainage of the face. B. Fingerpad contact can also be used for the submandibular region.

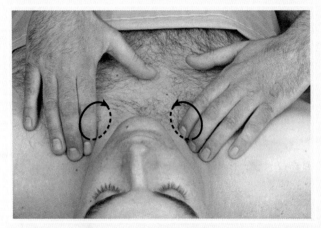

**Figure 8-12** A series of strokes down the neck ends near the junction of the venous and lymphatic systems. Direct pressure inferiorly under the clavicle and medially toward the "terminus." This sequence clears the most proximal portion of the lymphatic system and begins any intervention. The practitioner should repeat this stroke several times.

superficial fascia in the general direction of lymphatic flow (see Figure 8-11), without engaging underlying muscle, by applying pressure in a direction that is parallel to the surface. You can obtain better results if the stroke shape is semielliptical or semicircular. In this way, stretch of the tissues occurs in two directions on the plane of the surface of the client's skin, while you maintain a general centripetal orientation.[27,31]

5. The working surface of your hand does not glide over the client's skin. Areas of the hand that are adjacent to the working surface may glide in small amounts.

6. Pause at the end of each slow, short stroke, when you have stretched the skin and superficial fascia in a manner that takes the slack out of these tissues. Then gradually release the pressure you exerted and allow the skin to return to its original position.

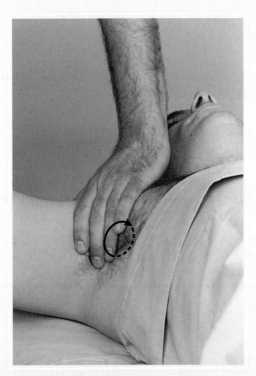

**Figure 8-14** Axillary and inguinal areas are treated prior to work on the related limb, and the therapist returns frequently to these areas during work on the client's limb. The hand directs pressure toward the midline of the arm and superiorly.

7. Your may keep your hands in one place and perform several strokes on the same location. In that situation, take care to ensure that you do not exert any **centrifugal** pressure when your hand follows the skin back to its original position (Figures 8-12, 8-14, 8-16, and

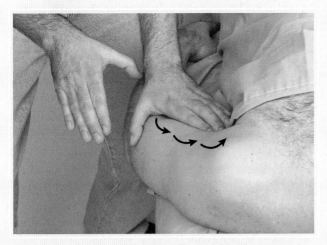

**Figure 8-15** The index finger, abducted thumb, and adjacent palm form a surface that can fit the arm well. The hands alternate and move proximally with each stroke. The sequence from elbow to axilla may be repeated several times. (A similar sequence uses the ulnar border of the palm to make contact.)

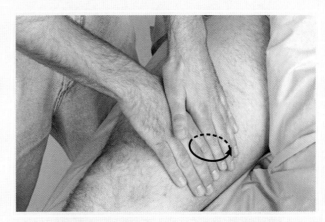

**Figure 8-16** Stationary ellipses on the anterior thigh. The return stroke (dotted line) must be applied without centrifugal pressure. Instead, the therapist's hand should follow the elastic recoil of the skin.

8-18). Alternatively, you may gently break contact with the client's body and move your hand(s) slightly proximally with each successive stroke, essentially "walking" your hands along the client's body segment (Figures 8-15 and 8-17). In either case, repeat strokes or series of strokes several times to overcome the inertial resistance of the fluid. Bear in mind that you must practice many, many hours to develop the fine control of pressure required by this technique.

8. The order of the intervention is important when you are using superficial lymphatic drainage techniques. Begin the intervention at the proximal junction between the lymphatic and venous systems (Figure 8-12), treat the client's neck, and drain the client's related trunk quadrant before proceeding to an affected limb. If time for the session is constrained, reduce the amount of time you spend treating the affected area, rather than the

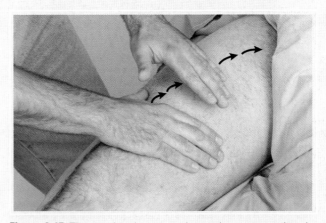

**Figure 8-17** The two hands can work together: one moving the lymph forward and the second holding the lymph as the first hand moves more proximally in preparation for the next stroke.

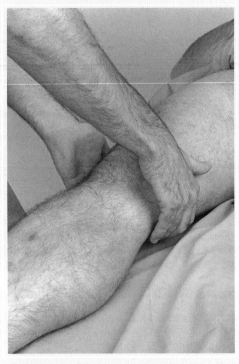

Figure 8-18   The popliteal nodes are treated with the client in supine.

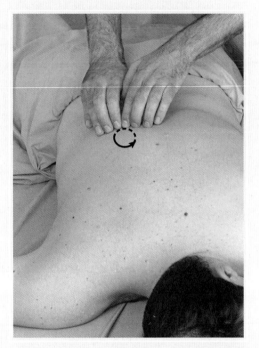

Figure 8-20   Fingerpad technique along the intercostal spaces; pressure is gently directed into the rib spaces and toward the spine to access deeper intrathoracic lymphatics.

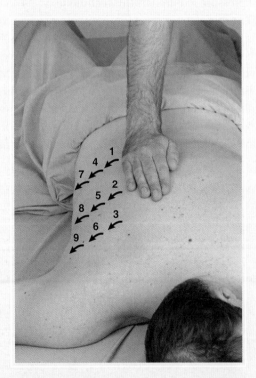

Figure 8-19   A series of strokes on the back directs pressure toward the axilla.

time you spend on the proximal areas.[33] Begin work on the limb by opening axillary or inguinal areas, whether or not the associated lymph nodes are intact (Figure 8-14). Furthermore, treat proximal portions of an affected region before distal portions. Finally, make frequent returns to the proximal areas that you cleared earlier in the intervention, thus making frequent movement back and forth from proximal areas to distal areas.

9. If the client's lymphatic vessels have been obstructed or recently irradiated, direct your strokes across normal lymphatic watersheds to the nearest group of nodes that have intact drainage. These are often the contralateral axillary or inguinal nodes or the ipsilateral abdominal nodes. First, drain these areas thoroughly in order to prepare them to receive lymph.[33]

10. Once you are familiar with the delicate contact required for performing superficial lymphatic drainage, strive to attain regularity of stroke rhythm to enhance the technique's sedative effect.

11. Superficial lymphatic drainage technique and its related complementary modalities are time consuming to deliver. During the initial stages of treatment, daily interventions of up to 45 to 90 minutes are often desir-

**Contact:** The entire relaxed palmar surface of the hand, heel of the hand, grouped fingers

**Pressure:** Minimal to light (5 mmHg, "the weight of a nickel")

**Engages:** Skin, superficial fascia, and fat only

**Direction:** Centripetal, in the direction of lymphatic pathways

**Amplitude/length:** Short, less than 2.5 cm (1 inch)

**Rate:** Slow, about 2.5 cm/second

**Duration:** 5 to 60 minutes or longer

**Intergrades with:** Superficial effleurage

**Combines with:** May be combined with varying amounts of compression (for fibrosed edema)

**Context:** Used alone for extended periods or alternated with superficial effleurage

able, depending on the client's condition and the severity of his or her edema.[31,33]

### ? Critical Thinking Question

In what ways are the components of superficial effleurage and superficial lymph drainage technique similar and different?

## *How superficial lymph drainage technique might work*

The light rhythmical pumping of superficial lymph drainage causes repeated pressure changes in the interstitium that stimulate the formation of lymph.[37] As with superficial effleurage, the light pressure deforms the most distal lymph vessels, mechanically pushing lymph forward through these vessels, which contain valves to prevent backflow.[7,9] Once a section of a vessel has been emptied, a suction effect also draws the fluid in the distal interstitial spaces proximally.[7,37] Light pressure also stimulates contraction of the smooth muscle of the collecting vessel segments called lymphangions,[37] which pumps lymph forward.[7,12,37] Finally, repetitive rhythmic pressure may entrain a relaxation response. (See the discussion of entrainment in the section titled How Superficial Stroking Might Work in Chapter 7, Superficial Reflex Techniques).

## THERAPIST'S POSITION AND MOVEMENT

1. Use the basic positions described in Chapter 6, Preparation and Positioning for Massage, in the sections on standing aligned, seated aligned, and lunge postures. Because superficial lymph drainage technique strokes are short, relatively little reaching is required.
2. Adjusting the manual contact to the contours of the client and the region of application requires flexibility in the movement of your shoulders and elbows. Consequently, you may use relatively large movements of the arm to achieve small manual movements.

## PALPATE

As you perform the technique, palpate the client for the following:

1. Skin texture
2. Skin temperature
3. Presence of perspiration and moisture
4. Stretch in skin and subcutaneous fascia. Because the rate of movement is slow, you can palpate the **end feel** of this gentle stretch of the superficial tissues. Work up to, but not through, this barrier.
5. Subcutaneous fatty lipomas, which are common on the back,[9] and floating, hard fibrositic nodules, which are common around the iliac crest and occiput. Both of these can be tender on palpation.
6. Surface contours
7. Increased pliability that reflects the reduction of viscosity of healthy superficial subcutaneous tissues, which normally occurs with continued application of the technique
8. Inertial resistance of the subcutaneous tissue that reflects its fluid content (interstitial fluid pressure)
9. Density of edematous tissue related to its degree of fibrosis
10. Resorption of fluid from edematous tissue, which is accompanied by changes in surface contours, tissue stretch, tissue density, and the viscosity and inertial resistance of the subcutaneous tissues

## OBSERVE

As you perform the technique, observe the client for the following signs of reduction of swelling.

1. Normalization of skin color and texture
2. Reduction of **trophic changes**

3. Reduction of surface contours
4. Visible reduction of swelling, which may often occur within 15 to 45 minutes. Cumulative reduction of swelling will occur during the course of the intervention, with resolution of an inflammatory process, or with resolution of circulatory and lymphatic dysfunction.

# COMMUNICATION WITH THE CLIENT

Get feedback on the client's level of comfort during the technique. Here are some issues that you need to address and examples of statements you can use.

1. "Let me know if this pressure becomes uncomfortable." When you are treating near areas of acute or subacute inflammation, ensure that the client finds the mechanical stimulus of the technique tolerable. This technique should be painless at all times.
2. Advise the client to urinate before the intervention, and inform her that she may still need to urinate during the intervention or soon after its conclusion.[36]
3. Explain to the client that it is not uncommon to experience fatigue after the first intervention. In addition, ask the client to report the occurrence of other sequelae such as more than mild nausea, shivering, or post-intervention pain, which suggest overtreatment.

## A Practice Sequence for Superficial Lymph Drainage

As with superficial effleurage, the best sequence of regions to facilitate return of lymph is to begin with proximal regions and proceed to distal ones. Because superficial lymph drainage technique is slow, a complete full-body sequence like the one below will take anywhere from 1.5 to 3 hours, depending on the amount of repetition that you use.

Apply the technique to each region in succession. Begin the strokes distally within each region and cover the entire region several times with short centripetal strokes, which gradually move proximally. For shorter practice periods, you can cover any region, preceded by the neck, within half an hour.

Supine: Neck, face, chest, arm, abdomen, anterior legs
Prone: Back, gluteals, posterior legs

Finding soft, comfortable, and relaxed hand contacts that best conform to the regional contours of the client's body can take some experimentation. Try variations that use:

- The full palmar surface
- The ulnar border of your hand
- The thumb, index, and included web space
- Flat hands, including the fingers

How would you apply the technique using only side-lying positions and working from proximal to distal regions?

# Superficial Lymph Drainage: Further Study and Practice

## NAMES AND ORIGINS

Superficial lymph drainage technique is a variant of superficial effleurage that was developed in the 20th century by Emil **Vodder** and subsequently elaborated on by several schools of **manual lymph drainage (MLD)**.[27–35,37] Superficial lymph drainage and superficial effleurage have in common the application of light pressure directed centripetally through the same tissue layer. During superficial effleurage, however, the clinician's hands glide over the skin—it is a faster and more general manipulation. Conversely, during superficial lymph drainage technique, the clinician very gently

stretches the client's skin, superficial fascia, and accompanying lymphatics to their elastic limit in the direction of lymphatic flow, without compressing deeper structures, and then carefully releases the stretched tissues.

Superficial lymph drainage technique is a principal technique of the various schools of MLD, which may also use superficial effleurage, compression, and other massage techniques in their interventions. It is used as part of a comprehensive intervention known as **complex** or **complete decongestive therapy** or **physiotherapy** (CDT, CDP, or CDMT). This intervention includes bandaging or **compression garments**, specific exercises, and education on hygiene.[33–35]

# OUTCOMES AND EVIDENCE

Local use of superficial lymph drainage technique can increase lymphatic return from the region to which clinicians apply it. When the clinician applies this technique to larger areas of the client's body, it can produce an increase in the volume of lymph that is returning to the venous system. The proposed mechanism for these effects is that the slow, delicate, rhythmic stretching of the tissues promotes the formation of lymph,[37] stimulates contraction of the lymphatic vessels,[12,27,31,37] propels lymph through the collapsible superficial lymphatics,[27,31,37,38] increases local blood flow,[39] and reduces the time required for alternative lymphatic pathways (anastomoses) to form after lymphatic pathways have been interrupted by damage. When clinicians perform this technique skillfully, it can result in **sedation** (parasympathetic activity), reduced pain (counterirritant analgesia), and improvement in general immune function.[27,37,40]

Complete decongestive therapy is a well-documented intervention that extensive research suggests is effective in the treatment of lymphedema,[41–59] particularly lymphedema that arises after surgical intervention in breast cancer.[34,43,60–74] There is currently debate about how much manual lymph drainage contributes to the effectiveness of this intervention.[44,75–80] Superficial lymph drainage is effective for traumatic edema,[81–84] venous insufficiency,[85,86] acne,[27,31] and a variety of other conditions,[87–94] but is not more effective than exercise for complex regional pain syndrome.[95] Table 8-1 summarizes the main outcomes for superficial lymph drainage.

## EXAMINING THE EVIDENCE

In 2004, the **Cochrane Database of Systematic Reviews** examined physical methods used to treat lymphedema including bandaging, compression sleeves, hosiery, and manual lymph drainage.[75] The research team selected for review **randomized clinical trials** indexed in major medical databases that had a follow-up period of more than 6 months. The three papers that met these criteria did not study the same intervention. In the single trial that considered massage, the effect of manual lymph drainage on lymphedema was no greater than that achieved with compression bandages. The review's major conclusion was that there is a clear need for well-designed, randomized trials of the whole range of ther-

apeutic interventions in order to determine the best approach to managing lymphedema.

This study was rigorous and well documented. Search strategies, selection criteria, and review procedures were detailed at length. The authors described 10 studies that initially met the inclusion criteria in detail and provided reasons for excluding seven of them. The end product of this rigor was that the authors were left with too few studies to perform a meta-analysis and could only conclude that more and better research is required.

Badger C, Preston N, Seers K, Mortimer P. Physical therapies for reducing and controlling lymphoedema of the limbs. *Cochrane Database Syst Rev.* 2004;4:CD00314183.

# CAUTIONS AND CONTRAINDICATIONS

Clinicians need clinical training and supervised practice to master the proper application of superficial lymph drainage technique. Advanced training may be advisable in certain situations, particularly when dealing with pathological conditions. The contraindications to the use of techniques with mechanical effects apply to the use of superficial lymph drainage (see Chapter 3, Clinical Decision Making for Massage).

The contraindications to the use of superficial lymph drainage technique include: acute systemic or local inflammation due to bacterial or viral infection, untreated metastatic disease, allergic reactions, recent thrombosis, and edema due to right-sided heart failure (the client may be massaged outside the area of the edema).[27–29,31,96,97] There are several cautions to the use of superficial lymph drainage technique. The clinician must exercise caution when the client presents with cardiac insufficiency or congestive heart failure, since an increase in venous return can compromise cardiac or pulmonary function. When the client presents with thyroid hyperactivity, avoid local application in the area of the thyroid. If the client has asthma, then treat between attacks, use shorter interventions, and avoid applying around the area of the sternum.

The clinician should avoid the client's abdomen during menstruation and reduce or omit treatment during pregnancy. If the client has low blood pressure, use caution and shorten interventions in early stages of treatment.[27,29,31] When treating traumatic edema, as with any condition, ensure that the application of superficial lymph drainage is painless and pleasant. If the client is unable to tolerate a local application of this technique, only apply it proximally.

Using superficial lymph drain-age technique on chronic inflammation may stimulate a transient acute inflammation.[29] Finally, the client may experience slight nausea or fatigue following full-body sessions.[31]

## Critical Thinking Question

What are the differences between superficial lymph drainage technique, manual lymph drainage, and complex decongestive therapy?

# USING SUPERFICIAL LYMPH DRAINAGE TECHNIQUE IN TREATMENT

Before you consider using superficial lymph drainage technique (manual lymph drainage) for treatment, you should be able to recognize the signs and symptoms of major vascular disease and major lymphatic dysfunction and understand their implications.

## Orthopedic Injuries

To treat edema secondary to trauma, use extended repetitive superficial lymph drainage technique proximal to the site of trauma. You can combine this with ice or the application of cold, elevation of the limbs to 30 or 45 degrees, and passive movements and gentle **joint mobilization** techniques to reduce pain. Encourage the client to perform deep dia-phragmatic breathing to assist lymphatic return. The post-intervention self-care intervention for orthopedic injuries (RICE) includes: rest, ice or the application of cold, compression, and elevation of injured limbs to 30 or 45 degrees.

## Lymphedema

The comprehensive treatment of lymphedema requires detailed, expert instruction on hygiene and skin care, regular use of compression bandages and garments, and specialized active exercises. Depending on the nature and extent of lymphedema, any of the following direct interventions may be indicated: gait, locomotion, balance, and posture awareness training; strengthening; and functional training in self-care and home management, including the use of assistive and adaptive devices.[2] Neuromuscular and connective tissue massage techniques may be useful for fibrosed edema.

## Venous Stasis

To treat edema associated with venous stasis, ensure that thrombus or thrombophlebitis are absent, and then apply the technique proximal to the site of stasis, avoiding ulcers or varicosities. Elevation of a limb during the intervention and raised leg exercises for homecare may be helpful.[26]

## Critical Thinking Question

Which types of edema can clinicians treat successfully with massage techniques? Which types of edema will not respond as well to massage techniques?

## Clinical Case

## History of Present Illness

A 45-year-old female with breast cancer in remission presents 1 month after mastectomy with chronic lymphedema of the right arm and hand. She has had 50% of axillary lymph nodes and some breast tissue removed and has had no radiation

## Subjective

- Complains of right-handed pain and swelling that interferes with function
- Complains of pain on activity
- Reports feeling self-conscious about appearance of her arm

# Objective

## Impairments

- Edema: Gross edema, pitting from shoulder to fingers; girth recorded
- Limb volume: Right > left; measured with volumetric analysis
- Strength: Grade 3—for shoulder, elbow, and wrist movements on right
- Range of motion:
  - Right shoulder: flexion = 85 degrees, extension = 5 degrees, abduction = 70 degrees, adduction = 10 degrees, external rotation = 30 degrees, internal rotation = 5 degrees
  - Right elbow: flexion = 95 degrees, extension = neutral, pronation = 45 degrees, supination = 30 degrees
  - Right wrist: flexion = 25 degrees, extension = 35 degrees, radial deviation = 5 degrees, ulnar deviation = 10 degrees
  - Right hand m.c.p.'s: flexion = 45 degrees, extension = neutral; i.p.'s: flexion = 50 degrees, extension = neutral

## Functional Limitations

- Unable to comb hair with right arm
- Difficulty dressing and performing self-care
- Unable to reach object placed above shoulder level
- Unable to carry objects in right hand

# Analysis

## Treatment Rationale

To reduce the patient's edema and address the secondary weakness, pain, distorted body image, and functional limitations

| Impairment | Outcomes and Role of Massage |
| --- | --- |
| Edema (impaired lymph drainage) | Decreased edema: right limb volume = left limb volume |
| | Primary treatment, direct effect on lymphatic drainage |
| Range of motion | Increased range of motion to within normal limits |
| | Primary treatment, direct effect since range is limited by edema |
| Strength | Increased strength to grade 5/5 throughout |
| | Possible secondary effect; weakness is primarily due to disuse; decreased edema may facilitate strengthening and will provide increased range for strengthening |
| Altered body image | Improved body image |
| | Possible primary and secondary effect since gross edema contributes to altered image |

| Activity Limitation | Functional Outcomes |
| --- | --- |
| Decreased ability to perform self-care activities | Patient will be able to carry a 10-lb object in her right hand while ambulating 100 ft, as required for carrying groceries |
| | Patient will be able to perform self-care activities (dressing, bathing, toileting) without adaptive equipment |

| *Activity Limitation* | *Functional Outcomes* |
|---|---|
| | ▥ Patient will be able to reach object placed 3 ft above head with her right hand, as required for hanging laundry on the clothesline |
| | ▥ Patient will be able to lift 1-lb object from overhead shelf with her right hand, as required for placing and removing groceries on an overhead kitchen shelf |
| ▥ Decreased social interaction | ▥ Patient will demonstrate increased social interaction with fewer complaints of self-consciousness regarding the appearance of her arm |

*Plan*

| Massage Techniques | Superficial effleurage, briefly, and then superficial lymph drainage technique. These are applied in sequence each session, thoroughly to the contralateral quadrant first (including intercostal and sternal areas), and then to proximal areas of the affected quadrant, especially to axillary, intercostal, and parasternal areas. The clinician gradually works more distally into the patient's arm and then alternates back and forth between proximal and distal segments. In addition, at the outset of each intervention, repetitive broad-contact compression delivered over the junctions of the right lymphatic and thoracic ducts with the vena cava may also be useful (see Chapter 9, Neuromuscular Techniques). |
|---|---|
| Other Appropriate Techniques and Interventions | Medical management, bandaging or pressure garments, skin hygiene, range-of-motion exercises, functional activity, strengthening exercises, adaptive equipment for short-term use |

*References*

1. Fritz S. *Mosby's Fundamentals of Therapeutic Massage.* 3rd ed. St. Louis: Mosby; 2004.
2. American Physical Therapy Association. *Guide to Physical Therapist Practice.* 2nd ed. Alexandria, VA: American Physical Therapy Association; 1999.
3. Benjamin PJ, Tappan FM. *Tappan's Handbook of Healing Massage Techniques.* 4th ed. Upper Saddle River, NJ: Pearson Prentice Hall; 2005.
4. Loving J. *Massage Therapy.* Stamford, CT: Appleton & Lange; 1999.
5. Salvo SG. *Massage Therapy: Principles and Practice.* 2nd ed. Philadelphia: WB Saunders; 2003.
6. de Domenico G, Wood EC. *Beard's Massage.* 4th ed. Philadelphia: WB Saunders; 1997.
7. Holey E, Cook E. *Evidence-Based Therapeutic Massage.* 2nd ed. Edinburgh: Churchill Livingstone; 2003.
8. Hollis M. *Massage for Therapists.* 2nd ed. Oxford, England: Blackwell Science; 1998.
9. Yates J. *A Physician's Guide to Therapeutic Massage.* 3rd ed. Toronto: Curties Overzet; 2004.
10. Tiidus PM, Shoemaker JK. Effleurage massage, muscle blood flow and long-term post-exercise strength recovery. *Int J Sports Med.* 1995;16:478–483.
11. Shoemaker JK, Tiidus PM, Mader R. Failure of manual massage to alter limb blood flow: measures by Doppler ultrasound. *Med Sci Sports Exerc.* 1997;29:610–614.
12. Schmid-Schonbein GW. Microlymphatics and lymph flow. *Physiol Rev.* 1990;70:987–1028.
13. Grieve GP. Episacroiliac lipoma. *Physiotherapy.* 1990;76:308–310.
14. Mason MP. The treatment of lymphoedema by complex decongestive physiotherapy. *Aust J Physiother.* 1993;39:41–45.
15. Groer M, Mozingo J, Droppleman P, et al. Measures of salivary secretory immunoglobulin A and state anxiety after a nursing back rub. *Appl Nurs Res.* 1994;7:2–6.
16. Labyak SE, Metzger BL. The effects of effleurage backrub on the physiological components of relaxation: a meta-analysis. *Nurs Res.* 1997;46:59–62.
17. Fischer RL, Bianculli KW, Sehdev H, Hediger ML. Does light pressure effleurage reduce pain and anxiety associated with genetic amniocentesis? A randomized clinical trial. *J Matern Fetal Med.* 2000;9:294–297.
18. Goldberg J, Sullivan SJ, Seaborne DE. The effect of two intensities of massage on H-reflex amplitude. *Phys Ther.* 1992;72:449–457.
19. Sullivan SJ, Seguin S, Seaborne D, et al. Reduction of H-reflex amplitude during the application of effleurage to the triceps surae in neurologically healthy subjects. *Physiother Theory Pract.* 1993;9:25–31.
20. Larsen JH. Infants' colic and belly massage. *Practitioner.* 1990; 234:396–397.
21. Emly M. Abdominal massage. *Nurs Times.* 1993:89:34–36.
22. Dunbar S, Redick E. Should patients with acute myocardial infarctions receive back massage? *Focus Crit Care.* 1986;13:42–46.

23. Tyler DO, Winslow EH, Clark AP, White KM. Effects of a one minute back rub on mixed venous saturation and heart rate in critically ill patients. *Heart Lung.* 1990;19:562–565.

24. Leduc A, Lievens P, Dewald J. The influence of multidirectional vibrations on wound healing and on regeneration of blood and lymph vessels. *Lymphology.* 1981;14:179–185.

25. Ueda W, Katatoka Y, Sagara Y. Effect of gentle massage on regression of sensory analgesia during epidural block. *Anesth Analg.* 1993;76:783–785.

26. Ciocon JO, Galindo-Ciocan D, Galindo DJ. Raised leg exercises for leg edema in the elderly. *Angiology.* 1995;46:19–25.

27. Wittlinger H, Wittlinger G. *Textbook of Dr Vodder's Manual Lymphatic Drainage, Volume 1: Basic Course.* 3rd ed. Heidelberg, Germany: Karl F Haug Verlag; 1982.

28. Kurz I. *Textbook of Dr. Vodder's Manual Lymph Drainage, Volume 2: Therapy.* 4th ed. Heidelberg, Germany: Karl F Haug Verlag; 1997.

29. Kurz I. *Textbook of Dr. Vodder's Manual Lymph Drainage, Volume 3: Treatment Manual.* 2nd ed. Heidelberg, Germany: Karl F Haug Verlag; 1990.

30. Kasseroller RG. The Vodder School: the Vodder method. *Cancer.* 1998;83:2840–2842.

31. Harris R. An introduction to manual lymph drainage: the Vodder method. *Massage Ther J.* 1992;winter:55–66.

32. Fritsch C, Tomson D. The usefulness of lymphatic drainage. *Schweiz Rundsch Med Prax.* 1991;80:383–386 (Abstract).

33. Casley-Smith JR, Boris M, Weindorf S, Lasinski B. Treatment for lymphedema of the arm—the Casley-Smith method: a noninvasive method produces continued reduction. *Cancer.* 1998;83 (Suppl 12):2843–2860.

34. Leduc O, Leduc A, Bourgeois P, Belgrado JP. The physical treatment of upper limb edema. *Cancer.* 1998;83(suppl 12):2835–2839.

35. Lerner R. Complete decongestive physiotherapy and the Lerner Lymphedema Services Academy of Lymphatic Studies (the Lerner School). *Cancer.* 1998;83(Suppl 12):2861–2863.

36. Kurz W, Kurz R, Litmanovitch YI, et al. Effect of manual lymph drainage massage on blood components and urinary neurohormones in chronic lymphedema. *Angiology.* 1981;32:119–127.

37. Foldi M, Strossenreuther R. *Foundations of Manual Lymph Drainage.* 3rd ed. St. Louis: Elsevier Mosby; 2005.

38. Francois A, Richaud C, Bouchet JY, et al. Does medical treatment of lymphedema act by increasing lymph flow? *VASA.* 1989;18:281–286.

39. Hutzschenreuter P, Brummer H, Ebberfeld K. Experimental and clinical studies of the mechanism of effect of manual lymph drainage therapy. *Z Lymphol (German).* 1989;13:62–64 (Abstract).

40. Hutzschenreuter P, Ehlers R. Effect of manual lymph drainage on the autonomic nervous system. *Z Lymphol (German).* 1986;10:58–60 (Abstract).

41. Liao SF, Huang MS, Chou YH, Wei TS. Successful complex decongestive physiotherapy for lymphedema and lymphocutaneous reflux of the female external genitalia after radiation therapy. *J Formos Med Assoc.* 2003;102:404–406.

42. Cheville AL, McGarvey CL, Petrek JA, Russo SA, Taylor ME, Thiadens SR. Lymphedema management. *Semin Radiat Oncol.* 2003;13:290–301.

43. Williams AF, Vadgama A, Franks PJ, Mortimer PS. A randomized controlled crossover study of manual lymphatic drainage therapy in women with breast cancer-related lymphoedema. *Eur J Cancer Care (Engl).* 2002;11:254–261.

44. Kriederman B, Myloyde T, Bernas M, et al. Limb volume reduction after physical treatment by compression and/or massage in a rodent model of peripheral lymphedema. *Lymphology.* 2002;35:23–27.

45. Kasseroller RG, Schrauzer GN. Treatment of secondary lymphedema of the arm with physical decongestive therapy and sodium selenite: a review. *Am J Ther.* 2000;7:273–279.

46. Ko DS, Lerner R, Klose G, Cosimi AB. Effective treatment of lymphedema of the extremities. *Arch Surg.* 1998;133:452–458.

47. Franzeck UK, Spiegel I, Fischer M, et al. Combined physical therapy for lymphedema evaluated by fluorescence microlymphography and lymph capillary pressure measurements. *J Vasc Res.* 1997;34:306–311.

48. Herpertz U. Outcome of various inpatient lymph drainage procedures. *Z Lymphol (German).* 1996;20:27–30 (Abstract).

49. Boris M, Weindorf S, Lasinski B, Boris G. Lymphedema reduction by noninvasive complex lymphedema therapy. *Oncology (Huntingt).* 1994;8:95–106.

50. Foldi M. Treatment of lymphedema. *Lymphology.* 1994;27:1–5.

51. Gillham L. Lymphedema and physiotherapists: control not cure. *Physiotherapy.* 1994;80:835–843.

52. Ruger K. Lymphedema of the head in clinical practice. *Z Lymphol (German).* 1993;17:6–11 (Abstract).

53. Barrellier MT. Lymphedema: is there a treatment? *Rev Med Interne (French).* 1992;13:49–57 (Abstract).

54. Lerner R. The ideal treatment of lymphedema. *Massage Ther J.* 1992;winter:37–39.

55. Clodius L, Foldi E, Foldi M. On nonoperative management of chronic lymphedema. *Lymphology.* 1990;23:2–3.

56. Cluzan R, Miserey G, Barrey P, Alliot F. Principles and results of physiotherapeutic therapy in mechanical lymphatic insufficiency of secondary or primary nature. *Phlebologie (French).* 1988;41:401–408 (Abstract).

57. Einfeld TH, Henkel M, Schmidt-Aufurth T, et al. Therapeutic and palliative lymph drainage in the treatment of face and neck edema. *HNO (German).* 1986;34:365–367.

58. Foldi E, Foldi M, Weissleder H. Conservative treatment of lymphoedema of the limbs. *Angiology.* 1985;36:171–180.

59. Kurz W, Wittlinger G, Litmanovitch YI, et al. Effect of manual lymph drainage massage on urinary excretion of neurohormones and minerals in chronic lymphedema. *Angiology.* 1978;29:764–772.

60. Howell D, Watson M. Evaluation of a pilot nurse-led, community-based treatment programme for lymphoedema. *Int J Palliat Nurs.* 2005;11:62–69.

61. Campisi C, Boccardo F, Zilli A, et al. Lymphedema secondary to breast cancer treatment: possibility of diagnostic and therapeutic prevention. *Ann Ital Chir.* 2002;73:493–498.

62. Enig B, Mogensen M, Jorgensen RJ. Lymphedema in patients treated for breast cancer. A cross-sectional study in the county of Ribe. The need of manual lymph drainage; risk factors. *Ugeskr Laeger (Danish).* 1999;161:3293–3298 (Abstract).

63. Johansson K, Albertsson M, Ingvar C, Ekdahl C. Effects of compression bandaging with or without manual lymph drainage patients with postoperative arm lymphedema. *Lymphology.* 1999;32:103–110.

64. Fiaschi E, Francesconi G, Fiumicelli S, et al. Manual lymphatic drainage for chronic post-mastectomy lymphoedema treatment. *Panminerva Med.* 1998;40:48–50.

65. Foldi E. The treatment of lymphedema. *Cancer.* 1998;83(Suppl 12): 2833–2834.

66. Johansson K, Lie E, Ekdahl C, Lindfeldt J. A randomized study comparing manual lymph drainage with sequential pneumatic compression for treatment of postoperative arm lymphedema. *Lymphology.* 1998;31:56–64.

67. Ferrandez JC, Laroche JP, Serin D, et al. Lymphoscintigraphic aspects of the effects of manual lymphatic drainage. *J Mal Vasc (French).* 1996;21:283–289 (Abstract).

68. Cluzan RV, Alliot F, Ghabboun S, Pascot M. Treatment of secondary lymphedema of the upper limb with CYCLO 3 FORT. *Lymphology.* 1996;29:29–35.

69. Mirolo BR, Bunce IH, Chapman M, et al. Psychosocial benefits of post-mastectomy lymphedema therapy. *Cancer Nurs.* 1995; 18:197–205.

70. Gruffaz J. Management by the angiologist of sequelae of radio-surgical treatment of breast cancer. *J Mal Vasc (French).* 1995; 20:150–152 (Abstract).

71. Bunce IH, Mirolo BR, Hennessy JM, et al. Post-mastectomy lymphoedema treatment and measurement. *Med J Aust.* 1994; 161:125–128.

72. Bertelli G, Venturini M, Forno G, et al. An analysis of prognostic factors in response to conservative treatment of post-mastectomy lymphedema. *Surg Gynecol Obstet.* 1992;175:455–460.

73. Casley-Smith JR, Casley-Smith JR. Modern treatment of lymphoedema. 1. Complex physical therapy: the first 200 Australian limbs. *Aust J Dermatol.* 1992;33:61–68.

74. Zanolla R, Monzeglio C, Balzarini A, Martino G. Evaluation of the results of three different methods of post-mastectomy lymphedema treatment. *J Surg Oncol.* 1984;26:210–213.

75. Badger C, Preston N, Seers K, Mortimer P. Physical therapies for reducing and controlling lymphoedema of the limbs. *Cochrane Database Syst Rev.* 2004;4:CD00314183.

76. McNeely ML, Magee DJ, Lees AW, Bagnall KM, Haykowsky M, Hanson J. The addition of manual lymph drainage to compression therapy for breast cancer related lymphedema: a randomized controlled trial. *Breast Cancer Res Treat.* 2004;86:95–106.

77. Harris R, Piller N. Three case studies indicating the effectiveness of manual lymph drainage on patients with primary and secondary lymphedema using objective measuring tools. *J Bodywork Movement Ther.* 2003;7:213–221.

78. Harris SR, Hugi MR, Olivotto IA, Levine M, Steering Committee for Clinical Practice Guidelines for the Care and Treatment of Breast Cancer. Clinical practice guidelines for the care and treatment of breast cancer. 11. Lymphedema. *CMAJ.* 2001;164:191–199.

79. Andersen L, Højris I, Erlandsen M, Andersen J. Treatment of breast-cancer-related lymphedema with or without manual lymphatic drainage: a randomized study. *Acta Oncol.* 2000; 39:399–405.

80. Johansson K, Albertsson M, Ingvar C, Ekdahl C. Effects of compression bandaging with or without manual lymph drainage treatment in patients with postoperative arm lymphedema. *Lymphology.* 1999;32:103–110.

81. Kessler T, de Bruin E, Brunner F, Vienne P, Kissling R. Effect of manual lymph drainage after hindfoot operations. *Physiother Res Int.* 2003;8:101–110.

82. Haren K, Backman C, Wiberg M. Effect of manual lymph drainage as described by Vodder on edema of the hand after fracture of the distal radius: a prospective clinical study. *Scand J Plast Reconstr Surg Hand Surg.* 2000;34:367–372.

83. Weiss JM. Treatment of leg edema and wounds in a patient with severe musculoskeletal injuries. *Phys Ther.* 1998;78:1104–1113.

84. Trettin H. Craniocerebral trauma caused by sports. Pathogenic mechanism, clinical aspects and physical therapy with special reference to manual lymph drainage. *Z Lymphol (German).* 1993;17:36–40 (Abstract).

85. Valentin J, Leonhardt D, Perrin M. Prevention of venous thromboses and cutaneous necroses using physical methods and pressure therapy in the surgery of chronic venous insufficiency of the lower limbs. *Phlebologie (French).* 1988;41:690–696 (Abstract).

86. Asdonk J. Physical lymph drainage and therapy of edema in chronic venous insufficiency. *Z Lymphol (German).* 1981;5: 107–111 (Abstract).

87. Chomard D, Habault P, Ledemeney M, Haon C. Prognostic aspects of TcPO2 in iloprost treatment as an alternative to amputation. *Angiology.* 1999;50:283–288.

88. Husmann MJ, Roedel C, Leu AJ, et al. Lymphoedema, lymphatic microangiopathy and increased lymphatic and interstitial pressure in a patient with Parkinson's disease. *Schweiz Med Wochenschr (German).* 1999;129:410–412 (Abstract).

89. Klyscz T, Bogenschutz O, Junger M, Rassner G. Micro-angiopathic changes and functional disorders of nail fold capillaries in dermatomyositis. *Hautarzt (German).* 1996;47:289–293 (Abstract).

90. Zahumensky E, Rybka J, Adamikova A. New aspects of pharmacologic and general prophylactic care of the diabetic foot. *Vnitr Lek (Russian).* 1995;41:531–534 (Abstract).

91. Bringezu G. Combating fatigue in sports physical therapy with reference to manual lymph drainage. *Z Lymphol (German).* 1994; 18:12–15 (Abstract).

92. Joos E, Bourgeois P, Famaey JP. Lymphatic disorders in rheumatoid arthritis. *Semin Arthritis Rheum.* 1993;22:392–398.

93. Trettin H. Neurologic principles of edema in inactivity. *Z Lymphol (German).* 1992;16:14–16 (Abstract).

94. Kaaja R, Tiula E. Manual lymph drainage in nephrotic syndrome during pregnancy. *Lancet.* 1989;21:990.

95. Uher EM, Vacariu G, Schneider B, Fialka V. Comparison of manual lymph drainage with physical therapy in complex regional pain syndrome, type I. A comparative randomized controlled therapy study. *Wien Klin Wochenschr.* 2000;112:133–137.

96. Preisler VK, Hagen R, Hoppe F. Indications and risks of manual lymph drainage in head-neck tumors. *Laryngorhinootologie (German).* 1998;77:207–212 (Abstract).

97. Herpertz U. Malignant lymphedema. *Z Lymphol (German).* 1990;14:17–23 (Abstract).

## Further Reading

Adcock J. Rehabilitation of the breast cancer patient. In: McGarvey CL III, ed. Physical *Therapy for the Cancer Patient.* New York: Churchill Livingstone; 1990:67–84.

Asdonk J. Effectiveness, indications and contraindications of manual lymph drainage therapy in painful edema. *Z Lymphol (German).* 1995;19:16–22 (Abstract).

Bauer WC, Dracup KA. Physiologic effects of back massage in patients with acute myocardial infarction. *Focus Crit Care.* 1987;14:42–46.

Bernas M, Witte M, Kriederman B, Summers P, Witte C. Massage therapy in the treatment of lymphedema: rationale, results, and applications. *IEEE Eng Med Biol Mag.* 2005;24:58–68.

Bertelli G, Venturini M, Forno G, et al. Conservative treatment of post-mastectomy lymphedema: a controlled study. *Ann Oncol.* 1991;2:575–578.

Browse NL. The diagnosis and management of primary lymphedema. *J Vasc Surg.* 1986;3:181–184.

Calnan JS, Pflug JJ, Reis ND, Taylor LM. Lymphatic pressures and the flow of lymph. *Br J Plast Surg.* 1970;23:305–317.

Campisi C, Boccardo F, Casaccia M. Post-mastectomy lymphedema: surgical therapy. *Ann Ital Chir.* 2002;73:473–478.

Carriere B. Edema: its development and treatment using lymph drainage massage. *Clin Manage.* 1988;8:119–121.

Casley-Smith JR. Changes in the microcirculation at the superficial and deeper levels in lymphoedema: the effects and results of massage, compression, exercise and benzopyrones on these levels during treatment. *Clin Hemorheol Microcirc.* 2000;23: 335–343.

Casley-Smith JR. Estimation of optimal massage pressure: is this possible? *Folia Angiol.* 1981;29:154–156.

Casley-Smith JR. Measuring and representing peripheral oedema and its alterations. *Lymphology.* 1994;27:56–70.

Chikly B. Post-mastectomy care and lymph drainage therapy. *J Bodywork Movement Ther.* 1999;3:11–16.

Drinker CK, Yoffey JM. *Lymphatics, Lymph, and Lymphoid Tissue: Their Physiological and Clinical Significance.* Cambridge, MA: Harvard University Press; 1941.

Dubois F. Use of a new specific massage technique to prevent the formation of hypertrophic scars. In: Cluzan RV, Pecking AP, Lokiec FM, eds. *Progress in Lymphology XIII, Exerpta Medica.* International Congress Series no. 994. Amsterdam: Elsevier Science Publishers BV; 1992:635.

Eliska O, Eliska M. Ultrastructure and function of the lymphatics in man and dog legs under different conditions—massage. In: Cluzan RV, Pecking AP, Lokiec FM, eds. *Progress in Lymphology XIII, Exerpta Medica.* International Congress Series no. 994. Amsterdam: Elsevier Science Publishers BV; 1992:97.

Enig B, Mogensen M, Jorgensen RJ. Lymphedema in patients treated for breast cancer. A cross-sectional study in the county of Ribe. The need of manual lymph drainage; risk factors. *Ugeskr Laeger.* 1999;161:3293–3298.

Evrard-Bras M, Coupe M, Laroche JP, Janbon C. Manual lymphatic drainage. *Rev Prat.* 2000;50:1199–1203.

Flowers KR. String wrapping versus massage for reducing digital volume. *Phys Ther.* 1998;68:57–59.

Foldi E. Massage and damage to lymphatics. *Lymphology.* 1995;28:1–3.

Foldi E, Sauerwald A, Hennig B. Effect of complex decongestive physiotherapy on gene expression for the inflammatory response in peripheral lymphedema. *Lymphology.* 2000;33:19–23.

Foldi M. Anatomical and physiological basis for physical therapy of lymphedema. *Experentia.* 1978;33(Suppl):15–18.

Francois A. Use of isoptic lymphography in the evaluation of manual lymphatic drainage effects in chronic lower limb edema. In: Partsch H, ed. *Progress in Lymphology XI, Exerpta Medica.* International Congress Series no. 779. Amsterdam: Elsevier Science Publishers BV; 1987:555.

Giardini D, Bohimann R. *Le Drainage Lymphatique Manuel.* Lausanne: Ed. Payot; 1991.

Gironet N, Baulieu F, Giraudeau B, et al. Lymphedema of the limb: predictors of efficacy of combined physical therapy. *Ann Dermatol Venereol.* 2004;131:775–779.

Gruffaz J. Le drainage lymphatique manuel. *J Mal Vasc (French).* 1985;10:187–191.

Herpertz U. Significance of radiogenic damage for lymphology. *Z Lymphol (German).* 1990;14:62–67.

Hurst PAE. Venous and lymphatic disease—assessment and treatment. In: Downie PA, ed. *Cash's Textbook of Chest, Heart and Vascular Disorders for Physiotherapists.* London: Faber and Faber; 1987:654–665.

Kaya TI, Kokturk A, Polat A, Tursen U, Ikizoglu G. A case of cutaneous lymphangiectasis secondary to breast cancer treatment. *Int J Dermatol.* 2001;40:760–761.

Kirshbgaum M. Using massage in the relief of lymphoedema. *Prof Nurse.* 1996;11:230–232.

Leduc A, Caplan I, Lievens P. Traitment Physique de l'Oedeme du Bras. Paris: Masson Editeurs; 1981.

Lindemayr H, Santler R, Jurecka W. Compression therapy of lymphedema. *Munch Med Wochenschr (German).* 1980;122:825–828 (Abstract).

Little L, Porche DJ. Manual lymph drainage (MLD). *J Assoc Nurses AIDS Care.* 1998;9:78–81.

Morgan RG, Casley-Smith JR, Mason MR, Casley-Smith JR. Complex physical therapy for the lymphoedematous arm. *J Hand Surg.* 1992;17:437–441.

Mortimer PS. Therapy approaches for lymphedema. *Angiology.* 1997; 48:87–91.

Mortimer PS, Simmonds R, Rezvani M, et al. The measurement of skin lymph flow by isotope clearance—reliability, reproducibility, injection dynamics, and the effect of massage. *J Invest Dermatol.* 1990;95:677–682.

Pastura G, Mesiti M, Saitta M, et al. Lymphedema of the upper extremity in patients operated for carcinoma of the breast: clinical experience with coumarinic extract from *Melilotus officinalis. Clin Ter.* 1999;150:403–408.

Reiss M, Reiss G. Manual lymph drainage as therapy of edema in the head and neck area. *Schweiz Rundsch Med Prax.* 2003;92:271–274.

Rinehart-Ayres ME. Conservative approaches to lymphedema treatment. *Cancer.* 1998;83(Suppl 12):2828–2832.

Robert L. *Therapie Manuelle des Oedemes.* Paris: Ed Spek; 1992.

Rubin A, Hoefflin SM, Rubin M. Treatment of postoperative bruising and edema with external ultrasound and manual lymphatic drainage. *Plast Reconstr Surg.* 2002;109:1469–1471.

Ruger K. Diagnosis and therapy of malignant lymphedema. *Fortschr Med (German).* 1998;116:28–30,32,34.

Stahel HU. Manual lymph drainage. *Curr Probl Dermatol.* 1999; 27:148–152.

Strossenreuther RH, Dax I, Emde C. Lymphedema: treatment. *MMW Fortschr Med.* 2004;146:28–30,32–3.

Swedborg I. Effectiveness of combined methods of physiotherapy for post-mastectomy lymphoedema. *Scand J Rehabil Med.* 1980;12:77–85.

Szuba A. Literature watch: the addition of manual lymph drainage to compression therapy for breast cancer related lymphedema— a randomized controlled trial. *Lymphat Res Biol.* 2005;3:36.

Thiadens SR. Current status of education and treatment resources for lymphedema. *Cancer.* 1998;83(Suppl 12):2864–2868.

Uher EM, Vacariu G, Schneider B, Fialka V. Comparison of manual lymph drainage with physical therapy in complex regional pain syndrome, type I. A comparative randomized controlled therapy study. *Wien Klin Wochenschr (German).* 2000;112:133–137 (Abstract).

Vasudevan SV, Melvin JL. Upper extremity edema control: rationale of the techniques. *Am J Occup Ther.* 1979;33:520–523.

Vignes S, Champagne A, Poisson O. Management of lymphedema: experience of the Cognacq-Jay Hospital. *Rev Med Interne.* 2002;23(Suppl 3):414s–420s.

Vodder E. Lymphdrainage. *Aesthet Med.* 1965;14:6.

Williams C. Compression therapy for lymphoedema from Vernon-Carus. *Br J Nurs.* 1998;7:339–343.

Woods M. The experience of manual lymph drainage as an aspect of treatment for lymphoedema. *Int J Palliat Nurs.* 2003;9: 336–342.

Worthington EL Jr, Martin GA, Shumate M. Which prepared-childbirth coping strategies are effective? *JOGN Nurs.* 1982;11:45–51.

Xujian S. Effect of massage and temperature on the permeability of initials. *Lymphology.* 1990;23:48–50.

# Chapter 9
## Neuromuscular Techniques

Neuromuscular techniques are those massage techniques that palpate muscle, affect the level of resting tension of muscles, and have additional psychoneuroimmunological effects. These techniques include broad-contact compression, petrissage, stripping, and specific compression. This chapter describes these techniques, how to perform them, and how to apply them in a practice sequence. A section on further study for each technique includes a discussion of relevant outcomes and evidence, cautions and contraindications, and how to use the technique in treatment.

| Table 9-1 | Summary of Outcomes for Neuromuscular Techniques | | | |
|---|---|---|---|---|
| | **Technique** | | | |
| **Outcome** | **Broad-Contact Compression** | **Petrissage** | **Stripping** | **Specific Compression** |
| Increased perceived relaxation and decreased levels of stress hormones | P | ✓ | P | ✓ |
| Decreased perceived anxiety and levels of stress hormones | P | ✓ | P | ✓ |
| Stimulated immune function | P | ✓ | P | P |
| Systemic sedation | P | ✓ | P | ✓ |
| Sensory arousal | P | ✓ | ? | ? |
| Analgesia | P | ✓ | ✓ | ✓ |
| Increased arterial supply (direct effect) | P | P | ? | ? |
| Increased venous return (direct effect) | P | P | ? | ? |
| Increased lymphatic return (direct effect) | P | P | ? | ? |
| Decreased edema (direct effect) | P | P | ? | ? |
| Normalized muscle resting tension and neuromuscular tone | ? | P | ✓ | ✓ |
| Decreased muscle spasm | ? | P | P | P |

*(continued)*

| Table 9-1 | continued | | | |
|---|---|---|---|---|
| | | **Technique** | | |
| **Outcome** | **Broad-Contact Compression** | **Petrissage** | **Stripping** | **Specific Compression** |
| Increased muscle extensibility | ? | ✓ | ✓ | ✓ |
| Enhanced muscle performance (secondary effect) | ? | ✓ | ✓ | ✓ |
| Balance of agonist/antagonist function | ? | P | P | P |
| Improved movement responses | ? | P | P | P |
| Decreased trigger point activity | ? | ✓ | ✓ | ✓ |
| Increased tissue mobility | ? | ✓ | ✓ | ✓ |
| Increased joint mobility | ? | ✓ | ✓ | ✓ |
| Separation and lengthening of fascia | ? | P | P | ? |
| Normalized postural alignment | ? | P | P | P |
| Decreased dyspnea | P | P | P | P |
| Increased rib cage mobility | P | P | P | P |
| Increased airway clearance/mobilization of secretions | ✓ | ? | ? | ? |
| Stimulated peristalsis | P | P | P | P |

✓: the outcome is supported by research summarized in this chapter. P: the outcome is possible. ?: the outcome is debatable (research results are absent or inconsistent).

## Broad-Contact Compression: Foundations

## DEFINITION

Broad-contact compression: A **nongliding** technique that therapists deliver with a broad-contact surface such as the palm. This technique engages the client's muscle, and the pressure and release of the stroke are perpendicular to the surface of the client's body.[1-8]

## USES

Therapists can use broad-contact compression to assess the general quality and level of **muscle resting tension** of larger skeletal muscles, to increase venous and lymphatic return, and to assist the client's expiration. Since it can be **sedating** or **stimulating**, therapists often use it in **sports massage** to prepare athletes for competition.

## PALPATION PRACTICE

1. With full palmar contact, slowly apply light and then moderate pressure to regions of your practice partner's body that have substantial muscle mass such as the chest; front of the shoulder; anterior and posterior arm and forearm; the back adjacent to the spine; anterior, posterior, and medial thighs; and calves. How much does the tissue **deform** with pressure? Do tissues tend to displace one way or another when you direct pressure into the body?

2. With full palmar contact, slowly apply light and then moderate pressure to major bony prominences of your practice partner's body such as the acromion, clavicles, ribcage, iliac crest, ischial tuberosity, lateral femur, and anterior tibia. How do related joints move during each compression?

3. Rest your hands on your supine partner's upper ribs, and describe the movement of this part of the rib cage during relaxed breathing. Now, have your partner perform full forced inspiration and expiration. Note the difference. Repeat both parts of this exercise with your hands placed on your partner's lateral ribs and then on your partner's lower ribs.

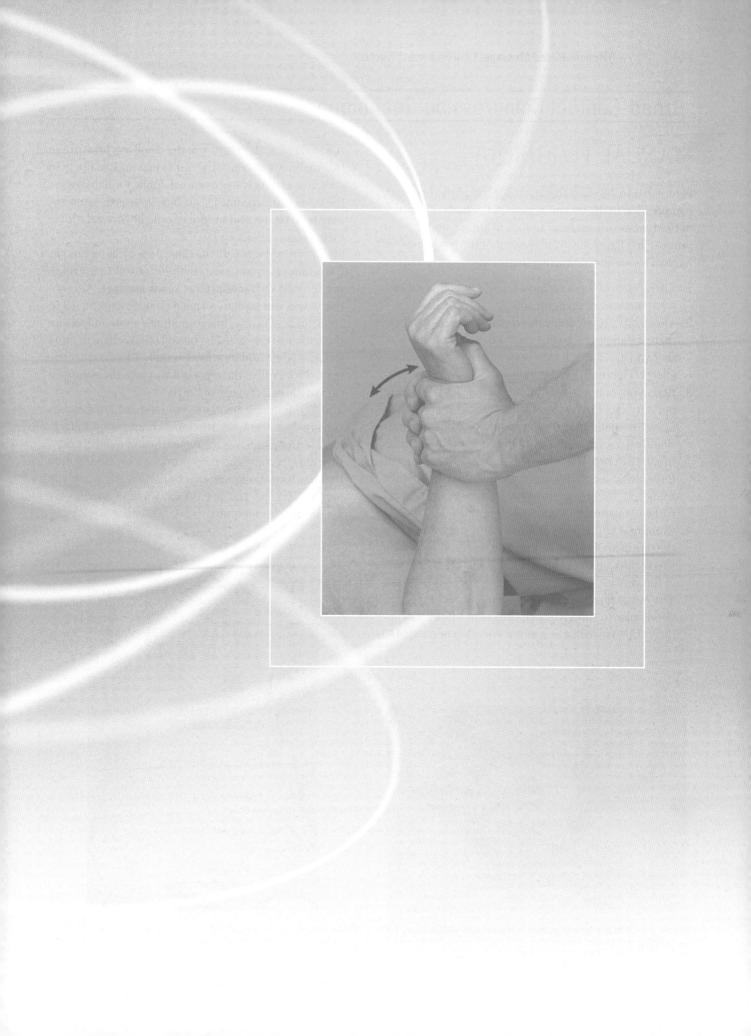

## Broad-Contact Compression: Technique

# MANUAL TECHNIQUE

Figures 9-1 to 9-8 show therapists applying broad-contact compression to the various regions of the body. The order of the figures is from head to foot in supine and then in prone. Each figure illustrates several of the guidelines for manual technique outlined in this section.

1. Therapists can best perform broad-contact compression with little or no lubricant.
2. Therapists usually apply this technique to areas where there is muscle tissue (Figures 9-4 to 9-7). Nevertheless, they can also apply it over bone to achieve specialized effects (Figures 9-1 and 9-3).
3. Relax your hands to facilitate palpation, and distribute pressure evenly over the entire contact surface. When using the palmar surface, spread your fingers apart slightly to increase the size of the contact surface (Figure 9-4). When you apply the stroke with significant force, avoid loading your wrist while it is extended by using your fist or your proximal forearm as the contact surface (Figures 9-5A and 9-5B, 9-6, and 9-7).
4. Compress and release gradually and smoothly when the rate of application is slow. You should still perform this technique smoothly when you increase the speed of the stroke.
5. The initial direction of application of pressure is perpendicular to the surface of the client's body. Do not direct the stroke in a horizontal direction or parallel to the surface of the client's body. Applying pressure in this manner will cause the individual muscle fibers to spread apart. As the pressure of application increases, the tissues in large muscle groups, such as the gluteals, may tend to roll and produce some horizontal movement (Figures 9-5A and 9-5B).
6. Stroke rate will vary with the clinical use of the technique. Clinicians often use a fast rhythmic rate (1 to 2 strokes per second) in **precompetition sports massage**. Alternatively, you can sustain a single compression for 10 to 20 seconds, allowing time to gradually apply and release the pressure (Figure 9-7). You will often achieve a more sedative effect and may more readily affect connective tissue elements of the muscle if you take the compression to the end of range of the tissues.
7. You can lift the client's tissues between each stroke when you are applying faster rhythmic compression to large muscle groups such as the hamstrings or quadriceps.
8. Rhythmic compression can produce a rocking motion that has its own clinical effects, particularly when you apply it around the pelvis (see Chapter 11, Passive Movement Techniques).

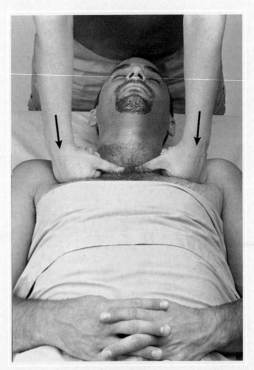

**Figure 9-2** Compression of the upper thorax to assist expiration.

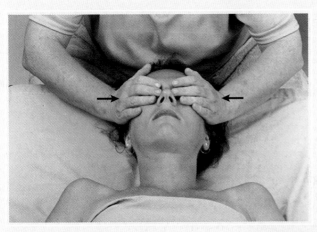

**Figure 9-1** Gentle bilateral palmar compression of the head can assist sinus drainage.

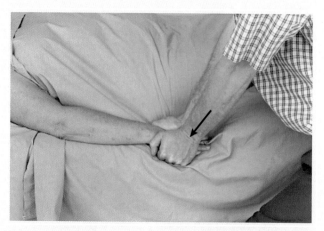

**Figure 9-3** Broad-contact compression to the distal extremity promotes general mobility.

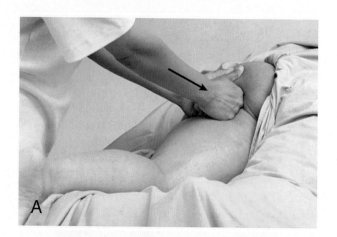

A

9. To enhance **venous and lymphatic return** from a limb, begin compression proximally at the junction between the limb and the limb girdle. Then apply a series of compression strokes that move from distal to proximal. From that point, begin each successive series of compressions distal to the previous series (Figure 9-8). When you are performing the technique to increase lymphatic return, consider waiting at least 8 seconds before compressing the same local area again.[9]

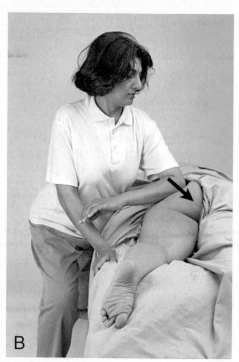

B

**Figure 9-5** A. Broad-contact compression of the glutei to produce sedation can be done either directly on the client's skin or through fabric. The practitioner has a choice of contact surfaces: reinforced or doubled fists or palms. B. Gluteal compression using the forearm in a lunge and lean posture. The practitioner uses her free hand to make the posture more stable.

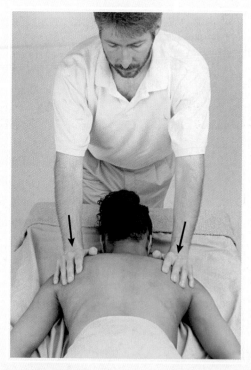

**Figure 9-4** Bilateral palmar compression of the shoulders using a standing controlled lean. The heels of the hands are in contact with the acromial portion of the upper trapezius muscle.

## How broad-contact compression might work

The mechanisms for cutaneous reflexes, **entrainment** to rhythm, and forward movement of fluid in valved vessels discussed for more superficial techniques in the earlier chapters also apply to broad-contact compression.[1,8] In addition, broad-contact compression spreads muscle fibers

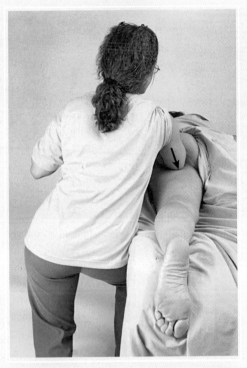

**Figure 9-6** Compression with the forearm or elbow is one of the few techniques that gives the therapist enough leverage to produce a mechanical effect on the superior attachment of the hamstring muscle. The technique must be executed carefully and should be done bilaterally to avoid producing a pelvic rotation in the client.

apart.[1,8] This spreading causes **proprioceptive** input that may reduce **neuromuscular tone**.[1,6] Furthermore, sustained pressure may produce connective tissue effects[6] by reducing both **collagen** cross-linking and increasing hydration of the **connective tissue matrix**.

# THERAPIST'S POSITION AND MOVEMENT

1. Use the basic positions described in Chapter 6, Preparation and Positioning for Massage, in the sections on standing **aligned** posture, standing controlled lean, **lunge** and lean, and **wide-stance knee bend** postures. You can increase the pressure you apply by shifting or rocking a stable **center of gravity** forward over the compressed segment of the client's body. Alternatively, you can bend both your knees to lower your upper body weight onto the client (Figures 9-4, 9-5B, 9-6, and 9-7).
2. Regardless of the working posture that you select, ensure that both of your feet remain flat on the floor, your hands and forearms remain as relaxed as possible,

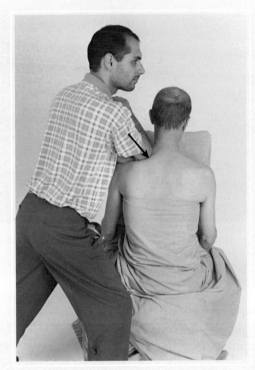

**Figure 9-7** Elbow or forearm compression with the client seated is an effective approach to soften a chronically indurated upper trapezius muscle. The therapist bends his knees, inclines his trunk slightly, and maintains relaxed shoulders to transfer his body weight to the client's body in a controlled manner.

**ON-LINE VIDEO**

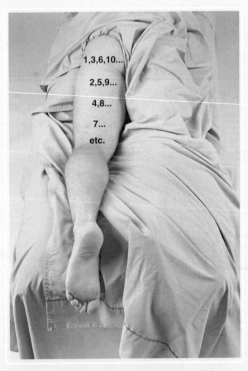

1,3,6,10...

2,5,9...

4,8...

7...

etc.

**Figure 9-8** The numbers indicate the sequence in which compressions are performed to enhance fluid return from the limb. (See Manual Technique, item #9, page 245, for description.)

Box 9-1

## Box 9-1  Components of Broad-Contact Compression

**Contact:** Whole palmar surface of the hand, heel of the hand, dorsal surface of proximal phalanges together (fist), or forearm

**Pressure:** Light to heavy

**Tissues engaged:** Muscle, associated tissues, and the underlying structures, such as the rib cage, that therapists reach through muscle. Therapists engage connective tissue elements when they sustain compression.

**Direction:** Perpendicular to surface of the client's body

**Amplitude/length:** NA

**Rate:** 5 to 10, or more, seconds per cycle of compression/release

**Duration:** 20 to 60 seconds or longer

**Intergrades with:** Petrissage, specific compression

**Combines with:** Can be combined with **rocking**, although neither technique is improved by this combination

**Context:** Can be used by itself extensively. Therapists often use it after effleurage and/or as a prelude to more specific **neuromuscular techniques**.

your elbows are flexed, and your shoulders are as relaxed as possible.

3. Use contact surfaces other than your hands for applying large amounts of pressure. When you do so, gauge how the client's compressed tissues are deforming under your body weight (Figures 9-4 to 9-7). This type of palpation might be termed "proprioceptive palpation," as opposed to strict manual palpation, since you are using proprioceptive sense to judge the movement of the client's tissues. The development of this "proprioceptive palpation" skill is essential to learning how to apply higher force neuromuscular and connective tissue techniques.

## PALPATE

When performing the technique, palpate the client's tissues for the following:

1. General resistance or resilience of soft tissues
2. Localized areas of hardness or tautness that may require the use of a more specific technique
3. Increased pliability that reflects the reduction in **viscosity** of healthy superficial subcutaneous tissues, which

normally occurs with continued application of the technique

4. Resorption of fluid from edematous tissue, which accompanies changes in surface contours, and the **viscosity** and **inertial resistance** of the subcutaneous tissues
5. Change in resting muscle tension with continued application of the technique
6. Change in the mobility of the rib cage when you apply the technique locally

## OBSERVE

When performing the technique, observe the client for changes in muscular tension, circulation, or breathing pattern. The signs listed below may signal this.

1. Reduction of **muscle resting tension**, as evidenced by softening of the tissue contours or broadening and flattening of body segments
2. If you are using the technique to treat respiratory conditions, note abnormalities in the client's usual breathing pattern and changes in these patterns with your application of the technique.
3. If you use the technique to treat **edema** and apply it proximal to the site of edema, visible reduction of swelling may often occur within 15 to 45 minutes. Cumulative reduction of **swelling** will occur during the course of the intervention, with resolution of an inflammatory process, or with resolution of circulatory and lymphatic dysfunction.
4. Normalizing of skin color and texture that reflects circulatory changes

## COMMUNICATION WITH THE CLIENT

Communicate to obtain feedback on the client's comfort during the application of techniques. Here are some examples of statements that you can use.

1. "Let me know if this starts to hurt." Ensure that the client finds the depth of the compression comfortable.
2. "Can you feel this pressure on your rib cage? Now breathe into my hand(s)." If you are applying the technique to the client's rib cage (Figures 9-2, 9-4), ensure that the resistance that you are providing with the compression stroke does not impede the client's breathing.

## A Practice Sequence for Broad-Contact Compression

Allow 30 minutes per person.

Allow 4 to 5 seconds per stroke, including the phases of gradual compression, hold, and gradual release. Synchronize the strokes with your breathing to achieve an even, relaxing tempo. Bend your knees and slowly rock your body weight over the contact surface to produce a deep, even compressive force. Use relaxed, broad contact.

### Supine

Partially rotate the client's head and gently apply techniques in the following manner:

1. Down the sides of his neck from the mastoid process to the clavicle. Note that this is a sensitive area on many people.
2. Across the upper chest from the sternum to the axilla inferior to the clavicle.
3. From the anterior deltoid down each arm. Then compress the hand as a unit.
4. Down the sternum. Use a narrower contact surface, such as the ulnar border of your hand, to avoid the client's breast tissue.

5. Across the lower ribs from midline toward the axilla. Avoid direct pressure on the xiphoid process when doing so.
6. Gently, with soft hands, around the abdomen in clockwise circles.
7. From the inguinal crease to just above the client's knee. Repeat to cover the anteromedial and anterolateral surfaces of the thigh.

### Prone

Gently apply techniques in the following manner:

1. Bilaterally along upper trapezius to the acromion process. Perform this while you are standing at the head of the table. Note: You can use considerable pressure here.
2. From the posterior deltoid, move down each arm.
3. Down either side of the spine from occiput to sacrum. Repeat, moving slightly more laterally on the back with each new series of compressive strokes.
4. Unilaterally and bilaterally on the lumbar musculature with broad palmar contact.
5. From the iliac crest on one side, down the gluteals, and distally to the knee. Repeat to cover the posteromedial and posterolateral surfaces of the thigh. If pressure on the posterior surface causes the client to report knee pain, place additional pillows under his ankles or lower legs from his knees to his feet.

# Broad-Contact Compression: Further Study and Practice

## NAMES AND ORIGINS

In other texts or massage-related systems, the technique that we call broad-contact compression is also known as "compression," "pressure," and "pressing."[1-8] Broad-contact compression owes its current classification as an independent technique largely to its applications in athletics.[1-3,5,10] The technique is not usually discussed in older texts[11-13] and is still omitted from some modern ones.[6,7] Nevertheless, this stroke is the technical foundation and prerequisite for many classical gliding techniques that **knead** muscle (see Petrissage, later in this chapter). Although broad-contact compression lacks the component of "**drag**" (horizontal tension) that characterizes petrissage, it is an extremely versatile technique in its own right.

## OUTCOMES AND EVIDENCE

Broad-contact compression is a useful introductory stroke that clinicians can use to assess the general quality and the level of resting tension of larger skeletal muscles. They can also use this technique to achieve effects on circulation, muscle resting tension, and rib cage mobility. Table 9-1 summarizes the main outcomes for broad-contact compression.

### Cardiopulmonary Effects

Although various texts state that the repetitive, rhythmic nature of broad-contact compression results in "increased circulation,"[1-8] this postulated direct **mechanical effect** may be an increase in **perfusion**, arterial supply, **lymphatic return**, or **venous return**. For example, broad-contact compression applied to the rib cage may assist systemic lymphatic return.[14] This is especially true in the region of the upper anterior and posterior ribs and over the junctions of the right lymphatic and thoracic ducts with the venous circulation.[14–16] In addition, when clinicians perform it on clients' soles or palms, it may assist lymphatic return from the limb.[15,16] The circulatory effects of broad-contact compression have not, however, been evaluated systematically in the research on massage. Furthermore, research on the effect of the similar compressive **petrissage** technique on fluid flow is inconclusive (discussed later in this chapter).[17]

Nevertheless, there are two extensive areas of related research that support circulatory effects of broad-contact compression that warrant consideration: closed-chest cardiac massage and pneumatic devices that apply compression. Vigorous compression of the rib cage in the context of closed-chest cardiac massage (CPR) produces forward blood flow.[18–20] Pneumatic devices that apply compression ("intermittent pneumatic compression," or "impulse compression") to clients' limbs increase venous return and are useful in the treatment of a variety of circulatory conditions.[21–26] Research also suggests that applying a moderate circumferential pressure on the limbs using a pneumatic cuff can increase circulatory supply[26] and lymphatic return.[27,28] In one study, the rate of lymphatic return increased with the pressure applied (up to 320 mmHg), and a wait of at least 8 seconds was required after each local compression to permit refilling of terminal lymphatics.[9] Compression of the rib cage is used in a variety of ways in cardiopulmonary rehabilitation. Rib cage compression is incorporated into breathing retraining techniques that improve breathing patterns and promote increased respiratory volume during inspiration and expiration.[29] When clinicians perform broad-contact compression vigorously and repetitively on the client's rib cage ("shaking" or "rib springing"), it facilitates the movement of secretions through the bronchial tree.[6,30,31] This technique can be used alone or combined with **postural drainage** (see Chapter 12, Percussive Techniques).

## Effects on Muscle Resting Tension

Texts are inconsistent on whether broad-contact compression increases or decreases muscle resting tension.[1–3,5] It is possible that broad-contact compression may result in a transient and marginal increase or decrease in muscle resting tension, depending on the rate and vigor of the application of the technique. Clinicians often use broad-contact compression in precompetition sports massage for several reasons: it has a possible effect on tone, it does

not require a lubricant or the removal of clothing, and it can be adapted to be either sedative or stimulating.[1–3,10] It is possible to perform effective full-body massage sequences that have specific effects on several of the clients' systems with the skillful use of only broad-contact compression.

# CAUTIONS AND CONTRAINDICATIONS

Clinicians need clinical training and supervised practice to master the proper application of broad-contact compression. Advanced training may be advisable when dealing with pathological conditions. All of the general and local contraindications noted for massage techniques apply to the use of broad-contact compression (see Chapter 3, Clinical Decision Making for Massage). There are also specific contraindications to the use of this technique, including clients with hemophilia and local sites of acute inflammation and infection and clients with confirmed or suspected thrombus, thrombophlebitis, or malignancy. If the clinician is applying broad-contact compression to the client's rib cage to mobilize the chest wall or to mobilize bronchial secretions and enhance airway clearance, some contraindications include a flail chest, an immobile rib cage, fractured or brittle ribs, and recent chest or spinal surgery.[6] The clinician should perform a careful examination and moderate her use of pressure with clients who have confirmed or suspected osteoporosis, clients with wounds that are in the early stages of healing, and clients who are taking anticoagulants. The clinician should also exercise caution when treating areas of **spasm**; areas of **hypotonia**; **active trigger points**; and the rib cage, when there is potential for bronchospasm.

# USING BROAD-CONTACT COMPRESSION IN TREATMENT

## Stress

Broad-contact compression is useful in general massage to address the effects of **stress**, whether clinicians use it alone or combine it with other techniques. It is probably most effective for **relaxation** when clinicians apply each stroke slowly and with considerable pressure, which they sustain for 2 seconds or more. In situations in which the client presents with a generalized elevation of resting muscle tension because of stress, use moist heat and **diaphragmatic breathing** or **progressive relaxation** as adjuncts to the intervention.

## Chest Wall Mobility

Broad-contact compression, especially when sustained, helps to improve chest wall mobility. Ensure that there are no contraindications, such as osteoporosis, especially in the elderly. Complementary methods that can be included during massage include:

1. Myofascial release applied to the upper body (see Chapter 10, Connective Tissue Techniques)
2. Direct fascial technique applied to the ribcage (see Chapter 10, Connective Tissue Techniques)
3. Breathing exercises that encourage full inspiration and expiration
4. Conventional upper body stretching

The client can also receive the latter two techniques as home care activities.

# Petrissage: Foundations

# DEFINITION

Petrissage: A group of related techniques that repetitively **compress**, **shear**, and release soft tissue—primarily muscle—with varying amounts of **drag**, **lift**, and glide.[1–8]

# USES

Petrissage is the workhorse of the **classical massage** techniques. Therapists use it to promote relaxation, reduce resting tension of skeletal muscle, and improve connective tissue **extensibility**. They can use it to treat many causes of musculoskeletal pain. Through its general relaxing effect, it also helps to reduce the perception of many other types of pain. Although the literature often states that petrissage increases local circulation, it is more accurate to say that it changes **perfusion** and, possibly, increases venous and lymphatic return. Its reflex effects on visceral function are less certain.

# PALPATION PRACTICE

Over a period of weeks, perform the following for each major skeletal muscle in the body:

1. Locate the attachments and borders of the chosen muscle on a practice partner, using an atlas as reference. Using your fingertips, palpate across the muscle fibers to confirm their direction.
2. With a washable marker, draw the muscle in place on one side of the body. Mark the fiber directions.
3. Observe your partner. How do the anatomical structures you have drawn influence the surface contours of the body?
4. Grasp the muscle and attempt to lift it off the underlying tissues. How easily does it lift? Does it lift away by itself, or do other muscles lift with it?
5. With the muscle lifted, attempt to bow it between your two hands. How easily does it bend?
6. Lastly, compress the muscle onto the underlying tissues. How much resistance do the tissues offer to the compression? What underlying structures provide the resistance to compression?

# Petrissage: Technique

## MANUAL TECHNIQUE: PETRISSAGE 1, MUSCLE SQUEEZING

Figures 9-9 to 9-15 show clinicians applying muscle squeezing to the various regions of the body. The order of the figures is from head to foot in supine and then in prone. Each figure illustrates most of the guidelines for manual technique outlined in this section.

1. Therapists can perform this **nongliding** technique best without lubricant, and they can apply it effectively through fabric (Figure 9-12).
2. Use one or both hands to grasp, lift, and squeeze a muscle, muscle group, or body segment, with minimal glide. It is easiest to perform on mid-sized body segments such as the calf (Figure 9-15), upper arm, upper trapezius (Figure 9-13), hand, and foot (Figure 9-12).
3. Therapists can squeeze smaller muscles, such as the sternocleidomastoid, between their thumb and index finger (Figures 9-9 and 9-10).
4. If you use two hands, you can add a bowing action to **shear** the muscle further.
5. Because this technique uses mostly hand and forearm strength, we do not recommend extended application. This is especially true if you are treating large muscle groups such as the quadriceps (Figure 9-11).

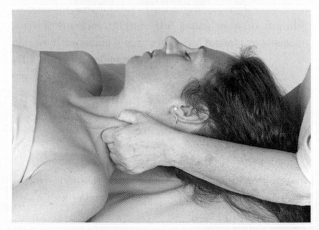

Figure 9-10 Squeezing either head of the sternocleidomastoid between thumb and index may elicit pain from latent myofascial trigger points (see later in this chapter). The therapist must be able to distinguish between the two divisions of the muscle.

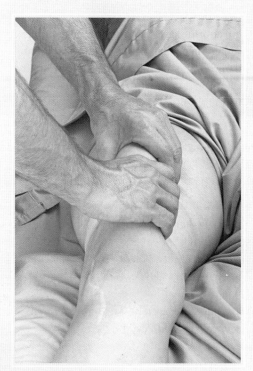

Figure 9-11 Two-handed squeezing of bulky muscle groups, such as the quadriceps, taxes the hands and should not be done for long periods.

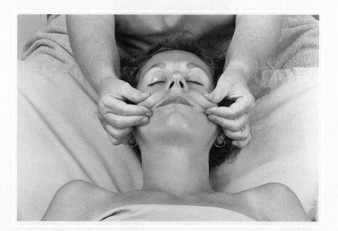

Figure 9-9 Gentle squeezing of facial muscles and superficial tissues between index and thumb.

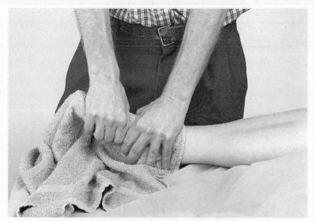

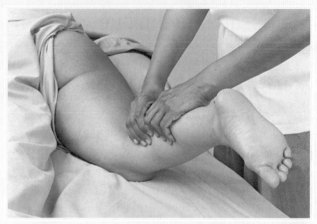

Figure 9-12  Squeezing the whole foot through the sheet or a towel often gives the practitioner a better grip and thus yields a deeper application of technique than working directly on the skin.

Figure 9-15  Two-handed squeezing of the posterior compartments of the leg can be combined with passive flexion/extension of the knee or with shaking of the ankle and foot.

## How petrissage might work

The mechanisms for cutaneous reflexes, **entrainment** to rhythm, and forward movement of fluid in valved vessels discussed for more superficial techniques in the earlier chapters also apply to petrissage. In addition, petrissage spreads muscle fibers apart, **shears** muscle layers between the contact surfaces, and applies **tension** (drag, stretch) to connective tissue in the muscle.[1–8] Spreading and shearing of muscle causes proprioceptive input that may reduce **neuro-**

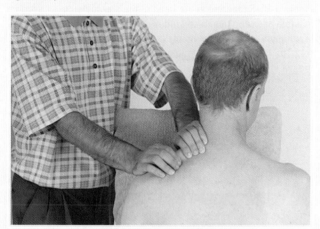

Figure 9-13  Squeezing of the upper trapezius muscle can be done with the client prone, supine, side-lying, or seated. An additional bowing force can be added.

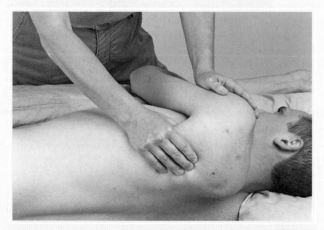

Figure 9-14  The muscles of the posterior axillary wall (teres major and latissimus dorsi) are easily accessible for squeezing when the client is in side-lying. One hand squeezes while the other hand positions the scapula, as desired, to increase accessibility of the muscles.

| Box 9-2 | **Components of Muscle Squeezing** |
|---|---|

**Contact:** The entire palmar surface, the thumb and index finger and the included web space

**Pressure:** Light to moderate

**Engages:** Muscle and associated **fascia**

**Direction:** Applied around the (partial) circumference of the muscle belly or limbs

**Amplitude/length:** N/A

**Rate:** 1 to 3 seconds or more per cycle of compression/release

**Duration:** 10 to 20 seconds or more

**Intergrades with:** Other forms of petrissage

**Context:** Usually used as an introductory muscular technique that is preceded by **superficial effleurage** and followed by more specific forms of petrissage. Can be used as a finishing stroke or by itself to address a region in a short time.

**muscular tone.**[1,4,6,8] Finally, slow rates of glide that maximize tension forces may produce connective tissue effects[4,8] by reducing **collagen** cross-linking and increasing hydration of the **connective tissue matrix**.

## Therapist's Position and Movement for Muscle Squeezing

1. Use the basic positions described in Chapter 6, Preparation and Positioning for Massage, in the sections on standing **aligned** posture and seated aligned posture.
2. Your position can be quite variable. When you are treating larger body segments, face the long axis of the muscle(s) you are going to squeeze (Figures 9-12 to 9-15).

# MANUAL TECHNIQUE: PETRISSAGE 2, WRINGING

Figures 9-16 to 9-22 show clinicians applying wringing to the various regions of the body. The order of the figures is from head to foot on the anterior surface and then the posterior surface. Each figure illustrates most of the guidelines for manual technique outlined in this section.

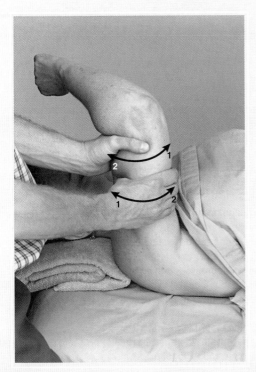

**Figure 9-16** On small body segments, such as the upper arm, wringing can be done with thumbs abducted. In this position, the client's arm must be completely relaxed.

 ON-LINE VIDEO

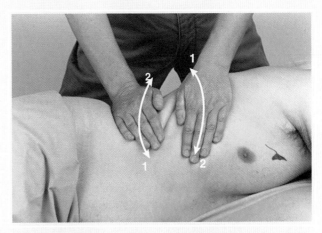

**Figure 9-17** Wringing the lower rib cage in prone, supine, or side-lying is an indirect way of loosening the respiratory diaphragm.

1. For large body segments, rest your hands on opposite sides of the circumference of the body segment you are going to wring and compress them toward each other (Figure 9-18A).
2. Maintaining compression, slide your hands toward each other, lifting and shearing the muscle between them as they pass each other (Figures 9-17, 9-18B, 9-20, and 9-22).
3. Continue to slide your hands, without exerting pressure, until they rest on opposite sides of the body segment on which they began (Figure 9-18C). Then initiate a new stroke. After two complete cycles, your hands will be in the positions in which they started.
4. Be careful to apply pressure gradually at the beginning of the strokes in order to avoid jerking.
5. To wring large body segments, such as the torso or quadriceps muscles, adduct your thumbs to avoid strain on your carpometacarpal joints (Figures 9-17, 9-18A to 9-18C, and 9-20). For smaller body segments, such as arms, hands, or feet, you can abduct your thumb so that the entire web space between your thumb and index finger remains in contact during the technique (Figures 9-16 and 9-19). Wringing with abducted thumbs places undue strain on the joints of your thumb and should be avoided except for short treatment periods.
6. As with other forms of petrissage that use the whole hand, begin wringing proximally on the limb and proceed in a distal direction. Return proximally with wringing or with superficial effleurage and repeat. Therapists believe that this will maximize **lymphatic return** by clearing proximal areas first.[32]
7. Areas of elevated resting tension can benefit from extended (5 or more minutes) periods of wringing, although this involves a lot of work on the part of the therapist.

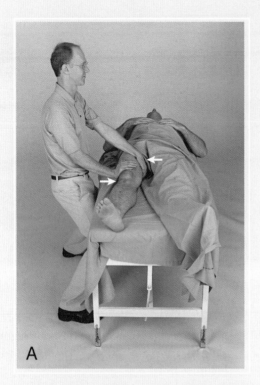

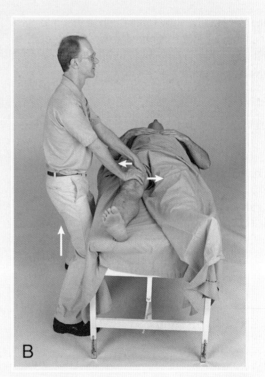

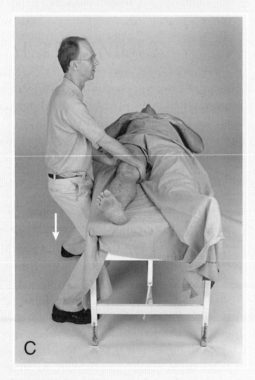

Figure 9-18  A. For bulky regions, such as the quadriceps, the hamstrings, and the back, effective wringing requires that the practitioner use correct body mechanics. At the start of the stroke, the hands are diametrically opposed. They then begin to compress together. The practitioner's posture is wide-stance ("horse stance") with bent knees. B. The practitioner's legs straighten, adding force to the lift and shear produced by the passing hands. C. The relaxation phase: the hands pass each other, release tissue, and move to a position opposite the starting position. Simultaneously, the knees bend again in preparation for the next stroke.

8.  Note: You need considerable pressure to lift and shear the bulk of large muscle groups between your hands. Do not produce a superficial effleurage that is oriented across the body segment and has no **mechanical effect** on the muscle itself.

## Therapist's Position and Movement for Wringing

For large body segments, such as the torso or thighs, you must perform wringing with correct leg movements in

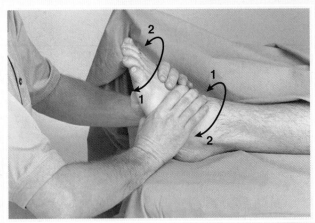

Figure 9-19 Wringing an entire foot or hand engages many structures with each stroke and is a good choice of technique when time is limited.

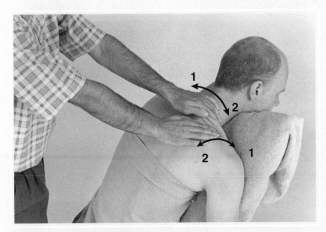

Figure 9-20 Wringing the upper trapezius with the client seated.

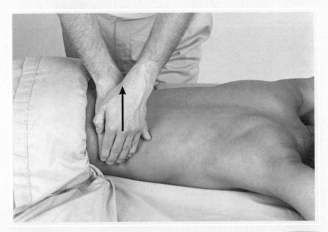

Figure 9-21 A variation of wringing involves one- or two-handed lifting of the torso in prone or supine. Gravity provides the opposing force.

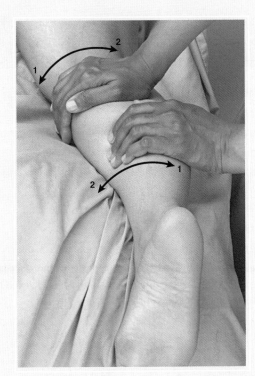

Figure 9-22 Wringing the calf.

order to generate sufficient force to compress, lift, and shear large masses between your hands. You can achieve this leg movement with the following steps:

1. Stand facing the long axis of the body segment you are going to wring (Figure 9-18A).
2. Begin in the wide-stance knee bend posture with your knees flexed between 30 and 45 degrees. The lowered position allows some palmar contact of your near hand while reducing extension of your wrist (Figure 9-18A).
3. During the **power stroke**, as your hands compress and slide toward each other, straighten your legs without hyperextending your knees (Figure 9-18B). During the **return stroke**, as your hands slide apart, flex your knees again (Figure 9-18C). Thus, for each stroke, you flex and extend your knees so that you generate most of the power for the application of the technique from the extension of your knees.
4. Coordination of your leg and arm movements takes practice. The reward is a secure, smooth, very deep, and effective technique.
5. Initially, your legs may fatigue or become sore. This will pass as your leg strength increases.

When wringing smaller body segments, you can use a variety of aligned postures that are described in Chapter 6, Preparation and Positioning for Massage.

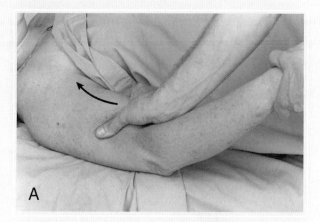

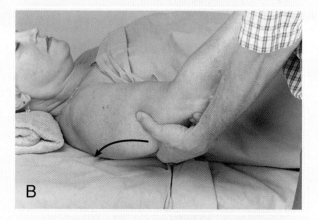

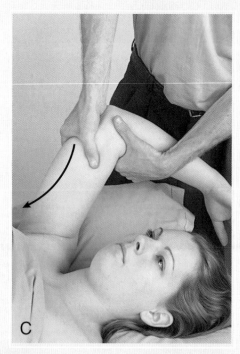

## Box 9-3 | Components of Wringing

**Contact:** Palmar surface of both hands

**Pressure:** Light to heavy

**Engages:** Muscle, associated fascia, and contained tissues

**Direction:** Across the long axis of the body segment

**Amplitude/length:** Half circumference of the body segment to which wringing is being applied

**Rate:** 1 to 3 seconds per cycle of compress/release

**Duration:** 20 to 60 seconds or more

**Intergrades with:** Other forms of general petrissage

**Context:** Usually used as an introductory muscular technique that is preceded by **superficial effleurage** and followed by more specific forms of petrissage

# MANUAL TECHNIQUE: PETRISSAGE 3, PICKING-UP ("C-KNEADING")

Figures 9-23 to 9-28 show clinicians applying picking-up to the various regions of the body. The order of the figures is from head to foot in supine and then in prone. Each figure illustrates most of the guidelines for manual technique outlined in this section.

A.  One-handed technique for smaller body segments such as the arms, forearms, and calves (Figures 9-23 to 9-24C)

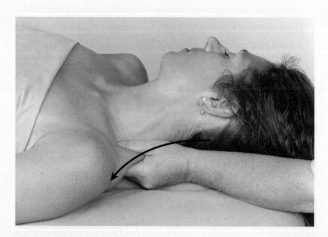

**Figure 9-23** Unilateral picking-up of upper trapezius muscle in supine.

**Figure 9-24** Upper arms are an ideal size for one-handed picking-up. A. The biceps brachii. B. The triceps brachii (with the glenohumeral joint in the loose-packed position). C. The triceps with the shoulder and elbow flexed. Apply pressure in a centripetal direction and lift the tissues away from the underlying bone.

 ON-LINE VIDEO

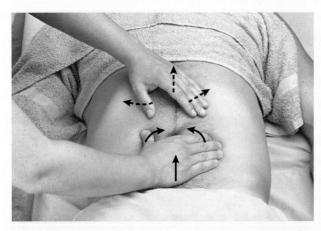

**Figure 9-25** Two-handed picking-up of rectus abdominis. Return stroke is shown in a dotted line. Practice is required to attain good contact during two-handed picking-up on flat surfaces like the abdomen or the back.

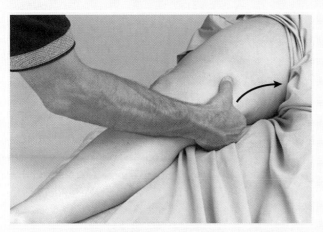

**Figure 9-26** One-handed picking-up of the adductors of the hip.

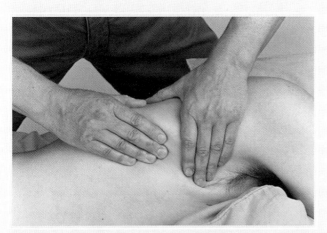

**Figure 9-27** Two-handed picking-up is a good technique for the lateral edge of the latissimus dorsi. The therapist can work her way down to the iliac crest. Placing the client's arm overhead also improves access to the abdominal obliques and quadratus lumborum muscles.

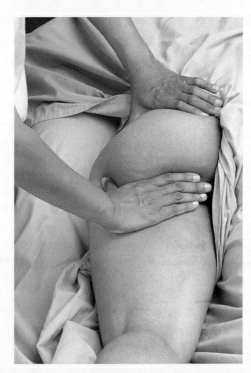

**Figure 9-28** Hand position to begin two-handed picking-up of the glutei.

1. Abduct your thumb so your hand forms a "C" shape, with the four fingers grouped together in adduction.
2. Grasp and squeeze while gliding your hand in a **centripetal** direction. Most of your hand remains in contact with the client's body, with the focus on your thumb, index finger, and web space. Squeeze the client's tissues through the closing web space for the power stroke, and abduct your thumb progressively toward the end of the stroke ("squeezing off the stroke").
3. During the power stroke, make an effort to lift the tissues off the underlying bone (Figures 9-24A to 9-24C).
4. Reopen your hand to a "C" shape as it glides back to its original position with minimal pressure (return stroke).
5. One author suggests using a four count as follows: compress on one, grasp and lift on two, release on three, and move/glide on four.[8]

B. Alternate two-handed technique for larger or flatter body segments such as the thighs and back (Figures 9-25, 9-27, and 9-28)

1. Place your two hands facing each other in an open "C" position as described in Step A4 (Figure 9-28).
2. The individual motion of each of your hands is similar to the one-handed technique described in

section A. The difference is that your hands work in contrary motion: one hand performs a short power stroke, while the other is performing a short return stroke. Deliver power strokes toward the opposing hand; with return strokes, move away from the opposing hand.

3. For optimal effectiveness, you should sustain some compression between your hands throughout the application of this technique. This results in a continuous lifting of the tissue between your hands.

4. On limbs, begin the sequence of strokes proximally, and gradually move the focus of the strokes distally.[32]

5. Coordination between your hands takes practice. Once you master it, it yields a technique that clients perceive to be very pleasant.

6. Picking-up (one- or two-handed) for more than a couple of minutes at a time is not advisable because of wear on the therapist's hands and forearms.

## Therapist's Position and Movement for Picking-Up

1. Use the basic positions described in Chapter 6, Preparation and Positioning for Massage, in the sections on standing aligned posture, **wide-stance knee bend**, and wide-stance knee bend with trunk rotation.

2. To generate more force during the application of one-handed forms, shift or lean forward into the client's body during the compression and lift portion of the stroke. Then shift or lean back during the release-and-move portion.

3. For the application of two-handed forms, face the long axis of the client's body segment in the wide-stance knee bend, as for wringing. Flexing your knees in this position may reduce hyperextension of your wrists by bringing you closer to the level of the client (Figure 9-27).

4. To generate more power for two-handed forms, rotate your ipsilateral shoulder to lean slightly into each power stroke (wide-stance knee bend with trunk rotation). This increases the force and effectiveness of the technique, minimizes hand and forearm fatigue, and results in a smooth upper body rhythm.

5. Do not let your shoulders elevate when applying the technique.

## MANUAL TECHNIQUE: PETRISSAGE 4, BROAD-CONTACT KNEADING AND DEEP EFFLEURAGE

Figures 9-29 to 9-36 show clinicians applying broad-contact kneading to the various regions of the body. The order of the figures is from head to foot in supine and then in prone. Each figure illustrates most of the guidelines for manual technique outlined in this section.

1. As with wringing and picking-up, there is a pressure stroke and a return stroke. Combine the pressure stroke and return stroke to form circles or ellipses that are ori-

---

| Box 9-4 | **Components of Picking-Up** |
| --- | --- |

**Contact:** Palmar surface, especially the web space between the thumb and index finger

**Pressure:** Light to moderate

**Engages:** Muscle and associated fascia

**Direction:** Parallel to the long axis of the body segment

**Amplitude/length:** 5 to 20 cm or more

**Rate:** 1 to 3 seconds per cycle of compression/release

**Duration:** 20 to 60 seconds or more

**Intergrades with:** Other forms of general petrissage

**Context:** Usually preceded by superficial effleurage and more general forms of petrissage and followed by more specific forms of petrissage

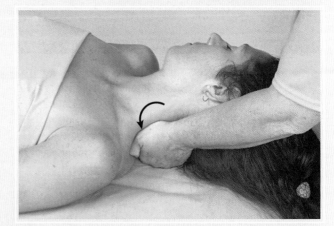

**Figure 9-29** Kneading the posterior triangle of the neck with the heel of the hand.

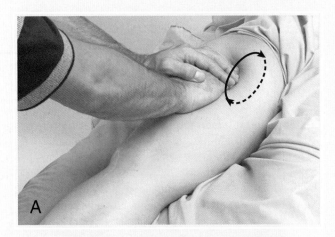

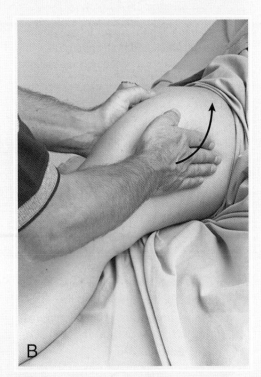

**Figure 9-30** A. Reinforced palmar kneading of the anterior thigh. Return stroke is shown in a dotted line. B. One version of "box-kneading." The hands can work in opposition, lifting tissue and/or pushing it proximally.

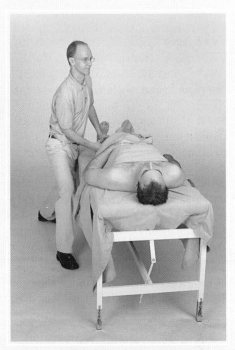

**Figure 9-31** Effective kneading requires correct application of the practitioner's body weight. This is especially true when kneading the iliotibial band, which is composed of dense connective tissue. The practitioner stabilizes his elbow against his iliac crest and carefully shifts his body weight toward the client.

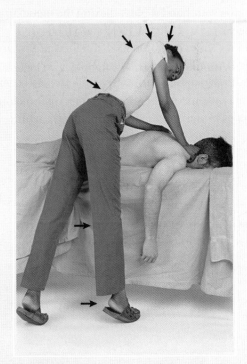

**Figure 9-32** This practitioner is committing at least five common errors of body mechanics while attempting a forceful kneading of trapezius. Common errors of body mechanics are detailed in Chapter 6, Preparation and Positioning for Massage.

ented along or across the fibers in the different muscle layers (Figures 9-30A and 9-30B and 9-33). Most often, the long axis of the stroke runs parallel to the long axis of the body segment or muscle to which you are applying the technique, especially when significant pressure is required (Figures 9-30A and 9-33). Elongating the ellipse results in "**deep effleurage**," provided the pressure is centripetal (Figures 9-33 and 9-34).

2. Maintain your wrist in neutral (no radial or ulnar deviation). This is critical to reduce joint stress during high-

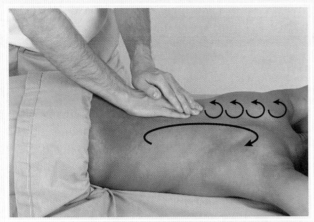

**Figure 9-33** Reinforced palmar kneading to the erector spinae muscles performed with a slightly arched hand. The strokes may take the form of smaller circles or of one long ellipse that covers the erector spinae muscles in a single stroke ("deep stroking" or "deep effleurage").

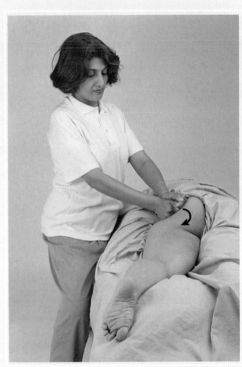

pressure applications of broad-contact kneading (Figures 9-29, 9-30A and 9-30B, 9-33, 9-35, and 9-36).

3. You may reinforce the dorsal surface of your hand or wrist with your other hand (Figures 9-30A and 9-33) or bring your hands together so that they reinforce each other (Figure 9-35).

**Figure 9-35** Reinforced fist kneading of the superior gluteal attachments is most effective when tissue is moved away from the sacrum or iliac crest.

4. More specific contact can be obtained by bridging or arching your hand slightly (flexing the metacarpophalangeal and interphalangeal joints). This produces two contact surfaces—broader at the heel and more specific at your fingertips (Figure 9-33).

5. As with the application of all types of petrissage, begin proximally and proceed in a distal direction while maintaining **centripetal** pressure to maximize lymphatic return.

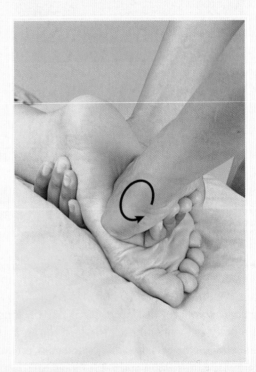

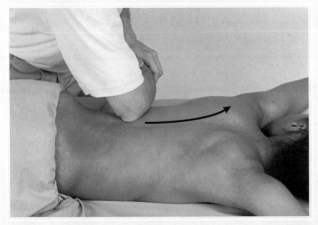

**Figure 9-34** Using the forearm along the erector spinae muscles. The therapist must be careful to avoid compressing the spinous processes. The return stroke is often omitted.

**Figure 9-36** Fist kneading to the sole of the foot is easier to control if the fist is rotated during the stroke. A deeper but less comfortable technique is obtained if the foot is passively dorsiflexed.

6. Variations: Some authors describe a form of circular **kneading** in which no glide occurs over the skin.[7] This technique engages muscle and is, in its effects, probably the same as kneading that glides over the skin.

7. Other variations: Some authors describe a two-handed form of kneading, termed **fulling** or broadening, in which your hands compress down and away from each other to spread or broaden the muscle belly and then lift the muscle up on the return stroke.[3,5]

8. Other variations: Some authors describe a two-handed form of kneading, termed **box kneading**, in which you position your hands so that they are diametrically opposed on the client's limb. You then compress them toward each other and finally move them proximally. This stroke is recommended to increase fluid return (Figure 9-30B).[7]

## Therapist's Position and Movement for Broad-Contact Kneading

1. Use the basic positions described in Chapter 6, Preparation and Positioning for Massage, in the sections on **lunge**, lunge and reach, lunge and lean, and standing **controlled lean**. In these positions, point your torso toward the point of contact (Figures 9-31 and 9-35).

2. To create the power portion of the stroke, hold your elbows partly extended, and drive forward with your legs during the lunge, or incline your body toward the contact point during the lunge and lean (Figures 9-31 and 9-35).

3. Use your shoulders and arms to transmit the force from the correct lower body movement, not to generate the force. You can generate much greater force for kneading through correct use of the lunge-and-lean posture.

4. Common errors that occur, especially when you are trying to generate more pressure, are:
   - Hyperextension of your elbows ("straight-arming")
   - Excessive elevation and/or protraction of your shoulders
   - Tilting of your head
   - Excessive leaning forward at your waist (Figure 9-32)

   All of these errors are more likely to occur if the table is too high.

| Box 9-5 | **Components of Broad-Contact Kneading** |
|---|---|

**Contact:** Full palmar surface of the hand, often reinforced on the wrist and/or metacarpals, fist/knuckles, or proximal forearm

**Pressure:** Light to heavy

**Engages:** Muscle and associated tissues. Slower strokes and greater **drag** (horizontal tension) will lengthen connective tissue elements of the muscle more.

**Direction:** Circular or elliptical. The long axis of ellipses is often oriented parallel to the long axis of muscles or muscle groups.

**Amplitude/length:** 10 cm or more

**Rate:** 10 to 25 cm/second

**Duration:** 20 to 60 seconds or more

**Intergrades with:** Superficial effleurage and other forms of petrissage. A notable, commonly used variation, sometimes called "deep effleurage" or "deep stroking," has the same long, gliding template of superficial effleurage but engages muscle with a considerable amount of pressure. This is not a superficial maneuver and has much in common with the broad-contact kneading described here. Nongliding forms using fingertip contact intergrade with **friction** (see Chapter 10, Connective Tissue Techniques).

**Context:** Usually preceded and followed by superficial effleurage, alternated with other general forms of petrissage, and followed by more specific forms of petrissage

## MANUAL TECHNIQUE: PETRISSAGE 5, SPECIFIC KNEADING (THUMBS, FINGERPADS, FINGERTIPS)

Figures 9-37 to 9-44 show clinicians applying specific kneading to the various regions of the body. The order of the figures is from head to foot in supine and then in prone. Each figure illustrates most of the guidelines for manual technique outlined in this section.

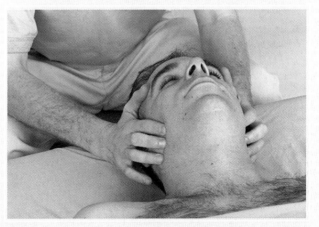

**Figure 9-37** Fingertips and fingerpads are ideal for petrissage of the face, which is usually done without applying lubricant. Fingerpad kneading of the masseter muscle.

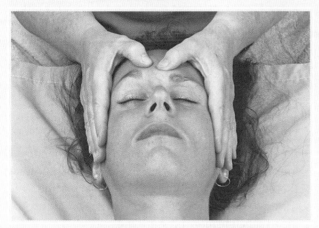

**Figure 9-38** Alternate thumb-kneading to the belly of the frontalis muscle.

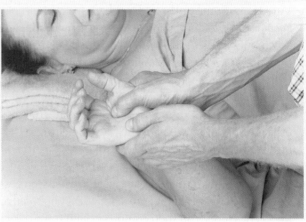

**Figure 9-41** Slow, rhythmic thumb-kneading of the thenar and hypothenar eminences is deeply relaxing. Because of the large number of structures in the hand (or the foot), thorough petrissage can take 30 minutes or longer.

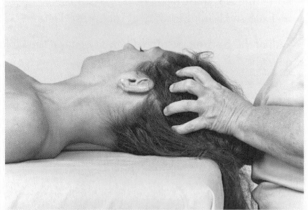

**Figure 9-39** Fingertip kneading of the scalp can be performed lightly with glide over the skin and through the hair or with more pressure and no glide.

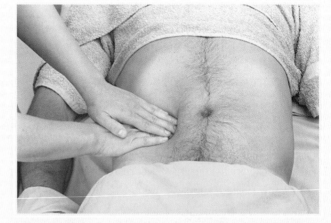

**Figure 9-42** Finger pad kneading to the lateral border of rectus abdominis.

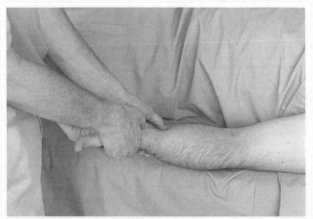

**Figure 9-40** Alternate thumb-kneading is a technique that fits onto forelimbs beautifully. Begin proximally, proceed distally, and return with a long centripetal stroke to the starting position. On the calf, the return stroke will "split" the heads of the gastrocnemius muscle.

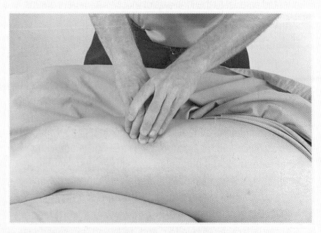

**Figure 9-43** Reinforced fingertip kneading of the quadriceps muscle.

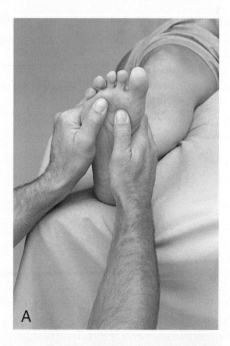

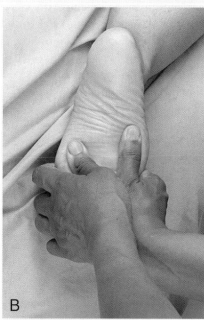

**Figure 9-44** A. The practitioner kneels at the foot of the table to perform alternate thumb-kneading to the sole of the foot in supine. B. The same technique in prone.

A. Fingertip and Fingerpad Technique (Figures 9-37, 9-39, 9-42, and 9-43)

1. Unless the surface you are kneading is relatively small (Figure 9-37), hold the fingers of your hand together (Figures 9-42 and 9-43). The heel or the entire rest of your hand may remain in contact with the client's body to provide stability (Figure 9-42).

When you require light pressure, as when you are kneading the face, you can omit this stabilization.

2. Perform repetitive circles, applying the pressure during the portion of the stroke that pushes away from your body. This potentially allows you to use your body weight to increase force.

3. You may use the other hand to reinforce across the carpals and metacarpals of your working hand in order to stabilize your wrist and enhance the force of the technique (Figure 9-43).

B. Thumb Technique (Figures 9-38, 9-40, 9-41, 9-44A, and 9-44B)

1. Place your hand close to or flat on the surface of the client's body, with your fingers parallel (Figure 9-38). Your fingertips remain loosely in contact with the client's body. Depending on the shape of the region you are kneading, the heel of your hand may also remain in partial contact (Figure 9-40).

2. Use the ventral surface of the distal thumb phalanx to deliver pressure in small ellipses. The long axes of these ellipses will be parallel to the long axis of your thumb. Do not abduct your thumbs widely during this motion (Figures 9-41 and 9-44A).

3. Ensure that you exert the pressure along, rather than across, the long axis of your thumb.

4. Usually, you use both thumbs in a technique known as alternate thumb kneading. One thumb performs a pressure stroke while the other performs a return stroke (Figures 9-38, 9-41, and 9-44A and 9-44B).

5. The technique described in Steps 1 to 3 may seem awkward at first, but it places a minimum amount of stress on the mobile, vulnerable joints of your thumb.

6. Perform specific kneading sparingly for short periods and alternate it frequently with other techniques that place different stresses on the joints of your hand.

## Therapist's Position and Movement for Specific Kneading

1. Use the basic positions described in Chapter 6, Preparation and Positioning for Massage, in the sections on standing, seated, or kneeling **aligned** posture. Face the body segment you are going to treat.

2. During thumb kneading, the movement of your thumbs is quite constrained, as described under Thumb Technique. Small movements at the carpometacarpal, carpal, and elbow joints create the force of the technique, which brings the weight of your forearm and upper arm into play.

3. During fingertip kneading, you can increase force by leaning slightly into the power stroke.

Box 9-6 **Components of Specific Kneading**

**Contact:** Fingertips, fingerpads, or thumbs form the working surface. In any case, the heel of the hand remains in contact to stabilize the hand.

**Pressure:** Light to moderate

**Engages:** Muscle and associated tissues. Slower strokes and greater drag (horizontal tension) will likely lengthen connective tissue elements of the muscle more than faster strokes.

**Direction:** Circular or elliptical. The long axis of ellipses is often oriented parallel to the long axis of muscles or muscle groups.

**Amplitude/length:** Up to 10 cm (determined by size of therapist's hand)

**Rate:** 0.5 to 2 seconds per cycle of compression/release

**Duration:** Up to 20 seconds at one time, provided the therapist does not experience hand fatigue

**Intergrades with: Stripping**

**Context:** Usually preceded by, alternated with, and followed by superficial effleurage and more general forms of petrissage such as wringing or palmar kneading

# PALPATE: FOR ALL FORMS OF PETRISSAGE

Palpate the client's skin and tissues for the following:

1. General resistance and resilience of soft tissues
2. Mobility of the interfaces between the muscles and muscle layers
3. Resistance to further stretch toward the end of the excursion of each stroke
4. Localized areas of hardness that may require use of more specific techniques
5. **Taut bands** in muscle, which may reflect **trigger point** activity (see later sections in this chapter)
6. **Fibrosis**, **adhesions**, and **indurations** within and between muscle layers, which can indicate **chronic inflammation**
7. Decrease in local fluid **viscosity** with continued application of the technique
8. The palpable softening of muscle tissue, which often results when the therapist applies petrissage for several minutes. This may reflect a decrease in the viscosity of superficial tissues caused by increased temperature; an increase in the hydration of the connective tissue matrix; a softening of taut bands, which is consistent with reduced

activity of trigger points; and a marginal systemic decrease in the level of resting tension of skeletal muscle, if the massage is relaxing.

In addition, slow the rate of petrissage when working in deep layers to facilitate palpation and to allow superficial tissues to move aside with each stroke.

# OBSERVE: FOR ALL FORMS OF PETRISSAGE

As you perform petrissage, observe the client for changes in the level of **muscle resting tension** and **edema**. Following are some of these signs:

1. Systemic reduction of muscle tension, as evidenced by softening of the tissue contours or broadening and flattening of body segments.
2. General consistency and resting level of tone. How fluid does the tissue appear as you move it?
3. Taut, visible bands in resting muscle. A muscle that has a visibly well-defined anatomical form when it is not in use is probably hypertonic.
4. Hyperemia. A **reactive hyperemia** may accompany the application of this technique.
5. If you are using petrissage to treat edema (proximal to the edema) or fibrosed edema (on-site), note the following signs of resorption of fluid from edematous tissue: changes in surface contours, reduction in size or hardness of edema, and changes in the viscosity and inertial resistance of the subcutaneous tissues.
6. The depth of the penetration of the stroke. As the client's muscles relax and the fluid viscosity of the tissues decreases, the same force will produce effects deeper into the client's tissues. Consequently, you do not always require greater force to achieve a greater penetration of effects; instead, simply the appropriate application of the technique for longer periods is required.

# COMMUNICATION WITH THE CLIENT: FOR ALL FORMS OF PETRISSAGE

Communicate to ensure the client's comfort during the application of the technique. Here are some examples of statements that you can use.

1. "Is this pressure okay?" "Would you like it deeper?" "Would you like less pressure?" "Which feels better, this

(adjust depth) or this?" Ensure that the depth of technique is comfortable for the client.

2. "Is it tender here?" "When I work here, do you feel it anywhere else?" In cases in which the client examination suggests that there is elevated muscle resting tension, slowly increase the depth of application of the technique while inquiring about tenderness and possible **referral** of pain.

## A Practice Sequence for Petrissage

First, attempt each technique individually until you are confident about the basics of the manual technique and body movement. You can then apply the following basic sequence, initially allowing 15 to 20 minutes for any region. You can adapt the same sequence, with minor variations, for all regions.

1. Apply a small amount of lubricant to the client's body using superficial effleurage.
2. Begin by applying **wringing** proximally on the region, and then move distally.
3. Once you reach the most distal part of the region, either apply wringing on the way back up or return with superficial effleurage.
4. Using a similar pattern, which begins proximally and proceeds distally, introduce in turn:
   - Muscle squeezing
   - Picking-up
   - Broad-contact kneading
   - Specific kneading

Whenever possible, maximize **centripetal** pressure. At the end, finish with wringing and then superficial effleurage. Regional modifications:

- Back: You can designate proximal and distal as being at either end of the client's back.
- Abdomen: Where possible, for example with effleurage and kneading, apply the techniques in a generally clockwise direction and sequence.
- Face: Use light pressure and no lubricant. You can apply most of the techniques as described with slight adaptations. Use only two fingers or finger and thumb for "smaller" versions of wringing, picking-up, and squeezing where you can lift the tissues. Fingertip kneading is the most useful technique.
- Hands and feet: You can address many small muscles, ends of tendons, and fascial sheaths individually with excellent results. As with the face, the amplitude of the techniques is smaller. You can, however, use considerable amounts of pressure because of the density of connective tissue in these regions.

## Critical Thinking Question

How would you apply and sequence the massage techniques described up to this point in the text in order to increase superficial **venous** and **lymphatic return**, deep venous and lymphatic return, and **arterial supply**?

# Petrissage: Further Study and Practice

## NAMES AND ORIGINS

Petrissage (from the French *petrir*, to knead)[3,6] is one of two techniques that are predominantly used in **classical** or **Swedish massage** (the other is effleurage). It is indispensable when the clinician is treating muscle. In other texts, the technique that we call petrissage is sometimes known as "kneading."[1-8] The term petrissage was formerly used to refer to techniques that repetitively grasp, lift, shear, and release muscle tissue between the hands (see sections on wringing, muscle squeezing, and picking-up earlier in this chapter). Other texts also defined related techniques that

repetitively compress, shear, and release muscle against underlying muscle and bone separately as "kneading," although sometimes these definitions were reversed. It is common now for both lifting and compressive forms of these techniques to be grouped under the single term of petrissage,[1,2,6-8] although slightly differing usages persist (one recent text drops the French term entirely[3]).

Authors generally agree that petrissage, in either **lifting** or **kneading** forms, repetitively compresses and releases muscle. Some authors,[3] however, follow **Kellogg's** usage[13] and classify other techniques that compress and release muscle as forms of "**friction**." We prefer to reserve the term friction for a precise, specific technique directed toward connective tissue (see Chapter 10, Connective Tissue Techniques).

Contemporary authors' opinions differ as to how much skin **glide** should occur when applying compressive or kneading forms of this technique.[2,6–8] Varying the amount of glide, rate, and pressure produces many varieties of petrissage that intergrade. Slowing the rate of application and using less lubricant will increase the amount of drag, or sustained horizontal force, that results and may produce greater effects on connective tissue.

A regrettable drawback of a lot of massage research is that researchers often give the most cursory descriptions of the **interventions** that they performed. Although this is changing, the word "petrissage" does not often show up in methodological descriptions, although it is often the predominant technique of classical (Swedish) massage and sometimes the only technique that is used. For this text, in situations in which the techniques performed in the intervention were not specifically mentioned or were characterized broadly as "massage," "standard massage," "Swedish massage," or "classical massage," we have assumed that clinicians have used petrissage (which, in our view, includes "deep effleurage" and "kneading") directed toward skeletal muscle. As a result, the discussion of the research base for petrissage and the list of related outcomes are larger for this technique than those for the other massage techniques. Note that some of the following discussion may be applicable to other techniques, especially the other **neuromuscular techniques** described in this chapter.

# OUTCOMES AND EVIDENCE

Much of the recent research on massage focuses on the **psychoneuroimmunological** effects of classical massage. Nevertheless, petrissage may also have physical effects on musculoskeletal, cardiopulmonary, and neurological systems and function. In addition, it may also affect **pain**, athletic performance, and specific clinical conditions. Finally, the effects of petrissage on circulation and reflex effects on visceral function are less certain. Table 9-1 summarizes the main outcomes for petrissage.

## Psychoneuroimmunological Effects

### Mood

Classical massage may reduce **anxiety** (measured by state-trait questionnaires and salivary **cortisol** levels), reduce stress, and improve relaxation.[33–43] Researchers have observed this anxiolytic effect in a wide variety of clinical settings and clinical conditions. In addition, petrissage may be useful in alleviating the behavioral symptoms of depression,[35,39,41,43–45] hyperactivity,[46] and other conditions with affective components.[38,42,46,47] Furthermore, the positive effects of petrissage on rehabilitation and mood have been consistently demonstrated in other contexts.[33–45,48–57]

### Immune Function

Several studies have shown improved immune function and positively altered allergic responses following the application of petrissage.[58–61]

## Musculoskeletal Effects

### Muscle Resting Tension

One cannot separate the effect of petrissage on the level of resting muscle tension from its psychological effects.[62] Anxiety has a well-documented generalized effect of increasing the level of resting tension of skeletal muscle.[63–65] As a result, interventions that reduce anxiety may have indirect effects on level of resting tension. Furthermore, some authors state that petrissage can reduce the level of muscle resting tension in the area to which clinicians apply it as a result of mechanical stress on proprioceptors.[1,3,5,6] Other researchers are equivocal about this effect or do not mention it at all.[2,7]

### Range of Motion

Research notes that increases in joint range of motion may occur after the application of petrissage[48,66,67] (with one dissent[68]).

### Position Sense

One recent study notes an increase in **joint position sense** after massage that included petrissage.[69]

### Tissue Extensibility

Texts[1,3,6,7] and research studies[49,50,70] list increased extensibility and mobility of connective tissue as effects of petrissage. Increased extensibility may be responsible for the ability of perineal massage to reduce the incidence of tears during labour.[70–75] However, it is unlikely that petrissage will lengthen connective tissue to the same degree as connective tissue techniques, which apply more sustained tensional load or drag (see Chapter 10, Connective Tissue Techniques).

## Neurological Effects

### Tone

Research suggests that petrissage decreases **motoneuron excitability** but only during the application of the technique.[76-83] This may be of limited clinical usefulness,[32,84] except when treating patterns of abnormal movement and abnormal neuromuscular tone (**spasticity**) that are associated with lesions of the brain or spinal cord.[78]

## Cardiovascular and Pulmonary Effects

### Pulmonary Function

The observed positive effects of petrissage on pulmonary conditions, such as asthma, chronic obstructive pulmonary disease (COPD), and cystic fibrosis, may be a result of the combined effects of decreased anxiety and increased **chest wall mobility**.[85-87]

### Circulation and Visceral Function

Although most texts state that petrissage increases venous return,[2,3,6,7] research suggests otherwise. This technique may have marginal effects on blood chemistry and local blood flow.[88-90] Furthermore, its effect on regional and systemic flow are likely to be both small and transient.[91-96] Consistent with the finding of a marginal effect of petrissage on blood flow is the observation that "**sports massage**" (including petrissage) does not always increase the rate of removal of **lactate** from muscle after exercise above the rate for passive rest.[97-102] Some research suggests that petrissage may have cardiac effects.[103,104] A more likely effect is an increase in lymphatic return. Most studies documenting this effect have, however, used repetitive compressive techniques produced by machines.[105-108] This may be the mechanism that explains the reduction of edema, which is a possible effect when the technique is applied proximal to the edema and around the periphery of swelling (if tolerable).

Finally, foreign studies intriguingly suggest that clinicians can use classical massage (including petrissage) to achieve reflex effects on circulation and visceral function that are absent in the English literature.[104,109-117]

## Multisystem Effects

### Pain

Clients who received petrissage reported a significant reduction in their perception of pain during labor,[118-120] after surgery,[121] with cancer,[122,123] with migraine,[124] and with chronic orthopedic conditions.[67,125-127] Petrissage may also be of value in the reduction of low back pain.[128,129] To date, the mechanisms of the analgesia that might result from the application of petrissage are not fully understood. Current theories include the **gating** of pain impulses, increased **serotonin** levels, improved **restorative sleep**, and reduction of **substance P**.[17,127,130,131]

### Athletic Performance

Although massage has experienced much recent popularity among athletes, recent reviews are generally skeptical about its ability to enhance many types of function in a sports context.[132-134] For example, research has not shown that petrissage before athletic activity can greatly enhance performance[135-137]; its effects on **delayed-onset muscle soreness** are equivocal[138-143]; and postperformance reports on repair of damage and recovery of function are mixed.[101,102,144-152] Conversely, reports on mood and perception of fatigue after exercise are more positive.[101,148,149,153]

## Use in Multimodal Interventions

Petrissage has been used in conjunction with a variety of other techniques in multimodal interventions for clinical conditions such as headaches, **trigger point syndromes**, low back pain, **fibromyalgia**, and emphysema.[51-57,129] In these situations, the positive effects of petrissage appear to be enhanced in programs that include the use of **modalities** and client participation.[52,56,129]

---

### EXAMINING THE EVIDENCE

The following elegant study[76] is unusual on a couple of counts: it studies petrissage alone, and it tests the mechanism by which petrissage reduces the **H-reflex**, which is a measure of spinal reflex excitability. Researchers monitored neurologically normal subjects (who acted as their own controls) at rest, during the application of petrissage, and during the application of petrissage with their skin anaesthetized. Reporting of the interrupted repeated-measures study protocol was very detailed and included a precise description of massage technique. The H-reflex was lower during petrissage, whether or not the skin was anaesthetized, compared with the level during rest periods. This suggests that deep mechanoreceptors, not superficial ones, mediate the inhibitory effect of petrissage on the H-reflex. We suggest that this finding may have clinical significance for treatment of spasm. However, researchers would have to repeat the protocol with subjects with spasm to test this hypothesis. Additionally, clinical significance may be limited because the H-reflex returned to normal as soon as massage stopped.

Morelli M, Chapman CE, Sullivan SJ. Do cutaneous receptors contribute to the changes in the amplitude of the H-reflex during massage? *Electromyogr Clin Neurophysiol.* 1999;39:441–447.

# CAUTIONS AND CONTRAINDICATIONS

Clinicians need clinical training and supervised practice to master the proper application of petrissage. Advanced training may be advisable when dealing with pathological conditions. All of the general and local contraindications noted for massage techniques apply to the use of petrissage (see Chapter 3, Clinical Decision Making for Massage). In addition, there are several specific contraindications to the application of petrissage: clients with hemophilia, local sites of acute inflammation and infection, confirmed or suspected thrombus,[117] thrombophlebitis, and potentially metastatic malignancy. Clinicians must conduct a careful examination and moderate the pressure with which they apply petrissage for clients who have confirmed or suspected osteoporosis, who have wounds in the early stages of healing, or who are taking anticoagulants. Furthermore, clinicians must exercise care when treating areas of **spasm**, **hypotonia**, and **active trigger points**. The use of excessive pressure may damage delicate terminal lymphatics, although this damage may facilitate the drainage of edema.[154] Finally, difficulties may arise with the application of any massage techniques to clients who have profound learning disabilities or dementia.[155,156]

# USING PETRISSAGE IN TREATMENT

## Psychosocial Stress

Clinicians can use petrissage by itself or in combination with other techniques in general massage to address the effects of psychosocial **stress**. It is often effective for relaxation when clinicians apply it slowly and rhythmically, gradually building up to short periods of higher pressure, which they alternate with periods of less pressure. In situations in which the client presents with a generalized elevation of resting muscle tension because of stress, clinicians can use moist heat and **diaphragmatic breathing** or **progressive relaxation** as adjuncts to petrissage.

## Orthopedic Injuries

Local application of petrissage is useful for treating orthopedic injuries in the subacute and chronic states. Depending on the severity and stage of the injury, clinicians can complement this technique with **superficial fluid techniques**, other neuromuscular techniques, **connective tissue techniques**, and **passive movement techniques**. Furthermore, petrissage is an excellent prelude to passive stretching, **proprioceptive neuromuscular facilitation** techniques, and **joint mobilization**.

## Postintervention Self-Care Instructions

1. Extensive deep petrissage may occasionally produce mild local soreness during a 24- to 48-hour period after treatment. A warm bath, a warm Epsom salts bath, or the application of moist heat may reduce this soreness.
2. Pain of increasing severity, persistent postintervention pain, or pain that arises in adjacent areas following treatment may indicate activation of a **latent** or **satellite trigger point** (see later sections in this chapter) or the generalized **reactive tightening** of antagonist muscle groups. Always instruct clients to contact you when more than mild, transient pain results from any massage intervention.
3. Depending on the clinical situation, use therapeutic exercise, **self-mobilization** techniques, diaphragmatic breathing, or progressive relaxation exercises.
4. You can teach clients self-massage of accessible areas.
5. Family members can be taught to perform basic petrissage and the cautions involved in applying this within a home program.[87]

# Stripping: Foundations

## DEFINITION

Stripping: A very slow and specific gliding technique that therapists apply from one attachment of a muscle to the other for the purpose of reducing the activity of myofascial trigger points. A trigger point is a hyperirritable area in skeletal muscle that is associated with a hypersensitive and palpable nodule located in a taut band. The area is painful on compression and can give rise to a variety of symptoms such as referred pain, referred tenderness, motor dysfunction, and autonomic phenomena.[1–8,157]

## USES

Therapists use stripping to reduce the activity, pain, and other symptoms of trigger points and to help restore the length and strength of the affected muscle.[157]

## PALPATION PRACTICE

The following muscles often harbor **latent trigger points**: upper trapezius, sternocleidomastoid, erector spinae, pectoralis minor, extensor digitorum, opponens pollicis, gluteus medius, the hamstrings, and tibialis anterior.

| Table 9-2 | Types of Trigger Points[145] |
|---|---|
| **Trigger Point Type** | **Description** |
| Active | Produces pain in a characteristic pattern at rest |
| Latent | Produces pain in a characteristic pattern only when palpated |
| Primary | Arises in response to trauma or acute or chronic overload |
| Key | Is responsible for activating (and inactivating) satellites |
| Satellite | Is activated by a key trigger point, by being in its area of referral, or by being its antagonist or synergist |
| Central | Is located near the center of muscle fibers |
| Attachment | Is located in a muscle's tendon or aponeurosis |

1. Review the attachments and fiber direction for these muscles.
2. Palpate some of the trigger point areas. Begin lightly, using digital contact, and work slowly across the fibers. Can you find a **taut band**? Taut bands run parallel to the muscle fiber direction, are often visible, and are often clearly palpable. The area will feel "hard," "hypertonic," "tight," "wiry," or "ropy." Do you notice any **twitch responses**?
3. Have an instructor confirm the taut bands that you find.

### Theory in Practice

#### Stripping

**Patient Profile**

Your patient is a 30-year-old male who is in good physical condition. He complains of persistent right "shoulder joint pain" when playing recreational football (quarterback), especially when he throws the ball. The pain began 2 years ago, during a long game when he passed the ball more than usual. His doctor has ruled out arthritis of the cervical spine and glenohumeral joints

**Clinical Findings**

Subjective:
Every time the patient plays football, the same pain reappears after several throws. He feels it deep in his right shoulder and over the entire deltoid. The pain increases in intensity with activity until it limits the force of his throwing and the length of time he is able to play. For a day after playing, his shoulder is stiff, sore, and bothers him if he sleeps on it.

Objective:
- Posture: His right shoulder appears internally rotated. His right scapula is further from the spine than his left scapula.
- Gait: His gait is normal.
- Range of Motion: Right active internal rotation is limited by 15 degrees. Other active and passive shoulder motions are within normal limits.
- Strength: Isometric resisted external rotation is weaker than the left.
- Palpation: Light and moderate palpation of the affected rotator cuff muscles produce local tenderness but no familiar referral. The upper fibers of the infraspinatus are extremely tender to *deep* palpation, and two points reproduce the patient's familiar "joint pain" that he associates with passing the ball.

**Treatment Approach**

At the time of the initial injury, the trigger points in the infraspinatus were overloaded during passing by the concentric wind-up and the eccentric contraction required to control the release. They are also reactivated each subsequent game.

The main initial outcomes are:
- To reduce the activity of the key trigger points in infraspinatus
- To restore full pain-free range of internal and external rotation
- To reduce and balance resting tension throughout the affected rotator cuff and shoulder girdle

With the patient in prone, warm up his upper back and shoulders for 10 minutes with broad-contact compression and the broad forms of petrissage and kneading. Then methodically strip the right infraspinatus, increasing the pressure as tolerated with each pass, until the patient reports no referral or tenderness. Stretch the infraspinatus passively while preventing the scapula from winging. Apply regional broad-contact petrissage for several minutes. Apply a hot pack to the area. Perform similar general, broad-contact neuromuscular techniques on the other shoulder for several minutes. Turn the patient supine, and have him perform *full* active movement of his affected shoulder. Finish with 5 to 10 minutes of general neck work.

You may have to repeat this basic intervention once or twice, with additional specific work for the synergists and antagonists of infraspinatus such as teres minor, the deltoids, subscapularis, and pectoralis major. Show the patient how to use heat and how to stretch infraspinatus properly (which requires preventing the scapula from winging). You may also show him how to perform self-massage of the infraspinatus using a small hard ball such as a squash ball or golf ball.

# Stripping: Technique

## MANUAL TECHNIQUE

Figures 9-45 to 9-52 show clinicians applying stripping to the various regions of the body. The order of the figures is from head to foot in supine and then in prone. Each figure illustrates most of the guidelines for manual technique outlined in this section. The manual technique presented largely follows Simons, Travell, and Simons.[157]

1. Place the client in a position that will comfortably allow full stretch of the target muscle. The target muscle should be neither slack nor tautly stretched.
2. If lubricant is not already present, apply a small amount (a drop or two) either to your hands or to the client's skin.
3. **Reinforce** your fingers or thumbs whenever possible by placing your hands together (Figures 9-46, 9-48, and 9-50) or using your fingers as a group, rather than individually (Figures 9-47 and 9-52). Whenever possible, use pushing strokes because they place less stress on the muscles of your hands, are easier to control than pulling strokes, and allow you to use more force when you need it (Figures 9-45 to 9-52). When stripping larger or deeper muscles, using your elbow as the contact surface allows you to use body weight to increase pressure (Figures 9-49 and 9-51). Your selected hand and body positions must be stable.
4. Beginning on one side of the trigger point, apply enough pressure to engage the taut band. Then, in one

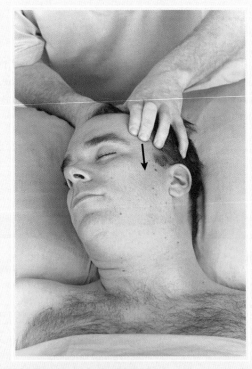

**Figure 9-45** Fingertip stripping of the temporalis muscle, a common contributor to temporal headaches.

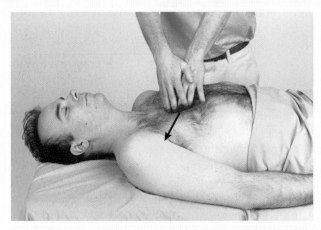

**Figure 9-46** Reinforced fingertip stripping of the sternal head of pectoralis major muscle in a cross body position. If the client finds the pulling of hair uncomfortable, the practitioner can add more lubricant or break the longer stroke into a series of shorter strokes, which follow the same line, at a comparable rate.

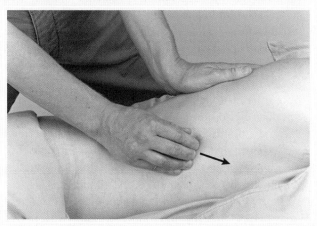

**Figure 9-47** This stroke—very much like stripping except in its orientation to the intercostal muscle fibers—follows the intercostal spaces and will improve chest wall mobility.

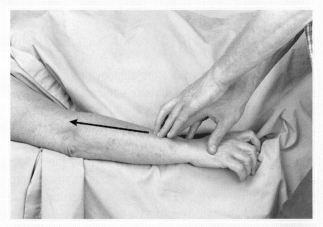

**Figure 9-48** Stripping of extensor digitorum with reinforced fingertips.

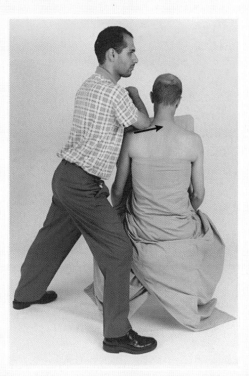

**Figure 9-49** The upper trapezius muscle, the most common cause of myofascial pain felt in the temple, is best addressed with the client seated. The client maintains an upright seated posture and pushes with his feet against the floor for support.

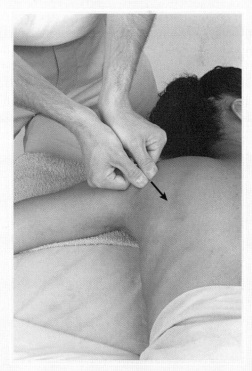

**Figure 9-50** Stripping the infraspinatus muscle. With this contact, the thumbs are doubly reinforced against each other and against the flexed index fingers.

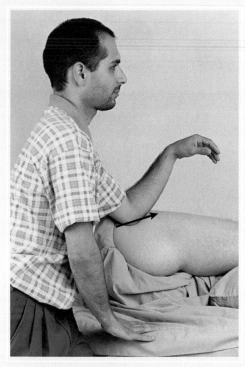

Figure 9-51 The elbow, a side-lying position, and considerable pressure may be needed when stripping the gluteus medius or minimus muscles. When trigger points are located near the iliac attachment (as with most gluteus medius trigger points), a superior-to-inferior path of application avoids pinching superficial tissue against the iliac crest.

continuous motion, glide slowly and with equal pressure along the band, across the trigger point, and all the way to the attachment of the muscle.[157,158] The next stroke glides in the opposite direction, across the trigger point, and toward the other attachment. If the taut band softens and the tenderness and pain referral diminish, you

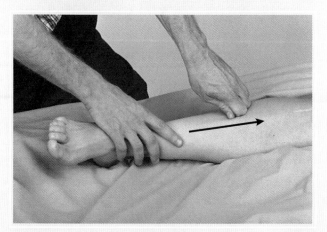

Figure 9-52 Stripping the tibialis anterior muscle with the knuckles. In addition to its effects on trigger point activity, stripping will likely lengthen the anterior fascial wall of the anterior compartment.

can repeat this procedure again with the same pressure. Alternatively, increase the pressure incrementally with each application of the technique.

5. The suggested rate of glide in the literature is 8 mm/second[158] or slowly enough to allow the nodule in the taut band to palpably release or soften beneath the advancing finger(s).[157] In either case, the rate of glide is much slower than that of standard petrissage.

6. You must maintain flawless control over the depth and pressure of this technique. During the initial pass along the taut band, you may find it necessary to reduce pressure quickly and smoothly as your contact surface passes over the trigger point so that you maintain a level of pressure that the client can tolerate.

7. Do not persist with the application of this technique if the taut band and referral are unchanged after two or three passes. Lack of response to treatment means that the trigger point may respond better to another technique or that the trigger point is a **satellite** and you need to treat the **key trigger point**.

8. Follow successful deactivation of a trigger point, as shown by an absence of pain referral on compression, right away with careful passive stretch for 30 seconds or more. Then, as soon as possible, ask the client to perform careful active movement through the full range of motion in order to produce an isotonic contraction of the muscle you have treated.[157] If it is not possible to have the client perform active movement while he is on the treatment table, then he should perform it at the end of the intervention. Finally, apply moist heat for several minutes.

9. When you treat several trigger points in an area, it may help to precede and follow stripping with petrissage and superficial effleurage. You can use a regional approach for a **myotactic unit** with multiple trigger points, especially if these trigger points are chronic or highly symptomatic.

## *How stripping might work*

An integrated hypothesis for the etiology of trigger points suggests that dysfunction at motor endplates causes sustained depolarization of the postsynaptic membrane, continuous release of calcium from the sarcoplasmic reticulum, and sustained shortening of sarcomeres in the region of the trigger point.[126,157,159] In addition, locally reduced blood flood and hypoxia sensitize nociceptors to produce the characteristic pain referrals.[157] Furthermore, two studies have shown that repeated deep massage of **fibrositic nodules** (trigger points) causes them to release myoglobin.[126,159] Simons and Travell support this theory by suggesting that the shortened sarcomeres of a trigger point "contrac-

| Box 9-7 | **Components of Stripping** |

**Contact:** Reinforced finger(s) and/or thumb(s), proximal interphalangeal joints (knuckles), olecranon process

**Pressure:** Light to heavy. Pressure varies with the muscle layer engaged and the sensitivity of that layer. The range of pressure can range from (A) scarcely more than the weight of the hand, when stripping a taut band harboring an active trigger point in a superficial muscle, to (B) controlled upper body weight reinforced with pressure from the legs, when stripping deep hamstring fibers.

**Tissues engaged:** Muscle and related fascia

**Direction:** Along or parallel to fibers

**Amplitude:** Length of muscle

**Rate:** Very slow. **Travell** and **Simons**[158] give the rate as 0.8 cm/second, or slow enough to obtain a palpable release[157]

**Duration:** 10 seconds to several minutes

**Intergrades with:** Specific petrissage and direct fascial technique

**Context:** Follow inactivation of a trigger point with passive stretch for 30 seconds and then with active range of motion to produce an isotonic contraction of the involved muscle. With severe or longstanding trigger points or those in deeper muscles, it is advantageous to apply regional **petrissage** before and after stripping.

tion knot" may be more susceptible to rupture by the pressure of a technique like stripping. They propose that the therapist's application of massage results in cell rupture. Following this rupture, the cell spills myoglobin, which probably destroys the involved neuromuscular junction as a functional structure, thus effectively terminating the contracture and associated energy crisis. As the technique eliminates more and more contraction knots within a nodule, the client will experience an increasing relief of symptoms.[157] Finally, stripping along the length of the muscle may apply a lengthening tension that restores the normal length of the sarcomere, the taut band, and the muscle as a whole.[157]

# THERAPIST'S POSITION AND MOVEMENT

1. Your posture must be very stable, especially when stripping an active trigger point, since inadvertent small deviations in pressure may produce large increases in pain referral from the trigger point. Figures 9-49 and 9-51 show two variations of a standing **controlled lean** that allow the therapist to transfer his body weight to the client in a controlled manner. Whatever position you choose, you must remain in perfect control of pressure, especially high pressure, at all times.[160]

2. Slight shifts in the direction of pressure can make a critical difference in whether you can access a trigger point. For example, stripping of iliocostalis lumborum trigger points may yield no increase in referred pain (or therapeutic effect) when you apply the pressure in a strictly anterior direction. On the other hand, a large increase in referred pain may occur when you direct the same amount of pressure along the same taut band in an anteromedial direction (see Figure 9-59).

# PALPATE

As you perform the technique, palpate the client's tissues for the following:

1. Taut bands. The direction of muscle fibers and the referral pattern will enable you to identify the involved muscle. The taut band will often show approximately even levels of tension along its length. Therefore, the therapist must develop an ability to identify layers of equal tension during palpation.
2. Local hardness. The trigger point itself may present as a very small area of local hardness (palpable nodule) in the taut band.
3. Twitch responses. You can palpate twitch responses in superficial muscles.
4. Jump sign. A client may produce a large involuntary contraction and other gross affective signs of pain when you palpate the trigger point.
5. Generalized hardness. If there are adjacent trigger points in overlapping layers as, for example, often occur between the scapulae, you may find it difficult to palpate anything other than a generalized hardness.
6. Softening of tissues. Softening of taut bands and regional hardness should occur with continued application of the technique.

As with petrissage, you also palpate for:

7. Tissue resistance. General resistance or resilience of soft tissues.

8. Tissue mobility. Mobility of the interfaces between muscles and muscle layers.
9. Signs of inflammation. Fibrosis, adhesions, and indurations within and between muscle layers, which are associated with chronic inflammation.

## OBSERVE

As you perform the technique, observe the client for signs of trigger point activity. The signs listed below may indicate trigger point activity or a positive response to treatment.

1. Taut bands in superficial muscles are often easily visible.
2. Twitch responses are transient events (1/4 second) that are often more easily seen than felt. They may occasionally appear as a "flutter" that cascades into adjacent muscles.
3. Softening of the contour of the taut band with continued application of the technique. Sometimes the contour of an entire muscle will soften and, more rarely, relaxation of the muscles throughout an entire region occurs as the activity of one trigger point diminishes.

As with petrissage, you may also observe:

4. Systemic reduction of muscle tension, as evidenced by softening of the tissue contours or broadening and flattening of body segments.
5. General consistency and resting level of tone.
6. Local hyperemia. A reactive hyperemia (caused by release of substance P)[161] may accompany the application of this technique.

## COMMUNICATION WITH THE CLIENT

Communicate to ensure the client's comfort during the application of the technique. Here are some examples of statements that you can use.

1. "As I pass over the trigger point, you may notice that it intensifies the pain you've been feeling in your. . . ." Explain to the client what a trigger point is, what pain referral means, and that his symptoms may be temporarily reproduced or intensified as you pass over the trigger point. It is very important for the client to understand that the discomfort of the technique has a therapeutic purpose.
2. "The pressure may feel somewhat uncomfortable, but it shouldn't be really painful. It should be tolerable. Tell me if at any time the discomfort is too great." Ensure that the pressure you apply is tolerable to the client. Although client discomfort is acceptable, outright pain is counterproductive. Recheck the client's tolerance with every increase in pressure. Obvious pain behavior indicates that you must reduce pressure. In addition, you can explain the use of a 10-point pain scale and ask that the client not let the pain of stripping exceed level 4. If the resting pain of an active trigger point already exceeds level 4, then the application of the technique should not increase the client's pain more than a point and should only do so if the client shows no obvious pain behavior and clearly agrees to the procedure.
3. "Does this bring back the exact pattern of pain you've been feeling in your . . . ?" When you locate a trigger point, you may pause over it briefly and allow the client to compare the pattern of pain referral of the trigger point with the presenting symptoms.

---

 **A Practice Sequence for Stripping**

Allow at least 30 minutes per person.
   Many people have latent trigger points in the fibers of the upper and middle trapezius and the rhomboids. If your client does not happen to have these, you can still practice stripping in this regional exercise.
   Before you start, assess the range and ease of motion of glenohumeral and scapular movements.

**Prone**
1. Apply a small amount of oil to the client's back, using superficial effleurage.
2. Perform regional petrissage to all of the muscles of the upper back and posterior shoulder girdle using a sequence similar to that described in the box titled "A Practice Sequence for Petrissage." Begin with broad-contact techniques that cover a wide area, and gradually proceed to more localized techniques such as fingertip kneading. Gradually progress deeper.

3. During this part of the massage, observe closely for muscles that appear to contain hard taut bands, twitch responses, and spots that are tender or produce pain referrals.
4. If you think you have found a trigger point, confirm this using palpation.
5. Progressively strip all of the fibers of the trapezius muscle, being attentive to the fiber directions. The muscle should be slightly stretched but not taut during this procedure. To strip the upper trapezius effectively in prone, you will have to sit at the head of the table and apply substantial, reinforced pressure in a caudal direction.
6. Periodically intersperse stripping with broader strokes like palmar kneading or picking-up.
7. On any active or latent trigger points, strip the taut band in alternating directions until the client's level of sensitivity decreases.

8. Repeat Steps 5 and 6, focusing on the rhomboids. You will have to use marginally more pressure for this. The fiber direction and the pain referral patterns will help you identify which layer you are on.
9. Conclude with regional petrissage and then superficial effleurage.
10. Get feedback on how your client feels. If your client has begun to experience a temporal headache, you have likely activated a latent trigger point in the upper trapezius muscle. In this case, return to Step 5. If your client has begun to experience a supraorbital headache, then the sternocleidomastoid is implicated and needs more treatment.
11. Reassess range and ease of movement of the scapular movements.

Many people also have latent trigger points in the pectoral muscles on the anterior surface. How would you adapt this sequence to address those?

# Stripping: Further Study and Practice

## NAMES AND ORIGINS

In other texts and massage-related systems, the technique that we call stripping is called "stripping massage," "deep stroking," "deep stroking massage," and "muscle stripping."[157] Travell and Simons first coined the term stripping massage.[158] Technically, it is related to specific petrissage (see previous sections in this chapter), because it involves the compression and release of muscle fibers, and to direct fascial technique (see Chapter 10, Connective Tissue Techniques), because of the slow rate of glide. In this text, we consider it separately because of its well-defined method and excellent effect on trigger point activity.

As defined by Chaitow[162] and others, "neuromuscular therapy" or "neuromuscular technique" is a complex system of techniques that includes, among other techniques, finger and thumb strokes that resemble stripping, which we defined earlier.

"Strumming" or "cross-fiber stripping" is a form of direct fascial technique that is directed along[163] or, more often, across[157,163] muscle fibers. This may sometimes resemble stripping and may have effects on trigger point activity.

## OUTCOMES AND EVIDENCE

A myofascial trigger point is a hyperirritable area in skeletal muscle that is associated with a hypersensitive and palpable nodule located in a taut band. The area is painful on compression and can give rise to a variety of symptoms such as referred pain, referred tenderness, motor dysfunction, and autonomic phenomena.[157] A trigger point has a characteristic response to palpation: a local twitch response of the taut muscle fibers and referred pain in a specific pattern for that muscle, which occurs or increases on direct compression of the trigger point.[157,158,163] There are two questions to answer when categorizing trigger points: 1) Is the trigger point active or latent? and 2) Is the trigger point primary (key) or a satellite? An active trigger point in a muscle will refer pain whether the muscle is working or at rest, can weaken a muscle, and can prevent it from lengthening fully. By contrast, a latent trigger point is painful only when you palpate it. The application of specific compression to a latent trigger point will evoke the characteristic pain referral pattern for that trigger point. A muscle containing a latent trigger point can also be shortened and weakened. Primary trigger points arise in response to trauma, acute and chronic overload (**tendinopathies** and **repetitive strain injuries**), **postural imbalance**, fatigue, and emotional stress. These trigger points are exacerbated by a variety of factors.[157,163] Satellite trigger points may develop in response to altered biomechanics, in the pain referral area of a primary trigger point, or in the synergist and antagonist muscle groups of the muscle that contains the primary trigger point.[157] Finally, key trigger points are responsible for activating satellites. Consequently, inactivation of a key trigger point will inactivate its associated satellites.[157]

Trigger points may also occur in connective tissue, such as fascia, ligaments, and periosteum, and produce a variety of symptoms.[157,163] Trigger points located in muscle are frequently the cause or the consequence of common musculoskeletal complaints such as tension headache, temporomandibular joint problems, spinal pain, chronic low back pain, disk herniation, chronic pelvic pain, painful rib syndrome, nonarticular pain, and other myofascial pain syndromes.[162–175] In addition, trigger points in muscle can cause **nerve entrapments**[157,164] and may also mimic nerve entrapments, radiculopathies, and visceral pathology.[157,164,175]

Clinicians can use stripping to reduce the activity, pain, and other symptoms of trigger points and to help restore the length and strength of the affected muscle.[157] It can be the preferred manual technique when trigger points are located near the center of a muscle. Since stripping applies similar forces to the same tissue layer as petrissage, stripping may have many of the effects of petrissage when clinicians systematically apply it to a region (see earlier sections in this chapter). Stripping may also share some effects with direct fascial technique (see Chapter 10, Connective Tissue Techniques). Table 9-1 summarizes the main outcomes for stripping.

### Critical Thinking Question

Describe the characteristics of trigger points. How do the treatment techniques for myofascial pain developed by Travell and Simons differ from traditional petrissage and broad-contact compression techniques?

### EXAMINING THE EVIDENCE

There are no clinical trials in the recent literature for stripping or for equivalent techniques such as "deep stroking" or "deep tissue massage." One case report[176] documents the use of **Active Release®** techniques for the treatment of shoulder pain, reduced range, and weakness in a client 2 years after surgical repair of a Bankart lesion. The Active Release system combines soft tissue techniques similar to stripping, as described earlier in this chapter, with active and passive movement into specific protocols for particular muscles. In this case, researchers provided "treatment directed to the muscles of the rotator cuff, with an emphasis on the subscapularis" twice a week for 2 weeks. The client's function, as measured by BIODEX isokinetic testing of shoulder rotation, improved significantly. This otherwise quite thorough case report contains no description of the protocols used for treatment, and it is probable that these are not readily available except by taking Active Release workshops. This begs the question: Can we assess evidence properly when critical information is withheld from the public domain?

Buchberger DJ. Use of Active Release techniques in the postoperative shoulder: a case report. *J Sports Chiropr Rehabil.* 1999; 13:60–66.

## CAUTIONS AND CONTRAINDICATIONS

Clinicians need clinical training and supervised practice to master the proper application of stripping. Advanced training may be advisable when dealing with pathological conditions. All of the general and local contraindications noted for massage techniques apply to the use of stripping (see Chapter 3, Clinical Decision Making for Massage).[1] Specific contraindications to the use of stripping include clients with hemophilia, local sites of acute inflammation and infection, confirmed or suspected thrombus,[117] thrombophlebitis, and potentially metastatic malignancies. Clinicians who are treating clients who have confirmed or suspected osteoporosis, who have wounds in early stages of healing, or who use anticoagulants may choose to use a noncompressive manual method of inactivating trigger points, such as the combination of ice and stretching.[157] In addition, clinicians should use care when treating muscles that are adjacent to areas of spasm or acute inflammation.

Simons, Travell, and Simons[157] state that clinicians must locate trigger points using palpation. Conversely, research suggests that clinicians may not reliably locate latent trigger points using palpation.[177] Consequently, clinicians must make every effort to locate the points with precision. In addition, because trigger points can cause entrapments[157,164] and may mimic entrapments, radiculopathies, and visceral pathology,[157,164,173] clinicians must take particular care with their differential examination and promptly refer the client to his physician if they suspect a more serious clinical condition.

Active trigger points can cause excruciating, debilitating pain and can be exquisitely sensitive to touch. In these cases, it is particularly important for clinicians to apply stripping with absolute respect for the client's pain tolerance. With long-standing or recurrent trigger points, clinicians must be careful to treat agonist, antagonist, and synergist muscle groups. They should also address the factors that may perpetuate the trigger points, such as structural asymmetry and repetitive ergonomic loading.[157,162,164,178] If an active trigger point remains after the correct application of treatment techniques, this may indicate that the trigger point is actually a satellite and that clinicians must treat the key trigger point first. Extensive application of massage techniques to one muscle or muscle group around a joint may cause **reactive tightening** (reactive cramping) in the antagonist or synergist muscle groups or on the opposite side during, or soon after, the intervention.[157] Postintervention pain, which differs markedly from the client's presenting symptoms, is often a result of the activation of a latent or satellite trigger point and may indicate a need for clinicians to treat the client's synergist and antagonist muscle groups more comprehensively.

# USING STRIPPING IN TREATMENT

## Trigger Points

There are several modalities that clinicians can use in a complementary manner to decrease trigger point activity. When treating acute trauma, apply cold packs to assist resolution of the acute inflammation, regardless of the effect that this has on the trigger points.[157] Once the clinically acute stage has passed, the following massage techniques may also be useful.

1. Petrissage
2. Specific compression (trigger point pressure release)[157,164]
3. **Connective tissue techniques** such as **skin rolling**,[157] **myofascial release**,[157,164] and **direct fascial technique**

Clinicians can also use the following related techniques to treat trigger points effectively.[157,164]

1. Sustained gentle passive stretch (required after trigger point inactivation)
2. Active range of motion to produce an isotonic contraction of the affected muscle (required after trigger point inactivation)
3. **Postisometric relaxation**
4. Contract-relax, hold-relax, and related muscle energy techniques
5. Moist heat application
6. Ice (or vapocoolant spray) and simultaneous passive stretch. Readers are referred to *Myofascial Pain and Dysfunction*[157] for the necessary comprehensive instructions.
7. **Therapeutic ultrasound**
8. High-voltage **galvanic stimulation**
9. **Transcutaneous electrical nerve stimulation**. While this is not a specific intervention for trigger points, it may provide temporary relief of pain.

A multidisciplinary approach to treatment that includes appropriate medical management is most effective for the treatment of myofascial pain syndromes and trigger points.[16,157,158] Clinicians can instruct clients in many of the aforementioned complementary modalities for home use. Of particular importance are:

1. Correct self-stretch techniques and postisometric relaxation
2. Gentle active range of motion through the full range of motion to produce an isotonic contraction of the affected muscle
3. Moist heat application to the trigger point (not the area of referral)
4. How to apply stripping in accessible areas, as appropriate
5. Ergonomic education related to posture or repetitive activity

## Specific Compression: Foundations

### DEFINITION

Specific compression: A nongliding technique that therapists apply with a specific contact surface to muscle, tendon, or connective tissue. Therapists apply compression and release in a direction that is perpendicular to the target tissue, and they often sustain the compression.

### USES

Specific compression is an effective manual technique for reducing the activity and symptoms of **myofascial trigger points**. It may also be a means of inhibiting the tone of the related muscle for a short time in conditions such as spasticity. In addition, it may be effective in softening adhesions and fibrosis in muscle, tendon, and fascia when therapists apply it in a slow and sustained manner. Finally, foot **reflexology**[3,5–7,178–180] and **Eastern-influenced massage systems**[181–184] use specific compression to influence pain and physiological function at sites that are remote from application of the technique. Table 9-1 summarizes the main outcomes for specific compression.

 **Critical Thinking Question**
    What are the similarities and differences between how therapists use specific compression in reflexology and acupressure?

### PALPATION PRACTICE

1. Begin by reviewing locations of some common trigger points.
2. With your instructor's help, locate one or more taut bands.
3. With fingers or thumbs, strip along the taut band very slowly. Look for twitch responses and/or jump signs.
4. Try to locate a trigger point precisely. The trigger point itself is not always distinctly palpable. You can identify it as a taut band, by local tenderness, by a twitch response or jump sign, and by the production of referred pain. Can you elicit a clear referral pattern? If not, then increase the pressure carefully and try again. When you find a trigger point, have your client give as clear a description of the pain referral as possible. Match the description with points shown in a larger text like *Myofascial Pain and Dysfunction.*[157]
5. Alternatively, you may try grasping and squeezing the taut band between your finger and thumb ("pincer palpation"). This method works well with muscles that are easy to pick up, like the sternocleidomastoid. Using a pincer grip on the upper trapezius requires considerable hand strength to elicit referral.
6. Passively stretch any muscle in which you found a trigger point for 30 seconds.

## Specific Compression: Technique

### MANUAL TECHNIQUE

Figures 9-53 to 9-60 show clinicians applying specific compression to the various regions of the body. The order of the figures is from head to foot in supine and then in prone. Each figure illustrates most of the guidelines for manual technique outlined in this section.

For all applications of specific compression:

1. The contact you choose depends on the relative size of the therapist and the client, the area to be treated, and the hardness of the tissue. It is important to choose a contact surface that fits the local "topography" of the client's body easily. Your thumb and fingers are better suited to working smaller muscles such as those in the rotator cuff, neck, and calves, and you should reinforce them as needed (Figures 9-53A and 9-53B, 9-54, 9-55, and 9-58). Your elbow is a good contact when the client's tissues are very hard and on larger muscles of the back, legs, and pelvis. This contact allows a greater use of upper body weight to sustain pressure and thus minimizes therapist fatigue (Figures 9-56 and 9-57). You may also use wooden or plastic tools (T-bars) that you grip in your hand. Figure 9-61 shows two of these tools.

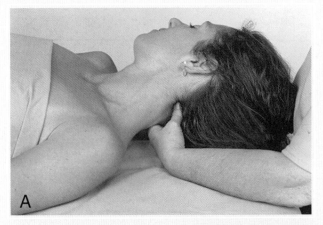

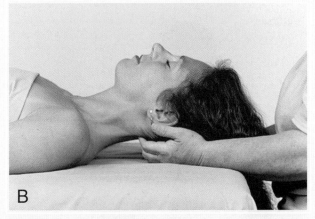

**Figure 9-53** Digital compression of occipital attachments is an effective nonspecific technique for tension headaches and neck tension. This can be done (A) using the thumb with the neck rotated or (B) on lined-up fingertips with the neck in neutral.

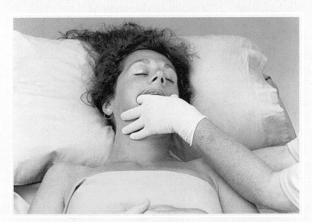

**Figure 9-54** The lateral pterygoid muscle may be implicated in temporomandibular joint dysfunction. Intraoral specific compression of this muscle demands excellent communication skills and great sensitivity of execution.

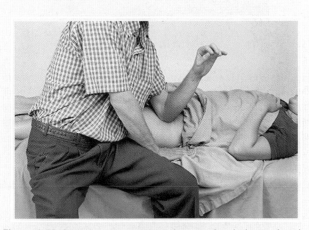

**Figure 9-56** Specific compression of tensor fascia lata using the elbow in a seated controlled lean.

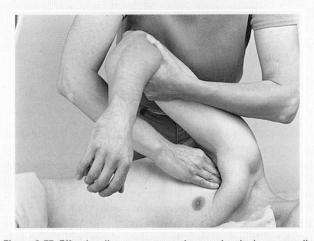

**Figure 9-55** Effective direct access to trigger points in the pectoralis minor muscle: slide under pectoralis major muscle, across the ribs, toward either the coracoid process or rib attachment. The approach must often be very slow because of tenderness. Your other hand stabilizes the arm (and scapula) laterally. You can also perform this technique with the client in supine.

2. Your chosen contact must be stable, and you must exercise exquisite control of both the direction and depth of pressure of application. For this reason, the client's skin must be free of excess lubricant to reduce slipping of your hands.

3. Apply pressure slowly, increase it gradually to the desired depth, sustain it evenly, and then release it gradually. The duration of compression will vary with the application from a few seconds to more than a minute.

When using specific compression to perform a trigger point pressure release:[157]

4. The pressure you apply must be enough to reproduce or marginally increase the referred pain from the trigger point, while remaining tolerable for the client. This amount of pressure will vary from being light, in the case of a highly active trigger point in a superficial

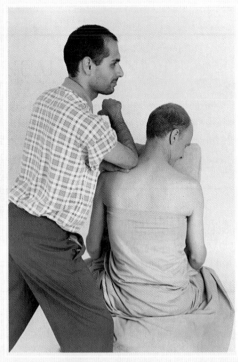

**Figure 9-57** While applying specific compression with the elbow to the upper trapezius muscle, ask the client to adjust the head position to obtain the strongest pain referral. The therapist is using his left hand to stabilize the point of contact and to palpate for softening of the taut band.

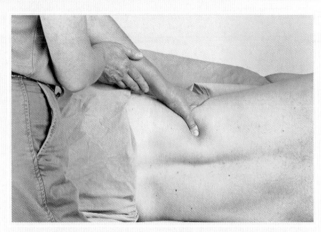

**Figure 9-59** Angle of approach is often important when applying specific compression to trigger points. Here the therapist directs pressure anteromedially onto the iliocostalis lumborum muscle. A single thumb and light pressure may be adequate to accentuate pain referral from an active trigger point; reinforced thumbs or an elbow and some body weight might be required to elicit pain referral from latent trigger points.

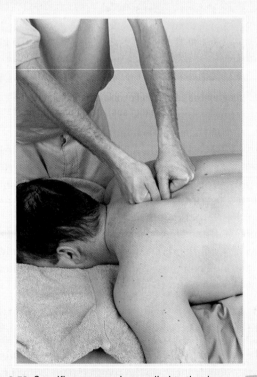

**Figure 9-58** Specific compression applied to the rhomboids/mid trapezius muscle area with reinforced double-thumb contact.

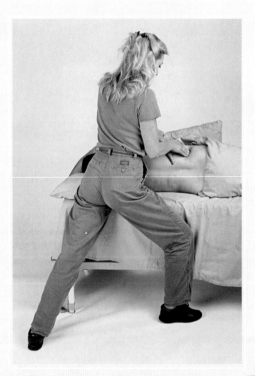

**Figure 9-60** The lateral edge of the quadratus lumborum is accessible to specific compression in side-lying only with correct positioning. The client's ipsilateral arm is fully abducted, and the ipsilateral leg has been passively stretched downward, to open space at the waist. Doubled thumbs, reinforced fingers, or even the tip of the elbow can be used. Take care to avoid the poorly supported 11th and 12th (floating) ribs.

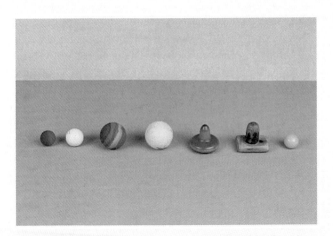

**Figure 9-61** Devices that can assist with self-administration of specific compression of trigger points include balls of various sizes and densities and wooden or plastic massage tools.

muscle, to being heavy, in a less active trigger point in a deep muscle such as the piriformis.

5. Once you have established a tolerable initial depth/pressure in consultation with the client, there are two approaches to progressing the specific compression of a trigger point.

*Progression using verbal client feedback:* This approach relies on frequent client feedback, and we recommend it for novice therapists. Maintain the compression at the initial depth of application until the referred pain subsides. For example: "Until you no longer feel pain, just the pressure of my thumb." Then increase the depth of application of the compression to a new level that reproduces a tolerable level of pain referral. Maintain the pressure of compression at that depth until the referral subsides, then repeat the application of the technique as needed. Gradually increase the depth of application in a series of stepwise increments, until the client reports that tenderness and pain referral have disappeared.

*Progression using feedback from palpation:* Alternatively, you can maintain the pressure of application at a constant level and exclusively use the barrier-release phenomenon to achieve the continuous increase of depth. As the trigger point releases and the tissues soften, the depth of penetration will gradually increase until the client reports that the referred pain has disappeared. This approach requires that you accurately feel the presence of the tissue barrier to compression and then sense and follow the release of the barrier into the client's tissue. This approach requires more refined palpation skills than the first method.[157]

In the verbal feedback or palpatory feedback methods of progression, it may be more practical for you to wait until the client reports that the pain referral has diminished substantially, rather than waiting for it to disappear completely. When you apply them correctly, both methods can provide clients with a demonstration of a correct and comfortable pressure of application that they can use at home.

6. There are differing opinions about how long to sustain specific compression of a trigger point, with lengths from 10 seconds to more than 1 minute.[157,164,185–187] For less experienced therapists, and especially when treating chronic or highly irritable trigger points, we recommend shorter, more frequent compressions that are sustained from 15 to 30 seconds and are interspersed with the application of petrissage, stripping, passive stretch, and other manual methods. This minimizes the possibility of overtreating the target muscle, activating latent satellites in synergist and antagonist muscle groups, or producing a biomechanical imbalance. Therapists with higher levels of manual skill can use their judgment on the degree to which they extend the period in which they apply compression.

7. It is not always easy to maintain specific compression on the precise spot that reproduces the client's pain referral, even when you have not applied lubricant. Consequently, you must determine whether a client's report of diminished pain referral reflects reduced trigger point activity or the movement of your contact off the trigger point. Stripping or stretching techniques may be better manual approaches for the treatment of "slippery" trigger points.

8. Following deactivation of the trigger point, perform a passive stretch of the treated muscle for 30 seconds. As soon as possible after passive stretching, ask the client to perform active range of motion carefully through the available range to produce an isotonic contraction of the affected muscle. Apply moist heat for several minutes.

9. When treating several trigger points within an area, you may find it useful to precede and follow specific compression with petrissage and superficial effleurage. Use a regional approach for a myotactic unit that has multiple trigger points, particularly if these trigger points are chronic or highly symptomatic.

## *How specific compression might work*

Ischemic compression may reduce the activity of trigger points through the same mechanism as stripping (see the discussion of stripping earlier in this chapter). This involves

---

**Box 9-8**     **Components of Specific Compression**

**Contact:** Reinforced fingers or thumbs, reinforced proximal interphalangeal joints, olecranon process

**Pressure:** Light to heavy

**Engages:** Muscle and/or connective tissue

**Direction:** Perpendicular to the target tissue layer. This is often, but not always, perpendicular to the surface of the body. Slight shifts in direction may facilitate access of individual trigger points

**Amplitude/length:** N/A

**Rate:** 5 to 30 seconds or more per compression

**Duration:** 5 minutes or more for a series of compressions applied to a muscle belly or region Intergrades with: Broad-contact compression, specific petrissage, stripping

**Context:** Follow inactivation of a trigger point with passive stretch for 30 seconds and then an active range of motion to produce an isotonic contraction of the involved muscle. If clinicians apply this technique repetitively in a small area or to a deep muscle, they should apply regional petrissage before and after their application of the technique. They should also follow specific compression, which they are using to inhibit abnormal neuromuscular tone, with the desired movement or functional activity. Boxes 9-9 and 9-10 describe contexts for **reflexology** and **acupressure**.

---

rupturing the shortened sarcomeres in the trigger point and destroying the dysfunctional neuromuscular junction, thereby terminating the trigger point and its symptoms.[157] It is important to follow specific compression for trigger points with a full passive stretch of the involved muscle to restore the normal length of the sarcomere, the taut band, and the muscle as a whole.[157] The mechanisms by which specific compression might produce reflex effects and effects distant to the site of its application are less clear and are discussed at length in Boxes 9-9 and 9-10 later in this chapter.

## THERAPIST'S POSITION AND MOVEMENT

1. The posture you select must be stable, comfortable, and sustainable.
2. The basic positions are described in Chapter 6, Preparation and Positioning for Massage, in the sections on lunge and lean (Figure 9-60), standing **controlled lean** (Figure 9-57),

and seated controlled lean (Figure 9-56). These positions allow controlled, sustained use of your upper body weight to increase pressure. Note that you should not use the client's body as a support when using these controlled leaning positions. Instead, incline your body toward the client in a controlled manner, and apply precisely the desired amount of upper body weight to the contact surface without becoming destabilized or unbalanced.

3. When you use your elbow as a contact (Figures 9-56 and 9-57), assess the degree of release that has occurred by gauging how the client's compressed tissue deforms under your upper body weight.

## PALPATE

As you perform the technique, palpate the client's tissues for the following:

1. Taut bands. The fiber direction and the pain referral pattern will enable you to identify the involved muscle.
2. Local hardness. The trigger point itself may present as a very small area of local hardness (palpable nodule) in the taut band. Apply compression slowly to this nodule until you reach the barrier to further compression.
3. Twitch responses. You can palpate twitch responses in superficial muscles.
4. Jump sign. A client may produce a large involuntary contraction and other gross affective signs of pain if you palpate the trigger point too forcefully.
5. Generalized hardness. If there are adjacent trigger points in overlapping layers as, for example, often occurs between the scapulae, you may find it difficult to palpate anything other than a generalized hardness.
6. As you sustain the pressure of application at the tissue barrier, the palpable nodule or contraction knot associated with the trigger point will soften or release. You may follow this release into the tissue without increasing the pressure of application.
7. Signs of inflammation. Fibrosis, adhesions, and indurations within and between muscle layers are associated with chronic inflammation.

## OBSERVE

As you perform the technique, observe the client for signs of trigger point activity. The signs listed below may indicate trigger point activity or a positive response to treatment.

1. Taut bands in superficial muscles are often easily visible.
2. Twitch responses are transient events ($\frac{1}{4}$ second) that are often more easily seen than felt. They may occa-

sionally appear as a "flutter" that cascades into adjacent muscles.
3. Softening of the contour of the taut band with continued application of the technique. Sometimes the contour of an entire muscle will soften and, more rarely, relaxation of the muscles throughout an entire region can occur as the activity of the key trigger point and its satellites diminishes.

As with petrissage, you also observe:

4. Systemic reduction of muscle tension, as evidenced by softening of the tissue contours or broadening and flattening of body segments
5. General consistency and resting tension of muscle
6. Local hyperemia. A reactive hyperemia may accompany the application of this technique.

# COMMUNICATION WITH THE CLIENT

Communicate to ensure the client's comfort during the application of the technique. Here are some examples of statements that you can use.

1. "As I compress the trigger point, you may notice that it intensifies the pain you've been feeling in your. . . ." Explain to the client what a trigger point is, what pain referral means, and that his symptoms may be temporarily reproduced or intensified as you pass over the trigger point. It is very important for the client to understand that the discomfort of the technique has a therapeutic purpose.
2. "The pressure may feel somewhat uncomfortable, but it shouldn't be really painful. It should be tolerable. Tell me if, at any time, the discomfort is too great." Ensure that the client can tolerate the pressure that you apply. Although client discomfort is acceptable, outright pain is counterproductive. Recheck the client's tolerance with every increase in pressure. Obvious pain behavior indicates that you must reduce pressure. In addition, you can explain the use of a 10-point **pain scale** and ask that the client not let the pain of stripping exceed level 4. If the resting pain of an active trigger point already exceeds level 4, then your application of the technique should not increase the client's pain by more than a point and should only do so if the client shows no obvious pain behavior and clearly agrees to the procedure.

3. "Does this bring back the exact pattern of pain you've been feeling in your . . . ?" When you locate a trigger point, you may pause to allow the client to compare the pattern of pain referral of the trigger point with her presenting symptoms.
4. "Let me know when the pain is gone and you can only feel the pressure of my thumb." Instruct the client to report when the pain referral disappears and she only feels the sensation of pressure.

---

 **A Practice Sequence for Specific Compression of Trigger Points (Trigger Point Pressure Release[157])**

Allow 30 to 40 minutes.
The following practice sequence begins like the sequence for stripping but substitutes specific compression for stripping at the point in the sequence when the trigger points are treated.

This sequence is for the hamstrings (another fairly common place to find latent trigger points) with the aim of performing the sequence with only one change of the client's position. Before you start, assess the length and strength of the client's hamstrings and consider how to perform the sequence with the minimum number of changes of position for the client.

1. Apply effleurage beginning "superficial" and progressing to "deep."
2. Apply regional petrissage to the posterior thigh with increasing depth and specificity.
3. Using palpation, search for and confirm the presence of trigger points.
4. Place the target muscle on a slight stretch and apply specific compression for 10 to 30 seconds.
5. Stretch the muscle passively for 30 seconds.
6. Repeat Steps 4 and 5 until the referral declines or disappears and the full length of the muscle is restored.
7. Apply regional petrissage that includes the antagonist and synergist muscle groups.
8. Repeat Steps 3 to 7 on other trigger points. Do not do more than three or four repetitions unless you also do a few minutes of broad-contact petrissage on the lower back, gluteals, and calves. Why do you have to do this?
9. Finish with petrissage and superficial effleurage.
10. You must treat the other leg for an equal time. Why is this?

Retest. Get feedback on how your client feels.

## Specific Compression: Further Study and Practice

# NAMES AND ORIGINS

In other texts and massage-related systems, the technique that we call specific compression is called "focal compression," "ischemic compression," "digital compression," "digital pressure," "sustained digital pressure," "direct pressure," "direct inhibitory pressure," "direct static pressure," "static friction," and "deep touch."[1–3,5–8,157,158,163] Along with static contact, specific compression is probably the most widespread of all massage techniques. It is either used alone or as a component of more elaborate methods and systems including: **positional release**,[185] **myotherapy**,[186,187] **trigger point pressure release**,[157] **Neuromuscular Technique**,[162] **Shiatsu**,[181,182] **acupressure**,[183,184] and **reflexology**.[1–3,6,7] Specific compression has been applied with a bewildering variety of rationales and names.

# OUTCOMES AND EVIDENCE

## Musculoskeletal Effects

Specific compression can be an effective manual technique for reducing the activity and symptoms of myofascial trigger points, especially for thin muscles that overlie bone.[157,158,164] For detailed definitions and descriptions relating to trigger points, see the preceding section on stripping or Table 9-2. During a "manual trigger point pressure release,"[157] clinicians apply specific compression to the trigger point itself (not to the area of referral) and follow it with passive stretch and active movement. Because clinicians can use it to reduce the activity of trigger points, specific compression has wide applicability when treating the effects of a variety of conditions. These conditions include: trauma; acute and chronic overload such as tendinopathies and repetitive strain injuries; postural imbalance; fatigue; emotional stress; common musculoskeletal complaints such as tension headache, temporomandibular joint problems, spinal pain, chronic low back pain, disk herniation, chronic pelvic pain, painful rib syndrome, and nonarticular pain; and other myofascial pain syndromes.[157,158,164–175,188] Our clinical observations suggest that specific compression may also be effective in softening adhesions and fibrosis in muscle, tendon, and fascia when clinicians apply it in a slow and sustained manner.

## Neurological Effects

Specific compression can also be used as a proprioceptive stimulation technique.[190–194] In addition, clinicians can also apply firm and moderate specific compression (inhibitory pressure) to tendons as a means of inhibiting the tone of the related muscle for a short time.[190] Furthermore, intermittent or sustained application of specific compression to tendons, but not muscle, will also cause a reduction of motor neuron excitability (H-reflex) but only during the application of the stimulus.[191–194] This application of specific compression for the purpose of inhibiting muscle contraction has been integrated into many therapeutic techniques that seek to facilitate movement in conditions associated with abnormal neuromuscular tone such as **spasticity**.

## Other Effects

Finally, foot reflexology[1–3,5–7,179,180,195] and Eastern-influenced massage systems[181–184] use specific compression extensively to influence pain and physiological function at sites that are remote from application of the technique. These systems suggest that the effects of treatment occur through postulated complex somatovisceral reflexes. Table 9-1 summarizes the main outcomes for specific compression.

### EXAMINING THE EVIDENCE

A recent **randomized clinical trial** with controls and a placebo, or **sham**, treatment examined the effects of foot **reflexology** on the symptoms of multiple sclerosis.[195] Once a week for 11 weeks, subjects (n = 53) received either 45 minutes of "full reflexology treatment" with calf massage or the placebo treatment of 45 minutes of "nonspecific calf massage." Significant improvement in paresthesias, urinary symptoms, and spasticity occurred in the reflexology group, and the improvement in paresthesia remained significant 3 months after treatment. The placebo that the researchers selected seems to be a reasonable control for **nonspecific treatment effects**. Unfortunately, the researchers only describe the treatment and placebo protocols very briefly in a single sentence. This raises questions such as: Were the two treatments applied with comparable pressure? The researchers sought to reduce the confounding variable of the skill of the clinicians by having each clinician treat one client in the treatment group and one in the control group. For the most part, this study is thoughtful and convincing.

Siev-Ner I, Gamus D, Lerner-Geva L, Achiron A. Reflexology treatment relieves symptoms of multiple sclerosis: a randomized controlled study. *Mult Scler*. 2003:9:356–361.

# CAUTIONS AND CONTRAINDICATIONS

Clinicians need clinical training and supervised practice to master the proper application of specific compression. Advanced training may be advisable when dealing with pathological conditions. As with other compressive neuromuscular techniques, all contraindications for massage techniques apply. (See Chapter 3, Clinical Decision Making for Massage, for a detailed discussion of contraindications.) Specific contraindications to the use of specific compression include clients with hemophilia; local sites of acute inflammation and infection; and confirmed or suspected thrombus, thrombophlebitis, and malignancy. Specific compression can be very useful when clinicians apply it on site in the subacute stage of trauma, provided that edema has resolved. In this situation, clinicians must reduce the force of application and ensure that the technique does not cause the client pain. Clinicians should not perform sustained specific compression directly over superficial nerves, such as the radial or common peroneal nerves, because a compression **neurapraxia** can result.[196] Further cautions to the application of specific compression are osteoporosis, early-stage wounds, anticoagulant therapy, and areas of spasm and hypotonia.[1,2,6,7]

Table 9-3 lists common errors when treating trigger points with specific compression. When clinicians use specific compression to treat trigger points, they must apply this technique with absolute regard for the client's pain tolerance

### Table 9-3 Common Errors When Treating Trigger Points with Specific Compression

| Error | Result |
|---|---|
| Pressure is applied too quickly | Client terminates technique Autonomic nervous system/sympathetic response |
| Pressure exceeds client's pain tolerance | Client terminates technique Autonomic nervous system/sympathetic response |
| Pressure is not maintained on the trigger point (sliding off) | No change in symptoms |
| Insufficient depth achieved | No change in symptoms |
| Too few repetitions of compression | No change in symptoms |
| Sustained accurate pressure does not diminish referral | Try a different trigger point |
| Passive stretch omitted | Recurrence of same trigger point symptoms |
| Perpetuating factors not addressed | Recurrence of same trigger point symptoms |
| Satellite and secondary trigger points not addressed | New symptoms appear |

and accompany the application of the technique with careful communication. In the case of long-standing or recurrent trigger points, clinicians can minimize the likelihood of recurrence of the trigger points by treating agonist, antagonist, and synergist muscle groups and addressing perpetuating factors such as structural asymmetry and repetitive ergonomic loading.[157,158,163,164] Postintervention pain that differs markedly from the client's presenting symptoms is most often due to the activation of a latent or satellite trigger point and indicates a need to address synergists and antagonists further.[157] Clinicians should be aware that specific compression may produce remote reflex effects that are out of proportion to the size of the area they treat and the force they apply.[7,162]

### ❓ Critical Thinking Question

What is the relationship between myofascial trigger points and the tender points of **fibromyalgia**?

# USING SPECIFIC COMPRESSION IN TREATMENT

## Trigger points

There are several modalities that the clinician can use in a complementary manner to decrease trigger point activity. When treating acute trauma, apply cold packs to assist resolution of the acute inflammation, regardless of the effect that this has on the trigger points.[157] Once the clinically **acute stage** has passed, the following massage techniques may also be useful.

1. Petrissage
2. Stripping[157,163]
3. Connective tissue techniques such as skin rolling,[157] myofascial release,[157,163] and direct fascial technique

The clinician can also use the following related techniques to treat trigger points effectively.[157,163]

1. Sustained gentle passive stretch (required after trigger point inactivation)
2. Active range of motion to produce an isotonic contraction of the affected muscle (required after trigger point inactivation)
3. Postisometric relaxation
4. Contract-relax, hold-relax, and related muscle energy techniques
5. Moist heat application
6. Ice (or vapocoolant spray) and simultaneous passive stretch. Readers should refer to *Myofascial Pain and Dysfunction*[157] for comprehensive instructions.
7. Therapeutic ultrasound
8. High-voltage galvanic stimulation
9. Transcutaneous electrical nerve stimulation. Although this is not a specific intervention for trigger points, it may provide temporary relief of pain.

A multidisciplinary approach to treatment that includes appropriate medical management is most effective for the treatment of myofascial pain syndromes and trigger points.[157,158,163,178] Clinicians can instruct the client in many of the aforementioned complementary modalities for home use. Of particular importance in the management of trigger points are:

1. Correct self-stretch techniques and postisometric relaxation
2. Gentle active range of motion through the full range of motion to produce an isotonic contraction of the affected muscle
3. Moist heat application to the trigger point (not the area of referral)

4. Self-administration of specific compression. Use balls of varying sizes and hardness or hand-held massage devices to demonstrate this (Figure 9-61). Clients must understand basic trigger point concepts prior to performing self-management programs. Advise clients not to repeat compression more than two to three times; to precede the application of compression with some preparation of the muscle, such as superficial stroking; and to follow the application of pressure with an isotonic contraction of the muscle and the appropriate stretching exercise. Above all, advise clients not to compress the same trigger point for minutes at a time even though it may feel good and afford temporary symptomatic relief.

5. An example of a conservative and effective self-management program for a single trigger point that produced significant decreases in trigger point sensitivity and perceived pain levels and increased frequency of self-care in adults with chronic myofascial neck pain follows.[275] This program has five primary components that clients perform once a day. The first is gentle superficial stroking of the muscle in which the trigger point occurs for 2 to 3 minutes. The second is the application of specific compression to the location of the trigger point with a hand-held massage device for 15 to 60 seconds. The third is gentle isotonic contraction of the affected muscle for five repetitions. The fourth is stretching of the affected muscle for two repetitions of 30 seconds. The fifth is gentle superficial stroking and kneading of the affected muscle for 2 to 3 minutes. In addition, the client may use the application of moist heat to the site of the trigger point as an adjunct to this self-management program.

6. Ergonomic education related to posture or repetitive activity

## Motor Control

When clinicians are using specific compression as a proprioceptive stimulation technique, there are several complementary techniques that are available for inhibiting or stimulating neuromuscular tone and facilitating movement responses.

1. Clinicians can apply prolonged cold, neutral warmth, and slow **superficial stroking** locally or over the posterior primary rami to inhibit neuromuscular tone and facilitate movement responses (see Chapter 7, Superficial Reflex Techniques).[190]

2. Clinicians can use **fine vibration**, joint approximation and traction, light brushing, and **static contact** ("maintained touch") with both light and firm contacts to increase neuromuscular tone and facilitate move-ment responses (see Chapter 7, Superficial Reflex Techniques).[190]

## Box 9-9 Reflex Effects of Specific Compression: Foot Reflexology

Foot reflexology is based on the premise that specific points on the feet (and hands) are reflexly related to other body segments or organs of the body (Figure 9-62).[2,3,6,7,179,180] In reflexology, pain, tenderness, or soft tissue hardening in particular areas of the foot is thought to reflect acute or chronic dysfunction of the related body segment or organ. On this basis, specific compression is applied to the reflex points on the foot to normalize function in the corresponding body segments or organs by "restoring lost balance" or "activating the movement of energy."[2]

The mechanisms for the effects of reflexology are unknown. Research and review on the subject are not common and often appear in untranslated European journals.[197–215] Results and opinions on the methods and effects of reflexology are not always positive,[207–213] but some research does support the possibility of specific effects on organ function.[199,201,205,214,215] Specific positive outcomes have been noted for infant colic,[216] multiple sclerosis,[195] and nausea and vomiting.[217] More general outcomes that may result from the application of foot reflexology include: reduced anxiety; increased relaxation; and improved mood, energy, and quality of life.[2,3,6,197,218,219,220] Foot reflexology is logistically simple to perform and requires no oil, towels, or significant disrobing of the client. Contraindications and cautions to the application of reflexology are relatively few. They are mostly local contraindications such as gout, peripheral vascular disease, and contagious or infectious foot conditions.[3] In addition, clinicians may have to shorten interventions for weak, convalescent, or elderly clients. A full intervention that consists only of the application of foot reflexology may take from 30 to 60 minutes. Alternatively, clinicians may use foot reflexology for 5 or 10 minutes to precede or follow a massage sequence that addresses another area of the body.

Following the client examination, a typical intervention might proceed in the following manner. After a brief foot bath, clinicians position clients comfortably in sitting or lying. Clinicians apply general, broad neuromuscular techniques such as wringing, compression, and passive joint movements of the ankles, metatarsals, and toes for several minutes.[2,6] Beginning with the toes and proceeding proximally,[6] clinicians apply specific compression systematically and thoroughly to all surfaces of the foot, using a slow, stable rhythm. Clinicians usually use their thumbs or knuckles for the plantar surface of the foot and their fingers for the dorsal surface.[2,3] They sustain pressure for several seconds on each point and can prolong it for an additional 15 to 30 seconds if a point is tender or hard.[3] The pressure is usually deep, but as with any massage technique, clinicians should moderate the pressure of application so that it feels pleasant or causes mild discomfort, as opposed to pain.[3] Clinicians can also use a short gliding stroke, similar to stripping or direct fascial technique.[2,3,6] More detailed descriptions of the technique of foot reflexology are offered in books that address this subject exclusively.[179,180]

## CLINICAL SIGNIFICANCE

At the very least, reflexology provides a method for performing a thorough foot massage with associated general benefits.[33,197] Clinicians who perform extended specific compression on the feet or hands should be mindful of its possible effects. Applying this type of massage technique on the client's feet or hands can produce systemic effects, which are far greater than the area of the feet or hands that they are treating might suggest. This occurs because altering patterns of tension and tenderness in the feet and hands may affect physiological processes elsewhere in the body.

(*Continued*)

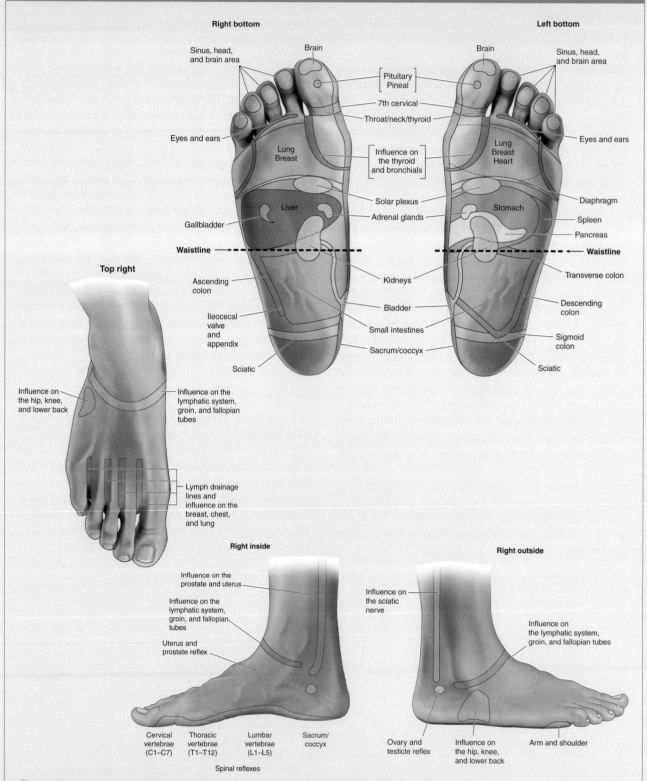

**Figure 9-62** Maps showing reflex areas of the bottom, top, and sides of the foot that correspond to distant body segments or organs. (From Williams, A. Spa Bodywork. Philadelphia, PA: Lippincott Williams & Wilkins: 2007: 159–160. Reprinted by permission of the publisher Lippincott Williams & Wilkins.)

Box 9-10 | **Reflex Effects of Specific Compression: Meridian Theory and Acupoints**

Traditional Chinese medicine is an ancient, vast, and sophisticated system of philosophy, clinical theory, and practice that has come to the attention of the West in recent decades primarily because of the evidence for the analgesic effects of **acupuncture**.[2,3,6,7,221,222] Fundamental to the system of Chinese medicine are several interrelated concepts that have no parallel concepts in Western medicine. In Chinese medicine, energy (qi, chi, ch'i) circulates through the body in well-defined cycles through conduits or channels called meridians.[2,223] There are 12 bilateral paired meridians and two median sagittal meridians.[1,2,222] Each meridian is associated with an "organ," for which it is named, and has associated physiological functions that do not correspond exactly to organ functions as defined in Western medicine. Each meridian also has a basic quality of energy that is characterized as being yin or yang.[1,2,223] Yin energy, metaphorically described as "female" and "negative," is ascending and is associated with hollow organs such as the stomach. Yang energy, metaphorically characterized as "male" and "positive," is descending and is associated with solid organs such as the liver.[1,2,223] Health is conceptualized as a dynamic balance between yin and yang energy flowing in precise diurnal patterns through the various meridians.[2,223] Pathways of the meridians do not consistently correspond to any material anatomical structure, although they sometimes follow intermuscular depressions and paths of major nerves.[2,7]

Strung along each meridian, at depths ranging from immediately below the surface up to 1 inch (2.5 cm) deep, are dozens of small points, or **acupoints**, which have lower electrical resistance and higher overlying skin temperature and show altered sensitivity during states of imbalance or disease (Figure 9-63).[2,223] While the position of most acupoints coincides with locations of nerves, trigger points, or motor points,[2,7] there is debate as to how these various entities might correspond to each other.[185,224,225] Acupoints can be activated by a variety of precise approaches to achieve remote effects on the meridian, its associated organ, and related physiological processes.[2,223] Each meridian has several points of unusual clinical importance including activating points, soothing points, and stabilizing points.[2,185,223] Activating and soothing points stimulate and sedate, respectively, the meridian and its related organ and functions. Stabilizing points link the functions of one meridian with those of others. Finally, a variety of other points show sensitivity or tenderness when there is a dysfunction in the related meridian.

Methods of stimulating acupoints include: needling (acupuncture), massage, electrical current, laser, and moxibustion.[7] Manual systems that stimulate acupoints, such as acupressure and Shiatsu, rely extensively on deep, sustained specific compression on the points themselves and may include small nongliding circular movements, tapping, and stretching.[181–184] Recent research suggests a variety of clinical effects of stimulation of acupoints with pressure. Most evidence suggests that sustained specific compression on individual acupoints (the pericardium-6 point, located in the middle of the ventral wrist crease) is an effective intervention for nausea, gagging, and vomiting associated with surgery, chemotherapy, pregnancy, or motion sickness[226–250] (with several dissents[251–254]). Acupressure may also be useful for anxiety,[255] various types of pain[256–261] (though possibly not postsurgical pain[251]), sleep disorders,[262–266] constipation,[267,268] COPD,[269,270] women's reproductive disorders,[271–273] and in palliative care.[274] Interventions aimed at restoring the harmonious flow of energy in the presence of imbalance or disease often involve the stimulation of multiple acupoints and the use of other interventions and complex diagnostic procedures. Acupuncture, acupressure, and related modalities rely on elaborate, sophisticated, and radically different conceptual **models** of body processes than those used in Western medicine. *Understanding the rationale of how to stimulate acupoints requires extensive study of these conceptual models* and is beyond the scope of this book. The interested reader can consult comprehensive texts.[221,222]

## CLINICAL SIGNIFICANCE

Clinicians who use specific compression extensively to treat trigger points should be aware of the following issues. Remote analgesic effects from specific compression may arise in patterns that do not always correspond to those suggested by trigger points. This may occur because clinicians are treating an acupoint, rather than a trigger point. In addition, patterns of pain and tension in the musculature, especially if they are recurrent, may reflect remote physiological and pathological processes. Always apply specific compression within the client's pain tolerance and expect a palpable tissue response to the application of the technique to occur quickly. Clinicians should avoid applying the technique if the client's tissues are extremely sensitive and should not persist with application if it fails to produce a quickly palpable tissue change. If the application of specific compression causes symptoms to abate for a short period followed by a recurrence of the symptoms, clinicians should identify the underlying causes of the symptoms before reapplying the technique.

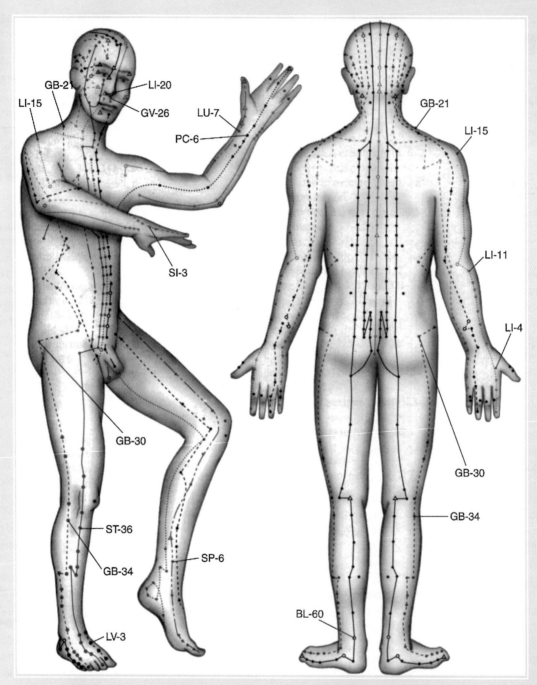

**Figure 9-63** A map showing meridians with acupoints strung along it. (From Tappan FM, Benjamin PJ. *Tappan's Handbook of Healing Massage Techniques.* 3rd ed. Upper Saddle River, NJ: Prentice-Hall, Inc.; 1998. Copyright 1998. Reprinted by permission of Prentice-Hall, Inc.)

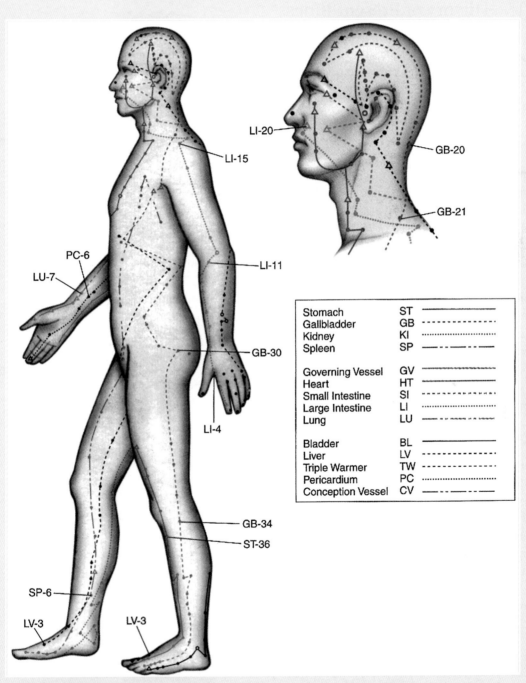

| Stomach | ST | ———————— |
| Gallbladder | GB | ------------ |
| Kidney | KI | ············ |
| Spleen | SP | —·—·—·—· |
| | | |
| Governing Vessel | GV | ———————— |
| Heart | HT | ———————— |
| Small Intestine | SI | —————————— |
| Large Intestine | LI | ············ |
| Lung | LU | ———————— |
| | | |
| Bladder | BL | ———————— |
| Liver | LV | ------------ |
| Triple Warmer | TW | ------------ |
| Pericardium | PC | ············ |
| Conception Vessel | CV | —·—·—·— |

**Figure 9-63** (*Continued*)

## History of Present Illness

A 40-year-old woman with a high-risk pregnancy who has been hospitalized at 28 weeks of gestation for evaluation and modification of pharmacologic management of premature onset of labor. Prior to hospitalization, she was bed bound for 6 weeks. Medication: terbutaline (β-adrenergic stimulant).

## Subjective

1. Complaints of muscle and joint achiness
2. Complaints of generalized weakness
3. Complaints of stress related to the high-risk pregnancy
4. Rating of perceived stress using a visual analog scale: 8/10
5. Reported stress-related symptoms
   - Physical: altered sleep patterns, fatigue, restlessness, headaches, achiness and tension in shoulder, neck, and back muscles
   - Emotional: Anxiety about the pregnancy, depression, and frustration; experiencing sudden shifts in mood
   - Mental: Forgetfulness, inability to concentrate
   - Behavioral: Frequent episodes of crying, disorganization, short temper, inability to sleep

## Objective

### Impairments

- Fetal monitor in situ
- Patient evaluated in lying. Sitting and standing evaluated at return visit during permitted ambulation to the bathroom.
- Range of motion: Within normal limits for neck and upper and lower extremity range of motion. Complaints of achiness during range of motion. Lumbar spine range of motion not assessed.
- Strength: Unable to assess formally; resisted movement is contraindicated. Risk of ongoing decrease in strength because of restricted activity level.
- Muscle resting tension: Increased level of muscle resting tension in neck, shoulder, and erector spinae muscles noted on palpation.

### Functional Limitations

- Bed mobility: Performed rolling side-to-side and scooting independently with use of monkey bar. Complaints of achiness and weakness.
- Transfers: Performed lying-to-sit, sit-to-stand, stand-to-toilet, and toilet-to-stand with contact guard assistance secondary to complaints of weakness and achiness
- Ambulation: 10 feet with minimal assistance of one person secondary to poor balance and complaints of weakness

# Analysis

## Treatment Rationale

Treatment is aimed at (1) preventing further deterioration of health status and functional level because of inactivity and (2) reducing stress-related symptoms as a means of increasing the patient's comfort level and facilitating maternal and fetal well-being.
Precautions:

- Monitor for maternal and fetal tachycardia and hypotension.
- Adhere to restrictions in physical activity: no sitting, standing, or ambulation (other than to the bathroom with assistance).
- Valsalva maneuver, resisted movements, and abdominal exercises are contraindicated.
- Ensure adequate hydration during treatment and encourage frequent emptying of the bladder.
- Side effects of β-adrenergic medication: Maternal and fetal tachycardia and hypotension

| Impairment | Outcomes and Role of Massage |
|---|---|
| Anxiety | Decreased anxiety |
|  | Primary treatment; direct effect of massage on reduction of perceived anxiety |
| Perceived stress | Decreased perceived stress |
|  | Primary treatment; direct effect of massage on increased perceived relaxation |
| Increased muscle resting tension | Decreased muscle resting tension |
|  | Primary treatment; localized primary effect of massage on reduction of level of muscle resting tension |
|  | Secondary effect of general increase in relaxation and reduction of anxiety |
| Muscle and joint pain ("achiness") | Decreased muscle and joint pain ("achiness") |
|  | Primary treatment; direct effect of massage on pain reduction through hyperstimulation analgesia and sedation |
| Fatigue | Decreased fatigue |
|  | Secondary treatment; possible indirect effect of massage through increased sensory arousal |
| Other stress-related symptoms | Decreased stress-related symptoms |
|  | Secondary treatment; possible indirect effect of massage through increase in perceived relaxation and reduction of perceived anxiety |
| Muscle weakness | Increased muscle strength |
|  | No effect |

| Activity Limitation | Functional Outcomes |
|---|---|
| Decreased ability to perform functional transfers and mobility tasks | Patient will maintain ability to perform rolling side-to-side and scooting independently with use of monkey bar |
|  | Patient will maintain ability to perform transfers lying-to-sit, sit-to-stand, stand-to-toilet, and toilet-to-stand with contact guard assistance |
| Decreased ambulation | Patient will maintain ability to ambulate 10 feet to bathroom with minimal assistance of one person |
| Complaints of pain and weakness during functional activity | Patient will report fewer complaints of achiness and weakness during functional activity |

- Complaints of decreased well-being and increased stress
- Patient will report increased sense of well-being and decreased stress-related symptoms

## *Plan*

Massage Techniques

General Issues:

The practitioner works in close consultation with the attending physician throughout treatment. At least initially during treatment, the application of techniques to the abdomen is contraindicated. Depth of application of techniques is limited to the most superficial muscle layer. Passive movement techniques such as rocking are not included in the intervention. Intervention is initially as brief as 15 minutes. When the patient tolerates this well, with no signs of fetal or maternal distress, the practitioner increases the intervention time in increments of 5 minutes, to up to 40 minutes. More areas of the patient's body are included as the intervention progresses.

Techniques:

The practitioner applies gentle superficial effleurage and broad-contact petrissage in a rhythmic and soothing manner to the limbs, back, and shoulders for the specific aim of producing and sustaining sedation during the course of the massage. She also applies rhythmic and gentle specific petrissage to the patient's hands, feet, and face. In areas of increased muscle tension, such as the shoulders, the practitioner applies more specific neuromuscular techniques, such as stripping and specific compression, in a manner that elicits a pleasurable response from the patient. She precedes or follows the application of massage techniques with diaphragmatic breathing. In addition, she applies massage techniques with gentle passive stretches of the muscles she treats. Finally, the practitioner uses relaxing music of the patient's choice during the intervention.

As the patient's impairments and mood improve, the practitioner instructs her on how to apply (nonmechanical) superficial reflex techniques, such as static contact and superficial stroking, to her own abdomen. She does this in the context of applying lotion for skin care and to improve the expectant mother's mood and her bonding with her child.

Other Appropriate Techniques and Interventions[29]

- Medical management
- Relaxation training (progressive muscle relaxation, guided imagery, meditation)
- Stress management instruction (coping skills)
- Therapeutic exercise in lying (stretching exercises and slow, smooth, active range of motion exercise for neck and upper and lower extremity muscles in lying), especially ankle pumping to promote lower extremity circulation
- Breathing training
- Positioning instruction
- Psychosocial counseling
- Self-monitoring for signs of medication side effects and labor
- Prenatal and postpartum education as required

## References

1. Fritz S. *Mosby's Fundamentals of Therapeutic Massage*. 3rd ed. St. Louis: Mosby; 2004.

2. Benjamin PJ, Tappan FM. *Tappan's Handbook of Healing Massage Techniques*. 4th ed. Upper Saddle River, NJ: Pearson Prentice Hall; 2005.

3. Salvo SG. *Massage Therapy: Principles and Practice*. 2nd ed. Philadelphia: WB Saunders; 2003.

4. Yates J. *A Physician's Guide to Therapeutic Massage*. 3rd ed. Toronto: Curties Overzet; 2004.

5. Loving J. *Massage Therapy*. Stamford, CT: Appleton & Lange; 1999.

6. de Domenico G, Wood EC. *Beard's Massage*. 4th ed. Philadelphia: WB Saunders; 1997.

7. Holey E, Cook E. *Evidence-Based Therapeutic Massage*. 2nd ed. Edinburgh: Churchill Livingstone; 2003.

8. Lowe WL. *Orthopedic Massage*. Edinburgh: Mosby; 2003.

9. McGeown JG, McHale NG, Thornbury KD. Effects of varying patterns of external compression on lymph flow in the hind limb of the anaesthetized sheep. *J Physiol*. 1988;397:449–457.

10. Benjamin PJ, Lamp SP. *Understanding Sports Massage*. Champaign, IL: Human Kinetics; 1996.

11. Murrell W. *Massotherapeutics or Massage as a Mode of Treatment*. Philadelphia: Blakiston; 1890.

12. Palmer MD. *Lessons on Massage*. 4th ed. London: Balliere Tindall and Cox; 1912.

13. Kellogg JH. *The Art of Massage: A Practical Manual for the Nurse, the Student and the Practitioner*. Battle Creek, MI: Modern Medicine Publishing; 1929.

14. Dery MA, Yonuschot G, Winterson BJ. The effects of manually applied intermittent pulsation pressure to rat ventral thorax on lymph transport. *Lymphology*. 2000;33:58–61.

15. DiGiovanna EL, Schiowitz S. *An Osteopathic Approach to Diagnosis and Treatment*. Philadelphia: Lippincott-Raven; 1997.

16. Greenman PE. *Principles of Manual Medicine*. 2nd ed. Baltimore: Williams & Wilkins; 1996.

17. Field TM. Massage therapy effects. *Am Psychol*. 1998;53:1270–1281.

18. Mair P, Kornberger E, Schwarz B, et al. Forward blood flow during cardiopulmonary resuscitation in patients with severe accidental hypothermia: An echocardiographic study. *Acta Anaesthesiol Scand*. 1998;42:1139–1144.

19. Boczar ME, Howard MA, Rivers EP, et al. A technique revisited: hemodynamic comparison of closed- and open-chest cardiac massage during human cardiopulmonary resuscitation. *Crit Care Med*. 1995;23:498–503.

20. Redberg RF, Tucker KJ, Cohen TJ, et al. Physiology of blood flow during cardiopulmonary resuscitation. A transesophageal echocardiographic study. *Circulation*. 1993;88:534–542.

21. Horiuchi K, Johnson R, Weissman C. Influence of lower limb pneumatic compression on pulmonary artery temperature: effect on cardiac output measurements. *Crit Care Med*. 1999;27:1096–1099.

22. Malone MD, Cisek PL, Comerota AJ Jr, et al. High-pressure, rapid-inflation pneumatic compression improves venous hemodynamics in healthy volunteers and patients who are postthrombotic. *J Vasc Surg*. 1999;29:593–599.

23. Liu K, Chen LE, Seaber AV, et al. Intermittent pneumatic compression of legs increases microcirculation in distant skeletal muscle. *J Orthop Res*. 1999;17:88–95.

24. Vanek VW. Meta-analysis of effectiveness of intermittent pneumatic compression devices with a comparison of thigh-high to knee-high sleeves. *Am Surg*. 1998;64:1050–1058.

25. Ricci MA, Fisk P, Knight S, Case T. Hemodynamic evaluation of foot venous compression devices. *J Vasc Surg*. 1997;26:803–808.

26. Allegra C, Bartolo M, Martocchia R. Therapeutic effects of Vascupump treatment in patients with Fontaine Stage IIB arteriopathy. *Minerva Cardioangiol*. 2001;49:189–195.

27. Valtonen EJ, Lilius HG, Svinhufvud U. The effect of syncardial massage produced without synchronization and with different pressure impulse frequencies. *Ann Chir Gynaecol Fenn*. 1973;62:69–72.

28. McGeown JG, McHale NG, Thornbury KD. The role of external compression and movement in lymph propulsion in the sheep hind limb. *J Physiol*. 1987;387:83–93.

29. Kisner C, Colby LA. *Therapeutic Exercise: Foundations and Techniques*. 4th ed. Philadelphia: FA Davis; 2002.

30. Frownfelter DL, Dean E. *Principles and Practice of Cardiopulmonary Physical Therapy*. 3rd ed. St. Louis: CV Mosby; 1996.

31. Frownfelter D, ed. *Chest Physical Therapy and Pulmonary Rehabilitation: An Interdisciplinary Approach*. Chicago: Year Book; 1978.

32. Lederman E. *The Science and Practice of Manual Therapy*. 2nd ed. Edinburgh: Elsevier Churchill Livingstone; 2005.

33. Hayes J, Cox C. Immediate effects of a five-minute foot massage on patients in critical care. *Intensive Crit Care Nurs*. 1999;15:77–82.

34. Ahles TA, Tope DM, Pinkson B, et al. Massage therapy for patients undergoing autologous bone marrow transplantation. *J Pain Symptom Manage*. 1999;18:157–163.

35. Field T, Hernandez-Reif M, Hart S, et al. Pregnant women benefit from massage therapy. *J Psychosom Obstet Gynecol*. 1999;20:31–38.

36. Richards KC. Effect of a back massage and relaxation intervention on sleep in critically ill patients. *Am J Crit Care*. 1998;7:288–299.

37. MacDonald G. Massage as a respite intervention for primary caregivers. *Am J Hospice Palliat Care*. 1998;15:43–47.

38. Field T, Schanberg S, Kuhn C, et al. Bulimic adolescents benefit from massage therapy. *Adolescence*. 1998;33:555–563.

39. Field T, Peck M, Krugman S, et al. Burn injuries benefit from massage therapy. *J Burn Care Rehabil*. 1998;19:241–244.

40. Field T, Hernandez-Reif M, Seligman S, et al. Juvenile rheumatoid arthritis: benefits from massage therapy. *J Pediatr Psychol*. 1997;22:607–617.

41. Field T, Ironson G, Pickens I, et al. Massage therapy reduces anxiety and enhances EEG pattern of alertness and math computations. *Int J Neurosci*. 1996;86:197–205.

42. Fraser J, Kerr JR. Psychophysiological effects of back massage on elderly institutionalized patients. *J Adv Nurs*. 1993;18:238–245.

43. Field T, Morrow C, Vaideon C, et al. Massage reduces anxiety in child and adolescent psychiatric patients. *J Am Acad Child Adolesc Psychiatry*. 1992;31:124–131.

44. Field T. Maternal depression effects on infants and early interventions. *Prev Med*. 1998;27:200–203.

45. Field T, Grizzle N, Scafidi F, Schanberg S. Massage and relaxation therapies effects on depressed adolescent mothers. *Adolescence*. 1996;31:903–911.

46. Field T, Quintino O, Hernandez-Reif M. Adolescents with attention deficit hyperactivity disorder benefit from massage therapy. *Adolescence*. 1998;33:103–108.

47. Field T, Lasko D, Mundy P, et al. Autistic children's attentiveness and responsivity improved after touch therapy. *J Autism Dev Disord*. 1997;27:329–334.

48. Leivadi S, Hernandez-Reif M, Field T, et al. Massage therapy and relaxation effects on university dance students. *J Dance Med Sci*. 1999;3:108–112.

49. Blackman PG, Simmons LR, Crossley KM. Treatment of chronic exertional anterior compartment syndrome with massage: a pilot study. *Clin J Sport Med*. 1998;8:14–17.

50. Field DA, Miller S. Cosmetic breast surgery. *Am Fam Phys*. 1992;45:711–719.

51. Gam AN, Warming S, Larsen LH, et al. Treatment of myofascial trigger-points with ultrasound combined with massage and exercise—a randomised controlled trial. *Pain*. 1998;77:73–79.

52. Gluck NI. Passive care and active rehabilitation in a patient with failed back surgery syndrome. *J Manipulative Physiol Ther*. 1996;19:41–47.

53. Hammill JM, Cook TM, Rosecrance JC. Effectiveness of a physical therapy regimen in the treatment of tension-type headache. *Headache*. 1996;36:149–153.

54. Inoue M, Ohtsu I, Tomioka S, et al. Effects of pulmonary rehabilitation on vital capacity in patients with chronic pulmonary emphysema. *Nihon Kyobu Shikkan Gakkai Zasshi (Japanese)*. 1996;34:1182–1188 (Abstract).

55. Pope MH, Phillips RB, Haugh LD, et al. A prospective randomized three-week trial of spinal manipulation, transcutaneous muscle stimulation, massage and corset in the treatment of subacute low back pain. *Spine*. 1994;19:2571–2577.

56. Waylonis GW, Perkins RH. Post-traumatic fibromyalgia. A long term follow-up. *Am J Phys Med Rehabil*. 1994;73:403–412.

57. Levoska S, Keinanen-Kiukaanniemi S. Active or passive physiotherapy for occupational cervico-brachial disorders? A comparison of 2 treatment methods with a 1 year follow-up. *Arch Phys Med*. 1993;74:425–430.

58. Ironson G, Field T, Scafidi F, et al. Massage therapy is associated with enhancement of the immune system's cytotoxic capacity. *Int J Neurosci*. 1996;84:205–217.

59. Zhao A. Study of effects of traditional Chinese massage. *Chin J Sports Med*. 1982;1:46–48,64.

60. Schachner L, Field T, Hernandez-Reif M, et al. Atopic dermatitis symptoms decreased in children following massage therapy. *Pediatr Dermatol*. 1998;15:390–395.

61. Shor-Posner G, Miguez MJ, Hernandez-Reif M, Perez-Then E, Fletcher M. Massage treatment in HIV-1 infected Dominican children: a preliminary report on the efficacy of massage therapy to preserve the immune system in children without antiretroviral medication. *J Altern Complement Med*. 2004;10:1093–1095.

62. Yates J. *A Physician's Guide to Therapeutic Massage*. 3rd ed. Toronto: Curties Overzet; 2004.

63. Hoehn-Saric R. Psychic and somatic anxiety: worries, somatic symptoms and physiological changes. *Acta Psychiatr Scand Suppl*. 1998;393:32–38.

64. Millensen JR. *Mind Matters: Psychological Medicine in Holistic Practice*. Seattle: Eastland Press; 1995.

65. Lundberg U. Muscle tension. *J Soft Tissue Manip*. 2006;13:3–9.

66. Crosman LJ, Chateauvert SR, Weisburg J. The effects of massage to the hamstring muscle group on range of motion. *Massage J*. 1985:59–62.

67. van den Dolder PA, Roberts DL. A trial into the effectiveness of soft tissue massage in the treatment of shoulder pain. *Aust J Physiother*. 2003;49:183–188.

68. Barlow A, Clarke R, Johnson N, Seabourne B, Thomas D, Gal J. Effect of massage of the hamstring muscle group on performance of the sit and reach test. *Br J Sports Med*. 2004;38:349–351.

69. Henriksen M, Højrup A, Lund H, Christensen L, Danneskiold-Samsøe B, Bliddal H. The effect of stimulating massage of thigh muscles on knee joint position sense. *Adv Physiother*. 2004;6:29–36.

70. Shipman MK, Boniface DR, Tefft ME, McCloghry F. Antenatal perineal massage and subsequent perineal outcomes: a randomised controlled trial. *Br J Obstet Gynaecol*. 1997;104:787–791.

71. Vendittelli F, Tabaste JL, Janky E. Antepartum perineal massage: review of randomized trials. *J Gynecol Obstet Biol Reprod (Paris)*. 2001;30:565–571.

72. Stamp G, Kruzins G, Crowther C. Perineal massage in labour and prevention of perineal trauma: randomised controlled trial. *BMJ*. 2001;322:1277–1280.

73. Eason E, Labrecque M, Wells G, Feldman P. Preventing perineal trauma during childbirth: a systematic review. *Obstet Gynecol*. 2000;95:464–471.

74. Labrecque M, Eason E, Marcoux S. Randomized trial of perineal massage during pregnancy: perineal symptoms three months after delivery. *Am J Obstet Gynecol*. 2000;182:76–80.

75. Shipman MK, Boniface DR, Tefft ME, McCloghry F. Antenatal perineal massage and subsequent perineal outcomes: a randomised controlled trial. *Br J Obstet Gynaecol*. 1997;104:787–791.

76. Morelli M, Chapman CE, Sullivan SJ. Do cutaneous receptors contribute to the changes in the amplitude of the H-reflex during massage? *Electromyogr Clin Neurophysiol*. 1999;39:441–447.

77. Morelli M, Sullivan SJ, Chapman CE. Inhibitory influence of soleus massage onto the medial gastrocnemius H-reflex. *Electromyogr Clin Neurophysiol*. 1998;38:87–93.

78. Goldberg J, Seaborne DE, Sullivan SI, Leduc BE. The effect of therapeutic massage on H-reflex amplitude in persons with a spinal cord injury. *Phys Ther*. 1994;748:728–737.

79. Goldberg J, Sullivan SI, Seaborne DE. The effect of two intensities of massage on H-reflex amplitude. *Phys Ther*. 1992;72:449–457.

80. Sullivan SJ, Williams LRT, Seaborne D, Morelli M. Effects of massage on alpha neuron excitability. *Phys Ther*. 1991;71:555–560.

81. Morelli M, Seaborne DE, Sullivan SJ. H-reflex modulation during manual muscle massage of human triceps surae. *Arch Phys Med Rehabil*. 1991;72:915–919.

82. Morelli M, Seaborne DE, Sullivan SJ. Changes in H-reflex amplitude during massage of triceps surae in healthy subjects. *J Orthop Sports Phys Ther*. 1990;12:55–59.

83. Dishman JD, Bulbulian R. Comparison of effects of spinal manipulation and massage on motoneuron excitability. *Electromyogr Clin Neurophysiol*. 2001;41:97–106.

84. Newham DJ, Lederman E. Effect of manual therapy techniques on the stretch reflex in normal human quadriceps. *Disabil Rehabil.* 1997;19:326–331.

85. Hernandez-Reif M, Field T, Krasnegor J, et al. Children with cystic fibrosis benefit from massage therapy. *J Pediatr Psychol.* 1999;24:175–181.

86. Beeken JE, Parks D, Cory J, Montopoli G. The effectiveness of neuromuscular release massage therapy in five individuals with chronic obstructive lung disease. *Clin Nurs Res.* 1998;7:309–325.

87. Field T, Henteleff T, Hernandez–Reif M, et al. Children with asthma have improved pulmonary functions after massage therapy. *J Pediatr.* 1998;132:854–858.

88. Ernst E, Matrai A, lmagyarosy I, et al. Massages cause changes in blood fluidity. *Physiotherapy.* 1987;73:43–45.

89. Arkko PJ, Pakarinen AJ, Kari-Koskinen O. Effects of whole-body massage on serum protein, electrolyte and hormone concentrations, enzyme activities and hematological parameters. *Int J Sports Med.* 1983;4:265–267.

90. Liu Y, Xu S, Yan J, et al. Capillary blood flow with dynamical change of tissue pressure caused by exterior force. *Sheng Wu Yi Xue Gong Cheng Xue Za Zhi.* 2004;21:699–703.

91. Shoemaker I, Tiduus M, Mader R. Failure of manual massage to alter limb blood flow: measures by Doppler ultrasound. *Med Sci Sports Exerc.* 1997;1:610–614.

92. Linde B. Dissociation of insulin absorption and blood flow during massage of a subcutaneous injection site. *Diabetes Care.* 1986;6:570–574.

93. Wyper DJ, McNiven DR. Effects of some physiotherapeutic agents on skeletal muscle blood flow. *Physiotherapy.* 1976; 62:83–85.

94. Hovind H, Nielsen SL. Effect of massage on blood flow in skeletal muscle. *Scand J Rehabil Med.* 1974;6:74–77.

95. Hansen TI, Kristensen JH. Effect of massage, shortwave diathermy and ultrasound upon $^{133}$Xe disappearance rate from muscle and subcutaneous tissue in the human calf. *Scand J Rehabil Med.* 1973;5:179–182.

96. Hinds T, McEwan I, Perkes J, Dawson E, Ball D, George K. Effects of massage on limb and skin blood flow after quadriceps exercise. *Med Sci Sports Exerc.* 2004;36:1308–1313.

97. Martin NA, Zoeller RF, Robertson RJ, Lephart SM. The comparative effects of sports massage, active recovery, and rest in promoting blood lactate clearance after supramaximal leg exercise. *J Athletic Train.* 1998;33:30–35.

98. Gupta S, Goswami A, Sadhukhan AK, Mathur DN. Comparative study of lactate removal in short term massage of extremities, active recovery and a passive recovery period after supramaximal exercise sessions. *Int J Sports Med.* 1996;17:106–110.

99. Dolgener FA, Morien A. The effect of massage on lactate disappearance. *J Strength Condition Res.* 1993;7:159–162.

100. Bale P, James H. Massage, warmdown and rest as recuperative measures after short term intense exercise. *Physiother Sport.* 1991;13:4–7.

101. Hemmings B, Smith M, Graydon J, Dyson R. Effects of massage on physiological restoration, perceived recovery, and repeated sports performance. *Br J Sports Med.* 2000;34:109–114.

102. Monedero J, Donne B. Effect of recovery interventions on lactate removal and subsequent performance. *Int J Sports Med.* 2000;21:593–597.

103. Boone T, Tanner M, Radosevich A. Effects of a 10-minute back rub on cardiovascular responses in healthy subjects. *Am J Chin Med.* 2001;29:47–52.

104. Anonymous. Trends in slow wave variability of the central circulation in healthy individuals in response to massage of the collar cervical region. *Vopr Kurortol Fizioter Lech Fiz Kult.* 2004;6:13–15.

105. Mortimer PS, Simmonds R, Rezvani M, et al. The measurement of skin lymph flow by isotope clearance—reliability, reproducibility, injection dynamics, and the effect of massage. *J Invest Dermatol.* 1990;95:677–682.

106. Yamazaki Z, Idezuki Y, Nemoto T, Togawa T. Clinical experiences using pneumatic massage therapy for edematous limbs over the last 10 years. *Angiology.* 1988;39:154–163.

107. Yamazaki Z, Fujimori Y, Wada T, et al. Admittance plethysmographic evaluation of undulatory massage for the edematous limb. *Lymphology.* 1979;12:40–42.

108. de Godoy JM, Batigalia F, Godoy Mde F. Preliminary evaluation of a new, more simplified physiotherapy technique for lymphatic drainage. *Lymphology.* 2002;35:91–93.

109. Aksenova AM, Teslenko OI, Boganskaia OA. Changes in the immune status of peptic ulcer patients after combined treatment including deep massage. *Vopr Kurortol Fizioter Lech Fiz Kult (Russian).* 1999;2:19–20 (Abstract).

110. Makarova MR, Kuznetsov OF, Markina LP, et al. The effect of massage on the neuromuscular apparatus and blood coagulating system of patients with chronic salpingo-oophoritis. *Vopr Kurortol Fizioter Lech Fiz Kult (Russian).* 1998;6:45–48 (Abstract).

111. Aksenova AM, Romanova MM. The effect of reflex muscle massage on the body regulator processes of peptic ulcer patients with concomitant diseases. *Vopr Kurortol Fizioter Lech Fiz Kult (Russian).* 1998;6:24–26 (Abstract).

112. Gusarova SA, Kuznetsov OF, Gorbunov FE, Maslovskaia SG. The characteristics of the effect of point and classical massage on the hemodynamics of patients with a history of transient ischemic attacks in the vertebrobasilar system. *Vopr Kurortol Fizioter Lech Fiz Kult (Russian).* 1998;5:7–9 (Abstract).

113. Kuznetsov OF, Makarova MR, Markina LP. The comparative effect of classic massage of different intensities on patients with chronic salpingo-oophritis. *Vopr Kurortol Fizioter Lech Fiz Kult (Russian).* 1998;2:20–23 (Abstract).

114. Aksenova AM. A new method for deep reflex muscular massage. *Vopr Kurortol Fizioter Lech Fiz Kult (Russian).* 1997;4:30–32 (Abstract).

115. Aksenova AM, Reznikov KM, Andreeva VV. The effect of deep massage and physical exercises on the cerebral circulation in osteochondrosis of the cervicothoracic spine. *Vopr Kurortol Fizioter Lech Fiz Kult (Russian).* 1997;3:19–21. (Abstract).

116. Gusarova SA, Kuznetsov OF, Maslovskaia SG. The effect of the massage of different areas of the body on the cerebral hemodynamics in patients with a history of acute disorders of the cerebral circulation. *Vopr Kurortol Fizioter Lech Fiz Kult (Russian).* 1996;1:14–16 (Abstract).

117. Richaud C, Bouchet JY, Bosson JL, et al. Manual fragmentation of deep vein thrombosis. *J Mal Vasc (French).* 1995;20:166–171 (Abstract).

118. Labrecque M, Nouwen A, Bergeron M, Rancourt JF. A randomized controlled trial of nonpharmacologic approaches

for relief of low back pain during labor. *J Fam Pract.* 1999; 48:259–263.

119. Field T, Hernandez-Reif M, Taylor S, et al. Labour pain is reduced by massage therapy. *J Psychosom Obstet Gynecol.* 1997; 18:286–291.

120. Yildirim G, Sahin NH. The effect of breathing and skin stimulation techniques on labour pain perception of Turkish women. *Pain Res Manag.* 2004;9:183–187.

121. Nixon N, Teschendorff J, Finney J, Karnilowicz W. Expanding the nursing repertory: the effect of massage on post-operative pain. *Aust J Adv Nurs.* 1997;14:21–26.

122. Ferrell-Tory AT, Glick OJ. The use of therapeutic massage as a nursing intervention to modify anxiety and the perception of cancer pain. *Cancer Nurs.* 1993;16:93–101.

123. Weinrich SP, Weinrich MC. The effect of massage on pain in cancer patients. *Appl Nurs Res.* 1990;3:140–145.

124. Akbayrak T, Citak I, Demirturk F, Akarcali I. Manual therapy and pain changes in patients with migraine: an open pilot study. *Adv Physiother.* 2001;3:49–54.

125. Puustjarvi K, Airaksinen O, Pontinen PJ. The effect of massage in patients with chronic tension headache. *Int J Acupunct Electrother Res.* 1990;15:159–162.

126. Danneskiold-Samsoe B, Christiansen E, Anderson RB. Myofascial pain and the role of myoglobin. *Scand J Rheumatol (Stockholm).* 1986;15:174–178.

127. Field T. Fibromyalgia pain and substance P decrease and sleep improves after massage therapy. *J Clin Rheumatol.* 2002; 8:72–76.

128. Ernst E. Massage therapy for low back pain: a systematic review. *J Pain Symptom Manage.* 1999;17:65–69.

129. Preyde M. Effectiveness of massage therapy for subacute low-back pain: a randomized controlled trial. *CMAJ.* 2000;162: 1815–1820.

130. Carreck A. The effect of massage on pain perception threshold. *Manipulative Physiother.* 1994;26:10–16.

131. Day JA, Mason RR, Chesrown SE. Effect of massage on serum level of beta-endorphin and beta-lipotropin in healthy adults. *Phys Ther.* 1987;67:926–930.

132. Tiidus PM. Manual massage and recovery of muscle function following exercise: a literature review. *J Orthop Sports Phys Ther.* 1997;25:107–112.

133. Callaghan MJ. The role of massage in the management of athletes: a review. *Br J Sports Med.* 1993;27:28–33.

134. Cafarelli E, Flint F. Role of massage in preparation for and recovery from exercise. *Physiother Sport.* 1993;16:17–20.

135. Harmer PA. The effect of pre-performance massage on stride frequency in sprinters. *Athletic Train.* 1991;26:55–59.

136. Boone T, Cooper R, Thompson WR. A physiologic evaluation of the sports massage. *J Athletic Train.* 1991;26:51–54.

137. Wiktorsson-Moller M, Oberg B, Ekstrand J, Giliquist J. Effects of warming up, massage, and stretching on range of motion and muscle strength in the lower extremity. *Am J Sports Med.* 1983;11:249–252.

138. Ernst E. Does post-exercise massage treatment reduce delayed onset muscle soreness? A systematic review. *Br J Sports Med.* 1998;32:212–214.

139. Weber MD, Servedis FJ, Woodall WR. The effects of three modalities on delayed onset muscle soreness. *J Orthop Sports Phys Ther.* 1994;20:236–242.

140. Smith LL, Keating MN, Holbert D, et al. The effects of athletic massage on delayed onset muscle soreness, creatine kinase, and neutrophil count: a preliminary report. *J Orthop Sports Phys Ther.* 1994;19:93–99.

141. Cheung K, Hume P, Maxwell L. Delayed onset muscle soreness: treatment strategies and performance factors. *Sports Med.* 2003;33:145–164.

142. Farr T, Nottle C, Nosaka K, Sacco P. The effects of therapeutic massage on delayed onset muscle soreness and muscle function following downhill walking. *J Sci Med Sport.* 2002; 5:297–306.

143. Hilbert JE, Sforzo GA, Swensen T. The effects of massage on delayed onset muscle soreness. *Br J Sports Med.* 2003; 37:72–75.

144. Rinder AN, Sutherland CJ. An investigation of the effects of massage on quadriceps performance after exercise fatigue. *Complement Ther Nurs Midwifery.* 1995;1:99–102.

145. Tiidus PM. Massage and ultrasound as therapeutic modalities in exercise-induced muscle damage. *Can J Appl Physiol.* 1999;24:267–278.

146. Rodenburg JB, Steenbeek D, Schiereck P, Bar PR. Warm-up, stretching and massage diminish harmful effects of eccentric exercise. *Int J Sports Med.* 1994;15:414–419.

147. Drews T, Kreider B, Drinkard B, et al. Effects of post-event massage therapy on repeated endurance cycling. *Int J Sports Med.* 1990;11:407.

148. Drews T, Kreider RB, Drinkard B, Jackson CW. Effects of post-event massage therapy on psychological profiles of exertion, feeling and mood during a 4-day ultra endurance cycling event. *Med Sci Sport Exerc.* 1991;23:91.

149. Weinberg R, Jackson A, Kolodny K. The relationship of massage and exercise to mood enhancement. *Sport Psychol.* 1988;2:202–211.

150. Robertson A, Watt JM, Galloway SD. Effects of leg massage on recovery from high intensity cycling exercise. *Br J Sports Med.* 2004;38:173–176.

151. Jonhagen S, Ackermann P, Eriksson T, Saartok T, Renstrom PA. Sports massage after eccentric exercise. *Am J Sports Med.* 2004;32:1499–1503.

152. Lane KN, Wenger HA. Effect of selected recovery conditions on performance of repeated bouts of intermittent cycling separated by 24 hours. *J Strength Cond Res.* 2004;18:855–860.

153. Tanaka TH, Leisman G, Mori H, Nishijo K. The effect of massage on localized lumbar muscle fatigue. *BMC Complement Altern Med.* 2002;2:9.

154. Eliska O, Eliska M. Are peripheral lymphatics damaged by high pressure manual massage? *Lymphology.* 1995;28:21–30.

155. Lindsay WR, Pitcaithly D, Geelen N, et al. A comparison of the effects of four therapy procedures on concentration and responsiveness in people with profound learning disabilities. *J Intellect Disabil Res.* 1997;41:201–207.

156. Brooker DJ, Snape M, Johnson E, et al. Single case evaluation of the effects of aromatherapy and massage on disturbed behaviour in severe dementia. *Br J Clin Psychol.* 1997;36:287–296.

157. Simons DG, Travell JG, Simons LS. *Travell and Simons' Myofascial Pain and Dysfunction: The Trigger Point Manual. Volume 1: Upper Half of Body.* 2nd ed. Baltimore: Williams & Wilkins; 1999.

158. Travell JG, Simons DG. *Myofascial Pain and Dysfunction. The Trigger Point Manual, Volume 1.* Baltimore: Williams & Wilkins; 1983.

159. Danneskiold-Samsoe B, Christiansen E, Lund B, Anderson RB. Regional muscle tension and pain ("fibrositis"): effect of massage on myoglobin in plasma. *Scand J Rehabil Med.* 1983; 15:17–20.

160. Hannon JC. The man who mistook his patient for a chair: a speculation regarding sitting mechanical treatment of lower back pain. *J Bodywork Movement Ther.* 1998;2:88–100.

161. Morhenn VB. Firm stroking of human skin leads to vasodilatation possibly due to the release of substance P. *J Dermatol Sci.* 2000;22:138–144.

162. Chaitow L. *Modern Neuromuscular Techniques.* New York: Churchill Livingstone; 1996.

163. Mannheim CJ. *The Myofascial Release Manual.* 3rd ed. Thorofare, NJ: SLACK Inc; 2001.

164. Travell JG, Simons DG. *Myofascial Pain and Dysfunction. The Trigger Point Manual, Volume 2.* Baltimore: Williams & Wilkins; 1992.

165. Murphy GJ. Physical medicine modalities and trigger point injections in the management of temporomandibular disorders and assessing treatment outcome. *Oral Surg Oral Med Oral Pathol Oral Radiol Endod.* 1997;83:118–122.

166. Fricton JR. Management of masticatory myofascial pain. *Semin Orthod.* 1995;1:229–243.

167. Clark GT, Seligman DA, Solberg WK, Pullinger AG. Guidelines for the treatment of temporomandibular disorders. *J Craniomandib Disord.* 1990;4:80–88.

168. Seaman DR, Cleveland C III. Spinal pain syndromes: nociceptive, neuropathic, and psychologic mechanisms. *J Manipulative Physiol Ther.* 1999;22:458–472.

169. Kovacs FM, Abraira V, Pozo F, et al. Local and remote sustained trigger point therapy for exacerbations of chronic low back pain. A randomized, double-blind, controlled, multicenter trial. *Spine.* 1997;22:786–797.

170. Ingber RS. Iliopsoas myofascial dysfunction: a treatable cause of "failed" low back syndrome. *Arch Phys Med Rehabil.* 1989; 70:382–386.

171. Morris CE. Chiropractic rehabilitation of a patient with S1 radiculopathy associated with a large lumbar disk herniation. *J Manipulative Physiol Ther.* 1999;22:38–44.

172. Hawk C, Long C, Azad A. Chiropractic care for women with chronic pelvic pain: a prospective single-group intervention study. *J Manipulative Physiol Ther.* 1997;20:73–79.

173. Hughes KH. Painful rib syndrome. A variant of myofascial pain syndrome. *AAOHN J.* 1998;46:115–120.

174. Antonelli MA, Vawter RL. Nonarticular pain syndromes. Differentiating generalized, regional, and localized disorders. *Postgrad Med.* 1992;91:95–98,103–104.

175. Gerwin RD. Myofascial pain syndromes in the upper extremity. *J Hand Ther.* 1997;10:130–136.

176. Buchberger DJ. Use of Active Release techniques in the post-operative shoulder: a case report. *J Sports Chiropr Rehabil.* 1999;13:60–66.

177. Lew PC, Lewis J, Story I. Inter-therapist reliability in locating latent myofascial trigger points using palpation. *Manual Ther.* 1997;2:87–90.

178. Han SC, Harrison P. Myofascial pain syndrome and trigger-point management. *Reg Anesth.* 1997;22:89–101.

179. Dougans I. *The Complete Illustrated Guide to Foot Reflexology.* Boston: Element Books; 1996.

180. Byers DC. *Better Health with Foot Reflexology: The Original Ingham Method.* St. Petersburg, FL: Ingham Publishing; 1996.

181. Masunaga S, Chashi W. *Zen Shiatsu: How to Harmonize Yin and Yang for Better Health.* Tokyo: Japan Publishers; 1977.

182. Yamamoto S, McCarty P. *The Shiatsu Handbook.* New York: Avery Publishing Group; 1996.

183. Tappan F. Finger pressure to acupuncture points. In: Tappan FM, Benjamin PJ, eds. *Tappan's Handbook of Healing Massage Techniques.* 3rd ed. Stamford, CT: Appleton & Lange; 1998:243–268.

184. Wolf JE, Teegarden IM. Jin shin do. In: Benjamin PJ, Tappan FM, eds. *Tappan's Handbook of Healing Massage Techniques.* 4th ed. Upper Saddle River, NJ: Pearson Prentice Hall; 2005: 363–376.

185. Chaitow L. *Positional Release Techniques.* New York: Churchill Livingstone; 1996.

186. Prudden B. *Pain Erasure: The Bonnie Prudden Way.* New York: M. Evans; 1980.

187. Prudden B. *Myotherapy: Bonnie Prudden's Complete Guide to Pain-Free Living.* New York: Ballantine Books; 1984.

188. Hou CR, Tsai LC, Cheng KF, Chung KC, Hong CZ. Immediate effects of various physical therapeutic modalities on cervical myofascial pain and trigger-point sensitivity. *Arch Phys Med Rehabil.* 2002;83:1406–1414.

189. Bodhise PB, Dejoie M, Brandon Z, Simpkins S, Ballas SK. Non-pharmacologic management of sickle cell pain. *Hematology.* 2004;9:235–237.

190. O'Sullivan SB. Strategies to improve motor control. In: O'Sullivan SB, Schmitz J, eds. *Physical Rehabilitation, Assessment and Treatment.* 2nd ed. Philadelphia: FA Davis; 1988.

191. Leone JA, Kukulka CG. Effects of tendon pressure on alpha motoneuron excitability in patients with stroke. *Phys Ther.* 1988;68:475–480.

192. Kukulka CG, Haberichter PA, Mueksch AE, Rohrberg MG. Muscle pressure effects on motoneuron excitability. A special communication. *Phys Ther.* 1987;67:1720–1722.

193. Kukulka CG, Beckman SM, Holte JB, Hoppenworth PK. Effects of intermittent tendon pressure on alpha motoneuron excitability. *Phys Ther.* 1986;66:1091–1094.

194. Kukulka CG, Fellows WA, Oehlertz JE, Vanderwilt SG. Effect of tendon pressure on alpha motoneuron excitability. *Phys Ther.* 1985;65:595–600.

195. Siev-Ner I, Gamus D, Lerner-Geva L, Achiron A. Reflexology treatment relieves symptoms of multiple sclerosis: a randomised controlled study. *Mult Scler.* 2003;9:356–361.

196. Herskovitz S, Strauch B, Gordon MJV. Shiatsu-induced injury of the median recurrent motor branch. *Muscle Nerve.* 1992; 15:1215 (Letter).

197. Stephenson NL, Weinrich SP, Tavakoli AS. The effects of foot reflexology on anxiety and pain in patients with breast and lung cancer. *Oncol Nurs Forum.* 2000;27:67–72.

198. Kesselring A. Foot reflexology massage: a clinical study. *Forsch Komplementarmed (German).* 1999;6(Suppl 1):38–40 (Abstract).

199. Sudmeier I, Bodner G, Egger I, et al. Changes of renal blood flow during organ-associated foot reflexology measured by color

Doppler sonography. *Forsch Komple-mentarmed (German)*. 1999;6:129–134 (Abstract).

200. Baerheim A, Algroy R, Skogedal KR, et al. Feet—a diagnostic tool? *Tidsskr Nor Laegeforen (Norwegian)*. 1998;118:753–755 (Abstract).

201. Kesselring A, Spichiger E, Muller M. Foot reflexology: an intervention study. *Pflege (German)*. 1998;11:213–218 (Abstract).

202. Kristof O, Schlumpf M, Saller R. Foot reflex zone massage—a review. *Wien Med Wochenschr (German)*. 1997;147:418–422 (Abstract).

203. Omura Y. Accurate localization of organ representation areas on the feet and hands using the bi-digital O-ring test resonance phenomenon: its clinical implication in diagnosis and treatment—part I. *Acupunct Electrother Res*. 1994;19:153–190.

204. Kesselring A. Foot reflex zone massage. *Schweiz Med Wochenschr Suppl (German)*. 1994;62:88–93 (Abstract).

205. Oleson T, Flocco W. Randomized controlled study of premenstrual symptoms treated with ear, hand, and foot reflexology. *Obstet Gynecol*. 1993;82:906–911.

206. Petersen LN, Faurschou P, Olsen OT. Foot zone therapy and bronchial asthma—a controlled clinical trial. *Ugeskr Laeger (Danish)*. 1992;154:2065–2068 (Abstract).

207. Brygge T, Heinig JH, Collins P, et al. Reflexology and bronchial asthma. *Respir Med*. 2001;95:173–179.

208. Mollart L. Single-blind trial addressing the differential effects of two reflexology techniques versus rest, on ankle and foot edema in late pregnancy. *Complement Ther Nurs Midwifery*. 2003;9:203–208.

209. Ross CSK, Hamilton J, Macrae G, Docherty C, Gould A, Cornbleet MA. A pilot study to evaluate the effect of reflexology on mood and symptom rating of advanced cancer patients. *Palliat Med*. 2002;16:544–545.

210. Stephenson N, Dalton JA, Carlson J. The effect of foot reflexology on pain in patients with metastatic cancer. *Appl Nurs Res*. 2003;16:284–286.

211. Tovey P. A single-blind trial of reflexology for irritable bowel syndrome. *Br J Gen Pract*. 2002;52:19–23.

212. White AR, Williamson J, Hart A, Ernst E. A blinded investigation into the accuracy of reflexology charts. *Complement Ther Med*. 2000;8:166–172.

213. Williamson J, White A, Hart A, Ernst E. Randomised controlled trial of reflexology for menopausal symptoms. *BJOG*. 2002;109:1050–1055.

214. Kannathal N, Paul JK, Lim CM, Chua KP, Sadasivan PK. Effect of reflexology on EEG: a nonlinear approach. *Am J Chin Med*. 2004;32:641–650.

215. Mur E, Schmidseder J, Egger I, et al. Influence of reflex zone therapy of the feet on intestinal blood flow measured by color Doppler sonography. *Forsch Komplementarmed Klass Naturheilkd*. 2001;8:86–89.

216. Bennedbaek O, Viktor J, Carlsen KS, Roed H, Vinding H, Lundbye-Christensen S. Infants with colic. A heterogenous group possible to cure? Treatment by pediatric consultation followed by a study of the effect of zone therapy on incurable colic. *Ugeskr Laeger*. 2001;163:3773–3778.

217. Yang JH. The effects of foot reflexology on nausea, vomiting and fatigue of breast cancer patients undergoing chemotherapy. *Taehan Kanho Hakhoe Chi*. 2005;35:177–185.

218. Hodgson H. Does reflexology impact on cancer patients' quality of life? *Nurs Stand*. 2000;14:33–38.

219. Kohara H, Miyauchi T, Suehiro Y, Ueoka H, Takeyama H, Morita T. Combined modality treatment of aromatherapy, footsoak, and reflexology relieves fatigue in patients with cancer. *J Palliat Med*. 2004;7:791–796.

220. Wright S, Courtney U, Donnelly C, Kenny T, Lavin C. Clients' perceptions of the benefits of reflexology on their quality of life. *Complement Ther Nurs Midwifery*. 2002;8:69–76.

221. Helms JM. *Acupuncture Energetics. A Clinical Approach for Physicians*. Berkeley, CA: Medical Acupuncture Publishers; 1995.

222. Porkert M, Hempen C-H, The China Academy. *Classical Acupuncture: The Standard Textbook*. Dinkelscherben, Germany: Phainon Editions and Media GmbH; 1995.

223. Kielkowska A. *Your Health in Your Hands*. Gdansk, Poland: Kolmio; 1995.

224. Melzack R. Myofascial trigger points: relation to acupuncture and mechanisms of pain. *Arch Phys Med Rehabil*. 1981; 62:114–117.

225. Melzack R, Stilwell DN, Fox EJ. Trigger points and acupuncture points for pain: correlations and implications. *Pain*. 1977;3:23.

226. Shenkman Z, Holzman RS, Kim C, et al. Acupressure—acupuncture antiemetic prophylaxis in children undergoing tonsillectomy. *Anesthesiology*. 1999;90:1311–1316.

227. Harmon D, Gardiner J, Harrison R, Kelly A. Acupressure and the prevention of nausea and vomiting after laparoscopy. *Br J Anaesth*. 1999;82:387–390.

228. Aikins, Murphy P. Alternative therapies for nausea and vomiting of pregnancy. *Obstet Gynecol*. 1998;91:149–155.

229. Stein DJ, Birnbach DJ, Danzer BI, et al. Acupressure versus intravenous metoclopramide to prevent nausea and vomiting during spinal anesthesia for cesarean section. *Anesth Analg*. 1997;84:342–345.

230. Ho CM, Hseu SS, Tsai SK, Lee TY. Effect of P-6 acupressure on prevention of nausea and vomiting after epidural morphine for post–cesarean section pain relief. *Acta Anaesthesiol Scand*. 1996;40:372–375.

231. Agarwal A, Pathak A, Gaur A. Acupressure wristbands do not prevent postoperative nausea and vomiting after urological endoscopic surgery. *Can J Anaesth*. 2000;47:319–324.

232. Collins KB, Thomas DJ. Acupuncture and acupressure for the management of chemotherapy-induced nausea and vomiting. *J Am Acad Nurse Pract*. 2004;16:76–80.

233. Cummings M. Hand acupressure reduces postoperative vomiting after strabismus surgery (n=50). *Acupunct Med*. 2001;19:53–54.

234. Dibble SL, Chapman J, Mack KA, Shih AS. Acupressure for nausea: results of a pilot study. *Oncol Nurs Forum*. 2000;27:41–47.

235. Eizember FL, Tomaszewski CA, Kerns WP 2nd. Acupressure for prevention of emesis in patients receiving activated charcoal. *J Toxicol Clin Toxicol*. 2002;40:775–780.

236. Harmon D, Ryan M, Kelly A, Bowen M. Acupressure and prevention of nausea and vomiting during and after spinal anaesthesia for caesarean section. *Br J Anaesth*. 2000;84:463–467.

237. Jewell D. Nausea and vomiting in early pregnancy. *Clin Evid*. 2003;9:1561–1570.

238. Klein J, Griffiths P. Acupressure for nausea and vomiting in cancer patients receiving chemotherapy. *Br J Community Nurs.* 2004;9:383–388.

239. Lu DP, Lu GP, Reed JF 3rd. Acupuncture/acupressure to treat gagging dental patients: a clinical study of anti-gagging effects. *Gen Dent.* 2000;48:446–452.

240. Norheim AJ, Pedersen EJ, Fonnebo V, Berge L. Acupressure treatment of morning sickness in pregnancy. A randomised, double-blind, placebo-controlled study. *Scand J Prim Health Care.* 2001;19:43–47.

241. Roscoe JA, Morrow GR, Hickok JT, et al. The efficacy of acupressure and acustimulation wrist bands for the relief of chemotherapy-induced nausea and vomiting. A University of Rochester Cancer Center Community Clinical Oncology Program multicenter study. *J Pain Symptom Manage.* 2003;26: 731–742.

242. Schlager A, Boehler M, Puhringer F. Korean hand acupressure reduces postoperative vomiting in children after strabismus surgery. *Br J Anaesth.* 2000;85:267–270.

243. Shin YH, Kim TI, Shin MS, Juon HS. Effect of acupressure on nausea and vomiting during chemotherapy cycle for Korean postoperative stomach cancer patients. *Cancer Nurs.* 2004; 27:267–274.

244. Slotnick RN. Safe, successful nausea suppression in early pregnancy with P-6 acustimulation. *J Reprod Med.* 2001;46: 811–814.

245. Steele NM, French J, Gatherer-Boyles J, Newman S, Leclaire S. Effect of acupressure by sea-bands on nausea and vomiting of pregnancy. *J Obstet Gynecol Neonatal Nurs.* 2001;30:61–70.

246. Stern RM, Jokerst MD, Muth ER, Hollis C. Acupressure relieves the symptoms of motion sickness and reduces abnormal gastric activity. *Altern Ther Health Med.* 2001;7:91–94.

247. Tiran D. Nausea and vomiting in pregnancy: safety and efficacy of self-administered complementary therapies. *Complement Ther Nurs Midwifery.* 2002;8:191–196.

248. Vachiramon A, Wang WC. Acupressure technique to control gag reflex during maxillary impression procedures. *J Prosthet Dent.* 2002;88:236.

249. White PF, Issioui T, Hu J, et al. Comparative efficacy of acustimulation (ReliefBand) versus ondansetron (zofran) in combination with droperidol for preventing nausea and vomiting. *Anesthesiology.* 2002;97:1075–1081.

250. Wright LD. The use of motion sickness bands to control nausea and vomiting in a group of hospice patients. *Am J Hosp Palliat Care.* 2005;22:49–53.

251. Sakurai M, Suleman MI, Morioka N, Akca O, Sessler DI. Minute sphere acupressure does not reduce postoperative pain or morphine consumption. *Anesth Analg.* 2003;96:493–497.

252. Samad K, Afshan G, Kamal R. Effect of acupressure on postoperative nausea and vomiting in laparoscopic cholecystectomy. *J Pak Med Assoc.* 2003;53:68–72.

253. Schultz AA, Andrews AL, Goran SF, Mathew T, Sturdevant N. Comparison of acupressure bands and droperidol for reducing post-operative nausea and vomiting in gynecologic surgery patients. *Appl Nurs Res.* 2003;16:256–265.

254. Windle PE, Borromeo A, Robles H, Ilacio-Uy V. The effects of acupressure on the incidence of postoperative nausea and vomiting in postsurgical patients. *J Perianesth Nurs.* 2001;16: 158–162.

255. Kober A, Scheck T, Schubert B, et al. Auricular acupressure as a treatment for anxiety in prehospital transport settings. *Anesthesiology.* 2003;98:1328–1332.

256. Brady LH, Henry K, Luth JF 2nd, Casper-Bruett KK. The effects of shiatsu on lower back pain. *J Holist Nurs.* 2001;19:57–70.

257. Chung UL, Hung LC, Kuo SC, Huang CL. Effects of LI4 and BL 67 acupressure on labor pain and uterine contractions in the first stage of labor. *J Nurs Res.* 2003;11:251–260.

258. Hsieh LL, Kuo CH, Yen MF, Chen TH. A randomized controlled clinical trial for low back pain treated by acupressure and physical therapy. *Prev Med.* 2004;39:168–176.

259. Kober A, Scheck T, Greher M, et al. Prehospital analgesia with acupressure in victims of minor trauma: a prospective, randomized, double-blinded trial. *Anesth Analg.* 2002;95:723–727.

260. Lee TA. Chinese way of easing pain: acupressure. *Int J Altern Med.* 2002;1:1.

261. Yip YB, Tse SH. The effectiveness of relaxation acupoint stimulation and acupressure with aromatic lavender essential oil for non-specific low back pain in Hong Kong: a randomised controlled trial. *Complement Ther Med.* 2004;12:28–37.

262. Chen ML, Lin LC, Wu SC, Lin JG. The effectiveness of acupressure in improving the quality of sleep of institutionalized residents. *J Gerontol A Biol Sci Med Sci.* 1999;54:M389–M394.

263. Shen P. Two hundred cases of insomnia treated by otopoint pressure plus acupuncture. *J Tradit Chin Med.* 2004;24: 168–169.

264. Tsay SL, Chen ML. Acupressure and quality of sleep in patients with end-stage renal disease: a randomized controlled trial. *Int J Nurs Stud.* 2003;40:1–7.

265. Tsay SL, Rong JR, Lin PF. Acupoints massage in improving the quality of sleep and quality of life in patients with end-stage renal disease. *J Adv Nurs.* 2003;42:134–142.

266. Wang XH, Yuan YD, Wang BF. Clinical observation on effect of auricular acupoint pressing in treating sleep apnea syndrome. *Zhongguo Zhong Xi Yi Jie He Za Zhi.* 2003;23:747–749.

267. Chen LL, Hsu SF, Wang MH, Chen CL, Lin YD, Lai JS. Use of acupressure to improve gastrointestinal motility in women after trans-abdominal hysterectomy. *Am J Chin Med.* 2003; 31:781–790.

268. Jeon SY, Jung HM. The effects of abdominal meridian massage on constipation among CVA patients. *Taehan Kanho Hakhoe Chi.* 2005;35:135–142.

269. Maa SH, Gauthier D, Turner M. Acupressure as an adjunct to a pulmonary rehabilitation program. *J Cardiopulm Rehabil.* 1997;17:268–276.

270. Maa SH, Sun MF, Hsu KH, et al. Effect of acupuncture or acupressure on quality of life of patients with chronic obstructive asthma: a pilot study. *J Altern Complement Med.* 2003;9: 659–670.

271. Beal MW. Acupuncture and acupressure. Applications to women's reproductive health care. *J Nurse Midwifery.* 1999; 44:217–230.

272. Chen HM, Chen CH. Effects of acupressure at the Sanyinjiao point on primary dysmenorrhoea. *J Adv Nurs.* 2004;48:380–387.

273. Taylor D, Miaskowski C, Kohn J. A randomized clinical trial of the effectiveness of an acupressure device (Relief Brief) for managing symptoms of dysmenorrhea. *J Altern Complement Med.* 2002;8:357–370.

274. Cho YC, Tsay SL. The effect of acupressure with massage on fatigue and depression in patients with end-stage renal disease. *J Nurs Res.* 2004;12:51–59.

275. Andrade C, Randall T, Swift T, Brescia N. The effect of a self-managed manual trigger point pressure program with a hand-held massage device on trigger point sensitivity, perceived pain levels, and frequency of self-care in adults with chronic myofascial neck pain. Project report. Oakland, CA: Samuel Merritt College; 1997.

## Further Reading

Airaksinen O. Changes in post-traumatic ankle joint mobility, pain and oedema following intermittent pneumatic compression therapy. *Arch Phys Med Rehabil.* 1997;70:341–344.

Airaksinen O, Partanen K, Kolari PJ, Soimalkallio S. Intermittent pneumatic compression therapy in post-traumatic lower limb edema: computed tomography and clinical measurements. *Arch Phys Med Rehabil.* 1991;72:667–670.

Aldridge S. Brain-injured turn to CAM therapies. *Massage Magazine.* 2003:28.

Allardice P. The no-surgery face lift. *Natural Way for Better Health.* 1997;3:22.

Alexander R, Bennet-Clerk HC. Storage of elastic energy in muscles and other tissues. *Nature.* 1977;265:114–117.

Angus S. Massage therapy for sprinters and runners. *Clin Podiatr Med Surg.* 2001;18:329–336.

Anonymous. Case problem: presenting conventional and complementary approaches for relieving nausea in a breast cancer patient undergoing chemotherapy. *J Am Diet Assoc.* 2000;100:257–259.

Anonymous. Physical therapy cures postpartum stress incontinence. *BMJ.* 2004;329:1296–1296.

Archer PA. Three clinical sports massage approaches for treating injured athletes. *Athletic Therapy Today.* 2001;6:14–20.

Ause-Ellias KL, Richard R, Miller SF, Finley RK Jr. The effect of mechanical compression on chronic hand edema after burn injury: a preliminary report. *J Burn Care Rehabil.* 1994;15:29–33.

Balke B, Anthony J, Wyatt F. The effects of massage treatment on exercise fatigue. *Clin Sports Med.* 1991;12:184–207.

Balla JI. The late whiplash syndrome. *Aust N Z J Surg.* 1980;50:610–614.

Barr JS, Taslitz N. The influence of back massage on autonomic functions. *Phys Ther.* 1970;50:1679–1691.

Bell GW. Aquatic sports massage therapy. *Clin Sports Med.* 1999;18:427–435.

Benjamin PJ. A look back: mechanical massage at the Battle Creek Sanitarium. *Massage Ther J.* 2004;43:138,140–142.

Birukov AA, Peisahov NM. Changes in the psycho-physiological indices using different techniques of sports massage. *Teoriya i Praktika Fizicheskoi Kult (Russian).* 1979;8:21–24. Translated in: Yessis M, ed. *Sov Sports Rev.* 1986;21:29.

Birukov AA, Pogosyan NM. Special means of restoration of work capacity of wrestlers in the periods between bouts. *Teoriya i Praktika Fizicheskoi Kult (Russian).* 1983;3:49–50. Translated in: Yessis M, ed. *Sov Sports Rev.* 1983;19:191–192.

Bodian M. Use of massage following lid surgery. *Eye, Ear, Nose Throat Monthly.* 1969;48:542–545.

Bonica JJ. Management of myofascial pain syndromes in general practice. *JAMA.* 1957;164:732–738.

Bork K, Korting GW, Faust G. Serum enzyme levels after a whole body massage. *Arch Dermatol Forsch (German).* 1971;240:342–348.

Braverman DL, Schulman RA. Massage techniques in rehabilitation medicine. *Phys Med Rehabil Clin N Am.* 1999;10:631–49.

Brown BR. Myofascial syndrome. In: Warfield CA, ed. *Principles and Practice of Pain Management.* New York: McGraw Hill; 1993:259–264.

Burovych AA, Samtsova IA, Manilov IA. An investigation of the effects of individual variants of sports massage on muscle blood circulation. *Sov Sports Sci Rev.* 1989;24:197–200.

Buskila D. Fibromyalgia, chronic fatigue syndrome, and myofascial pain syndrome. *Curr Opin Rheumatol.* 2001;13:117–127.

Cady SH, Jones CE. Massage therapy as a workplace intervention for reduction of stress. *Percept Motor Skills.* 1997;84:157–158.

Cailliet R. *Soft Tissue Pain and Disability.* Philadelphia: FA Davis; 1996.

Carrier EB. Studies on the physiology of capillaries: reaction of human skin capillaries to drugs and other stimuli. *Am J Physiol.* 1922;11:528–547.

Cawley N. A critique of the methodology of research studies evaluating massage. *Eur J Cancer Care (Engl).* 1997;6:23–31.

Chaitow L. What is NMT? *J Bodywork Movement Ther.* 1999;3:1–2.

Cheung K, Hume P, Maxwell L. Delayed onset muscle soreness: treatment strategies and performance factors. *Sports Med.* 2003;33:145–164.

Chor H, Cleveland D, Davenport HA, et al. Atrophy and regeneration of the gastrocnemius-soleus muscles: effects of physical therapy in monkeys following section and suture of sciatic nerve. *JAMA.* 1939;113:1029–1033.

Chor H, Dolkart RE. A study of simple disuse atrophy in the monkey. *Am J Physiol.* 1936;117:4.

Curties D. Could massage therapy promote cancer metastasis? *J Soft Tissue Manip.* 1994;April–May:3–7.

Danneskiold-Samsøe B, Christiansen E. The effect of massage on muscle infiltrations as assessed by myoglobin in the blood. *Ugeskr Laeger.* 1985;147:269–271.

Danneskiold-Samsøe B, Christiansen E, Lund B, Anderson RB. Regional muscle tension and pain ("fibrositis"): effect of massage on myoglobin in plasma. *Scand J Rehabil Med.* 1982;15:17–20.

Davidson K, Jacoby S, Brown MS. Prenatal perineal massage: preventing lacerations during delivery. *J Obstet Gynecol Neonatal Nurs.* 2000;29:474–479.

Dejung B. Manual trigger point treatment in chronic lumbosacral pain. *Schweiz Med Wochenschr Suppl (German).* 1994;62:82–87.

Delaney GA, McKee AC. Inter- and intra-rater reliability of the pressure threshold meter in measurement of myofascial trigger point sensitivity. *Am J Phys Med Rehab.* 1993;72:136–139.

Delaney JPA, Leong KS, Watkins A, Brodie D. The short-term effects of myofascial trigger point massage therapy on cardiac autonomic tone in healthy subjects. *J Adv Nurs.* 2002;37:364–371.

DeLany JPW. Neuromuscular therapy management: hamstring muscle strain. *J Bodywork Movement Ther.* 1996;1:16–18.

Drust B, Atkinson G, Gregson W, French D, Binningsley D. The effects of massage on intra muscular temperature in the vastus lateralis in humans. *Int J Sports Med.* 2003;24:395–399.

Dubrovsky VI. Changes in muscle and venous flow after massage. *Teoriya i Praktika Fizicheskoi Kult (Russian)*. 1982;4:56–57. Translated in: M Yessis, ed. *Sov Sports Rev*. 1980;18:134–135.

Dunn C, Sleep J, Collett D. Sensing an improvement: an experimental study to evaluate the use of aromatherapy, massage and periods of rest in an intensive care unit. *J Adv Nurs*. 1995;21:34–40.

Edgecombe W, Bain W. The effect of baths, massage and exercise on the blood-pressure. *Lancet*. 1899;1:1552.

Eichelberger G. Study on foot reflex zone massage: alternative to tablets. *Krankenpfl Soins Infirm*. 1993;86:61–63.

Elkins EC, Herrick JF, Grindlay JH, et al. Effects of various procedures on the flow of lymph. *Arch Phys Med*. 1953;34:31.

Elliott M. What future, medical massage? *Massage Bodywork*. 1999;14:128.

Evans RW. Some observations on whiplash injuries. *Neurol Clin*. 1992;10:975–997.

Felhendler D, Lisander B. Effects of non-invasive stimulation of acupoints on the cardiovascular system. *Complement Ther Med*. 1999;7:231–234.

Fernandez de las Penas, C., Sohrbeck Campo M, Fernandez Carnero J, Miangollara Page JC. Manual therapies in myofascial trigger point treatment: a systematic review. *J Bodywork Movement Ther*. 2005;9:27–34.

Field T, Hernandez-Reif M, Shaw KH, et al. Glucose levels decreased after giving massage therapy to children with diabetes mellitus. *Diabetes Spectrum*. 1997;10:23–25.

Field T, Quintino O, Henteleff T, et al. Job stress reduction therapies. *Altern Ther Health Med*. 1997;3:54–56.

Field T, Seligman S, Scafidi F, Schanberg S. Alleviating posttraumatic stress in children following Hurricane Andrew. *J Appl Dev Psychol*. 1996;17:37–50.

Field T, Sunshine W, Hernandez-Reif M, et al. Chronic fatigue syndrome: massage therapy effects on depression and somatic symptoms in chronic fatigue. *J Chron Fatigue Syndrome*. 1997;3:43–51.

Fire M. Providing massage therapy in a psychiatric hospital. *Int J Altern Complement Med*. 1984;June:24–25.

Fischer AA. Documentation of myofascial trigger points. *Arch Phys Med*. 1988;69:286–291.

Fishbain DA, Goldberg M, Steele R, et al. DSM-III diagnoses of patients with myofascial pain syndrome (fibrositis). *Arch Phys Med Rehab*. 1989;70:433–438.

Foda MI, Kawashima T, Nakamura S, Kobayashi M, Oku T. Composition of milk obtained from unmassaged versus massaged breasts of lactating mothers. *J Pediatr Gastroenterol Nutr*. 2004;38:484–487.

Fricton JR. Clinical care for myofascial pain. *Dent Clin North Am*. 1991;35:1–26.

Fricton JR, Kroening R, Haley D. Myofascial pain syndrome: a review of 168 cases. *Oral Surf*. 1982;60:615–623.

Gardener AMN, Fox RH, Lawrence C, et al. Reduction of post-traumatic swelling and compartment pressure by impulse compression of the foot. *J Bone Joint Surg*. 1990;72:810–815.

Goats GC. Massage—the scientific basis of an ancient art: part 1. The techniques. *Br J Sports Med*. 1994;28:149–152.

Goats GC. Massage—the scientific basis of an ancient art: part 2. Physiological and therapeutic effects. *Br J Sports Med*. 1994;28:153–156.

Goldman LB, Rosenberg NL. Myofascial pain syndrome and fibromyalgia. *Semin Neurol*. 1991;11:274–280.

Graff-Radford SB, Reeves JL, Baker RL, Chiu D. Effects of transcutaneous electrical nerve stimulation on myofascial pain and trigger point sensitivity. *Pain*. 1989;37:1–5.

Grimsby D, Grimsby K. Electromyographic and range of motion evaluation to compare the results of two treatment approaches: soft tissue massage versus a segmental manipulation off the cervical spine. *Ned Tijdschr Manuele Ther*. 1993;12:2–7.

Guan Z, Zheng G. The effects of massage on the left heart functions in patients of coronary heart disease. *J Tradit Chin Med*. 1995; 15:59–62.

Gulla J, Singer AJ. Use of alternative therapies among emergency department patients. *Ann Emerg Med*. 2000;35:226–228.

Gunn CC. *Treating Myofascial Pain: Intramuscular Stimulation for Myofascial Pain Syndromes of Neuropathic Origin*. Seattle: University of Washington; 1989.

Gusarova SA, Kuznetsov OF, Gorbunov FE, Maslovskaia SG. The use of point massage in patients with circulatory encephalopathy. *Vopr Kurortol Fizioter Lech Fiz Kult (Russian)*. 1997;6:11–13.

Hack GD, Robinson WL, Koritzer RT. Previously undescribed relation between muscle and dura. Proceedings of the Congress of Neurological Surgeons. Phoenix, AZ, February 14–18, 1995.

Hartman PS. Management of myofascial dysfunction of the shoulder. In: Donatelli RA, ed. *Physical Therapy of the Shoulder*. New York: Churchill Livingstone; 1991.

Hawk C, Long CR, Reiter R, Davis CS, Cambron JA, Evans R. Issues in planning a placebo-controlled trial of manual methods: results of a pilot study. *J Altern Complement Med*. 2002;8: 21–32.

Hemphill L, Kemp J. Implementing a therapeutic massage program in a tertiary and ambulatory care VA setting: the healing power of touch. *Nurs Clin North Am*. 2000;35:489–497.

Hernandez-Reif M, Field T, Hart S. Smoking cravings are reduced by self-massage. *Prev Med*. 1999;28:28–32.

Hernandez-Reif M, Field T, Theakson J, Field T. Multiple sclerosis patients benefit from massage therapy. *J Bodywork Move Ther*. 1998;2:168–174.

Hernandez-Reif M, Martinez A, Field T, Quintero O, Hart S, Burman I. Premenstrual symptoms are relieved by massage therapy. *J Psychosom Obstet Gynaecol*. 2000;21:9–15.

Hey LR, Helewa A. Myofascial pain syndrome: a critical review of the literature. *Physiol Can*. 1994;46:28–36.

Hinz B. Perineal massage in pregnancy. *J Midwifery Womens Health*. 2005;50:63–64.

Hobbs S, Davies PD. Critical review of how nurses research massage therapy: are they using the best methods? *Complement Ther Nurs Midwifery*. 1998;4:35–40.

Holmes MH, Lai WM, Mow VC. Compression effects on cartilage permeability. In: Hargens AR, ed. *Tissue Nutrition and Viability*. New York: Springer-Verlag; 1986.

Hondras MA, Linde K, Jones AP. Manual therapy for asthma. *Cochrane Database Syst Rev*. 2000;2:CD001002.

Hong CZ, Simons DG. Pathophysiologic and electrophysiologic mechanisms of myofascial trigger points. *Arch Phys Med Rehabil*. 1998;79:863–872.

Huang FY, Huang LM. Effect of local massage on vaccination: DTP and DTPa. *Chung Hua Min Kuo Hsiao Erh Ko I Hsueh Hui Tsa Chih*. 1999;40:166–170.

Hulme J, Waterman H, Hillier VF. The effect of foot massage on patients' perception of care following laparoscopic sterilization as day case patients. *J Adv Nurs.* 1999;30:460–468.

Issel C. The roots of reflexology. *Massage Bodywork.* 2003;18:52.

Jacobs M. Massage for the relief of pain: anatomical and physiological considerations. *Phys Ther Rev.* 1960;40:93–98.

Jami L. Golgi tendon organs in mammalian skeletal muscle: functional properties and central actions. *Physiol Rev.* 1992;73:623–666.

Janda V. On the concept of postural muscles and posture in man. *Aust J Physiother.* 1983;20:83–84.

Jimenez AC, Lane ME. Serial determinations of pressure threshold tolerance in chronic pain patients. *Arch Phys Med Rehab.* 1985;66:545–546.

Jones DA, Round JM. *Skeletal Muscle in Health and Disease.* Manchester, United Kingdom: Manchester University Press; 1990.

Jones NA, Field T. Massage and music therapies attenuate frontal EEG asymmetry in depressed adolescents. *Adolescence.* 1999; 34:529–534.

Jordan KD, Jessup D. The recuperative effects of sports massage as compared to rest. *Massage Ther J.* 1990;Winter:57–67.

Katz J, Wowk A, Culp D, Wakeling BA. A randomized, controlled study of the pain- and tension-reducing effects of 15 minute workplace massage treatments versus seated rest for nurses in a large teaching hospital. *Pain Res Manage.* 1999;4:81–88.

Katz J, Wowk A, Culp D, Wakeling H. Pain and tension are reduced among hospital nurses after on-site massage treatments: a pilot study. *J Perianaesth Nurs.* 1999;14:128–133.

Kelley D. Neuromuscular therapy for headache. *J Bodywork Movement Ther.* 1997;1:73–175.

Kinney BM. External fatty tissue massage (the "Endermologie" and "silhouette" procedures). *Plast Reconstr Surg.* 1997;100:1903–1904.

Kniazeva TA, Minenkov AA, Kul'chitskaia DB, Apkhanova TV. Effect of physiotherapy on the microcirculation in patients with lymphedema of lower extremities. *Vopr Kurortol Fizioter Lech Fiz Kult.* 2003;1:30–32.

Kolich M, Taboun SM, Mohamed AI. Low back muscle activity in an automobile seat with a lumbar massage system. *Int J Occup Saf Ergon.* 2000;6:113–128.

Kraus H, ed. *Diagnosis and Treatment of Muscle Pain.* Chicago: Quintessence; 1988.

Krilov VN, Talishev FM, Burovikh AN. The use of restorative massage in the training of high level basketball players. *Sov Sci Rev.* 1985;20:7–9.

Kristof O, Schlumpf M, Saller R. Foot reflex zone massage: a review. *Wien Med Wochenschr.* 1997;147:418–422.

Kristof O, Schlumpf M, Saller R. Foot reflex zone massage: general practice and evaluation. *Fortschr Med.* 1998;116:50–54.

Labrecque M, Eason E, Marcoux S. Perineal massage in pregnancy: such massage significantly decreases perineal trauma at birth. *BMJ.* 2001;323:753–754.

Labrecque M, Eason E, Marcoux S. Women's views on the practice of prenatal perineal massage. *BJOG.* 2001;108:499–504.

Ladd MP, Kottke FJ, Blanchard RS. Studies of the effect of massage on the flow of lymph from the foreleg of the dog. *Arch Phys Med.* 1952;33:604–612.

Lee YH. The effects of a foot-reflexo-massage education program on foot care in diabetic patients. *Taehan Kanho Hakhoe Chi.* 2003;33:633–642.

Lett A. The scope and limitations of treatment. An interview with Ann Lett, principle, British School: reflex zone therapy of the feet. *Complement Ther Nurs Midwifery.* 2001;7:146–149.

Le-Vu B, Dumortier A, Guillaume MV, et al. Efficacy of massage and mobilization of the upper limb after surgical treatment of breast cancer. *Bull Cancer (French).* 1997;84:957–961.

Li Z, Liu J, Wu Y, et al. Effect of massotherapy on the in vivo free radical metabolism in patients with prolapse of lumbar intervertebral disc and cervical spondylopathy. *J Tradit Chin Med.* 1995;15:53–58.

Linde B, Philip A. Massage-enhanced insulin-absorption—increased distribution or dissociation of insulin? *Diabetes Res.* 1989:11: 191–194.

Lipton SA. Prevention of classic migraine headache by digital massage of the superficial temporal arteries during visual aura. *Ann Neurol.* 1986;19:515–516 (Letter).

Losito JM, O'Neil J. Rehabilitation of foot and ankle injuries. *Clin Podiatr Med Surg.* 1997;14:533–557.

Lowe JC, Honeyman-Lowe G. Facilitating the decrease in fibromyalgic pain during metabolic rehabilitation: an essential role for soft tissue therapies. *J Bodywork Move Ther.* 1998;2:208–217.

Lucas KR, Polus BI, Rich PA. Latent myofascial trigger points: their effects on muscle activation and movement efficiency. *J Bodywork Movement Ther.* 2004;8:160–166.

Lund I, Lundeberg T, Kurosawa M, Uvnas-Moberg K. Sensory stimulation (massage) reduces blood pressure in unanaesthetized rats. *J Auton Nerv Syst.* 1999;78:30–37.

Lynn J. Using complementary therapies: reflexology. *Prof Nurse.* 1996;11:321–322.

Manyam BV, Sanchez-Ramos JR. Traditional and complementary therapies in Parkinson's disease. *Adv Neurol.* 1999;80:565–574.

McCaffrey R, Taylor N. Effective anxiety treatment prior to diagnostic cardiac catheterization. *Holist Nurs Pract.* 2005;19:70–73.

McCain GA. Treatment of fibromyalgia and myofascial pain syndromes. In: Rachlin ES, ed. *Myofascial Pain and Fibromyalgia.* St. Louis: Mosby Year Book; 1994:31–44.

McCain GA, Scudds RA. The concept of primary fibromyalgia (fibrositis): clinical value, relation and significance to other chronic musculoskeletal pain syndromes. *Pain.* 1988;33:273–287.

McCandlish R. Perineal trauma: prevention and treatment. *J Midwifery Womens Health.* 2001;46:396–401.

McPartland JM. Travell trigger points: molecular and osteopathic perspectives. *J Am Osteopath Assoc.* 2004;104:244–249.

Miller L H, Smith AD, Mehler BL. Stress Audit. Brookline, MA: Biobehavioral Associates; 1987.

Molea D, Mucek B, Blanken C, et al. Evaluation of two manipulative techniques in the treatment of post exercise muscle soreness. *J Am Osteopath Assoc.* 1987;87 477–483.

Morelli M, Chapman CE, Sullivan SJ. Do cutaneous receptors contribute to the changes in the amplitude of the H-reflex during massage? *Electromyogr Clin Neurophysiol.* 1999;39:441–447.

Morhenn VB. Firm stroking of human skin leads to vasodilatation possibly due to the release of substance P. *J Dermatol Sci.* 2000;22:138–144.

Nguyen HP, Le DL, Tran QM, et al. CHROMASSI: a therapy advice system based on chrono-massage and acupression using the method of ZiWuLiuZhu. *Medinfo* 1995;8:998.

Nordschow M, Bierman W. The influence of manual massage on muscle relaxation: effect on trunk flexion. *J Am Phys Ther Assoc.* 1962;42:653–657.

Nussbaum EL, Downes L. Reliability of clinical pressure-pain algometric measurements obtained on consecutive days. *Phys Ther.* 1998;78:160–169.

Oates-Whitehead R. Nausea and vomiting in early pregnancy. *Clin Evid.* 2004;11:1840–1852.

Omura Y. Simple and quick non-invasive evaluation of circulatory condition of cerebral arteries by clinical application of the "bidigital O-ring test." *Acupunct Electrother Res.* 1985;10:139–161.

Ortego, NE. Acupressure: an alternative approach to mental health counseling through body-mind awareness. *Nurse Pract Forum.* 1994;5:72–76.

Oschman JL. Acupuncture and related methods: energy review part 1B. *J Bodywork Movement Ther.* 1996;1:40–43.

Paikov VB. Means of restoration in the training of speed skaters. *Sov Sports Rev.* 1988;20:7–12.

Partsch H, Mostbeck A, Leitner G. Experimental studies on the efficacy of pressure wave massage (Lymphapress) in lymphedema. *Z Lymphol (German).* 1981;5:35–39.

Petermans J, Zicot M. Musculo-venous pump in the elderly. *J Mal Vasc.* 1994;19:115–118.

Pfaffenrath V, Rehm M. Migraine in pregnancy: what are the safest treatment options? *Drug Safety.* 1998;19:383–388.

Potapov IA, Abisheva TM. The action of massage on lymph formation and transport. *Vopr Kurortol Fizioter Lech Fiz Kult (Russian).* 1989;5:44–47.

Poznick-Patewitz E. Cephalic spasm of head and neck muscles. *Headache.* 1976;15:261–266.

Rachlin ES. Musculofascial pain syndromes. *Med Times.* 1984:34–47.

Rachlin ES. Trigger point management. In: Rachlin ES, ed. *Myofascial Pain and Fibromyalgia.* St. Louis: Mosby Year Book; 1994:173–195.

Rachlin I. Therapeutic massage in the treatment of myofascial pain syndromes and fibromyalgia. In: Rachlin ES, ed. *Myofascial Pain and Fibromyalgia.* St. Louis: Mosby Year Book; 1994: 173–195.

Reeves JL, Jaeger B, Graff-Radford SB. Reliability of the pressure algometer as a measure of myofascial trigger point sensitivity. *Pain.* 1986;24:313–321.

Rubin D. Myofascial trigger point syndromes: an approach to management. *Arch Phys Med Rehabil.* 1981;62:107–110.

Sa'adah S. Perineal massage to prevent perineal trauma during pregnancy. *J Fam Pract.* 1999;48:494–495.

Sander M, Siegert R, Gundlach KK. Results of physiotherapy for patients with myofacial dysfunction. *Dtsch Zahnarztl Z (German).* 1989;44:S12–S14.

Sandler S. The physiology of soft tissue massage. *J Bodywork Movement Ther.* 1999;3:118–122.

Schneider W, Dvorak J. Functional treatment of diseases and injuries of the cervical spine. *Orthopade (German).* 1996;25:519–523.

Schuler L. A new fix for old injuries. *Men's Health.* 1999;14:80.

Scifres C. Neuromuscular therapy for groin strain. *J Bodywork Movement Ther.* 1998;2:148–154.

Scifres C. Neuromuscular therapy management of tenosynovitis. *J Bodywork Movement Ther.* 1997;1:150–154.

Scudds RA, Trachsel LCE, Luckhurst BJ, Percy JS. A comparative study of pain, sleep quality and pain responsiveness in fibrositis and myofascial pain syndrome. *J Rheum.* 1989;16(Suppl 19):120–126.

Severini V, Venerando A. The physiological effects of massage on the cardiovascular system. *Eur Medicophys.* 1967;3:165–183.

Simons DG. Muscular pain syndromes. In: Fricton JR, Awad EA, eds. *Advances in Pain Research and Therapy.* Volume 17. New York: Raven Press; 1990.

Simons DG, Mense S. Diagnosis and therapy of myofascial trigger points. *Schmerz.* 2003;17:419–424.

Simons DG, Simons LS. Chronic myofascial pain syndrome. In: Tollison CD, ed. *Handbook of Chronic Pain Management.* Baltimore: Williams & Wilkins; 1989:509–529.

Sinyakov AF, Belov ES. Restoration of work capacity of gymnasts. *Gymnastika.* 1982;1:48–51.

Snyder-Mackler LS, Bork C, Bourbon B, Trumbore D. Effect of helium-neon laser on musculoskeletal trigger points. *Phys Ther.* 1986;66:1087–1090.

Sola AE. Trigger point therapy. In: Robers JR, Hooges JR, eds. *Clinical Procedures in Emergency Medicine.* Philadelphia: WB Saunders; 1985.

Sola AE, Rodenberger MS, Gettys BB. Incidence of hypersensitive areas in posterior shoulder muscles: a survey of two hundred young adults. *Am J Phys Med.* 1955;34:585–590.

Stamp GE, Kruzins GS. A survey of midwives who participated in a randomised trial of perineal massage in labour. *Aust J Midwifery.* 2001;14:15–21.

Stamp G, Kruzins G, Crowther C. Perineal massage in labour and prevention of perineal trauma. *BMJ.* 2001;322:1277.

Stephenson NL, Dalton JA. Using reflexology for pain management. A review. *J Holist Nurs.* 2003;21:179–191.

Strong TH Jr. Alternative therapies of morning sickness. *Clin Obstet Gynecol.* 2001;44:653–660.

Sullivan SJ, Blumberger J, Lachowicz C, Raymond D. Does massage decrease laryngeal tension in a subject with complete tetraplegia. *Percept Motor Skills.* 1997;84:169–170.

Sunshine W, Field T, Schanberg S, et al. Massage therapy and transcutaneous electrical stimulation effects on fibromyalgia. *J Clin Rheumatol.* 1997;2:18–22.

Suskind MI, Hajek NA, Hines HM. Effects of massage on denervated skeletal muscle. *Arch Phys Med.* 1946;27:133–135.

Takeuchi H, Jawad MS, Eccles R. The effects of nasal massage of the "yingxiang" acupuncture point on nasal airway resistance and sensation of nasal airflow in patients with nasal congestion associated with acute upper respiratory tract infection. *Am J Rhinol.* 1999;13:77–79.

Travell J. Pain mechanisms in connective tissue. In: Ragan C, ed. *Connective Tissues, Transactions of the Second Conference, 1951.* New York: Josiah Macy Jr Foundation; 1952:90,92–94,105, 119,121.

Travell JG, Rinzler SH. The myofascial genesis of pain. *Postgrad Med.* 1952;11:425–434.

Tunnell PW. Protocol for visual assessment: postural evaluation of the muscular system through visual inspection. *J Bodywork Movement Ther.* 1996;1:21–27.

Urba SG. Non-pharmacologic pain management in terminal care. *Clin Geriatr Med.* 1996;12:301–311.

Valtonen EJ. Syncardial massage for treating extremities swollen by traumata, vein diseases or idiopathic lymphedema. *Acta Chir Scand.* 1967;133:363–367.

Wakim KG, Martin GM, Krusen FH. Influence of centripetal rhythmic compression on localized edema of an extremity. *Arch Phys Med.* 1955;36:98.

Wakim KG, Martin GM, Terrier JC, et al. Effects of massage on the circulation in normal and paralyzed extremities. *Arch Phys Med.* 1949;30:135–144.

Walling AD. Perineal massage during labor offers limited benefit. *Am Fam Physician.* 2001;64:1888.

Watson S, Watson S. The effects of massage: an holistic approach to care. *Nurs Stand.* 1997;11:45–47.

Weerapong P, Hume PA, Kolt GS. The mechanisms of massage and effects on performance, muscle recovery and injury prevention. *Sports Med.* 2005;35:235–256.

Weiss JM. Pelvic floor myofascial trigger points: manual therapy for interstitial cystitis and the urgency-frequency syndrome. *J Urol.* 2001;166:2226–2231.

Wilkinson S, Aldridge J, Salmon I, Cain E, Wilson B. An evaluation of aromatherapy massage in palliative care. *Palliat Med.* 1999; 13:409–417.

Williams PE, Goldspink G. Changes in sarcomere length and physiological properties of immobilised muscle. *J Anat.* 1978;127: 459–468.

Yunus MB. Fibromyalgia syndrome and myofascial pain syndrome: clinical features, laboratory tests, diagnosis, and pathophysiologic mechanisms. In: Rachlin ES, ed. *Myofascial Pain and Fibromyalgia.* St. Louis: Mosby Year Book; 1994:3–29.

Yunus MB, Kalyan-Raman UP, Kalyan-Raman K. Primary fibromyalgia syndrome and myofascial pain syndrome: clinical features and muscle pathology. *Arch Phys Med Rehab.* 1988;69:451–454.

Yunus MB, Masi AT, Aldag JC. A controlled study of primary fibromyalgia syndrome: clinical features and association with other functional syndromes. *J Rheumatol.* 1989;16(Suppl 19):62–71.

Zalessky M. Coaching, medico-biological and psychological means of restoration. *Legkaya Atletika (Russian).* 1979;2:20–22.

Zalessky M. Restoration for middle, long-distance, steeplechase and marathon runners and speed walkers. *Legkaya Atletika (Russian).* 1980;3:10–13.

Zeitlin D, Keller SE, Shiflett SC, Schleifer SJ, Bartlett JA. Immunological effects of massage therapy during academic stress. *Psychosom Med.* 2000;62:83–84.

# Chapter 10

## Connective Tissue Techniques

Connective tissue techniques are those massage techniques that palpate, lengthen, and promote remodeling of connective tissue. These techniques include: skin rolling, myofascial release, direct fascial technique, and friction. This chapter describes these techniques, how to perform them, and how to apply them in a practice sequence. A section on further study for each technique discusses relevant outcomes and evidence, cautions and contraindications, and how to use the technique in treatment.

### Table 10-1 Summary of Outcomes for Connective Tissue Techniques

| Outcomes | Technique | | | |
| --- | --- | --- | --- | --- |
| | **Skin Rolling** | **Myofascial Release** | **Direct Fascial Technique** | **Friction** |
| Decreased resting muscle tension or neuromuscular tone | ? | P | P | ? |
| Separation/lengthening of fascia | P | ✓ | P | P |
| Promotion of dense connective tissue remodeling | ? | P | P | P |
| Increased muscle extensibility | ? | ✓ | P | P |
| Increased joint range of motion | P | ✓ | ✓ | ✓ |
| Systemic sedation/decreased anxiety | ? | P | ✓ | ? |
| Increased rib cage mobility | ? | P | P | ? |
| Decreased trigger point activity | ? | ✓ | P | P |
| Pain reduction | P | ✓ | ✓ | ✓ |
| Normalized structural alignment | ? | ✓ | ✓ | ? |
| Balance of agonist/antagonist function | ? | P | ✓ | ? |
| Improved quality and quantity of movement | ? | P | ✓ | P |
| Enhanced muscle performance | ? | P | ✓ | ? |

✓: the outcome is supported by research summarized in this chapter. P: the outcome is possible. ?: the outcome is debatable (research results are absent or inconsistent).

## Skin Rolling: Foundations

# DEFINITION

Skin rolling: A gliding stroke in which the therapist grasps the tissues superficial to the investing layer of deep fascia and continuously lifts and rolls it over underlying tissues in a wave-like motion.[1–3]

# USES

Therapists use skin rolling to assess and treat restrictions in the mobility of the client's skin and **superficial fascia**. These superficial restrictions may be the result of burns, wounds, surgery, orthopedic injuries,[3–5] chronically elevated levels of resting muscle tension, **segmental vertebral dysfunction**, or organic pathology.[5–7]

# PALPATION PRACTICE

1. For different areas of the body, using fingertips and very light pressure, **drag** the skin in various directions. How far does the skin move before you have taken up all the slack and begin to **glide**? Why is there more skin mobility in some areas than others? If you can, repeat the same exercise with an elderly partner.
2. For all regions of the body, using fingertip palpation, estimate and record the thickness of the tissue layer that is superficial to the **investing layer of deep fascia** and that consists of the skin, superficial fascia, and subcutaneous fat. Compare the thickness in different regions and on different models.
3. Using adducted fingers opposing your thumb, grasp and lift the layer superficial to the investing layer of deep fascia. You can reduce pinching by having 1 to 2 inches between your fingers and thumb before you grasp. How easily does the tissue lift? Once you have lifted a fold or roll of superficial tissue, gently attempt to pull the tissue in various directions without releasing your grasp. How far does it go? Does it go more easily in some directions than others? Compare all the regions, and compare several models. For example, what might explain the consistent difference between mobility of the superficial tissues on the dorsal and palmar surfaces of the hand?

 Critical Thinking Question

Which characteristics and effects of skin rolling result in therapists sometimes classifying it as a form of petrissage?

---

**Theory in Practice 10-1**

### Connective Tissue Techniques

**Patient Profile**

Your patient is a 30-year-old avid, accomplished recreational downhill skier who fractured his left lower tibia (a boot top fracture) 2 years ago. The fracture healed to the orthopedist's satisfaction. After cast removal, the patient completed several months of physical therapy that emphasized **strength** training. He returned to skiing the following season.

**Clinical Findings**

Subjective:
- Low-grade **pain**, fatigue, and **stiffness** in the left lower leg after skiing for more than 2 hours
- Reports that the leg "hasn't felt 100%" since the injury

Objective:
- Posture: Standing posture is within normal limits. The left lower leg appears to be slightly larger than the right.
- Girth: The left leg is 2 cm larger in circumference than the right leg at the level of the fracture.
- Gait: Gait is within normal limits.
- Palpation: The swelling in the region of the fraction does not feel fluid or watery. There is tenderness to deep palpation throughout the left lower leg.
- Range of Motion: Mild reduction in active and passive motion of the left ankle (10%), with stiffness at the end of range.
- Strength: Grade 5 strength throughout the lower extremities.

**Treatment Approach**

- Despite the time that has elapsed since his injury, this patient presents with signs of chronic inflammation. Clients who have sustained a serious trauma may present with residual impairments that are associated with poor modeling of connective tissue. In this case, the initial treatment outcome is to reduce the connective tissue restriction (**consolidated edema**), which is a likely result of the inflammatory process from 2 years ago.

■ You can achieve this treatment goal by using all four connective tissue techniques described in this chapter. In doing so, you will apply them from superficial layers to deep layers and focus on the client's affected lower leg. You may also find it beneficial to perform specific and deep direct fascial technique and friction throughout the area of swelling and at the fracture site on the tibia. In addition, you can use deep petrissage, stripping, and specific compression throughout the region.

■ If you are able to achieve therapeutic depth for these techniques, then you may need only 1 to 2 hours to restore full mobility to the client's affected leg. Finally, you must also allot a certain portion of each session to the other leg and the back in order to maintain comparable levels of resting tension, **myofascial balance**, and symmetry.

■ The patient's homecare should include: stretching of lower leg muscles, resumption of his prior strength training program for a couple of weeks, and *careful, incremental* increase of his skiing activity.

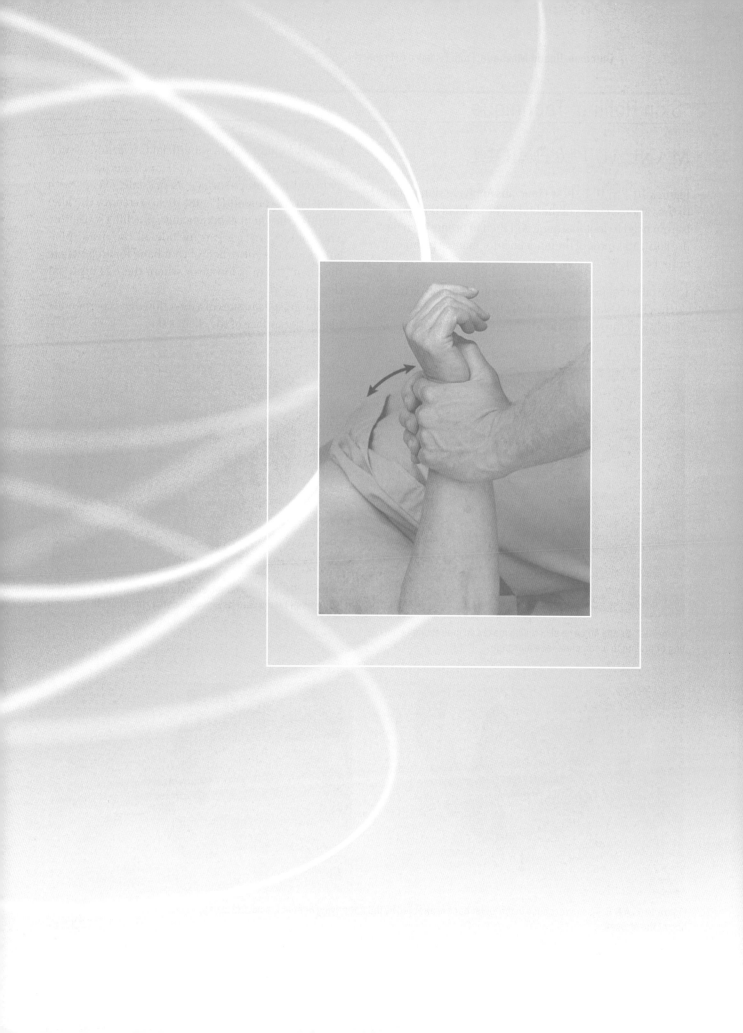

## Skin Rolling: Technique

# MANUAL TECHNIQUE

Figures 10-1 to 10-6 show clinicians applying skin rolling to the various regions of the body. The order of the figures is from head to foot in supine and then in prone. Each figure illustrates most of the guidelines for manual technique outlined below.

1.  No oil is required. Remove all previously applied oil from the client's skin. You can apply this technique reasonably well through fabric.

2.  Grasp the client's skin, superficial fascia, and associated fat between your thumb(s) and fingertips(s). Use as broad a contact surface as possible, except with small body segments (Figure 10-1), to reduce the likelihood of the client experiencing a pinching sensation. The contact surface can include all the distal phalanges and the entire heel of your hand for areas where the client's skin is looser or where there is more fat (Figure 10-5).

3.  Lift the grasped tissues in a direction that is perpendicular to the surface of the client's skin.

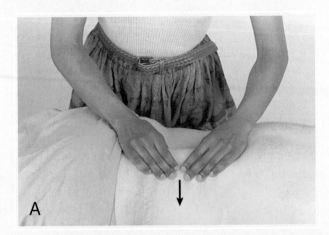

**Figure 10-1**  Gentle fingertip skin rolling makes an interesting beginning or ending to a complete face massage.

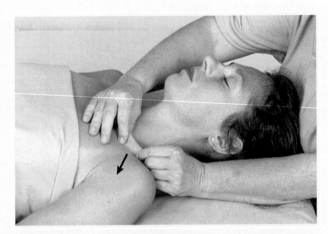

**Figure 10-2**  Skin rolling over the clavicle and anterior neck engages the superficial fascia with its embedded platysma muscle.

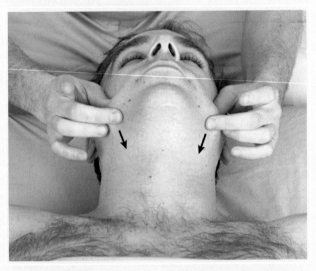

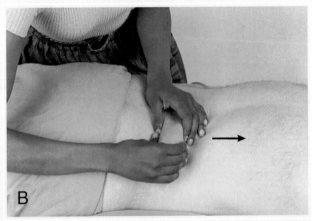

**Figure 10-3**  A & B. Tissue response in the lower back is affected by the underlying lumbar fascia and usually varies with the direction of the strokes.

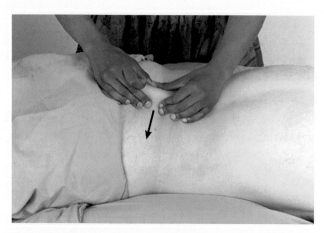

**Figure 10-4** Skin and superficial fascia in the region of the sacrum lie over dense fascial attachments and lift less easily.

4. Simultaneously maintain the stretch on the client's tissues and roll the superficial tissues along the surface in a slow wave. There are two concurrent stretching forces: one perpendicular to the skin, and the other parallel to the skin. A gliding motion occurs as you simultaneously gather and release the client's tissues while maintaining the grasping and lifting motion. Glide and roll the tissue towards or away from yourself. Do not release the roll of tissue until the end of the stroke.

5. Two-handed and single-handed skin rolling are both possible. Skin rolling is easier to perform two-handed with hands side-by-side and working together.

6. You can perform skin rolling in a variety of different directions. Since skin attaches to superficial fascia differently in the various parts of the body, it may be consistently easier to perform skin rolling in a particular direction in a given region (Figures 10-3, 10-4, and 10-6).

7. In an intervention, perform skin rolling over an entire region once, then return to adherent or sensitive spots for additional passes, performing the technique in different directions, until the client's subcutaneous tissues lift easily and any reported sensitivity has decreased.

8. When applied at a slow rate (less than 1 cm/second) and with moderate lifting force, skin rolling can produce a **creep** of the client's superficial fascia—an effect that can affect the underlying investing layer of the deep fascia.

9. Even when therapists apply skin rolling with the broadest hand contact, clients may not be able to tolerate it. If clients are very sensitive to the pressure of skin rolling, you can use a superficial **myofascial release** across the client's skin or a **direct fascial technique** applied with a light pressure and a broad contact surface to obtain similar results.

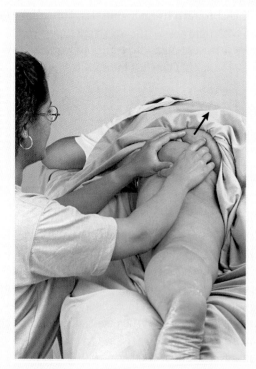

**Figure 10-5** In fatty areas, such as the glutei, a heel-and-fingers contact will include more tissue.

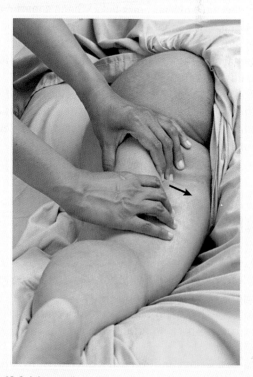

**Figure 10-6** It is usually easier to perform skin rolling around, rather than along, the limbs.

## Box 10-1 | Components of Skin Rolling

**Contact:** Distal phalanges of finger(s) plus your thumb, thenar eminence, or heel of your hand

**Pressure:** Sufficient to allow lifting of the superficial tissues

**Tissues engaged:** Skin, superficial fascia, fat; indirectly engages deeper layers of fascia

**Amplitude/length:** Variable, at the discretion of the therapist

**Rate:** Slow, less than 1–4 cm/second

**Duration:** 30 seconds or greater

**Intergrades with:** Direct fascial technique, petrissage

**Context:** Apply alone to mobilize surface connective tissue restrictions such as **scars**. Apply before and after direct fascial technique or myofascial release to evaluate tissue mobility.

## How skin rolling might work

The mechanical effects of skin rolling are a result of the **tension** that this technique applies to the connective tissue in superficial fascia. In cases of sustained tension, as during slower rates of application, this fascia probably lengthens through a controlled (minor) rupture of **collagen** molecules and **collagen cross-links**.[8] Since superficial and **deep fascia** are continuous,[3–5,8] using a greater, or more sustained, force in skin rolling will transmit tension to the deeper layers of fascia and may produce a smaller lengthening effect there.

The mechanisms for the **somatovisceral reflex** effects,[1,5] which some therapists postulate for this technique, are unclear. See the discussion on **connective tissue zones**[1,5] later in this chapter.

## THERAPIST'S POSITION AND MOVEMENT

1. Use the basic positions described in Chapter 6, Preparation and Positioning for Massage, in the sections on **aligned** standing or sitting positions.
2. Since your hands produce the entire force of skin rolling, you can use any comfortable aligned standing or seated position.
3. Use of a seated position will reduce wrist hyperextension when you are grasping the client's tissues between your fingers and the heels of your hands (Figure 10-4).

## PALPATE

As you perform the technique, palpate the client's skin and tissues for the following:

1. Temperature and texture of the skin.
2. Texture and thickness of superficial fat. **Lipomas** and **fibrositic deposits** are discrete, denser areas of tissue that move readily with the tissue layer. They are common on the back and around the pelvic girdle.
3. Tightness of the superficial fascia. You will perceive this as a resistance to stretching the client's tissues perpendicular to the skin surface; resistance to stretching the tissues parallel to the skin surface; or resistance to ease of rolling the tissues during the stroke.
4. **Viscoelastic** stretch of the tissues. If you perform skin rolling slowly, it may be possible to palpate a slow viscoelastic stretch or "creep" of the client's superficial tissues

## OBSERVE

As you perform the technique, observe the client for the following signs:

1. General appearance of skin, specifically circulatory or **trophic changes**.
2. Visible chronic tension in muscles. This can be associated with tightness of the overlying superficial fascia.
3. Reactive hyperemia. Skin rolling often quickly produces a hyperemia that can last for minutes.

## COMMUNICATION WITH THE CLIENT

Obtain feedback on the client's level of comfort and concerns about the effects of the technique. The following are some examples of statements that you can use.

1. "Let me know if you feel a burning sensation as I roll your skin." Initially, skin rolling produces an unpleasant "burning" sensation as you stretch the client's tight superficial fascia. You cannot completely avoid producing this sensation; therefore, moderate the degree of lift you use in response to the client's feedback or change to a broader connective tissue technique.
2. Reassure the client that skin rolling will not produce stretch marks and that it will not temporarily or permanently slacken healthy skin in any visible way.

**A Practice Sequence for Skin Rolling**

Practice Time: 30 minutes per person.

**Prone**

Undrape half of the client's posterior torso, from the shoulder down to the gluteal fold. Ensure that spinous processes are accessible.

1. Beginning at the shoulder: Lift the client's skin and as much of the subcutaneous fat as possible and roll the tissue down the back and, if possible, buttock in one long uninterrupted movement.
2. Return to the shoulder: Move laterally or medially and make successive passes in the same direction until you have treated all of the exposed area. During application, mentally note where tissue restrictions occur.

3. Cover the same area with similar long parallel "strokes," this time working in a superior direction. Again, mentally note where tissue restrictions occur.
4. Cover the same area with shorter parallel "strokes," this time working from medial to lateral and then lateral to medial. Note differences in the response of the tissue.
5. Return to the areas that appeared to present with greater restriction. Apply the technique repeatedly in a variety of directions.
6. Reassess the quality of the tissue restrictions. You may wish to have the client stand and actively move before you compare the two sides of the body.

Perform a comparable sequence on the other side of the client's body. At the end, investigate how you can apply skin rolling to other areas of the body such as the scalp, hands, feet, and around joints.

Home study: Devise and apply comparable routines for other regions.

# Skin Rolling: Further Study and Practice

## NAMES AND ORIGINS

In other texts or massage-related systems, the technique that we call skin rolling is also known as "rolling" and "tissue rolling."[1-3] "Subcutaneous tissue rolling" would be a more accurate name for this technique; however, the literature consistently uses the term "skin rolling."[1,4-6]

Clinicians often classify this unusual technique as a form of petrissage because it grasps and lifts the tissues (see Chapter 9, Neuromuscular Techniques). Skin rolling is, however, fundamentally different from petrissage in that it is not applied to muscle, but rather to the more superficial subcutaneous tissues.[1-11] The resistance to stretch that clinicians can palpate during the application of this technique is due to tightness in the skin and superficial fascia. That tightness may, in turn, stem from underlying tension in the fascia and muscle. When clinicians apply skin rolling slowly, it produces a **viscoelastic** stretch of the superficial fascia that results in clinical effects and a feel on palpation that is similar to that of other connective tissue techniques described later in this chapter (see Box 10-2).

## OUTCOMES AND EVIDENCE

Skin rolling is a useful technique for both client examination and treatment. The clinician can use skin rolling to assess restrictions in the mobility of the client's skin and superficial fascia, which may be the chronic stage result of burns, wounds, surgery, and orthopedic injuries.[3-5] A client's complaints of pain and palpable tissue resistance during skin rolling may indicate an underlying chronic elevation of **muscle resting tension**, segmental vertebral dysfunction, or organic pathology.[5-7]

As a treatment technique, the clinician can use repetitive applications of skin rolling to improve the mobility of skin and subcutaneous connective tissues and thus to increase joint range of motion.[1-5,12] When the clinician applies skin rolling slowly and with a greater force, the anatomical continuity of fascial layers may result in the mechanical lengthening effects of this technique penetrating to deeper fascial layers. Finally, a common (side) effect of skin rolling is the production of a significant reactive hyperemia.[12]

## EXAMINING THE EVIDENCE

There are few references in the literature on the use of skin rolling as a technique for assessment or treatment. In one simple study, chiropractic researchers assessed the usefulness of skin rolling to identify "segmental spinal dysfunction."[13] One clinician identified areas in the thoracic paraspinal muscles of 25 chiropractic students that were tender upon skin rolling. The clinician also measured sensitivity to pressure in these tender areas and selected nontender areas using a pressure **algometer**. A second clinician used specific joint challenges, to identify spinal segments that showed reduced mobility, in the same set of subjects. The researchers then correlated tender and nontender areas with mobile and nonmobile areas. They found that dorsal spine skin roll tenderness was a "moderately good indicator" of joint fixation within one vertebrae above or below the level of tenderness. By contrast, areas that showed tenderness during skin rolling were highly correlated with underlying areas that were tender to pressure, as measured by an algometer. The latter finding would be more credible if different clinicians had measured the tenderness during skin rolling and performed the algometry testing.

Taylor P, Tole G, Vernon H. Skin rolling technique as an indicator of spinal joint dysfunction. *J Can Chiropr Assoc.* 1990;34: 82–86.

## CAUTIONS AND CONTRAINDICATIONS

Clinical training and supervised practice are important when learning skin rolling. Advanced training may be advisable when dealing with pathological conditions. All of the general and local contraindications noted for mechanical techniques apply to the use of skin rolling (see Chapter 3, Clinical Decision Making for Massage).[4,8,10] As for all of the connective tissue techniques, clinicians should not use skin rolling in areas of acute inflammation, around hypermobile or unstable joints, or if the client's skin is fragile due to age or drug use.[4] Clinicians can apply skin rolling with reduced force over tissues that are in the subacute (**fibroplastic**) phase of inflammation if swelling has resolved and the client can tolerate treatment. Clinicians should use this technique with caution in the presence of **connective tissue diseases**. In addition, in the **osteopathic** tradition, the presence of persistently or recurrently immobile skin overlying a particular spinal segment indicates underlying imbalance, or pathology, in the viscera supplied by that segment.[5,12] In areas of fascial binding, skin rolling can be painful; consequently, clinicians must consider the client's pain tolerance when they apply this technique.

## USING SKIN ROLLING IN TREATMENT

### Mobilizing Chronic-Stage Scars

Skin rolling is the most superficial of the connective tissue techniques. For this reason, clinicians use it as a first technique for mobilizing **scars** in skin and subcutaneous fascia in their **chronic stage**. You can also apply myofascial release and direct fascial technique with light force to mobilize scars in these tissues. You can work more vigorously on scars that have matured than on scars in the early chronic stage, as long as you pay close attention to client feedback. Several sources suggest that the clinically chronic stage of scarring usually begins from 2 to 3 weeks after injury[14–16] and continues through **consolidation** and **maturation** phases for up to a year.[14] The determination of the clinical stage of scarring requires a thorough client examination.[14,15] Scars deep to superficial layers are mobilized with myofascial release, direct fascial technique, and friction. Depending on the situation, you can apply other massage techniques locally to damaged tissues earlier in the healing processes to reduce edema and pain and prevent the formation of poorly modeled scar tissue.

For homecare, teach the client how to perform self-administered skin rolling in accessible areas and stretching for 30 seconds or longer to help mobilize restrictions in the superficial fascia.

# Myofascial Release: Foundations

## DEFINITION

Myofascial release: A technique that combines a nongliding fascial traction with varying amounts of orthopedic stretch to produce moderate, sustained tension on the muscle and its associated fascia and that results in palpable viscoelastic lengthening or "creep."[1–3]

## USES

Therapists use myofascial release to lengthen fascial layers, restore fascial mobility, and decrease the effects of scars and **adhesions** on the locomotor system. They also find it useful for treating postural conditions and the chronic after-effects of trauma.

## PALPATION PRACTICE

1. If necessary, review the anatomy of major skeletal muscles. Palpate the borders, attachments, and fibers, and draw these with a marker on your partner.

2. Select a major muscle or muscle group in the lower limb such as the hamstrings. Test and record its length, and observe its appearance with your partner standing. Apply a conventional stretch technique to the muscle on one side for 2 to 3 minutes, while your partner practices diaphragmatic breathing; be sure to increase the stretch as the muscle relaxes. Have your partner stand for observation. What differences do you see and feel between the two sides? Perform the stretch on the other side and repeat the evaluation.

3. Choose a healthy joint on your partner (a single MCP joint or the wrist complex works well for this exercise). Stabilize securely with one hand proximal to the joint and one hand distal. **Distract** the joint with just enough force to take the slack out of the capsule. Maintain the same traction force for up to a minute, while you palpate with your eyes closed. You (and your partner) can usually feel the joint "give" slightly farther as the connective tissue in the capsule begins to **creep**. See Box 10-2.

---

**Box 10-2**  **How Connective Tissue Responds to Stretching Forces**

There is extensive research about how dense connective tissue responds to stretching forces.[17–24]
    Some relevant concepts are:

**Tension/tensile force:** Any force that is oriented in a manner so that its effect is to lengthen a structure.

**Elastic:** Behaves like a spring. Elastic stretch disappears when one releases the tensile force.

**Viscous/plastic:** Behaves like putty. Plastic stretch remains once one releases the tensile force.

**Viscoelastic:** Shows both viscous/plastic and elastic behavior. For a viscoelastic stretch, some of the length that the tissue gains during the stretch will remain when one releases the tensile force.

**"Creep" (viscoelastic "creep"):** Gradual lengthening of connective tissue that occurs with sustained tensile force and that reflects the viscous or plastic behavior of dense connective tissue under tension. Therapists can palpate "creep" during manipulations that place connective tissue under sustained tension.

    The elastic and plastic response of connective tissue to tensile forces can vary with the rate and duration of the force that is applied. The best way to lengthen connective tissue structures permanently, without compromising their structural integrity, is to apply prolonged low-intensity forces.

# Myofascial Release: Technique

## MANUAL TECHNIQUE[25,26]

Figures 10-7 to 10-14 show clinicians applying myofascial release to the various regions of the body. The order of the figures is from head to foot in supine and then in prone. Each figure illustrates most of the guidelines for manual technique outlined. Arrows indicate the direction of the applied force. No glide occurs between the therapist's hands and the client's skin.

1. Place the client so that you stretch the tissues you are going to treat, for example a muscle or an entire limb, to a point just short of tautness or at the point of tautness.

2. Place the chosen contact surfaces at opposite ends of the target tissues that are to be stretched (Figures 10-7, 10-9, and 10-14). Contact surfaces commonly chosen are the entire palmar surface of your hand, the heel of your hand, or your forearm.

3. Compress the client's tissues enough to engage the investing layer of deep fascia (or deeper), and then exert a light to moderate horizontal drag or traction force in opposite directions. This motion stretches the tissues between your hands in a direction parallel to the line of the muscle fibers. The contact surfaces should not glide over the client's skin.

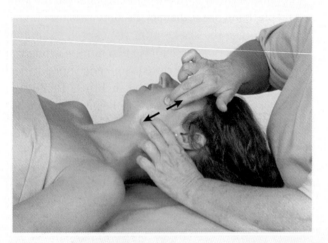

**Figure 10-7** Fingertip contact is used to stretch small muscles such as the masseter.

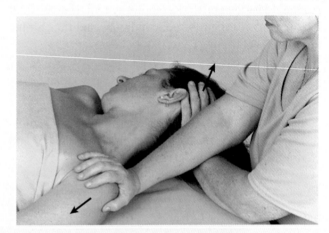

**Figure 10-9** Unilateral stretching of upper trapezius from a superior position using crossed hands.

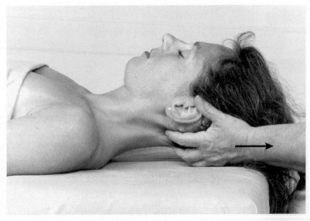

**Figure 10-8** Stretching of the posterior cervical myofascial units in supine.

ON-LINE VIDEO

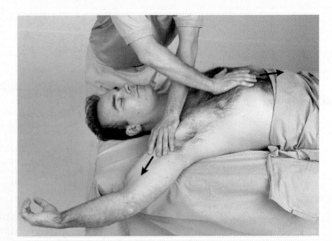

**Figure 10-10** Crossed-hand stretching of the lower fibers of pectoralis major.

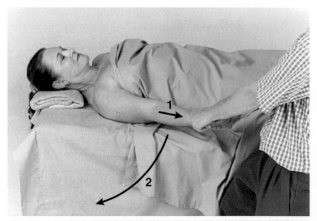

**Figure 10-11** Sustained traction can be performed with the client's arm (or leg) in almost any position. The practitioner maintains traction and moves the client's arm slowly and progressively into full abduction. This maneuver can be done in varying degrees of internal or external rotation.

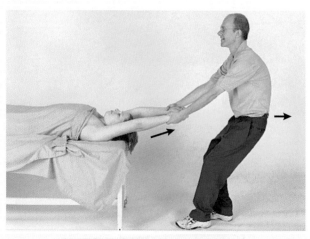

**Figure 10-12** Double-arm traction can be performed with the client in prone or supine. Starting from this basic position, the practitioner can use small shifts in position to direct the lengthening force to virtually any long muscle group in the upper body. A second practitioner can simultaneously provide double-leg traction and thus further expand the effects of the technique.

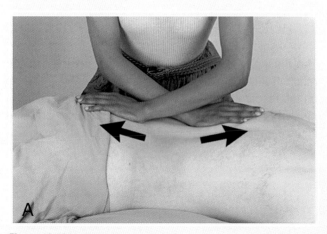

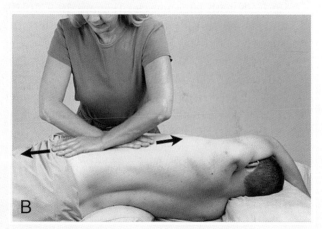

**Figure 10-13** A. Unilateral crossed-hand stretching of the lumbar region in prone. Extended gentle application of the technique can be required to address the barriers within the dense, many-layered lumbosacral fascia. Hands can also be positioned centrally and oriented across the body in order to cover the paraspinal musculature on both sides of the client's spine and produce a bilateral stretch. B. Unilateral crossed-hand stretching of the lumbar region in side-lying. To facilitate a stretch of the quadratus lumborum, position the client's arm over his head and place a pillow under his opposite side.

4. Sustain the horizontal drag or stretching force at a constant level as the client's tissues begin to lengthen slowly.

5. Take up the slack as the tissues lengthen. For example, if you have placed your hands at opposite ends of a muscle, they spread apart very slowly without gliding over the skin (Figures 10-7, 10-9, 10-10, 10-13A, 10-13B, and 10-14). When the client's body weight stabilizes one end of the stretch, both of your hands will move away from the point that gravity is stabilizing (Figures 10-8, 10-11, and 10-12). One author suggests that a minimum of 90 seconds is necessary for a myofascial release and advises therapists to hold initial releases for 3 to 5 minutes so that lengthening can proceed through a succession of fascial barriers.[26]

6. If you do not observe a palpable or visible stretch after 90 seconds, ask the client to consciously "breathe into" the area being stretched or to cough.[25,26] Adjust

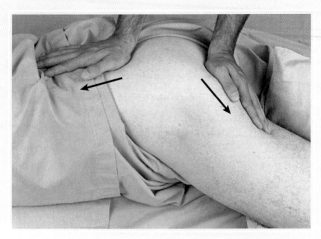

**Figure 10-14**  Myofascial release of the gluteus maximus.

the angle of stretch slightly, lighten the pressure, or change the target tissue entirely to produce an effective release.

7. Crossed-hand positions permit comfortable leverage, especially with large muscles (Figures 10-9, 10-10, 10-13A, and 10-13B). However, when used for prolonged periods of time, these may be stressful on the therapist's wrists.

8. You can exert variable amounts of compression into the client's tissues prior to initiating the lengthening traction; however, it is advisable to begin with a light compression. This is necessary because contact that

initially appears to engage only superficial tissue layers may affect deeper fascial layers once the myofascial release occurs. It is not primarily the amount of force applied, but the duration of sustained force that results in a stretch of connective tissue (see Box 10-2). In addition, the use of greater force is more likely to result in the client experiencing pain, guarding, and apprehension; therefore, do not use more than moderate force.

9. You can sustain the force of the stretch for 3 to 5 minutes, or longer, while the client's tissues release through a series of fascial barriers. Alternatively, you can maintain the stretch for a shorter period, and then reposition the client's body segment in a position of greater stretch and repeat the procedure until the tissues are adequately elongated. With the latter approach, you may alter the force on successive stretches in order to engage different layers and fibers of muscle and fascia.

10. Apply and release pressure gradually.

## How Myofascial Release Might Work

The mechanical effects of myofascial release are the result of the sustained tension that this technique exerts on the fascia associated with superficial and deep muscles. This tension probably lengthens fascia by creating minor ruptures of **collagen** molecules and **collagen cross-**

---

| Box 10-3 | **Components of Myofascial Release** |
|---|---|

**Contact:** All or part of both hands or forearms are used.

**Pressure:** Light to moderate

**Tissues engaged:** Fascia. The fascial response is the primary object of palpation, although this technique also engages the associated muscle.

**Direction:** Typically, force is oriented in a direction that is parallel to the long axis of muscles and the muscle fibers. The resulting stretch will occur in the same direction.

**Amplitude/length:** Length increase for a sustained stretch in a long myofascial unit may approach 3 cm.

**Rate:** Rate of "creep" is very slow, and region, amount, and health of tissues under stretch will also influence the rate.

**Duration:** 90 seconds to 5 minutes or greater

**Intergrades with:** Static contact, direct fascial technique, and conventional orthopedic stretching

**Combines with:** Combine with specific compression to treat trigger points.

**Context:** Commonly applied alone or alternated with direct fascial technique. Broad myofascial release can precede or follow specific neuromuscular or connective tissue technique.

links.[3] In addition, it may produce changes in the volume and level of **hydration** of the **ground substance**.[3,25,26] The rebalancing of tension throughout the connected **myofascial network** of the body, which may follow a myofascial release, may cause postural shifts[25,26] and associated changes in the client's awareness and body image.[25] Furthermore, changes in proprioception in the tissues whose length has changed may, in turn, facilitate new patterns of muscular use in the client.

There is no clear explanation for how this manual intervention might alter the function of the autonomic nervous system and increase relaxation.

## Critical Thinking Question

What are the mechanisms for connective tissue "creep" that occurs during connective tissue techniques? Consider possible mechanical and neurological mechanisms in your response.

## THERAPIST'S POSITION AND MOVEMENT

1. Use the basic positions described in Chapter 6, Preparation and Positioning for Massage, in the sections on standing aligned, seated aligned, and other postures.
2. Select a posture that is both efficient and comfortable because you may need to sustain it for several minutes. By using hand and forearm contacts, you can improve body mechanics and avoid prolonged stress to your wrists.
3. Alter the **ergonomic** load on your body by using small shifts of foot position and center of gravity as the release progresses.
4. You can perform whole-limb and full-body releases with the assistance of a second (or even a third) therapist.[25]
5. When you have to sustain a position for a long period with relatively little body movement, breathe using your diaphragm.

## PALPATE

As you perform the technique, palpate the client's tissues for the following:

1. Viscoelastic stretch or creep of the tissues. This is relatively easy to palpate during correct performance of myofascial release because the contact surfaces do not move over the client's skin. After you set up the stretch

position and carry the initial **elastic** stretch of the tissues to its endpoint, gradual separation of the contacts will reflect creep. Creep has a slow, soft, "hydraulic" feel (like pulling taffy or putty) that may be due in part to the constrained movement of fluid out of the extracellular matrix under pressure.
2. Location of layers of fascia. Attempt to engage the same fascial layer with both hands so that your hands "communicate." This will enable each hand to sense small changes in the amount and direction of the force that the other hand is exerting, as though they were pulling on opposite ends of a connected sheet. Developing the ability to isolate and palpate layers of fascia is a skill that requires practice.
3. Rhythm and motion of the stretch. Successful application of myofascial release depends on you noting the inherent rhythm and motion of each stretch as it progresses. Closing your eyes can help to focus attention on your hands and the results of palpation; this is especially useful when learning the technique.
4. **Cranial rhythm**. Small, palpable shifts in the orientation of the stretch force that seem to occur on their own may reflect the client's cranial rhythm or the untwisting of asymmetrically shortened fascial sheaths. Therapists can perform myofascial release in its simplest form without reference to cranial rhythm. We refer therapists who wish to refine the technique of attending to cranial rhythm during myofascial release to the work of Upledger and Vredevoogd.[27] Even at earlier stages of learning, however, you should be prepared to palpate the small, three-dimensional movements that can accompany the developing release.

## OBSERVE

As you perform the technique, observe the client for changes in muscle tension and tissue lengthening. The following signs may signal this.

1. Local lengthening. During the release, you may observe small amounts (millimeters to 1 or 2 centimeters) of local tissue lengthening, depending on the size of the area under stretch.
2. Lowered muscle tension. After you release the force of the stretch, local tissue contours may soften and flatten, reflecting lowered muscle tension.
3. **Thixotropic** rehydration. The thixotropic rehydration of the ground substance of tissues may contribute to a further softening of local tissue contours after you release the force of the stretch.

4. Changes in other body segments. Lengthening and positional shifts may appear in proximal, distal, or adjacent segments during the application of myofascial release. You must cultivate the habit of continually evaluating adjacent body segments for changes with the client on and off the table.

5. Structural alignment. Therapists can best assess changes in structural relationships of the client's body segments by inspection of standing static alignment and gait, both during and at the end of the session.

6. Signs of a shift in autonomic function towards relaxation such as decreased breathing rate, peristaltic noises, and changes in voice tone.

# COMMUNICATION WITH THE CLIENT

Encourage general relaxation and an awareness of tissue lengthening. Following are some examples of statements that you can use.

1. "Deepen your breathing without forcing it in any way." Conscious deep diaphragmatic breathing aids release; while lack of it impedes release. Occasionally, coughing can also facilitate release.

2. "Close your eyes and let your awareness move to . . ." Ask the client to close her eyes in order to better focus on the sensation of tissue lengthening.

3. "Let me know if you begin to feel uncomfortable." Both the pressure and the sensation of lengthening usually feel pleasant and, at all times, should be tolerable.

4. Ask the client to compare areas that you have treated with areas that you have not treated. For example, ask the client to compare the left and right sides. Clients may find changes more apparent when they are sitting or walking. Giving clients enough time to observe and report the ongoing effects of the technique is a useful teaching tool, particularly in the case of clients with poor postural habits.

5. "Does anything feel out of place?" "Do your left and right sides match?" "Can you describe the difference between the left and the right sides of your body?" Ensure that the client feels balanced at the end of a session.

6. "It's normal to feel a bit clumsy for a day or so after the treatment." Clients are often aware of altered **proprioception** and biomechanics for a day or two after undergoing a substantial release. While these changes are not painful, the client may find them uncomfortable. Consequently,

advise clients that this discomfort may occur and that they can reduce it by simple daily activities such as walking.

7. "Please phone if you experience anything unusual after the treatment, especially if you have persistent pain." When a significant shift in **agonist/antagonist balance** occurs, the client may experience transient muscle soreness in areas other than those that were treated. This occurs because of an increased loading of antagonists, synergists, or other muscles in the **kinetic chain**. Therefore, advise the client to report any postintervention soreness that is more than mild or that lasts longer than 2 days.

## A Practice Sequence for Myofascial Release

Practice Time: 40 minutes per person.
You can extend the following sequence for the more superficial lumbar and pelvic muscles by allowing each stretch to develop for longer than a minute and by pausing more often to take up the slack in the tissues. It is advisable to allocate a comparable amount of time for each of the stretches (90 seconds or more), so that a balanced intervention results. Before practice, review the fiber directions for the myofascial units to be treated and review static alignment and gait.

Before initiating the intervention, scan the client for static alignment and gait. In particular, pay attention to the relationship between the client's lumbar vertebrae and pelvis.

1. Begin with the client in prone over an abdominal pillow. Apply several crossed-hand stretches across the lumbar portion of the latissimus dorsi.

2. Turn the client to side-lying. Stretch the ipsilateral leg and open the space between the twelfth rib and the iliac crest (the lateral fascial portion of the obliques).

3. With the client's leg in the same position, apply myofascial releases between origins and insertions of gluteus medius and minimus.

4. Have the client draw the legs up into a semi-fetal position. In this position, lengthen the lower portion of the erector spinae and then gluteus maximus.

5. Turn client to the other side and repeat Steps 2, 3, and 4.

6. Turn the client to supine. Apply myofascial releases to the tensor fascia lata and rectus femoris on both sides. Allow the leg to hang over the side of the table if necessary.

7. Apply a conventional psoas stretch to both sides.

8. To finish, apply gentle sustained traction to each leg. Then apply a gentle sustained spinal traction from the neck and then from the sacrum.

# Myofascial Release: Further Study and Practice

## NAMES AND ORIGINS

Other texts or massage-related systems, name the technique that we call myofascial release as "myofascial stretching."[25] In addition, other texts use the term "myofascial release" as a synonym for the technique we call "**direct fascial technique**," which has a component of glide (see the discussion later in this chapter).

Clinicians sometimes use myofascial release as part of a wider system of treatment, known by the same name, which may incorporate a variety of craniosacral, osteopathic, and other soft tissue techniques.[25,26] Some authors[7,25] describe both "direct" and "indirect" applications of myofascial release. "Direct," in this sense, means that the clinician directs the force of the technique toward, and then through, the primary tissue restriction. In other word, the clinician applies the motion through and beyond the restrictive fascial barrier. This is in contrast to "indirect" techniques in which clinicians apply the force, or move the client, away from the fascial barrier or restriction of motion.[7,28] This book does not cover indirect applications of myofascial release.

Myofascial release is one of several approaches that clinicians have developed over the last 50 years to influence structure, as opposed to function, using massage. It owes a large conceptual debt to Ida **Rolf** and shows the influences of osteopathy and traditional stretching techniques.

## OUTCOMES AND EVIDENCE

Clinicians can use myofascial release to lengthen fascial layers, restore mobility between fascial layers, and decrease the effects of adhesions on the locomotor system. Consequently, myofascial release is appropriate for a variety of conditions in which chronic fascial shortening results in limited joint range and ease of movement such as postural conditions (kyphosis, lordosis, scoliosis, elevated shoulders, and anterior head posture), chronic after-effects of trauma, chronic fascial compartment syndromes, and neurological or circulatory compression syndromes such as thoracic outlet syndrome.[26,28–36] In these situations, myofascial release contributes to improved alignment,[37] balanced muscle function, enhanced quality and quantity of movement, and pain reduction through its direct treatment of the underlying dysfunction.[7,25,26] Myofascial release also has analgesic effects when combined with other modalities.[38–41] This technique may also help to resolve trigger point (TrP) syndromes,[42] counteract the effects of stress,[43] and facilitate athletic performance.

### EXAMINING THE EVIDENCE

A randomized controlled trial of 119 subjects, with a complex design, examined the effect of several methods on the immediate reduction of pain caused by active upper trapezius trigger points.[42] Researchers first tested the effect of "ischemic compression" (specific compression in Chapter 9, Neuromuscular Techniques) on trigger point activity by comparing two different pressures and treatments of three different durations. They found that a longer application (90 seconds) at a higher (but still tolerable) pressure was most effective. In the second stage, researchers tested the effect of various protocols on trigger point activity. The control group received only hot packs and active range of motion exercises. The other treatment groups received the control treatment plus various combinations of specific compression, TENS, stretch and spray, interferential current, and myofascial release. Several multimethod protocols showed a significant reduction of trigger point pain and increase in cervical range of motion. The most effective protocol included hot pack, active range of motion, interferential current, and myofascial release. Unfortunately, the authors' description of the myofascial release procedure was short and did not include even approximate times for its duration. Other than that, this study was unusually thorough in its design, execution, and reporting.

Hou CR, Tsai LC, Cheng KF, Chung KC, Hong CZ. Immediate effects of various physical therapeutic modalities on cervical myofascial pain and trigger-point sensitivity. *Arch Phys Med Rehabil*. 2002;83:1406–1414.

# CAUTIONS AND CONTRAINDICATIONS

Clinicians need clinical training and supervised practice to master the proper application of myofascial release. Advanced training may be advisable when dealing with pathological conditions. All of the general and local contraindications noted for mechanical techniques apply to the use of myofascial release (see Chapter 3, Clinical Decision Making for Massage).[4,8,10] As was the case for the connective tissue techniques, there are several cautions and contraindications to the use of myofascial release. These include malignancy,[44] cellulitis, fever, systemic or local infection, acute circulatory conditions, osteomyelitis, aneurysm, obstructive edema, acute rheumatoid arthritis, open wounds, sutures, hematomas, healing fractures, osteoporosis, anticoagulant therapy, advanced diabetes, and hypersensitivity of the skin.[26] In addition, clinicians should use extreme caution when performing myofascial release in the area of flaccid paralysis, lax or unstable joints, or diseased joints that are supported by **fascial** "**splinting**." Finally, clinicians should use myofascial release with caution and only in the nonacute stages of connective tissue diseases.

Clinicians need to appreciate the broader impact of myofascial release on the client's system as a whole. Although the force with which the clinician performs myofascial release is not particularly great, significant changes in the client's myofascial balance can occur quickly. Since the client's interwoven myofascial network demonstrates "whole-system" behavior,[3,25,26,45–52] the mechanical effects of myofascial release are not just local or even always predominantly local. Familiarity with fascial anatomy, as described in Myers' book **Anatomy Trains**,[47,48] can help clinicians gain an understanding of how fascial work performed in one location may "travel" to affect other locations. Furthermore, this technique can produce strong autonomic effects, reflex effects, and **somatoemotional release**, especially when clinicians use it for long periods.[25,53] This necessitates a conservative approach, careful observation, and continuous communication with the client during the application of the technique.

In light of the effects of myofascial release, clinicians should ensure that they are able to accurately perform a basic visual postural analysis before they begin to apply myofascial release during an intervention.[45,46,51,52] Furthermore, clinicians learning to perform myofascial release should initially limit their use of this technique to less than 10 minutes in any given session and should periodically conduct at least a visual reassessment of the client. In addition, clinicians should ensure that the client looks and feels "balanced" at the end of a session, especially if they have performed unilateral work around the client's legs or pelvis. Finally, clinicians must strive to maintain balanced function of the client's agonist, antagonist, and synergist muscle groups and to use a rigorous analysis of possible treatment effects. Specific strategies for extensive use of fascial techniques, such as myofascial release, are beyond the scope of this book and are the subject of several recent specialized texts.[47,49,50]

# USING MYOFASCIAL RELEASE IN TREATMENT

## To Increase Fascial Extensibility

You can apply myofascial release with specific reference to the **craniosacral rhythm** and integrate it with craniosacral technique and direct fascial technique.[1,25,26] Other massage techniques that increase connective tissue extensibility include skin rolling, **friction**, and probably petrissage, if it is applied slowly and with a high component of drag, as well as conventional stretching that is held for 30 seconds or longer. Self-stretching is particularly useful for client homecare. Also of benefit are **muscle energy techniques**, **joint mobilization** and **joint manipulation**, and spinal **traction** performed from the head or pelvis.[26]

In controlled laboratory conditions, the precise heating of tissue facilitates elongation of dense connective tissue without major structural damage.[21,24,54] In clinical practice, however, heating connective tissue prior to any sustained loading can increase the risk of large-scale rupture of collagen. Consequently, the clinician should avoid the application of either heat or cold before performing connective tissue techniques, unless his aim is specifically to rupture or denature collagen.[54] Heat applied after the use of myofascial release can enhance the temporary increase in the pliability of myofascial tissue.

## For Postural Conditions

Any of the techniques described earlier in this chapter may be relevant when attempting to lengthen areas of postural shortness. After postural change has occurred, then postural awareness training, neuromuscular education, and movement awareness training may be of benefit.[11] You may use systems of comprehensive postural awareness and movement training, such as the **Alexander technique**,[55] in these situations. Ergonomic retraining related to the client's work environment may be required. Clinicians can use strength training and endurance training for areas of postural weakness. These may be assisted with electrotherapeutic modalities such as biofeedback and electrical muscle stimulation.[11] Chronic conditions may require correction for bony asymmetry.

# Direct Fascial Technique: Foundations

## DEFINITION

Direct fascial technique: A slow, gliding technique that applies moderate, sustained tension to the superficial fascia or to the deep fascia and associated muscle. It results in palpable viscoelastic lengthening (creep).[1,3–9,26,49,50,56]

## USES

As was the case for myofascial release, use direct fascial technique to lengthen fascial layers, to restore fascial mobility, and to decrease the effects of scars and adhesions on the locomotor system. Therapists find it particularly useful for treating postural conditions and the chronic aftereffects of trauma. In addition, they sometimes use it for analgesia, to balance autonomic function, and, in Europe, for **somatovisceral** effects.

## PALPATION PRACTICE

1. Locate, trace on a partner's body, and palpate major superficial fascial structures such as the galea aponeurotica, lumbosacral fascia, retinacula of the wrist and ankle, intermuscular septa of the upper arm and thigh, iliotibial band, anterior compartment, and palmar and plantar aponeuroses. What is the texture and consistency of these tissues?
2. Palpate bones where they underlie the skin with no intervening muscle. How thick is the tissue that covers the bone? In what regions can you follow a fascial layer that overlies bone into adjacent muscle?
3. Attempt to find the **investing layer of the deep fascia** that lies superficial to muscle tissue and below the superficial layer of fat. How well can you distinguish between the investing layer of deep fascia and the muscle fibers that are deep to it?

## Direct Fascial Technique: Technique

# MANUAL TECHNIQUE

Figures 10-15 to 10-23 show clinicians applying direct fascial technique to the various regions of the body. The order of the figures is from head to foot in supine and then in prone. Each figure illustrates most of the guidelines for manual technique outlined here.

1. Fascia is most accessible for treatment at locations where it is exposed and has the least associated muscle bulk, such as at joints, on retinacula, and around bony prominences such as the sacrum and the occipital ridge (Figures 10-15 to 10-18, 10-22, and 10-23). These areas often receive less attention during **classical massage** because they have no muscle bulk, yet they are of great importance when using direct fascial technique. Most systems that use direct fascial technique emphasize the importance of working on the dense lumbosacral fascia at each session, either at the beginning of the session, as

in **Connective Tissue Massage (CTM)**, or the conclusion of the session, as in **Structural Integration**[57–59] (Figure 10-21, the lower arrow).

2. No oil is required. Remove previously applied oil. To prevent binding, you may need to apply a drop or two of cream or lotion to the working surface of your hands or forearms, but it should be a very small amount. Anything that facilitates glide also reduces your ability to apply tension to the fascia, thereby reducing the effectiveness of the technique.

3. There are two basic steps to directing the force. First, compress into the client's tissues to engage the most

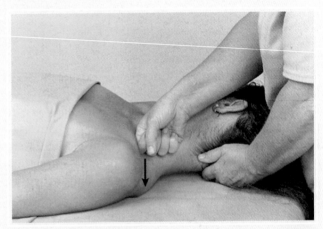

**Figure 10-16** A fist usually fits well into the space above the clavicle. Strokes in a posterolateral direction that follow the clavicle can release the scalenes.

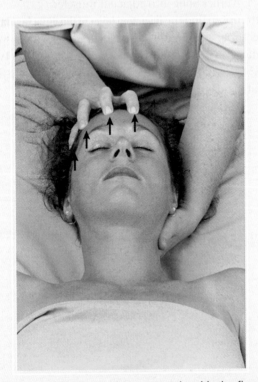

**Figure 10-15** Lifting the scalp aponeurosis with the fingertips. Slow strokes begin at the brow and cross the forehead to the hairline. On the scalp, short interconnected strokes can reduce pulling of the hair. Attempt to generate an equal amount of force with all fingers.

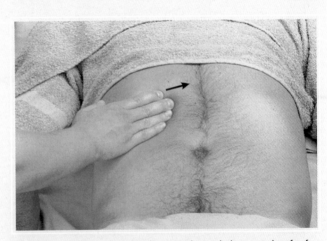

**Figure 10-17** The entire anterior costal margin is an anchor for fascia from above and below. This costal margin must be treated when lengthening the front of the torso. Avoid the xiphoid process.

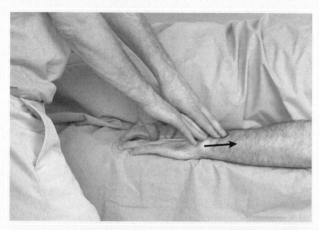

**Figure 10-18** Direct fascial technique applied to the retinacula of the wrist (or ankle) can have a lengthening effect throughout the related girdle. Note the desired neutral position of the practitioner's joints.

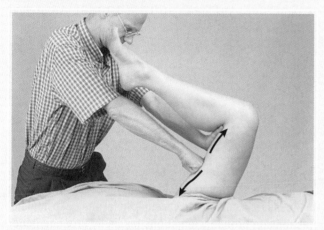

**Figure 10-19** Lengthening the fascial sheaths over and between the hamstrings can be done in supine or prone. Individual knuckles can be inserted into the intermuscular septae. On heavier clients, the technique illustrated may require the use of the practitioner's elbow.

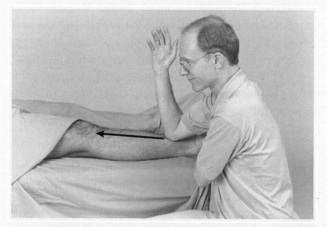

**Figure 10-20** The anterior compartment is surprisingly dense and requires use of body weight. Here, the therapist's body weight is transferred from a controlled kneeling posture.

superficial layer of restriction. Then slowly glide horizontally, while maintaining the same compressive force, to exert traction on the fascial layer you have engaged. The rate of glide is approximately 5 to 15 cm/second.

4. You can produce strokes of any length that freely cross joint lines to follow continuous fascial layers

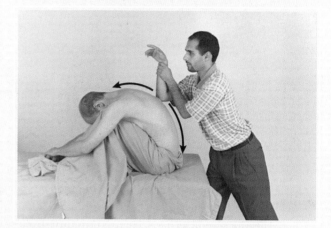

**Figure 10-21** Fascia associated with the erector spinae can be treated with the client's back in many positions, from neutral to fully flexed in prone, seated, or side-lying. Here, the therapist slides in the spinal groove along the medial surface of longissimus, taking care to avoid the spinous processes.

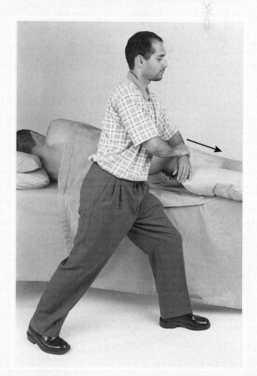

**Figure 10-22** The dense iliotibial band requires a forearm or elbow with judicious use of body weight. Include the superior iliac attachments.

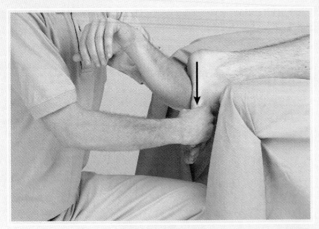

**Figure 10-23** The olecranon and the fist are easily-tolerated contact surfaces for applying direct fascial technique to the plantar fascia. The client's foot should be dorsiflexed to at least neutral and further increasing dorsiflexion will expose the fascia to more pressure.

(Figure 10-18). Shorter strokes may be more tolerable in hairy areas. At the end of the stroke, break contact and pause for several seconds. There is no return stroke.

5. You may direct the horizontal force in any direction in relation to muscle fibers: parallel to them or across them. Experiment with a variety of directions for each location, and evaluate the results of each stroke continuously by inspection and palpation, bearing in mind that the goal of the technique is to achieve an overall increase in tissue length and pliability.

6. Remain in contact with the chosen layer, as far as possible. Since this layer may not always be readily palpable, you can aim to maintain the same compressive force throughout a given stroke, and/or you can stay on the layer of tissue that feels equal in hardness, density, or resistance.

7. Repeat the stroke again, focusing on a less mobile portion of the client's tissues, or cover the original area from a different direction. If you can drag the superficial layer of fascia horizontally in all directions with relative ease, then you can increase compression in order to engage a deeper layer prior to repeating the stroke.

8. The order in which treatment proceeds is important. Work initially with broad surfaces and a general approach to free superficial layers of fascia before working the deeper layers. The benefits of direct fascial technique will accumulate incrementally when you free the fascial layers in an orderly succession from superficial to deep.[58] As a result, it is incorrect to attempt to use great amounts of pressure to move

deeper layers of fascia before ensuring that the superficial layers of fascia are thoroughly mobile at least regionally.

9. After two or three strokes, change the location of application regardless of whether or not there is palpable or visible tissue response. There are several actions you can take if shortened tissues do not seem to respond: change the stroke direction; work on the same layer proximally, distally, or across the midline; or work in a different area, such as the antagonists and synergists, before returning to the area of the unresponsive tissue. Cultivate the habit of thinking about presenting problems in a global manner; because the fascial system is interconnected, what you perceive to be a local problem may be a more generalized issue.

10. When using your hands as contacts, position them so that you avoid hyperextension of any of the joints of your fingers (Figures 10-17 and 10-18). An arched hand position, with the metacarpophalangeal and interphalangeal joints slightly flexed, is acceptable for pushing strokes that require the use of your fingers.

## *How Direct Fascial Technique Might Work*

The mechanical effects of direct fascial technique are the result of the sustained tension that this technique exerts on the fascia associated with superficial and deep muscle. This tension probably lengthens fascia by creating minor ruptures of collagen molecules and collagen cross-links.[3] In addition, it may produce changes in the volume and level of hydration of the ground substance.[3,25,26,49,50] It may also affect the activity of contractile cells located within the fascia.[60] The rebalancing of tension throughout the connected **myofascial network** of the body, which may follow a myofascial release, may cause postural shifts and associated changes in the client's awareness and body image.[26,49,50] Furthermore, changes in proprioception in the tissues whose length has changed may, in turn, facilitate new patterns of muscular use in the client.

There is no clear explanation for how direct fascial technique might alter the function of the autonomic nervous system and increase relaxation. (How does working near the vagus nerve at the occiput[49] or near parasympathetic outflow at the sacrum increase activity of the parasympathetic nervous system?) Nor is there a suggested mechanism for the **somatovisceral reflex** effects that some therapists attribute to this technique.

> ## Box 10-4 | Components of Direct Fascial Technique
>
> **Contact:** Fingers (adducted together, may be reinforced), knuckles, fist, elbow, ulnar border of your forearm
>
> **Pressure:** Light to heavy
>
> **Tissues engaged:** Fascia. Although this technique also engages associated muscle, the fascial response is the primary object of palpation.
>
> **Direction:** Varies. The force of application is often, but not necessarily, oriented in a direction that is parallel to the long axis of the myofascial units.
>
> **Amplitude/length:** Less than 5 to 50 cm
>
> **Rate:** Slow; less than 5 to 15 cm/second
>
> **Duration:** 5 seconds or greater
>
> **Intergrades with:** Stripping, frictions, myofascial release
>
> **Combines with:** You can enhance the lengthening effects of this technique dramatically by having the client perform simultaneous slow active movement, which further lengthens the treated tissues.
>
> **Context:** Commonly applied alone or alternated with myofascial release by experienced therapists. It is advisable for the less experienced therapists to precede or follow direct fascial technique with regional broad-contact petrissage (see Chapter 9, Neuromuscular Techniques).

## Critical Thinking Question

How does direct fascial technique, applied to the lumbar fascia, change the tension of the deeper fascial layers that are adjacent to the viscera?

# THERAPIST'S POSITION AND MOVEMENT

1. Use the basic positions described in Chapter 6, Preparation and Positioning for Massage. Since little body movement occurs during the slow strokes, any position that is efficient, stable, and comfortable is appropriate. Standing, seated, and kneeling positions that allow a controlled lean are all useful because they enable you to use your body weight in a controlled manner to engage deeper fascial layers. Figures 10-19, 10-20, 10-22, and 10-23 show good body mechanics in some of these positions.
2. Especially when using body weight to increase the force of the technique, you must use slow and controlled movements. Furthermore, use of body weight must not obstruct your ability to palpate subtle lengthening in the client's fascial sheaths.
3. The treatment of chronic restrictions in soft tissue may require the use of a fair amount of body weight; never-

theless, you must always be relaxed, poised, and alert to signs of overexertion. Common signs of physical and mental overexertion include: elevated shoulders; excessive hand and forearm tension; and uncontrolled leaning. The therapist's posture in Figure 10-21 shows the beginnings of an uncontrolled lean.

# PALPATE

As you perform the technique, palpate the client's tissues for the following:

1. Fascial structures. The palpation of the major fascial structures, such as the iliotibial tract, retinacula, occipto-frontal aponeurosis, clavipectoral fascia, and large intermuscular septae, is relatively easy.[45,57] By contrast, it can be virtually impossible to palpate minor fascial sheaths in areas where there is associated muscle bulk.
2. Fascial texture. Although scarring due to surgery or **consolidated edema** resulting from a major trauma can produce obvious palpable fascial thickening, it requires practice to detect less obvious restrictions in connective tissue. With the application of direct fascial technique, discrete connective tissue structures can become palpably softer and hard and fibrous areas may feel fuller, softer, hydrated, and less fibrous.

3. Fascial "layers." Although you may sometimes clearly palpate the movement of an entire fascial sheath from the point of contact, don't take the term "layer" too literally. In many ways, "layer" is a metaphor to help you focus your attention on a useful object of palpation. As with myofascial release, you must develop the ability to palpate the behavior of an entire layer of connective tissue while it is under sustained horizontal traction and the contact surface is gliding (a very refined skill). In addition, a shift to nonlocal palpation will be challenging if you have much prior practice of classical (Swedish) massage, which focuses attention on the qualities of the tissues that are immediately underhand.

4. Resistance to sustained lengthening. Resistance to a sustained lengthening force may arise from any location in the fascial layer that is under traction. With practice, you may be able to identify resistance to lengthening that comes from a point distant to the point of contact.

5. Viscoelastic stretch or creep. Creep occurs during direct fascial technique, although it is more difficult to identify than when it occurs during myofascial release since the glide of the contact surface occurs at the same time as the creep of the tissue that is under traction.

6. Adhesions or **trigger points**. During treatment, you may glide over adhesions or trigger points, which may soften with continued application of regional direct fascial technique. If this does not occur, then you may choose to change to a more specific technique such as specific compression or friction.

## OBSERVE

As you perform the technique, observe the client for changes in tissue length and quality. The following signs may signal this.

1. Hyperemia. A reactive hyperemia may accompany the application of this technique.

2. Local tissue contours. Observe areas that are drawn in, flattened, elevated, atrophied, or hypertrophied.[57] Tissue contours may change following the application of direct fascial technique.

3. Thixotropic rehydration. The thixotropic rehydration of the ground substance may contribute to a further softening of local tissue contours after you release the force of the technique.

4. Changes in other body segments. Lengthening and positional shifts may appear in proximal, distal, or adjacent segments during the application of myofascial release. You must cultivate the habit of continually evaluating adjacent body segments for changes with the client on and off the table.

5. Structural alignment. You can best assess changes in structural relationships of the client's body segments by inspection of standing static alignment and gait, both during and at the end of the session.

## COMMUNICATION WITH THE CLIENT

Encourage general relaxation and an awareness of tissue lengthening. The following are some examples of statements that you can use.

1. "Let me know if you begin to feel uncomfortable." In general, once a client overcomes the initial strangeness of direct fascial technique, it should feel pleasant. You need to inform the client about the different types of sensations that may arise. Clients frequently experience a burning sensation when stretching of superficial fascial layers first occurs. When you use specific contact surfaces, such as the fingers, a cutting or scratching sensation may occur,[57] which is not caused by nails. The client may experience local discomfort when there is a significant local fascial restriction. In general, ensure that the client understands that the amount of pressure used must be tolerable and is under control of the client, not the therapist.

2. "Notice what's occurring in your body. It's not unusual to experience sensations some distance from the location of my hands." Clients frequently report sensations that occur some distance from the therapist's hands and may need to be reassured that this is normal. These sensations are generally of two types: a transient referral from a latent trigger point that you pass over, or direct mechanical pulling of some distant part of the fascial layer that is currently under traction.

3. "Deepen your breathing without forcing it in any way." "As you breathe in, imagine the breath flowing into your. . . ." Conscious diaphragmatic breathing facilitates fascial release, and lack of it impedes release. It can help to have the client imagine their breath flowing into and out of the area that you are treating.

4. "Can you describe the difference between the left and the right sides of your body?" Ask the client to compare areas that you have treated with areas that you have not treated. For example, ask the client to compare the left

side to the right side. Clients may find changes more apparent when they are sitting or walking. Giving clients enough time to observe and report the ongoing effects of the technique is a useful teaching tool, particularly in the case of clients with poor postural habits.

5. "Does anything feel out of place?" "Do your left and right sides match?" "Can you live with this until your next session?" Ensure that the client feels balanced at the end of a session.

6. "It's normal to feel a bit clumsy for a day or so after the treatment." Clients are often aware of altered proprioception and biomechanics for a day or two after undergoing a substantial release. While these changes are not painful, the client may find them uncomfortable. Consequently, you should advise clients that this discomfort may occur and that they can reduce it by simple daily activities such as walking.

7. "Please phone if you experience anything unusual after the treatment, especially if you have persistent pain." When a significant shift in agonist/antagonist balance occurs, the client may experience transient muscle soreness in areas other than those that were treated. This occurs because of an increased loading of antagonists, synergists, or other muscles in the kinetic chain. You should advise the client to report any postintervention soreness that is more than mild or that lasts longer than 2 days.

8. When the client presents with a history of past physical or emotional trauma, it is possible, although uncommon, for spontaneous autonomic rebalancing to accompany somatoemotional release. The facilitation of somatoemotional release requires sensitivity and presence on your part. Chapter 4, Interpersonal and Ethical Issues for Massage, discusses this further.

 ### A Practice Sequence for Direct Fascial Technique

Practice Time: 45 minutes per person.

The shoulder girdle, with a focus on the arms, is a good place to begin learning direct fascial technique. Since individuals' forearms and hands are often tense, you can eas-

ily observe length changes. In addition, these changes will not affect the dynamics of the weight-bearing lower kinetic chain.

Several factors are important to keep in mind throughout the intervention.

- Use minimal lubricant.
- Contact connective tissue and apply traction to tissue layers in a horizontal direction.
- Work with a slow rate of glide, pause between strokes, and get frequent feedback from your client. Observe tissues for lengthening in addition to using palpation.
- Visually inspect the client's upper body structure.

**Supine**
1. Apply short fingertip strokes in several directions: over the retinacula of the wrist; repeatedly over the palmar fascia and both thenar and hypothenar eminences; and around the joints and bones of the fingers.
2. Observe the effect that this has on the entire shoulder girdle.
3. Use a broader contact surface such as your forearm, palm, or fist, on both ventral and dorsal surfaces of the client's forearm.
4. Using more specific finger or thumb contact, try to enter the space between the muscles to work on the intermuscular fascial layers. Again, observe the results.
5. Use broad and then more specific contact to treat the client's upper arms, as you did for the treatment of the forearms. Include the fascia over the deltoid, and the lateral and medial intermuscular septae.

Reassess.

Give equal treatment to the client's other arm.

To finish, apply each of the following strokes several times.

- Supine. Reach under the client to the mid-thoracic level, and then drag the tips of your flexed fingers up the erector spinae on either side of the client's spine from the mid-thorax to the occiput.
- Head turned. Use a broad surface like the heel of your hand moving anterior to posterior across the scalenes. Treat one side at a time.
- Seated with trunk flexion. Apply long descending strokes along the erector spinae with your wrist or forearm

Visually reassess.

# Direct Fascial Technique: Further Study and Practice

## NAMES AND ORIGINS

In other texts and massage-related systems, the technique we call direct fascial technique is called "fascial technique," "connective tissue technique," "connective tissue massage," "myofascial massage," "deep tissue massage," "deep stroking," "myofascial manipulation," "soft tissue mobilization," or "direct release myofascial technique."[1,3–9,11,26,49,50,56]

"Direct," used in relation to fascial technique, means that clinicians direct the force of the technique toward, and then through, the tissue restriction. In other words, they apply the motion through, and beyond, the restrictive fascial barrier. This is in contrast to "indirect" techniques, such as counterstrain or positional release, in which clinicians apply the force, or move the client, away from the fascial barrier or restriction of motion.[7,28] This book does not cover indirect techniques.

At a glance, direct fascial technique sometimes resembles modern neuromuscular techniques, such as stripping, that engage muscle while producing a sustained unidirectional drag in one plane. When clinicians apply direct fascial technique over the client's muscle belly, it may achieve some of the effects of neuromuscular techniques. However, this technique differs substantially from neuromuscular techniques in terms of the focus during palpation, location of application, intention, and effect on connective tissue.

Direct fascial technique is one of the most influential massage innovations of this century, popularized initially through the work of Ida **Rolf** in the United States and Elizabeth **Dicke** in Germany, who developed and elaborated on the technique for two distinctly different purposes.[46,57,58] Clinicians of the various schools of **Structural Integration** or Structural Bodywork, who seek to comprehensively realign bodies, apply direct fascial techniques to superficial and deep fascial layers and throughout the musculature within the framework of a 10-session series. These schools include: **Rolfing**[61–64] and its various descendents such as Heller Work, SOMA (Greek word meaning body and mind), Neuromuscular Integration and Structural Alignment (NISA), and Postural Integration.[4,9,46,65] In Dicke's Bindegewebsmassage (**Connective Tissue Massage [CTM]**), clinicians apply direct fascial technique in precise sequences to the skin and superficial fascial layers to elicit specific physiological reflex effects.[1,57,66] The CTM system also uses skin rolling and short strokes, which do not glide but nonetheless exert specific subdermal traction to fascia.[1] This system has a much larger following in Europe than North America.

## OUTCOMES AND EVIDENCE

Direct fascial technique has general clinical effects that are similar to those of myofascial release, including lengthening and restoring mobility between fascial layers. In addition, clinicians can use direct fascial technique within comprehensive systems of treatment, such as Structural Integration or Connective Tissue Massage, to address different outcomes. Like myofascial release, clinicians can use direct fascial technique in the treatment of conditions in which chronic fascial shortening results in limited joint range and ease of movement. These conditions include: postural conditions (kyphosis, lordosis, scoliosis, elevated shoulders, and anterior head posture), chronic after-effects of trauma, chronic fascial compartment syndromes, repetitive strain injury, neurological or circulatory compression syndromes such as thoracic outlet syndrome, chronic low back dysfunction, and mild spasticity.[26,46,57–59,61–69] In these situations, direct fascial technique contributes to normalized structural alignment, balance of agonist/antagonist muscle function, improved quality and quantity of movement between and across body segments, and improved energy consumption.[46,65,68–72] These effects, in combination with the enhanced muscle performance that follows increased muscle extensibility, may make the technique useful for athletic performance. In addition, direct fascial technique has complex direct and indirect effects on pain through endorphin-mediated analgesia, the restoration of mobility, and the reduction of anxiety.[59,67,70–83] Finally, this technique also often results in a local reactive hyperemia and may indirectly affect local circulation.[1,57]

Within the context of **Structural Integration** interventions, direct fascial technique has other clinical effects. First, it appears to produce an increase in parasympathetic activity,[59,71] and when applied during a series of sessions, it can result in a lasting reduction in anxiety states.[72–74] Studies on the use of direct fascial technique in Connective Tissue Massage (CTM) interventions have, however, reported less consistent autonomic effects, although the literature on CTM suggest that it is useful for treating autonomic imbalance.[1,57,60,75,84]

When direct fascial technique (or any other massage technique) affects autonomic activity, it can produce generalized, indirect visceral effects. CTM, however, takes this notion further to suggest that clinicians can achieve a direct regulating effect on a client's organ function, via **somatovisceral reflexes**, by detecting and freeing tightness in somatic connective tissue.[66,84–91] The scientific basis for this theory is uncertain. The literature states that the skin can develop predictable areas of hypersensitivity (Head's zones) and that muscles and related fascia can exhibit predictable areas of increased tone (MacKenzie's zones) in response to specific visceral pathology.[58,84] Unfortunately, there is a scarcity of English-language research to support the existence of direct somatovisceral paths of influence on organ function. This is a consequence of the lack of English translations of the potentially substantiating German and Russian literature, even as journal abstracts.[92–95] Review articles in English-speaking journals suggest that there is no empirical evidence for the concept of somatovisceral reflexes.[96] Consequently, advocates of CTM have recently acknowledged that the scientific basis for somatovisceral reflexes requires clarification and research.[84,95] Perhaps, clinicians may look forward to receiving greater clarity on the basic notions about the psyche–soma–viscera relationship in the future.

## EXAMINING THE EVIDENCE

A recent pilot study[81] with a **pretest, posttest design** examined the effects of a manual therapy program, composed of hot pack, classical massage, and connective tissue manipulation, on 30 female clients with migraine headaches. The researchers evaluated the subjects before and after 20 sessions of treatment that they delivered over a 4-week period. They noted statistically significant decreases in pain intensity, frequency of headache, and frequency of four accompanying symptoms (nausea, vomiting, photophobia, and difficulty concentrating). Decreases in all symptoms were still significant after 6 months. In light of the long follow-up time, these results are promising, but the study lacked a control. In addition, the authors did not describe the massage methods they used in a manner that would permit a clinician to reproduce them. For example, they describe the protocol for the connective tissue manipulation but not for the classical massage; they do not report treatment times for the two massage approaches; and session times varied from 45 to 60 minutes. Finally, this study examined an intensive intervention that is likely to be beyond the means of many clients or facilities to fund.

Akbayrak T, Citak I, Demirturk F, Akarcali I. Manual therapy and pain changes in patients with migraine: an open pilot study. *Adv Physiother*. 2001;3:49–54.

## CAUTIONS AND CONTRAINDICATIONS

Clinicians need clinical training and supervised practice to master the proper application of direct fascial technique. Advanced training may be advisable when dealing with pathological conditions. All of the general and local contraindications noted for mechanical techniques apply to the use of direct fascial technique (see Chapter 3, Clinical Decision Making for Massage).[4,8,10] As for all of the connective tissue techniques, there are several cautions and contraindications to the use of direct fascial technique. These include malignancy, cellulitis, fever, systemic or local infection, acute circulatory conditions, osteomyelitis, aneurysm, obstructive edema, acute rheumatoid arthritis, open wounds, sutures, hematomas, healing fractures, osteoporosis, anticoagulant therapy, advanced diabetes, and hypersensitivity of the skin.[26] In addition, clinicians should use extreme caution when performing direct fascial technique in areas of flaccid paralysis, lax or unstable joints, or diseased joints that are supported by fascial "splinting." Finally, clinicians should use direct fascial technique with caution and only in the nonacute stages of systemic connective tissue disorders.

Clinicians need to appreciate the broader impact of direct fascial technique on the client's system as a whole. Although the force with which the clinician performs direct fascial technique is not particularly great, significant changes in the client's **myofascial balance** can occur quickly. Since the client's interwoven myofascial network demonstrates "whole-system" behavior,[3,25,26,45–52] the mechanical effects of direct fascial technique are not just local or even always predominantly local. Familiarity with fascial anatomy, as described in Myers' book **Anatomy Trains**,[47,48] can help clinicians gain an understanding of how fascial work performed in one location may "travel" to affect other locations. Furthermore, this technique can produce strong autonomic effects, reflex effects, and somatoemotional release, especially when clinicians use it for long periods.[25,53] This necessitates a conservative approach, careful observation, and continuous communication with the client during the application of the technique.

In light of the effects of direct fascial technique, clinicians should ensure that they are able to accurately perform a basic visual postural analysis before they begin to apply direct fascial technique during an intervention.[45,46,51,52] Furthermore, clinicians learning to perform direct fascial technique should initially limit their use of this technique to less than 10 minutes in any given session and should periodically conduct at least a visual reassessment of the client. In addition, clinicians should ensure that the client looks and feels "balanced" at the end of a session, especially if they have performed unilateral work around the client's legs or pelvis. Finally, clinicians must strive to maintain balanced function of the client's agonist, antagonist, and synergist muscle groups and to use a rigorous analysis of possible treatment effects. Specific strategies for extensive use of fascial techniques, such as direct fascial technique, are beyond the scope of this book and are the subject of several recent specialized texts.[47,49,50]

# USING DIRECT FASCIAL TECHNIQUE IN TREATMENT

## To Increase Fascial Extensibility

Clinicians can integrate direct fascial technique with craniosacral technique and myofascial release.[1,25,26] Other massage techniques that can be used to increase connective tissue extensibility include skin rolling, friction, and probably petrissage, if it is applied slowly and with a high component of drag, as well as conventional stretches that are held for 30 seconds or longer. Self-stretching is particularly useful for client homecare. Also of benefit are neuromuscular or muscle energy techniques, joint mobilization, joint mobilization and manipulation, and spinal traction performed from the head or pelvis.[26]

In controlled laboratory conditions, the precise heating of tissue facilitates a greater elongation of collagenous structures without resulting in significant structural damage.[21,24,54] In clinical practice, however, the application of heat prior to any sustained loading of connective tissue can increase the risk of large-scale collagenous rupture. Consequently, the clinician should avoid the application of either heat or cold before performing connective tissue techniques, unless his aim is specifically to rupture or denature collagen.[54] Heat applied after the use of direct fascial technique can enhance the temporary increase in the pliability of myofascial tissue.

## For Postural Conditions

Any of the techniques described earlier in this chapter may be relevant when attempting to length areas of postural shortness. When the client experiences significant shifts in posture, postural awareness training, neuromuscular education, and movement awareness training may be of benefit.[11] The clinician may use systems of comprehensive postural awareness and movement training, such as the **Alexander technique**,[55] in these situations. Ergonomic retraining related to the client's work environment may be required. Strength training and/or endurance training is indicated for areas of postural weakness; this may be assisted by electrotherapeutic modalities such as biofeedback and electrical muscle stimulation.[11] Chronic conditions may require correction for bony asymmetry.

# Friction: Foundations

# DEFINITION

Friction: A repetitive, nongliding technique where a specific contact, such as the fingertips or thumb, is used to penetrate dense connective tissue and produce small movements between its fibers.[1–11]

# USES

Use friction to increase the extensibility of connective tissue by promoting the realignment and remodeling of its constituent collagen fibers.[97] This is often required when treating adhesions associated with chronic-stage orthopedic injuries, scars, and repetitive strain injuries.

# PALPATION PRACTICE

As time allows:

1. Locate and thoroughly palpate from end to end the following ligaments: three lateral and one medial ankle ligaments, and the collateral ligaments of the knee and elbow. Ask your partner if he or she has ever sprained

---

| Box 10-5 | **How Connective Tissue Responds to Immobility** |

Immobilization of connective tissue, which commonly occurs after orthopedic injury, produces a succession of important biochemical changes.[98–102] These include:

Decreased concentration of **hyaluronic acid** in the **matrix**

Decreased water-bonding capacity of the matrix

Decreased water content of the matrix

Approximation of collagen fibers

Increased collagen cross-linking

These in turn may contribute to the clinical impairments of:

Increased tissue **stiffness**

Decreased tissue mobility and extensibility

Restrictions of joint capsule and ligaments

Impaired joint mobility

Pain

Damaged tissue that receives carefully applied stress during the healing process, by appropriate movement or massage, shows improved hydration of the extracellular matrix and more orderly deposition of collagen. This results in stronger, more mobile, and more functional scar tissue.

---

any of these ligaments. If so, compare the texture and sensitivity of the damaged and undamaged ligaments bilaterally, if possible.

2. Fully stretch each ligament listed in Step 1. Palpate the ligament again in this stretched position.

3. Locate and thoroughly palpate from end to end the following tendons: Achilles, tendons of biceps femoris and quadriceps femoris, the four tendons that make up the rotator cuff, the two "common" tendons at the elbow, and the "snuffbox" tendons at the wrist. Ask your partner if he or she has ever had tendinitis at any of these sites. If so, compare the texture and sensitivity of the damaged and undamaged tendons (bilaterally, if possible).

4. Fully stretch each tendon listed in Step 3. Palpate the tendon again in this stretched position.

5. Resist a midrange isometric contraction of the muscle(s) attached to each tendon listed in Step 3.

# Friction: Technique

## MANUAL TECHNIQUE[97,103–106]

Figures 10-24 to 10-31 show clinicians applying friction to the various regions of the body. The order of the figures is from head to foot in supine and then in prone. Each figure illustrates most of the guidelines for manual technique outlined here.

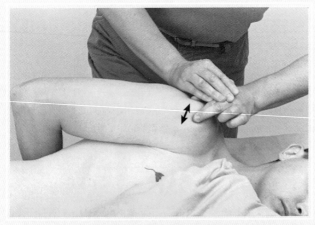

**Figure 10-24** To expose the supraspinatus tendon for friction, the client's arm is extended, adducted, and internally rotated. The insertions of the tendons of the rotator cuff muscles lie beneath the thick, coarse-fibered deltoid muscle. Lesions in the rotator cuff muscles are located using the client's response to deep palpation.

1. Prior to performing friction, clip or file your nails so that they are very short (at least 2 mm shorter than the end of your fingertips).
2. No oil is required. If oil is present, remove it using alcohol or witch hazel to prevent slippage.
3. Position the body segment you will be treating so that there is enough tension in the target tissues for the force of the friction to be isolated to it without affecting the surrounding normal tissues.[97,103–106] Target tissues are exact portions of the ligament or tendon that are too dense, not the overlying or adjacent tissues. If the target tissues are slack, the contact surface will tend to slide over them, and the force of the friction will fall on adjacent healthy tissue and cause inflammation there. On the other hand, if the target tissues are overstretched, they become hard to penetrate. A useful rule of thumb is that the more superficial the tissue, the more stretch that should be exerted on the body segment. For example, if the lesion is in a synovial sheath, place the related tendon on the fullest tolerable stretch. For ligaments, use a position between neutral and a full stretch, depending on the desired depth for the friction (Figure 10-29). For tendons, use a position between partial and full stretch. If the lesion is deep in the muscle, slacken the superficial tissues to allow access to the lesion. Finally, the degree of stretch that

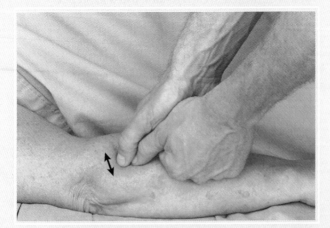

**Figure 10-25** Lesions in the common extensor tendon ("tennis elbow") can develop anywhere between the tenoperiosteal and musculotendinous junctions. The therapist must pretreat local trigger points and avoid damaging the radial nerve with the friction.

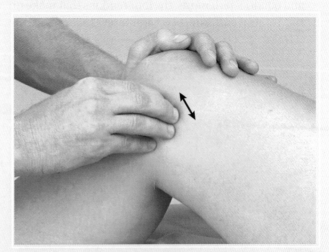

**Figure 10-26** Friction to the medial collateral ligament of the knee. The knee is positioned to exert a moderate stretch on the ligament. Friction for sprains should be given at the maximum allowable flexion and extension.[69]

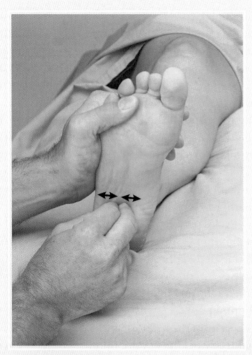

**Figure 10-27** The foot must be dorsiflexed when applying friction to the dense plantar fascia, particularly when treating plantar fasciitis. If digital contact is difficult for the client to tolerate, precede the use of friction with a more general stroke such as kneading.

is most effective can also vary with the hardness of the target tissue (Figures 10-24, 10-27, and 10-30).

4. Use focused and specific contact. Usually this involves holding some combination of the first three digits together tightly and reinforcing them. You can reinforce on top of the index finger with the middle finger, or you can reinforce the index finger between your thumb and third digits (Figures 10-24 to 10-29 and

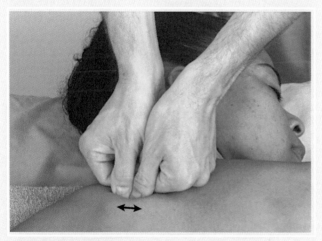

**Figure 10-28** The clinician should differentiate the fibrosis commonly found at the lower attachment of the levator scapulae from a trigger point before treating it with friction.

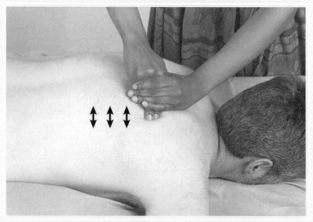

**Figure 10-29** The tendinous slips of iliocostalis thoracis are prone to become "ropy" or "stringy" due to chronic inflammation, especially if a client is hyperkyphotic. This local lack of tissue resilience can be improved with friction.

10-31). When the lesion is deep or large and requires the use of body weight to access it, substitute the olecranon process for your fingers (Figure 10-30). When the target tissues are very dense and hard, a wooden or plastic T-bar may be necessary (see Figure 9-62).

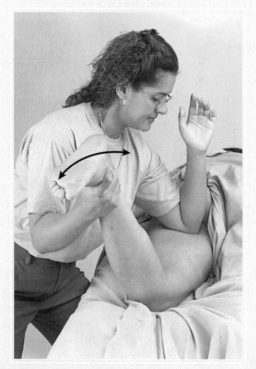

**Figure 10-30** This friction of the hamstring just distal to its attachment on the ischial tuberosity begins with deep specific compression on the tendon using the therapist's body weight and the elbow. The therapist then uses the client's lower leg to internally and externally rotate the femur in order to control the cross-fiber movement between the contact surface and the target tissue.

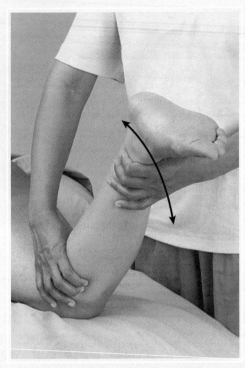

**Figure 10-31** The first two fingers of the practitioner's right hand contact the pes anserinus. Controlled movement of the contact surface over the bursa or tendinous insertions can be accomplished easily by flexing and extending the client's knee.

Regardless of the contact surface that you use, frequent change of contact surfaces will reduce the likelihood of repetitive strain.

5. Do not glide over the client's skin. Your hand does not move in relation to any of the tissues that are superficial to the target tissue because these tissues move with your hand. The aim of friction is to penetrate dense, immobile connective tissue with your fingertips and then to make small motions that move one part of the target tissue with respect to another. This is like using your fingertips to tease apart the fibers of a tightly wound ball of string. It requires good palpation skills and very careful control of pressure.

6. Begin by working on the most superficial layer of the connective tissue that needs remodeling. If the problem is superficial, this may not require much pressure. If, however, the lesion is located beneath layers of muscle, you may need to use some bodyweight, even after first softening the intervening tissues (Figures 10-24, 10-29, and 10-30).

7. Use short strokes (less than 2 cm) to move the superficial part of the target tissues back and forth over the deeper part. Do not slip off or bump over the target tissues, since this may damage adjacent healthy tissue.

Although Cyriax[105,106] suggests applying friction with "sufficient sweep," using short strokes will improve your control. If the target tissue is less than 2 cm across, you can cover it with one stroke (Figures 10-24 to 10-26). If it is more than 2 cm across, you will need to use two or more strokes side by side.

8. The direction of the stroke is typically across fibers when treating ligament, tendon, or muscle. When treating fascia or scar tissue where the collagen has a less regular organization, you can alternate directions or use a circular stroke.

9. Therapists typically apply friction at a rate of one to two cycles per second.[97] Two cycles per second is the maximum rate for an experienced therapist working on a superficial lesion. A more modest rate of one cycle per second is effective, facilitates palpation, and reduces the possibility of overtreatment.

10. Maintain contact with the same tissue layer while you perform the friction until a palpable softening of that tissue occurs or for 2 minutes, whichever comes first.

11. Take frequent breaks of several seconds to change contact surfaces. Take care to locate the lesion accurately and to re-establish a similar depth of friction once you reinitiate treatment.

12. If the client gives positive feedback (see following Communication with the Client section), you can increase pressure to engage a deeper layer of the target tissue or shift very slightly to an adjacent area and then perform another cycle of friction.

13. If the lesion is located on a limb, it may be easier for you to maintain static specific compression on the target tissue with one hand, while moving the client's limb with the other to produce the required motion between the target tissue and your hand (Figures 10-30 and 10-31). This technique is often also more tolerable to the client.

14. Depending on the client's feedback about level of comfort, you can apply friction to one area for a maximum of 6 minutes in the first intervention.[97] You can increase the duration by increments of 2 or 3 minutes per session,[97] with an upper limit (rarely required) of 15 to 20 minutes.[97,103]

## How friction might work

Friction may break some of the cross-links that bind adjacent collagen molecules and adjacent fibers (adhesions and fibrosis), allowing more relative movement between

| Box 10-6 | **Components of Friction** |
|---|---|

**Contact:** Reinforced finger(s), thumb, knuckle, olecranon

**Pressure:** Light to heavy, depending on location of lesion

**Tissues engaged:** Dense connective tissue (ligament, tendon, fascia, extraneous deep connective tissue, scar tissue, or fibrosis in muscle)

**Direction:** Strokes lie in a plane parallel to the body's surface. Currently, therapists most commonly use friction across fibers for ligaments and tendons. Nevertheless, circular friction may be useful, and parallel friction was common in the past.

**Amplitude/length:** Short; 1 to 2 cm

**Rate:** Slow; 1 Hz is recommended, 2 Hz is maximum

**Duration:** 30 seconds, up to a maximum of 15 minutes delivered in shorter segments

**Intergrades with:** Petrissage, specific compression, direct fascial technique

**Context:** May be performed alone. Another option is to precede friction with regional petrissage, myofascial release, or direct fascial technique. You can follow friction with superficial effleurage and passive or active stretches. Apply a cold pack afterwards only if overtreatment has occurred.

the fibers.[2,97] As a result, these fibers occupy more space and the matrix holds more water (hydrates). Furthermore, the tissues become more pliable, which enables them to absorb and transmit the tensional loads caused by movement better.[97] This, in turn, promotes more orderly modeling of collagen fibers in the long term, as the fibroblasts align along new lines of stress.[16] Finally, friction may also exert a long-term effect on tissue organization by stimulating fibroblast activity.[107]

### Critical Thinking Question

How do friction and myofascial release reduce the negative effects of immobilization on connective tissue?

## THERAPIST'S POSITION AND MOVEMENT

1. Use the basic positions described in Chapter 6, Preparation and Positioning for Massage.
2. Effective friction demands a careful use of the therapist's body weight. Do not rely on hand and arm strength alone, except when treating small, superficial lesions. In a standing or seated controlled lean position, you can hold your hand and arm stable and use a slight rocking

of the body to produce sufficient force and the required movement of the contact surface.
3. Use of your elbow in standing or seated controlled lean demands skilled **proprioceptive palpation** (Figure 10-30).

## PALPATE

As you perform the technique, palpate the client's skin and tissues for the following:

1. Contours. Chronic orthopedic injuries often appear to be "swollen" or enlarged. Soft (fluid-filled) edema cannot, however, be present when you apply friction.
2. Density or hardness of the target tissue. Compare the target tissues with healthy tissue that is adjacent or on the opposite side to form an impression of what normal bulk and texture are for that individual.
3. Fiber direction. Note the fiber direction of discrete structures such as tendon or ligament prior to treatment.
4. Location of target tissue. You must accurately locate the desired target tissue throughout the application of friction.
5. Softening of tissue. Taut bands or hardened slabs of tissue may soften as a result of rehydration of the ground substance or rupture of collagen fibrils. A reduction of tenderness and improvement of the client's key symptoms should accompany this palpable softening.

6. Reduction of hypertrophy. A single session of friction can reduce hypertrophied structures.
7. Resistance to stretch. The resistance to stretch of both contractile and noncontractile tissues should decline as treatment progresses.

# OBSERVE

As you perform the technique, observe the quality of the target tissue and for signs of the client's comfort. The following signs may signal this.

1. Surface contours reflect the bulk, tautness, and hardness of the target tissues.
2. Reactive hyperemia. Rapid reddening of the client's skin may indicate an abrasion caused by nails that are too long.
3. Client's facial expression should reflect relaxation and comfort.

# COMMUNICATION WITH THE CLIENT

Friction involves the localized application of a repetitive force to a very small area. Consequently, it presents the highest risk for producing local tissue damage of all the massage techniques. If you communicate carefully, you can avoid overtreatment and increasing inflammation. Beyond the production of a transient hyperemia, the point of friction is not to increase inflammation in already damaged tissue, although this may result from overzealous or unskilled application. You can use the following protocol, adapted from Kessler and Hertling,[97] to test the tissues and obtain frequent feedback, thereby reducing the risk of overtreatment.

1. Immediately before applying friction, test the sensitivity of the target tissues in one of two ways: with **contractile tissues**, palpate the tissues while performing resisted isometric movements; with **inert tissues**, palpate the tissues while performing a passive stretch. You can also ask the client to rate current pain on a **10-point scale** to obtain a more objective measure of how sensitive the lesion is to mechanical stress. These **key signs** provide an essential baseline for measuring progress and grading the dosage of friction applied during the session.
2. "Where is it most tender to touch?" You must use orthopedic testing to determine the structure that requires friction. However, you can use client feedback in response to palpation to identify the exact location of the lesion within the implicated structure.
3. Begin the friction at a level that the client finds tolerable, with discomfort rated at no more than 4 on a 10-point scale. The client should not demonstrate signs of pain such as inhibited breathing or grimacing or more subtle signs of sympathetic arousal. Assure the client that the initial discomfort (if any) usually declines as the friction proceeds, and direct the client to speak up right away if discomfort increases during the friction.
4. Towards the end of the first cycle (up to 2 minutes), ask the client if the discomfort caused by the friction is more or less than it was at the beginning of the cycle. If the discomfort has lessened, you can move to an adjacent location or increase the pressure based on the client's tolerance and proceed for another 2 minutes.
5. At the end of three cycles (up to 6 minutes), retest key signs. If the lesion is less sensitive during testing, you may continue to use friction if it is not the first intervention.
6. If, at any time, the client reports that the discomfort caused by the friction has increased or if the lesion is more painful on retesting, you must stop applying friction for that session. Use superficial effleurage to drain towards the nearest lymph nodes and apply ice to the area until visible vasoconstriction (blanching) occurs.

---

 **A Practice Sequence for Friction**

Practice Time: 30 minutes per person.
To acquire a feel for this technique, practice around large joints where connective tissue is easily accessible. The ankle is a good choice since it is a common location of sprains and is often the site of residual fibrosis. The joint chosen for practice should show no signs of instability.

Connective tissue is remarkably tough, and a stable, healthy joint can certainly withstand up to 5 minutes of properly applied friction without showing signs of negative effects. Respect your client's pain tolerance; do not apply friction to any given spot (for practice purposes) for more than a minute, and avoid "endangerment sites," such as the locations of major nerves (the radial nerve at the elbow).

Ensure that your nails are very short!

1. Begin by applying 5 minutes of petrissage to the major muscles that cross the joint (see Chapter 9, Neuromuscular Techniques). This is particularly useful when treating lesions in contractile tissue.
2. Remove residual lubricant completely.

3. Evaluate for (hypothetical) key signs using passive and/or contractile testing, and thoroughly palpate around the joint for tenderness.

4. Beginning superficially, apply friction for a minute to five or six different locations around the client's joint: on the tendon (also around the tendon), the ligament, and the retinaculum. A minute of friction is generally long enough to detect a palpable change; the tissue to which you applied friction should feel slightly spongy. If you are not sure of tissue change, do a bilateral comparison. If there is no detectable change, increase the pressure slightly and try a different location for a minute.

5. Retest key signs.
6. Have the client stretch the treated area.
7. Drain towards the regional lymph nodes with superficial effleurage or superficial lymph drainage technique.
8. Ensure that the client shows no signs of overtreatment, although it is unlikely to occur with treatment this brief.

Home study: Superior gluteal insertions are a common site of fibrosis. Devise a comparable sequence for that area that uses knuckle or elbow contact to deliver the friction. Apply this sequence bilaterally.

# Friction: Further Study and Practice

## NAMES AND ORIGINS

In other massage texts, the technique we call friction is also called "transverse friction," "deep friction," "deep transverse friction," "cross-fiber friction," "Cyriax friction," and "circular friction."[1-11]

Various forms of this connective tissue technique differ in the direction and the amount of force that is applied. Nevertheless, the treatment aims, clinical effects, focus of palpation, and many aspects of the manual technique are similar, whether the force is directed transverse or parallel to the fiber direction of well-defined structures, such as tendons or ligaments, or to less well-defined dense connective tissue formations such as adhesions and fibrosis.

Historically, the term "friction" has a broad, ambiguous usage that has embraced virtually any manner of rubbing between two surfaces. Some authors describe a "superficial friction" that is a fast chafing of the body's surface.[8,9] Other authors have used the term "friction" to refer to nongliding techniques that repetitively move one layer of muscle over another, which are similar to petrissage in terms of their shearing forces and clinical effects (see Chapter 9, Neuromuscular Techniques).[4,9] In this text, the term "friction" is reserved for the specific connective tissue technique described earlier in this chapter.

Clinicians can apply a much less forceful version of the technique, described earlier in this chapter, to clients with subacute orthopedic injuries as a means of preventing the formation of adhesions.

## OUTCOMES AND EVIDENCE

Friction maintains, or increases, the extensibility of connective tissue by promoting the realignment and remodeling of its constituent collagen fibers.[97] Consequently, clinicians can use friction to treat any condition in which mobility may be compromised by irregular tissue remodeling that occurred during the consolidation and maturation stages of connective tissue healing. Use friction for the rehabilitation of virtually all **chronic-stage** orthopedic conditions, including sprains (with one dissenting opinion[108]), strains, fractures, and adhesive capsulitis.[97,103-112] In these situations, friction may result in maintained or increased joint range, capsular mobility, and accessory movement.[97,103,108,112-114] Opinions differ, however, regarding the effectiveness of friction in increasing the extensibility of hypertrophic scar tissue.[115,116] Cross-fiber friction has often been regarded as the manual intervention of choice for **repetitive strain injuries** such as tendinitis, tenosynovitis, bursitis, and plantar fasciitis,[97,103,117-121] in which there is ongoing microtrauma, low-grade inflammation, and tissue remodeling. By contrast, recent reviews[122,123] note a lack of evidence to support its use in the treatment of tendinitis. Finally, like many other massage techniques, application of friction may result in analgesia and transient postintervention hyperemia.[2,97,106]

A **randomized clinical trial** compared patients' early response to two different treatment protocols for adhesive capsulitis.[112] Researchers randomized 40 clients into two treatment groups. One group received hour-long sessions, which included Cyriax deep friction massage, manipulation, active stretching, and pendulum exercises, three times a week. The other group received hour-long sessions, which included hot pack (20 minutes), short-wave diathermy (20 minutes), and similar active stretching and pendular exercises, five times a week. Both groups received the same daily home exercise program of passive range of motion and pendulum exercises. Nineteen clients in the group who received massage and 13 clients in the nonmassage group achieved 80% of full passive range of motion at the end of the second week. However, the improvement in range and decreases in pain with motion were significantly better in the massage group after the first week of treatment. This study focused specifically on early responses to the two methods, so the researchers' lack of follow-up is understandable. One limitation is that the authors give no information, beyond a reference to Cyriax, about the methods they used during the 40-minute treatments of friction and manipulation. While the protocol the authors described for this promising treatment certainly allows for clinician discretion, it is too vague for clinicians to reproduce.

Guler-Uysal F, Kozanoglu E. Comparison of the early response to two methods of rehabilitation in adhesive capsulitis. *Swiss Med Wkly.* 2004;134:353–358.

# CAUTIONS AND CONTRAINDICATIONS

Clinicians need clinical training and supervised practice to master the proper application of friction. Advanced training may be advisable when dealing with pathological conditions. All of the general and local contraindications noted for mechanical techniques apply to the use of friction (see Chapter 3, Clinical Decision Making for Massage).[4] As for all of the connective tissue techniques, there are several cautions and contraindications to the use of friction. These include hemophilia, thrombus, malignancy, vascular insufficiency, cellulitis, phlebitis, fever, systemic or local infection, acute circulatory conditions, osteomyelitis, aneurysm, obstructive edema, acute rheumatoid arthritis, open wounds, sutures, hematomas, healing fractures, osteoporosis, advanced diabetes, hypersensitivity of the skin, and client's use of local or systemic analgesic, anti-inflammatory, or anticoagulant drugs (see Chapter 3, Clinical Decision Making for Massage).[4,8,10,26] All signs of acute inflammation such as spasm, pain at rest, heat, redness, and unconsolidated edema must be absent prior to the use of friction.[97] Clinicians should not perform friction in the area of hematomas, calcifications, peripheral nerves, or fragile skin.[103] Clinicians should use extreme caution when applying friction around hypermobile or unstable joints such as recurrent sprains or dislocations; in clients with systemic connective tissue disorders; and in clients with osteoporosis. Finally, the clinician should use care when applying friction in hypotonic regions or in the vicinity of active trigger points.

# USING FRICTION IN TREATMENT

## To Decrease Adhesions and Fibrosis and Increase Connective Tissue Extensibility

The massage techniques for increasing connective tissue extensibility include skin rolling, myofascial release, direct fascial technique, friction, and conventional stretches that are held for 30 seconds or longer. Petrissage may be appropriate when applied slowly and with a high component of drag. Self-stretching is particularly useful for client homecare. Neuromuscular or muscle energy techniques, joint mobilization, joint mobilization and manipulation, and spinal traction performed from the head or pelvis may be useful depending on the situation.[26]

In controlled laboratory conditions, the precise heating of tissue facilitates a greater elongation of collagenous structures without resulting in significant structural damage.[21,24,54] In clinical practice, however, the application of heat prior to any sustained loading of connective tissue can increase the risk of large-scale collagenous rupture.

Consequently, the clinician should avoid the application of either heat or cold before performing connective tissue techniques, unless his aim is specifically to rupture or denature collagen.[54] This may be the case when using friction to treat a large or dense adhesion. Heat applied after the use of friction can enhance the temporary increase in the pliability of myofascial tissue.

If the client reports increased tenderness after you apply friction, immediately apply a cold pack until vasoconstriction (blanching) occurs. Instruct the client to apply a cold pack to the area for 10 to 14 minutes at intervals for the next 24 hours.

## For Contractile Lesions

For repetitive strain injuries involving muscle or tendon and for chronic-stage strains, a local application of myofascial release or direct fascial technique prior to the application of friction may reduce the need for extensive or prolonged use of friction. Preapplication of ultrasound has also been recommended.[103] Gentle pain-free passive stretch of the target tissues for 30 seconds and active movement in the pain-free range of motion can be beneficial following friction.[103] Teach the client to perform these several times a day between interventions. Instruct the client who has a repetitive strain injury to avoid aggravating activities, resistance exercise, and intensive stretching until later in the healing process. At that point, the client may engage in more aggressive stretching and strengthening. Splints, taping, and ergonomic or neuromuscular retraining may be useful in reducing repetitive strain or preventing recurrence of accident.[11]

If the client reports increased tenderness after you apply friction, immediately apply a cold pack until vasoconstriction (blanching) occurs. Instruct the client to apply a cold pack to the area for 10 to 14 minutes at intervals for the next 24 hours.

## Clinical Case

## History of Present Illness

A 40-year-old male computer programmer has right-sided lateral epicondylitis (repetitive strain injury) secondary to keyboarding, poor posture, and poor ergonomics.

## Subjective

1. Complaints of pain at rest and while keyboarding
2. Complaints of inability to keyboard for greater than 10 minutes without severe pain
3. Complaints of dropping objects held in his right hand during work and self-care activities because of pain and a feeling of weakness
4. Complaints of mild swelling after work
5. Visual analog scale pain rating = 8.5
6. Reports lack of ergonomic modifications to work station
7. Poor knowledge of ergonomics and self-care

## Objective

*Impairments*

- Pain elicited on resisted R wrist and finger extension
- Grip strength: Right grip less than left on testing with JAMAR dynamometer
- Palpation: Fascial shortening in area of the right common extensor origin and forearm musculature
- Posture: Kyphotic, forward head posture

## Functional Limitations

- Unable to keyboard for greater than 10 minutes or perform job requirements as a computer programmer secondary to pain
- Compromised ability to perform work and self-care due to pain and weakness; drops objects held in his right hand
- Unable to perform recreation activity of racquetball secondary to pain

# Analysis

## Treatment Rationale

To reduce the pain and inflammation associated with lateral epicondylitis and to provide education on self-care and ergonomics to prevent future exacerbations of this condition

| Impairment | Outcomes and Role of Massage |
|---|---|
| Pain | Decreased pain |
| | Primary treatment; direct effect since the pain is secondary to inflammation of the tissues at common extensor origin |
| | Primary treatment; direct effect resulting from counterirritant analgesia |
| Inflammation | Decreased inflammation |
| | Primary treatment; reduction of inflammation is a direct effect |
| Fascial shortening | Normalized fascial extensibility |
| | Primary treatment; fascial lengthening is a direct effect |
| Postural malalignment | Normalized postural alignment |
| | Primary treatment; direct effect resulting from fascial lengthening |
| Decreased strength | Increased strength |
| | Secondary effect since decreased strength is largely due to pain and inflammation. |

| Activity Limitation | Functional Outcomes |
|---|---|
| Decreased ability to keyboard | Patient will be able to keyboard with the use of ergonomic modifications for 1 hour with appropriate stretching and rest periods without complaints of pain. |
| Decreased ability to perform household tasks | Patient will be able to carry 10-lb weight in his right hand for 25 feet without complaints of pain or dropping the weight as needed for performing household chores. |
| Decreased ability to perform athletic tasks | Patient will be able to play racquetball for 20 minutes following the appropriate warm-up without complaints of pain. |

| Plan | |
|---|---|
| Massage Techniques | Petrissage, myofascial release, and direct fascial technique applied to shortened muscles related to kyphosis and forward head posture |
| | Superficial effleurage, petrissage, myofascial release, and direct fascial technique applied to the entire forearm, especially muscles of the extensor compartment. |

       ▣ Some work on the contralateral arm may be required to maintain right-left balance.

       ▣ Friction to the common extensor origin.

**Other Appropriate Techniques and Interventions**

Ice after friction if signs of overtreatment are present; wrist and hand stretches; wrist and hand strengthening exercises; postural stretches; postural education; ergonomic examination; education in ergonomics; and self-care

## References

1. Holey E, Cook E. *Evidence-Based Therapeutic Massage*. 2nd ed. Edinburgh: Churchill Livingstone; 2003.
2. Yates J. *A Physician's Guide to Therapeutic Massage*. 3rd ed. Toronto: Curties Overzet; 2004.
3. Cantu RI, Grodin AJ. *Myofascial Manipulation: Theory and Clinical Application*. 2nd ed. Gaithersburg, MD: Aspen Publishers; 2001.
4. Fritz S. *Mosby's Fundamentals of Therapeutic Massage*. 3rd ed. St. Louis: Mosby; 2004.
5. Chaitow L. *Palpation and Assessment Skills*. Edinburgh: Churchill-Livingston; 2003.
6. Maigne R. Low back pain of thoracolumbar origin. *Arch Phys Med Rehabil*. 1980;61:389–395.
7. Greenman PE. *Principles of Manual Medicine*. 2nd ed. Baltimore: Williams and Wilkins; 1996.
8. Benjamin PJ, Tappan FM. *Tappan's Handbook of Healing Massage Techniques*. 4th ed. Upper Saddle River, NJ: Pearson Prentice Hall; 2005.
9. Salvo SG. *Massage Therapy: Principles and Practice*. 2nd ed. Philadelphia: WB Saunders; 2003.
10. de Domenico G, Wood EC. *Beard's Massage*. 4th ed. Philadelphia: WB Saunders; 1997.
11. American Physical Therapy Association. *Guide to Physical Therapist Practice*. 2nd ed. Alexandria, VA: American Physical Therapy Association; 1999.
12. Chaitow L. *Modern Neuromuscular Techniques*. New York: Churchill-Livingston; 1996.
13. Taylor P, Tole G, Vernon H. Skin rolling technique as an indicator of spinal joint dysfunction. *J Can Chiropr Assoc*. 1990; 34:82–86.
14. Tillman LJ, Chasan NP. Wound healing: injury and repair of dense connective tissues. In: Hertling D, Kessler RM, eds. *Management of Common Musculoskeletal Conditions*. 4th ed. Philadelphia: Lippincott Williams and Wilkins; 2006:15–26.
15. Kisner C, Colby LA. *Therapeutic Exercise: Foundations and Techniques*. 4th ed. Philadelphia: F. A. Davis Company; 2002.
16. Lederman E. *The Science and Practice of Manual Therapy*. Edinburgh: Elsevier Churchill Livingstone; 2005.
17. Tillman LJ, Cummings GS. Biologic mechanisms of connective tissue mutability. In: Currier DP, Nelson RM, eds. *Dynamics of Human Biologic Tissues*. Philadelphia: FA Davis; 1992:1–44.
18. Taylor DC, Dalton JD, Seaber AV, Garret WE. Visco-elastic properties of muscle-tendon units: the biomechanical effects of stretching. *Am J Sports Med*. 1990;18:300–309.
19. Frank C, Amiel D, et al. Normal ligament properties and ligament healing. *Clin Orthop*. 1985;196:15–25.
20. Dunn MG, Silver FH. Visco-elastic behavior of human connective tissue: relative contribution of viscous and elastic components. *Connective Tissue Res*. 1983;12:59–70.
21. Sapega AA, Quedenfeld TC. Biophysical factors in range of motion exercise. *Physician Sports Med*. 1981:9:57–65.
22. Light KE, Nuzik S, Personius W, Barstrom A. Low load prolonged stretch vs high load brief stretch in treating knee contractures. *Phys Ther*. 1984;64:330–333.
23. Hooey CJ, McCrum NG, et al. The visco-elastic deformation of tendon. *J Biomech*. 1980:13:521–529.
24. Warren CG, Lehmann JF, et al. Heat and stretch procedures: an evaluation using rat tail tendon. *Arch Phys Med Rehabil*. 1976;57:122–126.
25. Mannheim CJ. *The Myofascial Release Manual*. 3rd ed. Thorofare, NJ: Slack Inc; 2001.
26. Barnes, JF. Myofascial release. In: Hammer WI, ed. *Functional Soft Tissue Examination and Treatment by Manual Methods*. 2nd ed. Gaithersburg, MD: Aspen; 1999:533–548.
27. Upledger J, Vredevoogd JD. *Craniosacral Therapy*. Seattle, WA: Eastland Press; 1983.
28. DiGiovanna EL, Schiowitz S. *An Osteopathic Approach to Diagnosis and Treatment*. 2nd ed. Philadelphia: Lippincott-Raven; 1997.
29. Sucher BM, Heath DM. Thoracic outlet syndrome—a myofascial variant: Part 3. Structural and postural considerations. *J Am Osteopath Assoc*. 1993;93:334,340–345.
30. Sucher BM. Thoracic outlet syndrome—a myofascial variant: Part 2. Treatment. *J Am Osteopath Assoc*. 1990;90:810–812, 817–823.
31. Sucher BM. Thoracic outlet syndrome—a myofascial variant: Part 1. Pathology and diagnosis. *J Am Osteopath Assoc*. 1990; 90:686–696,703–704.
32. Sucher BM. Myofascial manipulative release of carpal tunnel syndrome: documentation with magnetic resonance imaging. *J Am Osteopath Assoc*. 1993;93:1273–1278.
33. Sucher BM. Myofascial release of carpal tunnel syndrome. *J Am Osteopath Assoc*. 1993;93:92–94,100–101.
34. Cisler TA. Whiplash as a total-body injury. *J Am Osteopath Assoc*. 1994;94:145–148.
35. Hanten WP, Chandler SD. Effects of myofascial release leg pull and sagittal plane isometric contract-relax techniques on passive straight-leg raise angle. *J Orthop Sports Phys Ther*. 1994;20: 138–144.
36. Radjieski JM, Lumley MA, Cantieri MS. Effect of osteopathic manipulative treatment on length of stay for pancreatitis: a randomized pilot study. *J Am Osteopath Assoc*. 1998;98:264–172.
37. Barnes MF, Gronlund RT, Little MF, Personius WJ. Efficacy study of the effect of a myofascial release treatment technique

on obtaining pelvic symmetry. *J Bodywork Movement Ther.* 1997;1:289–296.

38. Konczak CR, Ames R. Relief of internal snapping hip syndrome in a marathon runner after chiropractic treatment. *J Manipulative Physiol Ther.* 2005;28:67 (Abstract).

39. Anonymous. Research: massage reduces headache frequency. *Massage Magazine.* 2003;109.

40. Crawford JS, Simpson J, Crawford P. Myofascial release provides symptomatic relief from chest wall tenderness occasionally seen following lumpectomy and radiation in breast cancer patients. *Int J Radiat Oncol Biol Phys.* 1996;34:1188–1189.

41. Moore MK. Upper crossed syndrome and its relationship to cervicogenic headache. *J Manipulative Physiol Ther.* 2004;27:414–420.

42. Hou CR, Tsai LC, Cheng KF, Chung KC, Hong CZ. Immediate effects of various physical therapeutic modalities on cervical myofascial pain and trigger-point sensitivity. *Arch Phys Med Rehabil.* 2002;83:1406–1414.

43. Anonymous. Massage offers respite for primary caregivers. *Massage Magazine.* 2001:68.

44. Anonymous. Tips for bodyworkers working with cancer patients. *Massage Bodywork.* 1999;14:19.

45. Schultz RL, Feitis R. *Fascial Anatomy and Physical Reality.* Berkeley, CA: North Atlantic Books; 1996.

46. Rolf I. *Rolfing: The Integration of Human Structures.* New York: Harper and Row; 1977.

47. Myers T. *Anatomy Trains.* Edinburgh: Churchill Livingstone; 2001.

48. Myers TW. The "anatomy trains": part 2. *J Bodywork Movement Ther.* 1997;1:134–145.

49. Stanborough M. *Direct Release Myofascial Technique.* Edinburgh: Churchill Livingstone; 2004.

50. Smith J. *Structural Bodywork.* Edinburgh: Elsevier Churchill Livingstone; 2005.

51. McCutcheon B. Fascial integration: a global approach for specific results. *J Soft Tissue Manipulation.* 2000;7:4–7.

52. McCutcheon B. Fascial gait analysis. *J Soft Tissue Manipulation.* 2000;7:3–7.

53. Erickson S. How to understand tissue memory and its implications. *Massage Ther J.* 2003;42:70–77.

54. Cummings GS, Tillman LJ. Remodeling of dense connective tissue in normal adult tissues. In: Currier DP, Nelson RM, eds. *Dynamics of Human Biologic Tissues.* Philadelphia: FA Davis; 1992:45–73.

55. Barlow W. *The Alexander Technique.* New York: Alfred A. Knopf; 1973.

56. Quality Assurance Committee of the College of Massage Therapists of Ontario. *Code of Ethics and Standards of Practice.* Toronto: College of Massage Therapists of Ontario; 2006.

57. Ebner M. *Connective Tissue Manipulations: Theory and Therapeutic Application.* 3rd ed. Malabar, FL: Krieger; 1985.

58. Rolf I. *Rolfing and Physical Reality.* Rochester, VT: Healing Arts Press; 1990.

59. Cottingham JT, Porges SW, Richmond K. Shifts in pelvic inclination angle and parasympathetic tone produced by Rolfing soft tissue manipulation. *Phys Ther.* 1988;68:1364–1370.

60. Schleip R. Fascial plasticity—a new neurobiological explanation: part 1. *J Bodywork Movement Ther.* 2003;7:11–19.

61. Jones TA. Rolfing. *Phys Med Rehabil Clin N Am.* 2004;15:799–809.

62. Myers TW. Structural integration: developments in Ida Rolf's "recipe." Part 3: an alternative form. *J Bodywork Movement Ther.* 2004;8:249–264.

63. Myers TW. Structural integration: developments in Ida Rolf's "recipe." Part 2. *J Bodywork Movement Ther.* 2004;8:189–198.

64. Myers TW. Structural integration: developments in Ida Rolf's "recipe." Part 1. *J Bodywork Movement Ther.* 2004;8:131–142.

65. Stillerman E. *The Encyclopedia of Bodywork.* New York: Facts on File; 1996.

66. Holey EA. Connective tissue massage: a bridge between complementary and orthodox approaches. *J Bodywork Movement Ther.* 2000;4:72–80.

67. Cottingham JT, Maitland J. A three-paradigm treatment model using soft tissue mobilization and guided movement-awareness techniques for a patient with chronic low back pain: a case study. *J Orthop Sports Phys Ther.* 1997;26:155–167.

68. Perry J, Jones MH, Thomas L. Functional evaluation of Rolfing in cerebral palsy. *Dev Med Child Neurol.* 1981;23:717–729.

69. Anonymous. World-class pianist recovers with rolfing. *Massage Magazine.* 1996:148.

70. Hunt VV, Massey W. Electromyographic evaluation of structural integration techniques. *Psychoenergetic Systems.* 1977;2:1–12.

71. Cottingham JT, Porges SW, Lyon T. Effects of soft tissue mobilization (Rolfing pelvic lift) on parasympathetic tone in two age groups. *Phys Ther.* 1988;68:352–356.

72. McKechnie AA, Wilson F, Watson N, Scott D. Anxiety states: a preliminary report on the value of connective tissue massage. *J Psychosom Res.* 1983;27:125–129.

73. Weinberg RS, Hunt VV. Effects of structural integration on state-trait anxiety. *J Clin Psychol.* 1979;35:319–322.

74. Silverman J, Rappaport M, Hopkins HK, Ellman G, Hubbard R, Belleza T, et al. Stress, stimulus intensity control, and the structural integration technique. *Confinia Psychiatrica.* 1973;16:201–219.

75. Reed BV, Held JM. Effects of sequential connective tissue massage on autonomic nervous system of middle-aged and elderly adults. *Phys Ther.* 1988;68:1231–1234.

76. Kisner CD, Taslitz N. Connective tissue massage: influence of the introductory treatment on autonomic functions. *Phys Ther.* 1968;48:107–119.

77. Kaada B, Torsteinbo O. Increase of plasma beta-endorphins in connective tissue massage. *Gen Pharmacol.* 1989;20:487–489.

78. Kaada B, Torsteinbo O. Vasoactive intestinal polypeptides in connective tissue massage. With a note on VIP in heat pack treatment. *Gen Pharmacol.* 1987;18:379–384.

79. Gross D. Physical therapy and rheumatism of soft tissues. *Schweiz Med Wochenschr (German).* 1982;112:1214–1218 (Abstract).

80. Frazer FW. Persistent post-sympathetic pain treated by connective tissue massage. *Physiotherapy.* 1978;64:211–212.

81. Akbayrak T, Citak I, Demirturk F, Akarcali I. Manual therapy and pain changes in patients with migraine: an open pilot study. *Adv Physiother.* 2001;3:49–54.

82. Brattberg G. Connective tissue massage in the treatment of fibromyalgia. *Eur J Pain.* 1999;3:235–244.

83. Enebo BA. Conservative management of chronic low back pain using mobilization: a single-subject descriptive case study. *J Chiropr Technique.* 1998;10:68.

84. Gifford J, Gifford L. Connective tissue massage. In: Wells PE, Frampton V, Bowsher D, eds. *Pain Management by Physiotherapy.* 2nd ed. London: Butterworth-Heinemann; 1994:213–227.

85. Holey LA. Connective tissue zones: an introduction. *Physiotherapy.* 1995;81:366–368.

86. Holey LA, Walston MJ. Inter-rater reliability of connective tissue zones recognition. *Physiotherapy.* 1995;81:369–372.

87. Holey LA. Connective tissue manipulation: towards a scientific rationale. *Physiotherapy.* 1995;81:730–739.

88. Michalsen A, Buhring M. Connective tissue massage. *Wien Klin Wochenschr (German).* 1993;105:220–227 (Abstract).

89. Goats GC, Keir KA. Connective tissue massage. *Br J Sports Med.* 19 91;25:131–133.

90. Palastanga N. Connective tissue massage. In: Grieve GP, ed. *Modern Manual Therapy for the Vertebral Column.* New York: Churchill-Livingston; 1986:827–833.

91. Ebner M. Connective tissue massage. *Physiotherapy.* 1978;64:208–210.

92. Gonin M, Gerster JC. Pigmentation disorders in systemic scleroderma. *Schweiz Rundsch Med Prax.* 1994;83:42–45.

93. Predel K. Physical therapy in gastroenterology. *Z Gesamte Inn Med (German).* 1987;42:112–114 (Abstract).

94. Sabir'ianov AR, Shevtsov AV, Sabir'ianova ES, et al. Effect of reflex-segmental massage on central hemodynamics in healthy people. *Vopr Kurortol Fizioter Lech Fiz Kult.* 2004;2:5–7.

95. Anonymous. Segmental-reflex massage in rehabilitation of patients with ischemic heart disease. *Vopr Kurortol Fizioter Lech Fiz Kult.* 2005;1:45–49.

96. Nansel D, Szlazak M. Somatic dysfunction and the phenomenon of visceral disease simulation: a probable explanation for the apparent effectiveness of somatic therapy in patients presumed to be suffering from true visceral disease. *J Manipulative Physiol Ther.* 1995;18:379–397.

97. Kessler RM, Hertling D. Friction massage. In: Hertling D, Kessler RM, eds. *Management of Common Musculoskeletal Conditions.* 3rd ed. Philadelphia: Lippincott-Raven; 1996:133–139.

98. Lagrana NA, Alexander H, Strauchler I, Mehta A, Ricci J. Effect of mechanical load in wound healing. *Ann Plastic Surg.* 1983;10:200–208.

99. Magonne T, DeWitt MT, Handeley CJ, et al. In vitro responses of chondrocytes to mechanical loading: the effect of short term mechanical tension. *Connect Tissue Res.* 1984;12:97–109.

100. Arem AJ, Madden JW. Effects of stress on healing wounds. I. Intermittent noncyclical tension. *J Surg Res.* 1976;20:93–102.

101. Woo S, Matthews JV, et al. Connective tissue response to immobility. *Arthritis Rheum.* 1975;18:257–264.

102. Akeson WH, Woo SL-Y, et al. The connective tissue response to immobilization: biochemical changes in periarticular connective tissue of the rabbit knee. *Clin Orthop.* 1973;93:356–362.

103. Hammer WI. Friction massage. In: Hammer WI, ed. *Functional Soft Tissue Examination and Treatment by Manual Methods.* 2nd ed. Gaithersburg, MD: Aspen; 1999:463–478.

104. Palastanga N. The use of transverse frictions for soft tissue lesions. In: Grieve GP, ed. *Modern Manual Therapy for the Vertebral Column.* New York: Churchill-Livingston; 1986:819–825.

105. Cyriax J, Coldham M. *Textbook of Orthopedic Medicine. Volume 2. Treatment by Manipulation, Massage and Injection.* 11th ed. London: Bailliere Tindall; 1984.

106. Cyriax J. Deep massage. *Physiotherapy.* 1977;63:60–61.

107. Lowe WL. *Orthopedic Massage.* Edinburgh: Mosby; 2003.

108. Walker JM. Deep transverse frictions in ligament healing. *J Orthop Sports Phys Ther.* 1984;62:89–94.

109. de Brujin R. Deep transverse friction; its analgesic effect. *Int J Sports Med.* 1984;5(Suppl):35–36.

110. Chamberlain GJ. Cyriax's friction massage: a review. *J Orthop Sports Phys Ther.* 1982;4:16–22.

111. Bajuk S, Jelnikar T, Ortar M. Rehabilitation of patient with brachial plexus lesion and break in axillary artery. Case study. *J Hand Ther.* 1996;9:399–403.

112. Guler-Uysal F, Kozanoglu E. Comparison of the early response to two methods of rehabilitation in adhesive capsulitis. *Swiss Med Wkly.* 2004;134:353–358.

113. Nilsson N, Christensen HW, Hartvigsen J. Lasting changes in passive range motion after spinal manipulation: a randomized, blind, controlled trial. *J Manipulative Physiol Ther.* 1996;19:165–168.

114. Nilsson N. A randomized controlled trial of the effect of spinal manipulation in the treatment of cervicogenic headache. *J Manipulative Physiol Ther.* 1995;18:435–440.

115. O'Sullivan S, Schmitz T. *Physical Rehabilitation, Assessment and Treatment.* 2nd ed. Philadelphia: F. A. Davis; 1988.

116. Patino O, Novick C, Merlo A, Benaim F. Massage in hypertrophic scars. *J Burn Care Rehabil.* 1999;20:268–271.

117. Sevier TL, Wilson JK. Treating lateral epicondylitis. *Sports Med.* 1999;28:375–380.

118. Hammer WI. The use of friction massage in the management of chronic bursitis of the hip or shoulder. *J Manipulative Physiol Ther.* 1993;16:107–111.

119. Fritschy D, de Gautard R. Jumper's knee and ultrasonography. *Am J Sports Med.* 1988;16:637–640.

120. Hunter SC, Poole RM. The chronically inflamed tendon. *Clin Sports Med.* 1987;6:371–388.

121. Woodman RM, Pare L. Evaluation and treatment of soft tissue lesions of the ankle and forefoot using the Cyriax approach. *Phys Ther.* 1982;62:1144–1147.

122. Brosseau L, Casimiro L, Milne S, et al. Deep transverse friction massage for treating tendinitis. *Cochrane Database Syst Rev.* 2002;4:CD003528.

123. Boisaubert B, Brousse C, Zaoui A, Montigny JP. Nonsurgical treatment of tennis elbow. *Ann Readapt Med Phys.* 2004;47:346–355.

## Further Reading

Adcock D, Paulsen S, Jabour K, Davis S, Nanney LB, Shack RB. Analysis of the effects of deep mechanical massage in the porcine model. *Plast Reconstr Surg.* 2001;108:233–240.

Akeson WH, Amiel D, et al. The connective tissue response to immobility: an accelerated aging response. *Exp Gerontol.* 1968;3:289–301.

Anonymous. Deep tissue massage and myofascial release. *Massage Bodywork.* 2003;18:105.

Anonymous. Clinical perspectives. Connective tissue perspectives: part 2. *J Bodywork Movement Ther.* 2002;6:220–227.

Archer PA. Three clinical sports massage approaches for treating injured athletes. *Athletic Therapy Today.* 2001;6:14–20.

Barnes JF. Myofascial release for craniomandibular pain and dysfunction. *Int J Orofacial Myology.* 1996;22:20–22.

Barnes JF. Myofascial release in treatment of thoracic outlet syndrome. *J Bodywork Movement Ther.* 1996;1:53–57.

Barnes MF. The basic science of myofascial release: morphologic change in connective tissue. *J Bodywork Movement Ther.* 1997; 1:231–238.

Barnes JF. The myofascial release approach. Part II: the mind/body connection. *Massage Magazine.* 1994:58.

Barnes JF. The myofascial release approach. Part III: the fascial cranium and intuitive therapy. *Massage Magazine.* 1994:84.

Barnes JF. The myofascial release approach. Part IV: therapeutic artistry. *Massage Magazine.* 1994:72.

Barnes JF. The myofascial release approach: the missing link. *Massage Magazine.* 1994:36.

Barnes JF. The myofascial release mind/body healing approach. *Massage Magazine.* 1998:91.

Bernau-Eigen M. Rolfing: a somatic approach to the integration of human structures. *Nurse Pract Forum.* 1998;9:235–242.

Cook JL, Khan KM. Overuse tendinosis, not tendinitis. *Phys Sportsmed.* 2000;28:31.

Cook JL, Khan KM. What is the most appropriate treatment for patellar tendinopathy? *Br J Sports Med.* 2001;35:291–294.

Crawford JS, Simpson J, Crawford P. Myofascial release provides symptomatic relief from chest wall tenderness occasionally seen following lumpectomy and radiation in breast cancer patients. *Int J Radiat Oncol Biol Phys.* 1996;34:1188–1189.

Cummings GS, Crutchfield CA, Barnes MR. *Soft Tissue Changes in Contractures.* Atlanta, GA: Stokesville Publishing; 1995.

Dalton E. Professional discovery through personal disaster. *Massage Magazine.* 2002:94.

Danto JB. Review of integrated neuromusculoskeletal release and the novel application of a segmental anterior/posterior approach in the thoracic, lumbar, and sacral regions. *J Am Osteopath Assoc.* 2003;103:583–596.

Davidson CJ, Ganion LR, Gehlsen GM, Verhoestra B, Roepke JE, Sevier TL. Rat tendon morphologic and functional changes resulting from soft tissue mobilization. *Med Sci Sports Exerc.* 1997;29:313–319.

Dicke E. *Meine Bindegewebsmassage.* Stuttgart: Hippokrates; 1953.

Dicke E, Schliack H, Wolff A. *A Manual of Reflexive Therapy of Connective Tissue.* Scarsdale, NY: Simon; 1978.

Fung YCB. Elasticity of soft tissues in simple elongation. *Am J Physiol.* 1967;213:1532–1544.

Gallagher A. The integrated approach. *Massage Aust.* 2003:28–35.

Glaser O, Dalicho AW. *Segmentmassage: Massage Reflektorischer Zonen, Verl.* Leipzig, Germany: Georg Thieme; 1955.

Hammer WI. How does friction massage help tendinitis heal? *J Soft Tissue Manipulation.* 1999;7:20–21.

Hardy MA. The biology of scar formation. *Phys Ther.* 1989;69:22–32.

Head H. On disturbance of sensation with especial reference to the pain of visceral disease. *Brain.* 1893;16:1–133.

Holey LA, Lawler H. The effects of classical massage and connective tissue manipulation on bowel function. *Br J Ther Rehabil.* 1995;2:627–631.

Hunter G. Specific soft tissue mobilization in the treatment of soft-tissue lesions. *Physiotherapy.* 1994;30:15–21.

James H. Tendon and ligament healing: a new approach through manual therapy. *Massage Magazine.* 2001:155.

Jamison CE, Marangoni RD, Glaser AA. Visco-elastic properties of soft tissue by discrete model characterization. *J Biomech.* 1968;1:33–46.

King RK. Myofascial breathwork: a regenerative bodywork approach. *J Bodywork Movement Ther.* 2002;6:224–225.

King RK. *Myofascial Massage Therapy: Towards Postural Balance.* Chicago, IL: Self-published training manual by Bobkat Productions; 1996.

LaBan MM. Collagen tissue: implications of its response to stress in vitro. *Arch Phys Med Rehabil.* 1962;43:461–466.

Latz J. CTM. *Massage Bodywork.* 2001;16:12.

Latz J. Key elements of connective tissue massage. *Massage Ther J.* 2003;41:46–50,52–53.

Leahy PM. Improved treatments for carpal tunnel. *Chiropractic Sports Med.* 1995;9:6–9.

Leahy PM, Mock LE. Myofascial release technique and mechanical compromise of peripheral nerves of the upper extremity. *Chiropractic Sports Med.* 1992;6:139–150.

Lowther DA. The effect of compression and tension on the behavior of connective tissue. In: Glasgow EF, Twomey LT, Scull ER, Klenhans AM, Edczek RM, eds. *Aspects of Manipulative Therapy.* 2nd ed. London: Churchill Livingstone; 1985:16–22.

MacKenzie J. *Symptoms and Their Interpretation.* London: Shaw and Sons; 1909.

Myers T. Some thoughts on intra-nasal work. *J Bodywork Movement Ther.* 2001;5:149–159.

Myers TW. A structural approach. *J Bodywork Movement Ther.* 1998;2:14–20.

Nilsson N. A randomized controlled trial of the effect of spinal manipulation in the treatment of cervicogenic headache. *J Manipulative Physiol Ther.* 1995;18:435–440.

Nilsson N, Christensen HW, Hartvigsen J. The effect of spinal manipulation in the treatment of cervicogenic headache. *J Manipulative Physiol Ther.* 1997;20:326–330.

Oschman JL. Structural integration (rolfing), osteopathic, chiropractic, feldenkrais, Alexander, myofascial release and related methods: energy review part 5B. *J Bodywork Movement Ther.* 1997;1:305–309.

Oschman JL. What is healing energy? Part 5: gravity, structure, and emotions: energy review part 5A. *J Bodywork Movement Ther.* 1997;1:297–309.

Pellechia GL, Hamel H, Behnke P. Treatment of infrapatellar tendinitis: a combination of modalities and transverse friction massage versus iontophoresis. *J Sport Rehabil.* 1994;3:135–145.

Rigby BJ. The effect of mechanical extension upon the thermal stability of collagen. *Biochim Biophys Acta.* 1964;79:634–636.

Rigby BJ. The mechanical behavior of rat-tail tendon. *J Gen Physiol.* 1959;43:265–283.

Riggs A. Deep tissue massage. *Massage Bodywork.* 2005;20:38–49.

Robertson A, Gilmore K, Frith PA, Antic R. Effects of connective tissue massage in subacute asthma. *Med J Aust.* 1984;140:52–53.

Smith FR. Causes of and treatment options for abnormal scar tissue. *J Wound Care.* 2005;14:49–52.

Stromberg DD, Weiderhielm DA. Visco-elastic description of a collagenous tissue in simple elongation. *J Appl Physiol.* 1969;26: 857–862.

Turchaninov R, Prilutsky B. Massage therapy: a beneficial tool in treating fibromyalgia. *Massage Bodywork.* 2004;19:82–93.

Weinstock D. Conscious bodywork. *Massage Bodywork.* 2000;15:24.

Wiltsie CW. Deep tissue massage: does therapy have an impact on body dimensions in the hips and thighs of women? *Massage Bodywork.* 1999;14:32.

Passive movement techniques are those massage techniques that primarily palpate the movement of tissues and structures, as opposed to palpating their substance. These techniques, such as shaking, rhythmic mobilization, and rocking, use passive motion to treat restrictions in tissues and structures. This chapter describes these techniques, how to perform them, and how to apply them in a practice sequence. A section on further study for each technique discusses relevant outcomes and evidence, cautions and contraindications, and how to use the technique in treatment.

## Table 11-1 Summary of Outcomes for Passive Movement Techniques

| Outcome | Technique | | |
| --- | --- | --- | --- |
| | Shaking | Rhythmic Mobilization | Rocking |
| Systemic sedation | P | P | P |
| Decreased perceived anxiety | P | P | P |
| Increased arousal | P | P | ? |
| Analgesia | P | ✓ | ✓ |
| Increased local muscle resting tension or neuromuscular tone | P | ? | ? |
| Decreased muscle resting tension | P | P | P |
| Increased joint mobility | ? | P | P |
| Increased accessory joint motion | ? | P | P |
| Increased rib cage mobility | ? | P | P |
| Increased airway clearance/mobilization of secretions | ? | ✓ | ? |
| Decreased dyspnea | ? | P | P |
| Stimulated peristalsis | P | P | P |
| Alteration of movement responses | ? | ✓ | ✓ |
| Increased ability to perform movement tasks | ? | ✓ | ✓ |

✓: the outcome is supported by research summarized in this chapter. P: the outcome is possible. ?: the outcome is debatable (research results are absent or inconsistent).

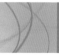

## Shaking: Foundations

## DEFINITION

Shaking: The technique moves soft tissue—primarily muscle—back and forth repetitively over the underlying bone, with minimal joint movement.

## USES

Therapists use shaking to reduce "holding," which is what Mense and Simon[1] call **unnecessary muscle tension**. Unnecessary muscle tension is an unintentional muscle contraction that is under voluntary control, which is often due to situational stress.[1] They also use shaking to reduce the muscle resting tension of skeletal muscles.[2,3] In addition, they often use shaking in pre-event and interevent **sports massage** because it may reduce tone while enhancing **arousal** (wakefulness).[4]

## PALPATION PRACTICE

1. Review regional myology as time permits by drawing the major skeletal muscles on a partner. Palpate the fiber directions, borders, and tendons of all superficial muscles.
2. Assess muscle resting tension through palpation. Attempt to describe the quality of resistance to pressure in detail (see Chapter 5, Client Examination for Massage). When the muscle it is at rest, what do muscle, fascia, fat, and fluid contribute to the firmness of each muscle that you feel? Use the discussion in Chapter 5, Client Examination for Massage, for assistance.
3. Grasp the long muscle groups of your partner's legs and arms and attempt to roll them around the bones to which they attach. How far do they go? At the limit of each muscle group's excursion, release the limb and watch the resulting motion as the tissues move back to their original position.

---

### Box 11-1    Components of Shaking

**Contact:** Whole relaxed palmar surface. Use variable levels of fingertip contact depending on the desired degree of stimulation.

**Pressure:** Light to moderate. Avoid constant heavy manual pressure since it dampens the wave of motion that is produced through tissues.

**Tissues engaged:** Hands engage to the depth of the superficial muscle layers. The motion produced by the stroke simultaneously engages all the tissues throughout the body segment that you are shaking, including muscle, fascia, tendon, ligament, and periosteum.

**Direction:** Direct your force around the circumference of the long axis of the body segment. As a result, the motion produced by the stroke will travel in waves along this long axis.

**Amplitude:** Depends on the region

**Rate:** 2 to 5 cycles per second

**Duration:** 5 seconds or longer

**Intergrades with:** Fine vibration

**Combines with:** You can apply broad and specific compression at the same time as shaking. At this point, because of the combination of compression and (nongliding) movement, it becomes a technique that resembles, although technically is not identical to, **petrissage**, which combines compression and gliding movement.

**Context:** Can be alternated with other techniques presented in this chapter in interventions that focus solely on movement. You can also alternate this technique with the **neuromuscular techniques** described in Chapter 9, Neuromuscular Techniques.

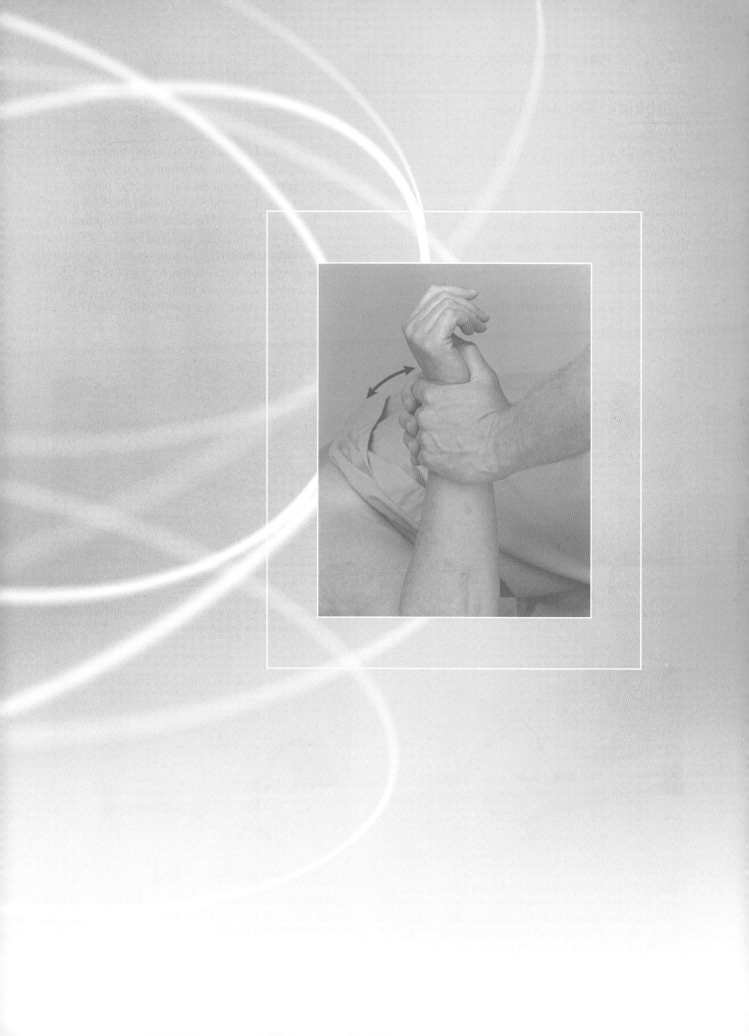

## Shaking: Technique

# MANUAL TECHNIQUE

Figures 11-1 to 11-8 show therapists applying shaking to the various regions of the body. The order of the figures is from head to foot in supine and then in prone. Each figure illustrates most of the guidelines for manual technique outlined below.

1. Shaking muscle over underlying bone can have a psychologically sedative or **stimulating** effect depending on the contact and rate of application therapists use when they are performing the technique.

A. For **sedation**: Use an even, relaxed, full palmar contact and a slower rate. Your hand contact is flat on the flat surfaces of the client's body (Figures 11-1 and 11-4). In this case, a relaxed hand contact that produces minimal tissue compression will produce the greatest tissue excursion. Arch your hand slightly for curved surfaces of the client's body, since this will lift the client's tissues into your palm (Figures

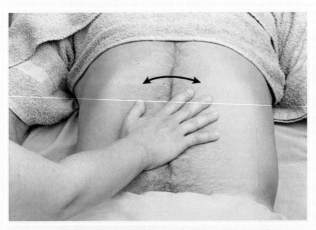

Figure 11-1 This superficial shaking of the abdomen does not cause movement of the pelvis or spine (compare with Figure 11-12). All types of abdominal shaking can be useful for constipation.

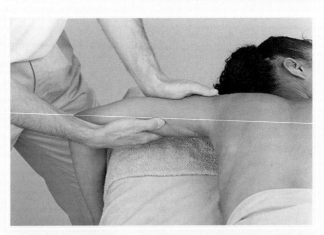

Figure 11-3 When shaking the deltoid, first lift the arm off the table to permit free movement of the client's tissues. If a client involuntary tenses her arm, draw her awareness to the tension and wait until the shoulder relaxes before beginning the shaking.

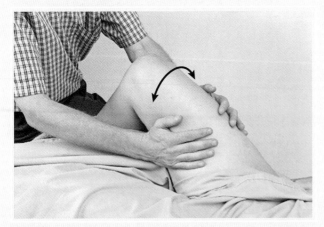

Figure 11-2 Two-handed shaking of the entire thigh with the knee flexed. Hands work together, rolling the tissue around the bone, first one way and then back to, and past, resting position. You can add varying amounts of compression to produce a more forceful and stimulating stroke.

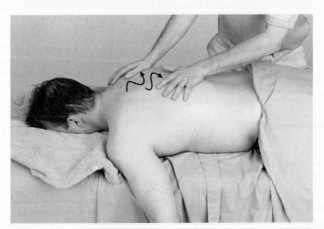

Figure 11-4 During shaking of the superficial tissues and muscles of the back, the two hands can be moved in the same, or in opposite, directions.

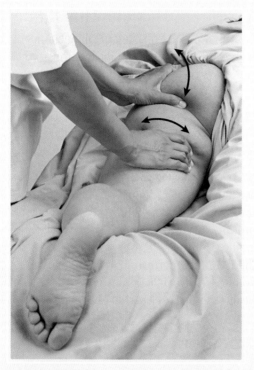

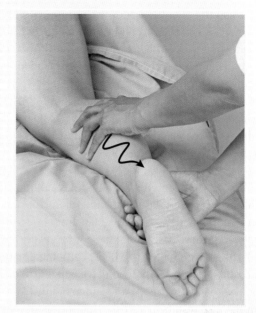

Figure 11-7   Shaking the calf.

Figure 11-5   Shaking of the gluteals can be done one-handed or two-handed and can simultaneously include the proximal hamstrings. Each hand shakes cross-fiber.

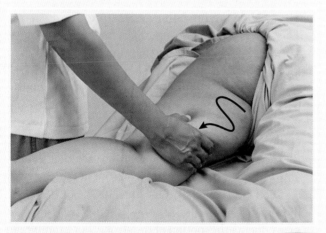

Figure 11-6   One-handed shaking of the adductors of the thigh in prone. You may release and regrasp, or you may maintain a loose grasp while shaking the client's limb and gliding distally to the knee (arrow).

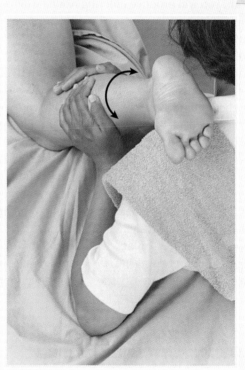

Figure 11-8   This two-handed "rolling" technique for the calf is also possible in supine (position as in Figure 11-2).

11-3 and 11-5). The client should perceive the pressure as being evenly distributed over the entire contact surface, an effect that is not easy for you to achieve. For each stroke, lift the client's tissues and then allow them to drop under their own weight. Maintain hand contact so that the strokes are con-nected. It takes practice to perform this technique with the full, comfortable contact that will allow you to apply it for longer periods.

B.   For stimulation: Focus your contact more specifically on your thumb and fingertips (Figure 11-6).

Grasp the client's tissues with more pressure and increase the rate. In addition, make a continuous effort to move the tissues back and forth, rather than allowing gravity or the **elastic recoil** of the tissue to perform the return stroke.

2. Let your wrist(s) remain relaxed as you move your hand(s) back and forth rhythmically. When you are on the client's limbs, move your hands perpendicularly to the long axis of the limb to produce waves of tissue motion that travel along, or parallel to, the long axis of the limb.

3. To achieve movement throughout a region, use a lighter contact and slide your hands along the region as you perform shaking (Figures 11-6 and 11-7). Alternatively, you can release your hand contact every few seconds, move your hands to a new position in the region, and establish a new hand contact. Changing hand positions every few seconds can reduce hand strain. This strategy also results in a stroke that the client may perceive as being more pleasant and less "machine-like."

4. Bear in mind that when you perform shaking with two hands, you will produce differing results when you use different approaches to coordinating the movement of your hands (Figures 11-2, 11-5, and 11-8).

5. "Rolling," or "rolling friction,"[5] is a useful two-handed version of shaking that you can perform on the client's limbs. Begin by resting your hands on opposite sides of the client's limb. Both of your hands will work together to roll the client's tissues around the circumference of the long axis of the limb, using the same motion as you would if you were rolling the cylinder of a rolling pin around its core. Then, reverse the direction of movement of your hands, rolling the tissue back to, and then past, its original position. Repeat these two motions in a rhythmic manner (Figures 11-2 and 11-8).

6. You can combine shaking with neuromuscular techniques by compressing into the client's tissues, or gripping and lifting these tissues, before beginning the shaking motion.

## How shaking might work

Shaking may help clients who are holding muscles tensely in response to situational stress to realize that this contraction is unnecessary by rapidly producing changes in muscle position.[2,6] In addition, the spreading and **shearing** of muscle that happens during shaking may cause proprioceptive input that reduces resting tension.[3,4,6] A similar mechanism occurs for petrissage.

### Critical Thinking Question

What are the physiological mechanisms by which shaking affects resting muscle tension?

## THERAPIST'S POSITION AND MOVEMENT

1. Use **standing aligned posture** and the other basic positions described in Chapter 6, Preparation and Positioning for Massage. You can avoid producing a choppy, irritating stroke by keeping your wrist, elbows, and shoulders relaxed.

2. When you are performing shaking for longer than 30 seconds, you can maintain a relaxed posture by periodically standing back to shake out your arms and hands briefly.

## PALPATE

While performing the technique, palpate the client's skin and tissues for the following:

1. The local skin temperature and texture.
2. The tone of the client's superficial muscles and tissues.
3. The excursion of the tissue that you are shaking. Try to form an impression of how far and how easily the tissues move during the application of the technique. In particular, identify how loose, dense, or tight the tissues feel under your hand and how this relates to the motion of the tissues.
4. Resistance to tissue movement. Note whether there is any resistance as you take the slack out of the tissues. In addition, note whether you can relate the resistance to movement to a specific tissue or structure that is involved in producing the motion of the stroke. For example, an adhesion at the proximal hamstring attachment can have a visible and palpable effect on the motion of the entire hamstring muscle during shaking.
5. The rhythmic response or **cadence** of the client's tissues during the stroke. Often, there is a rate and amplitude of shaking that the client finds the most pleasant. This varies with the person, body structure, level of muscle tone, region, and the type of shaking that you are using. It is critical, especially if sedation is the desired effect, to palpate for this optimal cadence and to adjust the rate and amplitude of the stroke to the client's needs.

6. The depth of penetration of the effect of the stroke. As the client's muscles relax and the **viscosity** of the tissues decreases, the same force will produce effects deeper into and further along the client's tissues. Consequently, as with petrissage, you will not need to apply greater force to achieve a greater penetration of effects; simply apply the technique for a longer duration.

## OBSERVE

As you perform the technique, observe the client to evaluate the degree of muscle movement you have achieved and to ensure that the **draping** maintains privacy. The following signs may signal this.

1. The degree of muscle movement. Movement of the client's muscles will be visibly less within areas of connective tissue hardening and elevated muscle resting tension. Even in normal tissue, movement will vary with different body shapes, proportions of body fat, and levels of conditioning.
2. Inappropriate draping. Since extended shaking can loosen draping, you may need to adjust or retuck a loosened drape to maintain discreet coverage of the client's body.

## COMMUNICATION WITH THE CLIENT

Communicate to ensure the client's comfort during the application of shaking. Here are some examples of statements that you can use.

1. "Is this pressure perfectly comfortable?" Alternatively, offer the client a choice: "Which feels better, this . . . or this?" This will enable you to ensure that your hand contact is comfortable for the client.
2. "Would it feel more relaxing if I slowed down a bit . . . like this?" Determine whether the rate and rhythm are comfortable for the client.
3. "Is everything okay?" "Are you feeling anything unusual?" When you are applying shaking continuously for longer than 2 minutes, find out whether the client is experiencing unpleasant symptoms of a sympathetic response such as irritation or nausea.
4. "Is this causing pain anywhere?" Use this statement periodically to check whether the client perceives that the intervention is causing pain. When the client presents with spasm or inflammation, the application of shaking to a distant area may result in pain by producing small motions at a distance from the point of contact.

---

 **A Practice Sequence for Shaking**

Practice time: 15 to 30 minutes per person or longer.
This sequence for anterior and posterior aspects of the legs uses no oil. You can easily perform it through loose clothes or draping, although the techniques are somewhat easier to apply on bare skin.

There are two basic ways of approaching movement sequences. One is to perform each technique in the sequence once for a longer period of time. An alternative, which tends to reduce therapist fatigue and tension, is to introduce all movements quickly, and then alternate frequently from one technique to the next, repeating the sequence as time permits. Strive for smooth continuous motion, without breaks between the various moves. Explore each motion and the infinite number of variations that are possible.

**Supine**
1. With one-hand contact, shake the quadriceps over the femur. Alternate your hands to reduce fatigue, and focus the technique more to the medial or lateral segment of the quadriceps. Move or slide the point of contact along the full length of the muscle group.
2. With your inner (table-side) hand, shake the adductors from their midpoint and distally.
3. Flex the client's knee to 90 degrees, sit on the foot (wrapped in the bottom sheet), and with two hands, contact the thigh on its medial and lateral surfaces. Roll the thigh back and forth repeatedly around the femur.
4. With the leg in the same position, grasp the calf with one hand and shake it while gliding your hand distally. Use whole-hand and fingertip contacts. Repeat.
5. With the leg in the same position, contact the medial and lateral surfaces of the calf with your entire hand. Roll the calf back and forth repeatedly around the tibia and fibula. Repeat this sequence two or more times.

Turn the client to **prone**.

6. Shake the gluteals over the pelvis with one of your hands, changing your hand positions to cover the entire muscle. Shake the gluteals with two hands, moving your hands towards each other and then apart, in contrary motion.

7. Flex the client's knee by placing one or two pillows under the ankle. Shake the hamstrings along their length with one hand and with two hands, in contrary motion.

8. With your inner (table-side) hand, shake the adductors from their midpoint and distally.

9. Rest the client's ankle on your toweled shoulder and roll the muscles of the posterior compartment between your palms.

10. Flex the knee to 90 degrees, grasp the heel and ankle, and shake the entire foot.

11. Repeat this sequence two or more times.

Home study: Devise a comparable supine and prone sequence for the arm.

# Shaking: Further Study and Practice

## NAMES AND ORIGINS

In other texts or massage-related systems, the technique that we call shaking is also known as "muscle shaking," "coarse vibration," "rolling friction," or "jostling."[2–9] Shaking is sometimes classified as a form of **petrissage** because both techniques focus force on skeletal muscle.[7,8] In this book, we present shaking in a separate chapter from petrissage because the method, effects, and uses differ from those discussed in Chapter 9, Neuromuscular Techniques. There is also a well-established tradition of presenting shaking as a technique in its own right.[9]

This book makes a distinction between the shaking of tissue over underlying bone, as defined earlier, and the shaking of entire structures such as the rib cage, limbs, and pelvis. The latter techniques involve the movement of joints and thus intergrade with more rigorous joint mobilization techniques (see Rhythmic Mobilization and Rocking later in this chapter). The manual techniques, effects, and uses of these other techniques are different enough to justify this distinction.

## OUTCOMES AND EVIDENCE

Traditionally, clinicians reported that shaking altered muscle resting tension through the stimulation of complex proprioceptive reflexes.[2–6] They also thought that it had a relaxing effect on skeletal muscle,[2–6] except for vigorous shaking, which might temporarily and marginally increase **muscle tone** via the stretch reflex.[9] Recently, clinicians have questioned whether it is possible for any passive technique, such as shaking, to substantially alter muscle

tone and suggest that active techniques are far more effective in this regard.[10]

Shaking has a variety of clinical applications. First, it can be an effective approach to reducing "holding," or **unnecessary muscle tension**.[2,3] In this case, reducing "holding" may be the primary goal. On the other hand, clinicians can use it as a preparatory technique used to reduce unnecessary muscular tension that may interfere with the execution of a technique such as high-grade **joint mobilization**. Second, clients often regard shaking as being pleasurable. Consequently, it is a useful technique for clinicians to use when they are seeking to achieve fully relaxed skeletal muscle. In addition, shaking is often used in precompetition and intercompetition **sports massage** to achieve systemic arousal and enhanced awareness of the muscle and, possibly, a temporary effect on muscle resting tension.[4,11–13] Finally, shaking has minor **mechanical effects** on connective tissue.[3] When it is applied gently in the fibroplastic stage of connective tissue repair, it may facilitate orderly remodeling of connective tissue. Table 11-1 summarizes the main outcomes for shaking.

### EXAMINING THE EVIDENCE

It is difficult to locate studies that evaluate the effects of shaking as an independent technique. Moreover, shaking is not often included in trials of massage that incorporate several techniques. A small study[14] (n = 14) examined the effect on **delayed-onset muscle soreness** (DOMS) of a 30-minute sports massage sequence, which included shaking, that clinicians performed 2 hours after eccentric exercise. Trend analysis showed significantly less DOMS, lower creatine kinase levels, and a higher neutrophil count for the massage group compared with the control group, who received a treatment consisting of the application of lubricant followed by 30 minutes of rest. The authors make interesting speculations regarding how massage might affect DOMS. This otherwise well-conceived study is hampered by its small sample. It also illustrates a common methodological quandary in massage research: How much discretion in applying the treatment protocol should researchers give the treating clinicians? In this case, researchers specified a fairly rigid sequence that was typical of those used to treat athletes after exercise. This protocol did not allow the clinician much freedom to adapt to each person's presenting issues, as usually happens in practice.

Smith LL, Keating MN, Holbert D, Spratt DJ, McCammon MR, Smith SS, et al. The effects of athletic massage on delayed onset muscle soreness, creatine kinase, and neutrophil count: a preliminary report. *J Orthop Sports Phys Ther*. 1994;19:93–99.

# CAUTIONS AND CONTRAINDICATIONS

Clinicians need clinical training and supervised practice to master the proper application of shaking. Advanced training may be advisable when dealing with pathological conditions. All of the general and local contraindications noted for massage techniques apply to the use of shaking (see Chapter 3, Clinical Decision Making for Massage). In particular, clinicians should avoid shaking any muscle that contains an acute injury, even if their hand position is remote from the site of injury. They can introduce less vigorous shaking at later stages, provided that they can perform it without causing the client pain. In addition, they should consider shaking a contraindication when the client exhibits spasm, hyperreflexia, or **spasticity**.

# USING SHAKING IN TREATMENT

## To Reduce Unnecessary Muscle Tension

First, focus the client's attention on an identified area of unnecessary muscle tension. Encourage deep breathing, relaxation, and a feeling of "letting go." Clients may find

simple visual images like "melting" or more complex guided imagery scripts[15] useful. Other manual techniques that move the client's body in space, such as rhythmic mobilization, rocking, joint mobilization, and passive relaxed movement, may assist the client in recognizing and releasing patterns of unnecessary muscle tension. Give the client positive feedback when he or she has released tension, since the client may not recognize that this has happened.

For homecare, you can instruct the client to self-administer shaking to accessible areas of the body, such as the arms and legs, and to perform active shaking movements to achieve muscle relaxation and facilitate ease of motion.[16] As an adjunct to the latter, suggest the use of any effective breathing and relaxation methods that are familiar to the client.[15]

## To Enhance Arousal (Wakefulness)

You can use shaking with other massage techniques that tend to wake clients quickly such as fast fingertip superficial stroking, fine vibration, and percussion. Commercially available machines can produce the latter two techniques. Cold, contrast hydrotherapy, and rubbing the skin with coarse cloth, bristle brushes, or salt also enhance arousal.[17]

## In Pre- and Intercompetition Sports Massage

Clinicians use this type of massage on the day of competition and, possibly, immediately before the event and vary how they use it depending on the sport and the athlete. In general, they avoid using deeper techniques close to the time of competition.[4] Alternate shaking and rhythmic mobilization with broad-contact compression, light petrissage, percussion, stretching, and passive range of motion. Keep sessions short (10 to 20 minutes for all included regions), maintain a fast tempo (70 to 90 Hz), and focus on the most important muscle groups the client will be using in the activity. See the clinical example at the end of this chapter.

### ? Critical Thinking Question

It seems paradoxical that you can use the same technique to both reduce muscle tension and increase wakefulness in a client. What are the mechanisms that enable you to achieve both of these effects with shaking?

## Rhythmic Mobilization: Foundations

# DEFINITION

Rhythmic mobilization: The technique repetitively moves entire structures, resulting in the movement of soft tissue over bone and the movement of the related joints and internal organs.

# USES

Therapists use rhythmic mobilization to help a client voluntarily release unnecessary muscle tension, to reduce muscle resting tension, to prepare a client for joint mobilization or **passive range of motion** techniques, and in precompetition massage for athletes. This technique may also cause passive joint motion that may help to mobilize stiff joints, stimulate joint healing, enhance a client's joint awareness, and mobilize bronchial secretions.[18-24] When therapists apply rhythmic mobilization skillfully, it can have a calming, soothing effect.[25]

# PALPATION PRACTICE

1. For each of your partner's extremity joints, perform and measure passive range of motion (the osteokinematic or angular motions at the joint). Explore the quality of the resistance to further movement that you feel at the end of the range.
2. While performing passive range of motion, have your partner alternately tense slightly and relax different muscle groups without warning you. Ensure that you can detect "holding" of skeletal muscles. This exercise works better when you are blindfolded.
3. Attempt to produce pendular motions at extremity joints; the knee and elbow work well. Apply a force in one direction once, and then let your partner's body segment oscillate at its own frequency. Determine the frequency with which the limb oscillates, and measure the time for the motion to stop. Compare frequencies and rates of decay at different joints. Compare the frequency and rate of decay at the same joint for different partners. How does your partner's build influence these parameters?

---

### Theory in Practice 11-1

## Passive Movement Techniques

### Patient Profile

Your patient is a middle-aged "type A" manager in a high-stress public relations position who spends 4 to 5 hours per day at a computer and the rest of her time on the phone, in meetings, or giving presentations. She is married and has two teenaged children. Her physician has referred her for treatment of tension headaches. She has no experience with manual therapy.

### Clinical Findings

Subjective:
- Constant tightness in her neck and shoulders
- Severe temporal headaches 2 to 3 times a week.
- An inability to relax due to her hectic schedule

Objective:
- Posture: Forward head, elevated shoulders bilaterally, and moderate kyphosis
- Range of motion: Active and passive cervical range of motion is limited by 20% in all directions, with stiffness at the end of range but no pain. Active and passive shoulder range of motion is limited by 10%, without pain.
- Resisted tests: Resisted isometric cervical motions do not cause pain.
- Palpation: There is point tenderness throughout the muscles of her neck. Maximal compression of her hard upper trapezius muscles reproduces the temporal headache pattern of **referred pain**.

### Treatment Approach

Important initial outcomes include:
- Reducing the muscle resting tension and **trigger point** activity throughout the neck and shoulders, especially in the upper trapezius
- Increasing her awareness of the posture of her head and shoulders and how it changes in response to stress

In the first session, perform most of the treatment in supine, focusing on the upper trapezius and the neck. Use rhythmic settling of the patient's shoulders (Figure 11-9) as the **framing general technique**. Begin by applying this technique for a few minutes. Intersperse it with the full range of neuro-muscular and fascial techniques to reduce muscle tension, trigger point activity, and fascial shortening in the neck, as tolerated (see Chapter 7, Superficial Reflex Techniques; Chapter 8, Superficial Fluid Techniques; and Chapter 9, Neuromuscular Techniques). Every time you palpate softening of tissue or see the shoulders relax downwards, return to rhythmic mobilization of the shoulders for a minute. Use rocking and settling of the patient's shoulders as a focus of the treatment because it helps her become aware of her increasing range of motion as it occurs during treatment. Augment the intervention with homecare methods such as

stretching, active movement, and postural awareness exercises.

As the patient's intervention proceeds, progress the depth of the neuromuscular and connective tissue techniques; introduce other areas of her body such as the chest, jaw, and back; and try approaches like **diaphragmatic breathing** and guided relaxation to encourage general relaxation. Given her personality and lifestyle, she will likely present with elevated shoulders often, and you can incorporate rhythmic mobilization of the shoulders as part of her treatment to help restore her awareness of her posture and muscle tension.

# Rhythmic Mobilization: Technique

## MANUAL TECHNIQUE

Figures 11-9 to 11-17 show therapists applying rhythmic mobilization to the various regions of the body. The order of the figures is from head to foot in supine and then in prone. Each figure illustrates most of the guidelines for manual technique outlined here.

1. Use a hand contact that is comfortable for both you and your client. Ensure that this contact is full and relaxed,

and use as much of your hand as possible (Figures 11-9 to 11-17). Your hand position for optimal manual contact will vary with the region you are treating, the size of the client, and your size.

2. Strive to maintain an uninterrupted rhythmic flow of movement, even when you are switching positions and techniques.

3. Since rhythmic mobilization has widely distributed **mechanical effects**, it can easily become too stimulating for the client. Consequently, you should aim to perform

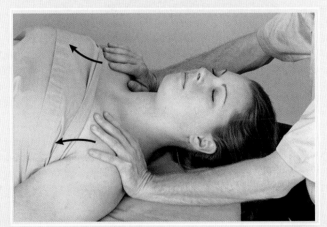

**Figure 11-9** Rhythmic settling of the shoulders. Depress the client's shoulder girdle and then allow the shoulders to rebound passively while maintaining hand contact. If the hands depress the shoulders simultaneously, the shoulders bounce up and down. If the hands alternately depress the shoulders, a lateral rocking results.

*ON-LINE VIDEO*

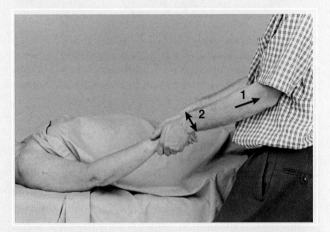

**Figure 11-10** Gentle traction, which the therapist produces by leaning backward, precedes longitudinal shaking of the arm. Perform this technique in the same manner as shaking a rope along its length. Do it gently and do not sustain it beyond one or two movements before releasing traction and reapplying. You can apply a similar technique to the leg.

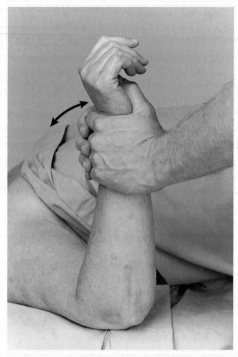

**Figure 11-11** Shaking of the entire hand can be vigorous. The illustrated contact allows the practitioner to control the flexion/extension movement at the client's wrist.

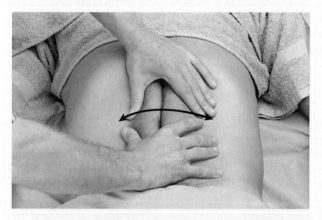

**Figure 11-12** Here, the rectus abdominis is gently gathered and lifted off the deeper muscles with a soft, broad contact. The hands maintain this contact, using it to sway the client's abdomen back and forth slowly.

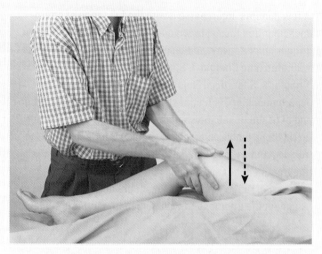

**Figure 11-13** The thigh is lifted and then allowed to fall rhythmically (dotted line). The hands can slide distally to deliver the lifting force to the lower leg as well.

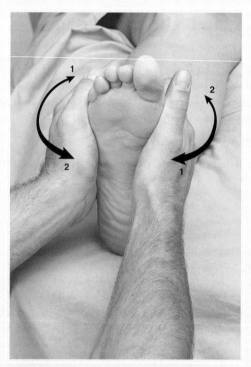

**Figure 11-14** Wrists and hands remain loose while rolling the client's entire foot briskly between the hands (two to three cycles per second). This pleasant stroke is a gentle, effective way to rouse sleeping clients.

the technique with a relaxed tempo that will produce reflex sedation. This requires that you maintain contact throughout the motion, while allowing the freest excursion of movement of the body segment you are treating.

4. The variety of possible rhythmic movements is limited only by your imagination. Here are some examples of these variations.
   A. To mobilize an entire limb from its distal end, with the client in prone or supine: Assume a very comfort-

able two-handed grip on the client's wrist or ankle. Simultaneously exert a gentle, long-axis **traction** on the client's limb and lift it so that it clears the table. Then, immediately perform one or two gentle shaking motions, using the same motion used to initiate vertical waves along a rope. The client's limb will look

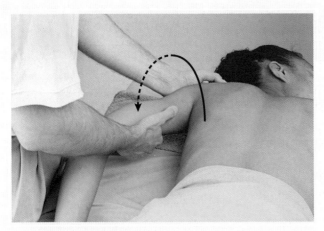

Figure 11-15 "Tossing" the shoulder rhythmically and repetitively. Maintain contact as the client's shoulders are allowed to fall back to the table under their own weight (dotted line). You may use a gentle force to distract the shoulder as it is being lifted.

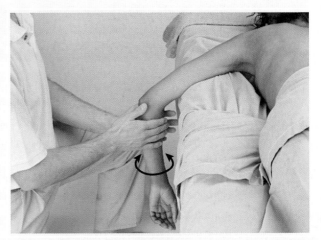

Figure 11-17 Rolling the dependent forearm between the hands. Hand contact slides proximally and distally on the forearm to focus the movement on different areas.

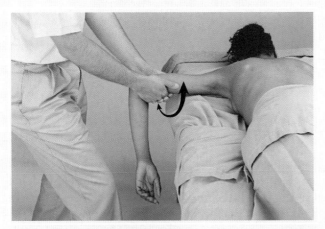

Figure 11-16 Swinging the dependent arm in prone: Rhythmic passive internal and external rotation performed in the midrange of abduction.

D. To swing the arm, with the client in supine: Grasp the client's wrist and hand, bend the elbow, lift until the upper arm clears the table, and swing the entire arm from the wrist. In this position, you can also bounce the proximal limb segment on the table surface.

E. To swing the leg, with the client in prone: Grasp the client's foot and ankle, bend the knee, lift until the thigh clears the table, and swing the entire leg from the ankle. In this position, you can also bounce the proximal limb segment on the table surface.

F. To shake or roll the client's entire hand or foot. Grasp the client's hand or foot with two hands and briskly shake or roll it (Figures 11-11 and 11-14). You can shake or roll individual digits using this technique. Shaking of the client's hand or foot is a useful technique for waking sleeping clients.

### Critical Thinking Question

How would you organize the rhythmic mobilization techniques shown in the figures in the chapter in reference to the anatomical planes and axes? Hint: Explore all possible rhythmic mobilization techniques for the glenohumeral joint, organize those, and then generalize to all joints.

## How rhythmic mobilization might work

There are multiple mechanisms for the effects of rhythmic mobilization. The compression and release of soft tissue that accompanies rhythmic mobilization may produce

and feel like a weighted rope during this maneuver, provided that you are using neither too much nor too little traction (Figure 11-10). Release the traction on the limb between repetitions of this technique.

B. For proximal limb segments such as the entire shoulder, with the client in prone or supine, or the thigh, with the client in supine: Position your hands between the client's limb and the table. Lift the client's limb segment and let it drop (Figures 11-13 and 11-15). Repeat this maneuver as needed.

C. To roll the upper arm, with the client in prone, or the thigh, with the client in supine: Roll the client's limb back and forth over the table surface. You may also lift and swing the client's proximal arm from the elbow (Figure 11-16) or roll the client's dependent forearm between your hands (Figure 11-17).

| Box 11-2 | **Components of Rhythmic Mobilization** |
|---|---|

**Contact:** Whole palmar surface of one or both hands with your hands as relaxed as possible

**Pressure:** Moderate. Enough to securely lift or move the body segment.

**Tissues engaged:** Your hands engage to the depth of the superficial muscle layers. The motion produced by the stroke simultaneously engages all of the joint tissues and soft tissues in the region that you are mobilizing.

**Direction:** Varies with the region you are treating. Often you repeatedly lift or move a body segment and allow it to drop or settle under the force of gravity

**Amplitude:** Depends on the region

**Rate:** 0.5 to 2 seconds per cycle

**Duration:** 5 seconds or longer

**Intergrades with:** Shaking, passive range of motion, joint mobilization, and manual traction

**Combines with:** Combine with broad-contact compression and muscle squeezing

**Context:** In interventions that focus solely on movement, you can alternate it with other techniques presented in this chapter. This technique often precedes or follows neuromuscular techniques such as those described in Chapter 9, Neuromuscular Techniques.

modest increases in **lymphatic and venous return** by squeezing vessels with valves. The rhythmic deformation of joint capsules moves synovial fluid through the capsule and facilitates joint nutrition and healing.[2,6] Stimulation of joint afferents[10] enhances joint awareness. In addition, when therapists apply mobilization to the rib cage, it physically shakes and moves mucus to a point where the client can cough it out.[9] Sedative effects of mobilization[6] may be due to **entrainment** to rhythm, which is a shift in the autonomic nervous system toward **parasympathetic** function that may occur with certain kinds of rhythmic sensory stimulation (see discussion and references in Chapter 7, Superficial Reflex Techniques). Finally, **vestibular reflexes** that are stimulated by rhythmic mobilization may cause a generalized decrease in postural tone.[3,6]

# THERAPIST'S POSITION AND MOVEMENT

1. You must be able to use all of the basic positions described in Chapter 6, Preparation and Positioning for Massage.

# PALPATE

As you perform the technique, palpate the client's skin and tissues for the qualities noted in the following list. In doing so, focus your attention on the qualities of the motion you produce with the technique and on the resistance of the client's tissues to this movement. Strive to palpate, simultaneously and from a distance, the different tissues and structures that influence the movement you produce. Diligent practice is required to refine your awareness of tissue resistance to movement.

1. The local skin temperature and texture of the client's skin.
2. The tone of the client's superficial muscles and tissues.
3. The movement of the joints you are shaking. Try to form an impression of the quality of the motion of the limb, or the body segment as a whole, and its constituent joints. In addition, note how the resistance to movement varies throughout the available range of the induced motion.
4. Resistance to tissue or joint movement. Determine whether you can relate the resistance to movement to a specific tissue or structure that is involved in producing the motion of the stroke. For example, elevated resting tension in one of the client's scapular stabilizers will have a visible and palpable effect on the manner in

which the entire shoulder moves when you swing or roll the upper arm on the table.

5. The rhythmic response or cadence of the client's tissue during the stroke. Even more so than with shaking, the client will have a rate and amplitude that she perceives to be the most pleasant for any given rhythmic movement.[26] This varies with the person, body structure, level of **muscle tone**, region, and the type of rhythmic mobilization that you are using. As a result, it is critical for you to palpate for this optimal cadence and adjust the rate and amplitude of the stroke to the client's needs in order to ensure sedation and avoid the unpleasant effects of a sympathetic response.

6. The depth of penetration of the effect of the stroke. As the client's muscles relax and the fluid **viscosity** of the tissues decreases, the same force will produce effects deeper into and further along the client's tissues. Consequently, as with petrissage, you will not need to apply greater force to achieve a greater penetration of the technique. You will simply have to apply it for a longer duration.

## OBSERVE

As you perform the technique, observe the client for:

1. The degree of muscle movement you achieve and how the stroke moves from the points of contact to adjacent areas of the client's body. This observation can provide you with information about the level of function of intervening tissues and joints. For example, when you are mobilizing the client's entire leg with traction, observe how the lumbar and thoracic spine respond.

2. The degree of muscle movement. Movement of the client's muscles will be visibly less within areas of connective tissue hardening and elevated muscle resting tension. Even in normal tissue, movement will vary substantially with different body shapes and proportions of body fat.

3. Inappropriate draping. Because rhythmic mobilization can loosen draping, you may need to adjust or retuck a loosened drape to maintain discreet coverage of the client's body.

## COMMUNICATION WITH THE CLIENT

Communicate to ensure the client's comfort during the application of rhythmic mobilization. Here are some examples of statements that you can use.

1. "Is this hand position comfortable?" Alternatively, offer the client a choice: "Which feels better, this . . . or this?" Ensure that your hand contact is comfortable for the client.

2. "Would it feel more relaxing if I slowed down a bit . . . like this?" "Is this motion comfortable, or is the movement too much?" Determine whether the rate and amplitude of motion are comfortable for the client.

3. "Is everything okay?" "Are you feeling anything unusual?" When you are applying rhythmic mobilization continuously for longer than 2 minutes, determine whether the client is experiencing unpleasant symptoms of sympathetic arousal such as irritation or nausea.

4. "Is this causing pain anywhere?" You can use this statement at intervals to check whether the client perceives that the intervention is resulting in pain. When the client presents with spasm or inflammation, the application of rhythmic mobilization to a distant area may produce small motions, at a distance from the point of contact, that result in pain.

## A Practice Sequence for Rhythmic Mobilization

Practice time: 15 to 30 minutes per person or longer.
Do not use oil for this sequence for the anterior and posterior aspects of the legs. You can easily perform it through loose clothing or draping, although the techniques are somewhat easier to apply on bare skin.

There are two basic ways of approaching movement sequences. One is to perform each technique in the sequence once for a longer period of time. The other is to introduce all movements quickly, and then alternate frequently from one technique to the next, repeating the sequence as time permits. This alternative tends to reduce therapist fatigue and tension.

Strive for a smooth continuous motion without breaks between the various moves. Explore each motion and the numerous variations that are possible.

### Supine

1. Repeatedly lift the client's thigh slightly and let it drop while working down the leg to the heel. Be careful not to hyperextend the knee.

2. Flex and extend the knee rhythmically in the midrange. The hip will also flex and extend. Be careful not to allow the knee to hyperextend. Perform this flexion and extension while gradually internally and externally rotating the hip.
3. With heel-of-hand contacts just proximal to both malleoli, shake the whole foot while the leg rests on the table.
4. Gently circumduct the ankle.
5. Grasp the foot and ankle securely, lift the leg, and apply gentle long-axis traction to the leg. Then shake the entire leg briefly, in the sagittal plane, like a rope. Repeat.
6. Hold the posterior ankle above the calcaneus. Lift the leg off the table slightly. Now rhythmically internally and externally rotate the hip joint and the entire leg. Continue this while slowly abducting and adducting the hip joint.

Repeat this supine sequence two or more times.

Turn client to **prone**.
7. Hold the client's ankle with two hands. Flex the knee to 90 degrees, lift the thigh off the table, and swing the entire leg from side to side.
8. With the knee flexed to 90 degrees and the thigh resting on the table, grasp the heel and shake the entire foot.
9. Grasp the foot and ankle. Lift the leg and apply gentle long-axis traction to the entire leg prior to shaking it in the sagittal plane like a rope.
10. Hold the foot and flex the knee to 45 degrees. Passively plantarflex and dorsiflex the ankle joint.
11. Hold the foot and flex the knee to 45 degrees. Make clockwise and counterclockwise circles of various sizes in the air with the heel.

Repeat this prone sequence two or more times.

Home study: Devise a comparable supine and prone sequence for the arm.

# Rhythmic Mobilization: Further Study and Practice

## NAMES AND ORIGINS

In other texts or massage-related systems, the technique that we call rhythmic mobilization is also known as "shaking."[9] Similar relaxed approaches to passive movement are featured prominently in the work of the American physician Milton Trager (**Trager Method of Psychophysical Integration**)[27,28] and the British osteopath **Eyal Lederman** (Harmonic Technique).[25]

Rhythmic mobilization involves the repetitive passive movement of entire structures—usually a limb, a segment of a limb, or the limb girdle—and all of the tissues that the treated body segment contains. At times, rhythmic mobilization may resemble **passive relaxed movements** or **joint play** or **joint mobilization** techniques, both of which other textbooks cover extensively. The techniques of rhythmic mobilization are, however, less specific than joint mobilization or passive relaxed movements. For example, when clinicians are treating areas around synovial joints with rhythmic mobilization, they do not attempt to isolate movement to anatomical planes, the joint capsule, or even to a single joint. A single movement by the clinician may result in simultaneous movements from several joints in a **kinetic chain**. Additionally, you can perform the movements in the midrange, rather than through the full osteokinematic range of the joint you are treating.

## OUTCOMES AND EVIDENCE

Some of the clinical indications and **outcomes** for rhythmic mobilization are similar to those for shaking, described earlier in this chapter. Like shaking, clinicians can use rhythmic mobilization to reduce holding and muscle tension, to prepare the client for joint mobilization or passive range of motion techniques, and in precompetition preparation for athletes. Since rhythmic mobilization results in passive joint motion, it may produce some of the effects of more rigorous passive range exercises such as the mobilization of stiff joints, the stimulation of joint healing, and neuromuscular re-education.[18-23] The repeated approximation and distraction of the joint surfaces that occur during the application of this technique may be used to enhance a client's joint awareness.[24] When it is used in the context of **Trager Psychophysical Integration**, rhythmic mobilization may also be of use in the treatment of headache,[29] chronic pain,[30] and neurological conditions that alter movement patterns such as cerebral palsy, muscular dystrophy, and multiple sclerosis.[31] Rhythmic mobilization of the rib cage ("shaking"), alternated with rapid repeated compression, percussion ("cupping" or "clapping"), and postural drainage, is a standard intervention for mobilizing bronchial secretions in chest physical therapy (see Chapter 12, Percussive Techniques). Finally, rhythmic mobilization may stimulate vestibular reflexes and result in a generalized decrease in postural tone, decreased arousal, and a calming, soothing effect.[10,24] Table 11-1 summarizes the main outcomes for rhythmic mobilization.

---

## EXAMINING THE EVIDENCE

Gentle, unforced, meditative, rhythmic mobilization and rocking are central to the method of Trager Psychophysical Integration. This small clinical trial tested the effect of 20 minutes of Trager on the EMG responses to passive movement in clients with Parkinson's disease, which were considered an indication of **rigidity**.[32] The sample of 30 patients was divided into four subgroups who were assigned to one of four treatment conditions that varied in terms of the treatment position (seated or supine) and the location of treatment (on the more rigid or less rigid side of the body). There was no control group, and the authors did not describe their process for assigning subjects to the groups. The authors observed a decrease in stretch responses immediately after treatment, and this decrease was still evident 11 minutes later. This effect was largest when the researchers applied the intervention with the client in supine and least when it was applied with the client seated. This research is promising. The authors discuss the study's limitations, such as the need for a longer monitoring period after treatment and the need to relate EMG results to a clinical assessment of rigidity. Hopefully, they will complete further studies with greater numbers of subjects and suitable control groups.

Duval C, Lafontaine D, Hèrbert J, Leroux A, Panisset M, Boucher JP. The effect of Trager therapy on the level of evoked stretch responses in patients with Parkinson's disease and rigidity. *J Manipulative Physiol Ther.* 2002;25:455–464.

---

# CAUTIONS AND CONTRAINDICATIONS

Clinicians need clinical training and supervised practice to master the proper application of rhythmic mobilization. Advanced training may be advisable when dealing with pathological conditions. All of the general and local contraindications noted for massage techniques apply to the use of rhythmic mobilization (see Chapter 3, Clinical Decision Making for Massage). One current list of contraindications for rhythmic mobilization includes metastatic cancer, acute nerve impingement or disk rupture, severe carotid artery disease, use of anticoagulant therapy, and high-risk pregnancies.[27] Clinicians should consider a flail chest, fractured or brittle ribs, and recent chest or spinal surgery to be contraindications to applying this technique to the rib cage for mobilizing bronchial secretions.[9] Avoid performing rhythmic mobilization on, or adjacent to, the site of acute orthopedic injuries.[27] Clinicians can introduce this technique at later stages of recovery provided that they can perform it without causing the client pain. Apply rhythmic mobilization with reduced force and great sensitivity when clients present with spasm, hyperreflexia, or spasticity. In general, clinicians can often move the client's hands and feet quite vigorously. Elsewhere, however, they need to perform rhythmic mobilization at a moderate rate, since it may be too stimulating for the client when they perform it rapidly. Clinicians should not use rhythmic mobilization when a client suffers from vertigo or motion sickness.[27]

# USING RHYTHMIC MOBILIZATION IN TREATMENT

## To Reduce Unnecessary Muscle Tension

First, focus the client's attention on an identified area of unnecessary muscle tension. Encourage deep breathing, relaxation, and a feeling of "letting go." Clients may also find simple visual images such as "melting" or more complex guided imagery scripts useful.[15] Other manual techniques that move the client's body in space, such as shaking, rocking, joint mobilization, and passive relaxed movement, may assist the client in recognizing and releasing patterns of unnecessary muscle tension. Provide positive feedback when the client has released tension because the client may not immediately realize that this has happened. In addition, use rhythmic mobilization as a precursor to traction, joint mobilization, or passive relaxed movement techniques to decrease unnecessary muscle tension that would interfere with your application of those techniques.

For homecare, you can instruct the client to perform active rhythmic mobilization movements to achieve muscle relaxation and facilitate ease of motion.[16] Encourage clients to use any effective breathing and relaxation methods that they knows.[15]

## To Enhance Arousal (Wakefulness)

Perform rhythmic mobilization at a faster tempo to wake clients. Other massage techniques that tend to wake clients quickly are fast fingertip superficial stroking, fine vibration, and percussion (use commercially available machines to produce the latter two techniques). In addition, cold, contrast hydrotherapy, and rubbing the skin with coarse cloth, bristle brushes, or salt also enhance arousal.[17]

## In Pre- and Intercompetition Sports Massage

Clinicians use this type of massage on the day of and immediately before competition. Their application of the technique will vary with the sport and the athlete. In general, they avoid deeper techniques as competition draws near[4] and alternate shaking and rhythmic mobilization with broad-contact compression, light petrissage, percussion, stretching, or passive range of motion. Finally, they use short (15 to 20 minutes for all regions), fast-tempo (70 to 90 Hz) sessions that focus on the most important muscle groups that the athlete will be using in the activity. See the clinical example at the end of this chapter.

## To Enhance Airway Clearance

When you are using rhythmic mobilization of the rib cage to mobilize bronchial secretions, use percussion (preferably cupping), postural drainage, steam inhalation, forced expiration, and coughing techniques in a complementary manner. You can also teach clients the last four methods for home use.

# Rocking: Foundations

## DEFINITION

Rocking: Gentle, repetitive oscillation of the pelvis or torso that therapists achieve by pushing the pelvis or torso from a midline resting position into lateral deviation and then allowing it to return to resting position. This repetitive movement results in waves of motion that travel along the body.

## USES

Rocking has a profoundly **sedative** effect that is useful in the treatment of stress-related autonomic dysfunction, generalized elevation of skeletal muscle tone, unnecessary muscle tension, insomnia, and fatigue. Therapists can also use the sedative effect of rocking to reduce the client's perception of pain indirectly.

## PALPATION PRACTICE

1.  Using the pads of your index and middle fingers, landmark adjacent spinous processes on your partner's spine. Have your partner perform active lumbar side flexion to the left and right, while you palpate the movement between adjacent vertebrae. Work your way down the spinal column from C2 to S1

2.  The following exercise shows how the natural oscillatory rhythm differs from person to person and suggests how rocking can be synchronized to each individual's body. In prone, move your partner's pelvis laterally 5 to 15 cm (2 to 6 inches) from the midline, then remove your hands and observe the result. Note how far the body rebounds past midline and how long the motion continues for one or two cycles. Try lateral pushes in several places like the ribs, waist, iliac crest, and greater trochanter, observing the motion in the same way as before. Repeat this palpation exercise on several people who have different body types. How does the natural rocking rate and amplitude compare for **ectomorphs**, **mesomorphs**, and **endomorphs**? Repeat the entire exercise again with several partners in supine.

3.  Put on a blindfold. Have your partner select an area of the body to consciously tense while you repeat Step 2 above. Can you identify the tensed area without someone telling you?

# Rocking: Technique

## MANUAL TECHNIQUE

Figures 11-18 to 11-24 show therapists applying rocking to the various regions of the body. The order of the figures is from head to foot in supine and then in prone. Each figure illustrates most of the guidelines for manual technique outlined here.

1. If the client can tolerate lying prone without lumbar support, remove the abdominal pillow, since its presence will significantly dampen the motion that rocking produces. Even clients with back pain, who often require an abdominal pillow when they are prone, may be able to tolerate lying with an increased lordosis as long as the rocking motion continues. You may need to replace the abdominal pillow after application of rocking. This may also be the case for using pillows under the client's knees in supine.
2. Use relaxed whole-hand contact, with your fingers spread, which will evenly distribute the pressure over the contact surface of your hand (Figures 11-18, 11-19, and 11-22 to 11-23B).

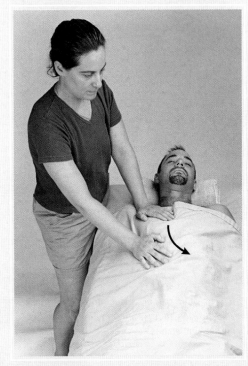

**Figure 11-19** As hand contact moves farther from the pelvis, the rocking motion naturally becomes attenuated. In this situation, you can maintain the rocking motion by using upper and lower rib hand contacts.

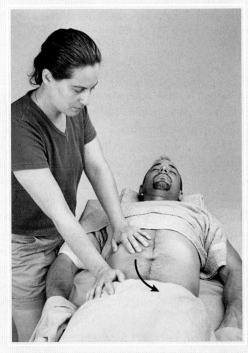

**Figure 11-18** Rocking in supine with hand contact on the lower ribs and anterior superior iliac spines.

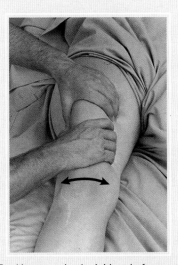

**Figure 11-20** Rocking can also be initiated after gently lifting a large muscle mass such as the quadriceps, hamstrings, or gluteals. The cadence at which rocking can be performed will be dictated by the passive response of the pelvis.

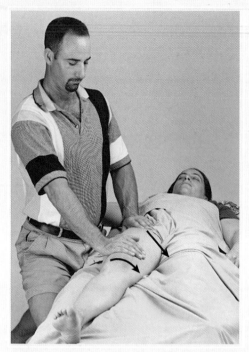

**Figure 11-21** The thigh can be rolled into internal rotation while the rocking motion is maintained from the anterior superior iliac spines.

ON-LINE VIDEO

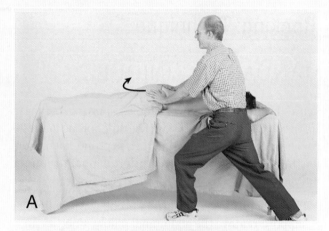

A

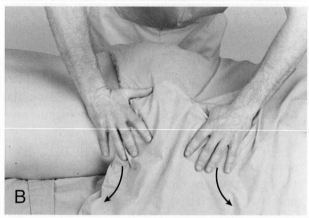

B

**Figure 11-23** A. Hand contact may be varied to different positions as the rocking motion is maintained. Here, the gluteals are gently stretched distally off their superior iliac attachments with the practitioner's left hand. B. Here, the gluteals are pushed away from the sacrum with both hands.

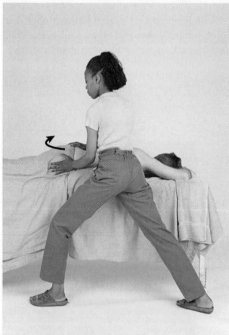

**Figure 11-22** Basic hand contact for rocking the back. Hands are placed on the sacrum and the greater trochanter. The therapist directs the force of the motion distally, to produce lumbar traction, and toward the client's contralateral knee. With each stroke, the therapist produces a lateral displacement of the client's pelvis and then allows the pelvis to fall back past the midline without breaking hand contact. The aim is to produce a succession of seamlessly interconnected strokes.

ON-LINE VIDEO

3.  Gently push the client's pelvis or torso laterally from the midline resting position in supine (Figures 11-18 to 11-21) or in prone (Figures 11-22 to 11-24); this motion will raise the center of gravity of the client's body. Then, allow the client's body to fall back toward the midline passively; momentum will carry the body past its resting position. Precisely at the end of the excursion of the motion of the pelvis or torso, repeat the application of the same pressure, and push the client's pelvis or torso past the midline once more. Ideally, rocking consists of a seamlessly interconnected series of pushes and releases (falls) that produce a continuous oscillation of the client's body. The maximum amplitude of the motion should occur around the client's iliac crest.

4.  Although it is preferable for you to maintain contact during the passive **return stroke**, you must do this without impeding the natural "falling" of the body back toward, and through, the resting position.

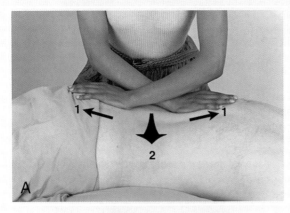

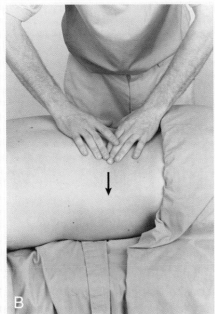

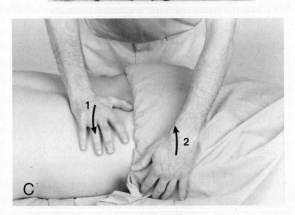

**Figure 11-24** A. Techniques for the erector spinae. Cross-handed contact permits a gentle traction of the erector spinae (1), while simultaneously performing the rocking motion (2). Hand contact is maintained as the pelvis is allowed to fall back past the midline. B. Techniques for the erector spinae. Two hands gather the erector spinae together while producing the rocking motion. C. Alternately, one hand draws the opposite innominate bone toward the practitioner, and then the other hand gently pushes the erector spinae away from the spinous processes.

5. Time the initiation of each push so that the rocking motion you produce is smooth and the client is scarcely aware of your hand pressure and the point at which you apply that motion.

6. Change your hand position every 5 to 10 seconds to avoid producing a motion that has a mechanical feel. Slide your hands easily from one contact position to another without interrupting the regular rhythm, so that you are moving your point of contact up and down the client's body.

7. As the application of rocking proceeds and the client relaxes, you will often note an increased amplitude and decreased rate of the rocking motion, with little increase in the amount of force you apply.

8. You may also position your hands on opposite sides of the client's body, so that they can alternately push and pull the client's body to generate the rocking motion (Figure 11-24C). Bear in mind that this approach eliminates the passive return of the client's body to its resting position. Consequently, it is more likely to be inharmonious with the body's natural rhythm and to produce a stroke that is less effective or that the client perceives as being unpleasant.

9. You may find it useful to intersperse rocking with gentle long-axis traction of the client's legs. This enhances the incremental lengthening of the spine that can result from longer applications of rocking.

## *How rocking might work*

The mechanism for the effects of rocking is similar to that of rhythmic mobilization. Compression and release of soft tissue, and the resulting passive motions, may produce modest increases in lymphatic and venous return by squeezing and stretching vessels with valves. The slight rhythmic deformation of joint capsules may help to propel synovial fluid through the capsule.[3,6] In addition, stimulation of joint afferents enhances joint awareness.[10] Sedative effects can be the result of entrainment to rhythm (see discussion and references in Chapter 7, Superficial Reflex Techniques). Finally, vestibular reflexes may cause a generalized decrease in postural tone.[3,6,25]

## PRACTITIONER'S POSITION AND MOVEMENT

1. Use the basic positions described in Chapter 6, Preparation and Positioning for Massage, in the sections on **standing aligned**, **lunge**, and **lunge-and-lean** postures.

---

### Box 11-3 — Components of Rocking

**Contact:** Entire palmar surface

**Pressure:** Light to moderate

**Tissues engaged:** Hands engage to the depth of the superficial muscle layers. The motion produced by the stroke simultaneously engages all the tissues throughout the body segments that you are rocking. This can include muscle, fascia, tendon, ligament, and periosteum.

**Direction:** Direct your force so that you produce a lateral deviation of the pelvis and/or spine from the midline. The resulting motion is propagated along the client's body.

**Amplitude and length:** Lateral deviation may reach 10 cm or more from midline, depending on the duration of application of the technique and the client's body size and type.

**Rate:** 1 to 2 seconds per cycle

**Duration:** 60 seconds to 15+ minutes

**Intergrades with:** Passive range of motion and joint mobilization techniques

**Combines with:** Combine with compression

**Context:** May be used alone for sedation. Therapists usually use it at the beginning or end of longer sequences that include other techniques.

---

2. Use a standing upright posture when beginning the application of rocking or when the amplitude of the movement is small.
3. Using a standing lunge-and-lean posture, shift your body weight backward and forward from your front leg to your back leg in a gentle rocking motion. Then transfer this motion through your arms to the client. This feels much better to the client than a rocking motion that you generate solely through exertion of your arm and shoulder muscles (Figures 11-19, 11-22, and 11-23A). As with other massage techniques, using your lower body and pelvis to generate the motion of the stroke, rather than your arms alone, will add a perceptible sureness and evenness to the stroke.
4. During the rhythmic lunge-and-lean movement, relax your shoulders and stretch out your arms without locking your elbows in extension ("straight-arming"). (Figures 11-22 and 11-23).
5. The more rhythmic and relaxed the movement of your body is, the more effective the rocking motion you produce.

## PALPATE

As you perform the technique, palpate the client's skin and tissues for the qualities noted in the following list. In doing so, focus your attention on the qualities of the motion you produce with the technique and the client's tissues' resistance to movement.

1. The local skin temperature and texture.
2. The tone of the client's superficial muscles and tissues.
3. The weight of the client's body as you set it into motion with rocking.
4. Resistance to tissue or joint movement. The initial resistance to movement from the midline resting position comes from the client's weight. As you push the client's body farther from the midline, additional resistance develops as various tissues are lengthened passively. The goal of rocking is not to achieve the fullest possible passive stretch, but rather to produce a repetitive, pleasurable motion within the inner and midranges of the available range of motion.
5. The inherent rhythm of rocking for the client's body. No two clients' bodies will respond to rocking in the same manner. Several factors can influence the inherent rhythm of the client's body: body type, the amount of body fat, levels of muscular tension, and the client's fascial structure. In general, rock clients with ectomorphic body types at a slightly faster rate and with less movement. Conversely, clients with endomorphic body types can tolerate more movement, and the rate will be correspondingly slower. Muscular tension, especially of the low back, can also reduce the amount of movement that the client can tolerate. You must identify the inher-

ent rhythm of each client's body at the time of treatment, rather than merely imposing the same motion on every client.

6. Changes in ease of application of the technique. As the application of rocking proceeds and the client relaxes, you will note an increased amplitude and a decreased rate of the rocking motion, with little increase in the amount of force you apply.

## OBSERVE

As you perform the technique, observe the client for the degree of movement you achieve and signs of relaxation or sedation. The following signs may signal this.

### Movement Achieved

1. Observation of the motion throughout the body during rocking. Careful observation can provide information about the client's body, including patterns of muscular tension, the relationship of body segments, and areas of connective tissue tightness due to past trauma. For example, when rocking the pelvis, observe the relative ease of motion of the various spinal segments.
2. Lengthening of the spine, as reflected by a reduction of the client's spinal curves, especially the lumbar lordosis.

### Relaxation or Sedation

1. Decrease in rate and depth of breathing
2. Deeper voice tone
3. Changes in skin color such as flushing. Pallor may indicate an undesirable sympathetic response.

4. Systemic reduction of muscle tone, as evidenced by softening of the tissue contours or broadening and flattening of body segments
5. Muscle twitches and jerks
6. Increases in peristaltic noises
7. Decreases in heart rate, as evidenced by change in the client's pulses that are visible at the neck, wrist, and foot
8. Agitation or sweating, which may indicate an undesirable **sympathetic response**

## COMMUNICATION WITH THE CLIENT

Communicate to ensure the client's comfort during the application of rocking. Here are some examples of statements that you can use.

1. "This technique should make you feel very relaxed, even sleepy. It should not feel abrupt." After you establish a motion that you perceive to be consistent with the inherent rhythm of the client's body, check that the motion feels comfortable, rather than forced or excessive in any way.
2. "Do you feel alert enough to drive home?" If you use rocking for long periods during the session or at the end of a session, observe the client's level of function and ensure that he or she is sufficiently alert to resume daily activities safely.
3. The relaxation, sensual pleasure, and motion of rocking may occasionally result in sexual arousal on the part of the client or prompt comments of a sexual nature. You must be prepared to maintain clear verbal and physical boundaries with the client in a mature manner, while neither denigrating nor facilitating the client's sexual response to the technique.

---

 **A Practice Sequence for Rocking**

Practice time: Allow 30 minutes per person.

Begin with the client in prone. Establish a stable rocking rhythm that is continuous and does not feel machine-like. Use light soft full palmar contact. Do not remove your hands between each application of pressure ("stroke") because this reduces the sedative effect. Slide your hands from one position to another while maintaining light contact.

Hand positions to try include:

■ Trochanter and sacrum
■ Trochanter and superior gluteal insertions
■ Crossed-hand lumbar traction position
■ Both sides of the iliac crest
■ Both sides of the waist
■ Pelvis and the erector spinae
■ Pelvis and rib cage
■ Both sides of the rib cage

Initially, check with the client several times to ensure that your hand contact, rate, and rhythm are comfortable. Experiment with moving your hand contacts as far up and down the body as you can, while still maintaining the basic rocking motion. Notice how the client's body responds differently over time: the amplitude of the initial rocking will be smaller until the client's body begins to relax. Periodically intersperse rocking with gentle traction of the client's legs in order to lengthen the client's back as the back muscles begin to relax. Many people will become drowsy or even fall asleep during this sequence. Continue for 15 minutes,

and give your client 5 minutes to return to the present before ending the session.

Home study: Devise and practice a comparable sequence for rocking in supine, using the trochanter, anterior thigh, iliac crest, anterior superior iliac spines, waist, and lower ribs as contact points. Note whether a supine rocking sequence has effects similar to the ones described earlier for prone.

# Rocking: Further Study and Practice

## NAMES AND ORIGINS

In other texts or massage-related systems, the technique that we call rocking is also known as "pelvic rocking" or "rocking vibration."[2-9] This form of rhythmic mobilization results in a lateral motion of the body, especially of the pelvis, lumbar region, and thoracic region. The distinctive elements of the manual technique of rocking and the technique's reflex effects merit an independent description.

Although every mother (and child) has known the effects of repetitive motion since time immemorial,[33-35] few people documented a rocking technique prior to the latter part of the 20th century. These relaxed movements figure prominently in the work of the American Milton Trager (Trager Psychophysical Integration)[27,28] and the British osteopath Eyal Lederman (Harmonic Technique).[25]

## OUTCOMES AND EVIDENCE

Rocking may produce a generalized decrease in postural tone and arousal as a result of stimulation of vestibular reflexes.[24] When clinicians perform rocking skillfully, it has a profoundly sedative effect. For this reason alone, this technique is worth mastering.[10,25] As a result of its sedative effect, clinicians find rocking useful for treating stress-related autonomic dysfunction; generalized elevation of skeletal muscle tone; "holding" or unnecessary muscle tension; insomnia; and mental, physical, or emotional fatigue. Furthermore, people intuitively use rocking motions to calm infants; consequently, clinicians incorporate it into infant massage.[33-35] They may also find it valuable for treating a variety of chronic musculoskeletal disorders in which clients present with muscular tension, provided

that the client is able to tolerate the motion of the technique.[27,29,30] Finally, clinicians can use the sedative effect of rocking to indirectly reduce the client's perception of pain.[29,30] Table 11-1 summarizes the main outcomes for rocking.

### EXAMINING THE EVIDENCE

To our knowledge, there are no clinical trials of the technique we call rocking. Several studies have examined the effects of rocking and rhythmic mobilization in the context of Trager Psychophysical Integration.[29-32] One text[25] describes many methods of rocking and rhythmic mobilization in detail. This rigorous text also includes chapters about the physics of motion and the effects of motion and passive movement on neurology, tissue and joint repair, fluid flow, and analgesia. It also includes relevant literature, including the theoretical background and related clinical trials, and several clinical examples, which resemble actual case studies.[25]

Lederman E. *Harmonic Technique.* Edinburgh: Churchill Livingstone; 2000.

## CAUTIONS AND CONTRAINDICATIONS

Clinicians need clinical training and supervised practice to master the proper application of rocking. Advanced training may be advisable when dealing with pathological conditions. All of the general and local contraindications previously noted for massage techniques and rhythmic mobilization apply to the use of rocking (see Chapter 3, Clinical Decision Making for Massage). Rocking sets the entire body in motion; therefore, it is contraindicated, or should be used with a reduced amplitude, for any condition in which movement will increase pain. The effects of rocking vary with the manner in which you perform the technique and the duration for which you use it. If clinicians perform rocking abruptly or too quickly, it can quickly produce unpleasant effects such as nausea. Consequently, they should not use rocking when a client suffers from vertigo or motion sickness.[27] When clinicians use rocking for more than 10 minutes in the intervention, it can induce a combination of deep relaxation and mild disorientation in the client that may temporarily reduce their competence to perform physical tasks such as driving. In this situation, they must ensure that the client is capable of functioning before allowing him or her to leave. If they have any doubt about the client's capabilities, they should return the client to the table; apply some deep, specific petrissage to the soles of the feet; and then let the client rest for 10 to 20 minutes before reassessing his or her level of mental function.

# USING ROCKING IN TREATMENT

## For Relaxation or Sedation

There are several modalities that you can use in a complementary manner with rocking to promote relaxation or sedation.

1. Use diaphragmatic breathing[15] prior to, or simultaneously with, rocking to enhance sedative effects.
2. Moist **hot packs** can enhance sedation and analgesia, if heat is appropriate for the client's condition.[17]
3. Some **craniosacral** techniques may have a calming effect on the client.[36]

4. Relaxing massage techniques include superficial stroking and rhythmic petrissage. These may produce greater effects if you apply them to the client's hands, feet, face, occiput, and sacrum.

Instruct the client to rest from 10 to 30 minutes and to resume activity slowly if he or she is experiencing the sedative effects of rocking.

For homecare, you can instruct the client in a form of self-rocking that she can use for relaxation. She will lie in supine, on a cushioned floor or firm bed, with her knees drawn up toward the chest with her hands. She will produce a rocking motion in the sagittal plane by pulling gently on the backs of her knees. During this movement, her thighs, pelvis, and lower back will flex and extend passively.

## To Reduce Unnecessary Muscle Tension

First, focus the client's attention on an identified area of unnecessary muscle tension. Encourage deep breathing, relaxation, and a feeling of "letting go." The client may find simple visual images like "melting" or more complex guided imagery scripts[15] useful. Other manual techniques that move the client's body in space, such as rhythmic mobilization, shaking, joint mobilization, and passive relaxed movement, may assist the client in recognizing and releasing patterns of unnecessary muscle tension. Give the client positive feedback when he releases tension because he may not realize immediately that this has happened.

For homecare, you can instruct the client to self-administer shaking to accessible areas of the body such as the arms and legs and to perform active shaking movements to achieve muscle relaxation and facilitate ease of motion.[16] You may also suggest the use of any effective breathing and relaxation methods that the client knows.[15]

### Critical Thinking Question

What are the differences in technique, effects, and uses of rocking versus rhythmic mobilization?

## Clinical Case

### History of Present Illness

A 25-year-old female professional pentathlete at competition, prior to the javelin throw.

## Subjective

- No complaints
- Wants to be physically and mentally prepared to perform optimally during the event

## Objective

### Impairments

- Likelihood of muscle tear during propulsive motion
- Less than optimal tissue extensibility
- Coordination may be less than optimal for peak performance
- Less than optimal ease of movement through range for peak performance in the javelin throw
- Less than optimal mental arousal for peak performance

### Functional Limitations

- Not sufficiently prepared physically and mentally to give peak athletic performance during the competitive javelin event without sustaining an injury

## Analysis

### Treatment Rationale

To prepare the athlete mentally and physically for peak performance during a competitive event.

| Impairment | Outcomes and Role of Massage |
|---|---|
| Risk of muscle tear | Decreased risk of muscle tear |
| | Primary treatment; decreased tissue viscosity and decreased resting level of tension are direct effects |
| Less than optimal tissue extensibility | Optimized tissue extensibility |
| | Primary treatment; increased tissue extensibility is a direct effect |
| Less than optimal coordination | Enhanced coordination |
| | Secondary effect; rhythmic mobilization facilitates neuro-muscular patterning |
| Less than optimal ease of movement | Enhanced optimal ease of movement |
| | Primary treatment, since increased tissue extensibility will facilitate ease of movement |
| Less than optimal mental arousal | Enhanced mental arousal |
| | Primary treatment; increased arousal is a direct effect of the faster movement techniques |

| *Activity Limitation* | *Functional Outcomes* |
|---|---|
| ▪ Less than optimal athletic performance | ▪ Client will demonstrate peak athletic performance during the javelin event without injury |

| *Plan* | |
|---|---|
| Massage Techniques | ▪ Rhythmic mobilization and fast shaking interspersed with repetitive, broad-contact compression and fast petrissage (see Chapter 9, Neuromuscular Techniques) |
| Other Appropriate Techniques and Interventions | ▪ Stretching, passive range of motion, and visualization her performance |

## References

1. Mense S, Simons DG. *Muscle Pain: Understanding Its Nature, Diagnosis, and Treatment.* Philadelphia: Lippincott Williams and Wilkins; 2001.
2. Benjamin PJ, Tappan FM. *Tappan's Handbook of Healing Massage Techniques.* 4th ed. Upper Saddle River, NJ: Pearson Prentice Hall; 2005.
3. Fritz S. *Mosby's Fundamentals of Therapeutic Massage.* 3rd ed. St. Louis: Mosby; 2004.
4. Fritz S. *Sports and Exercise Massage.* St. Louis: Elsevier Mosby; 2005.
5. Salvo SG. *Massage Therapy: Principles and Practice.* 2nd ed. Philadelphia: WB Saunders; 2003.
6. Yates J. *A Physician's Guide to Therapeutic Massage.* 3rd ed. Toronto: Curties Overzet; 2004.
7. Hollis M. *Massage for Therapists.* 2nd ed. Oxford, England: Blackwell Science; 1998.
8. Holey E, Cook E. *Evidence-Based Therapeutic Massage.* 2nd ed. Edinburgh: Churchill Livingstone; 2003.
9. de Domenico G, Wood EC. *Beard's Massage.* 4th ed. Philadelphia: WB Saunders; 1997.
10. Lederman E. *The Science and Practice of Manual Therapy.* 2nd ed. Edinburgh: Churchill Livingstone; 2005.
11. Pike G. *Sports Massage for Peak Performance.* New York: Harper Perennial; 1999.
12. Benjamin PJ, Lamp SP. *Understanding Sports Massage.* Champaign, IL: Human Kinetics; 1996.
13. Bob Karcy Productions. *A Soigneur's Sports Massage. The Massage Therapy Video Library: Sports Massage Series, Volume 4.* New York: View Video; 1988.
14. Smith LL, Keating MN, Holbert D, Spratt DJ, McCammon MR, Smith SS, et al. The effects of athletic massage on delayed onset muscle soreness, creatine kinase, and neutrophil count: a preliminary report. *J Orthop Sports Phys Ther.* 1994;19:93–99.
15. Payne R. *Relaxation Techniques.* 3rd ed. Edinburgh: Elsevier Churchill Livingstone; 2005.
16. Trager M, Guadagno-Hammond C. *Trager Mentastics: Movement as a Way to Agelessness.* Barrytown, NY: Station Hill Press; 1987.
17. Nikola RJ. *Creatures of Water.* Salt Lake City, UT: Europa Therapeutic; 1997.
18. Salter RB. The biologic concept of continuous passive motion of synovial joints. The first 18 years of basic research and its clinical application. *Clin Orthop.* 1989;242:12–25.
19. Akeson WH, Amiel D, Woo S-Y. Physiology and therapeutic value of passive motion. In: Helminien JH, Kivaranka I, Rammi M, eds. *Joint Loading—Biology and Health of Articular Structures.* Bristol, United Kingdom: John Wright; 1987:375–394.
20. Levick JR. Synovial fluid and transsynovial flow in stationary and moving normal joints. In: Helminien JH, Kivaranka I, Rammi M, eds. *Joint Loading—Biology and Health of Articular Structures.* Bristol, United Kingdom: John Wright; 1987: 149–186.
21. Frank C, Akeson WH, Woo SL-Y, et al. Physiology and therapeutic value of passive joint motion. *Clin Orthop.* 1984;185: 113–125.
22. Korcok M. Motion, not immobility, advocated for healing synovial joints. *JAMA.* 1981;246:2005–2006.
23. Gelberman RH, Menon J, Gonsalves M, Akeson WH. The effects of mobilization on vascularisation of healing flexor tendons in dogs. *Clin Orthop.* 1980;153:283–289.
24. O'Sullivan SB. Strategies to improve motor control. In: O'Sullivan SB, Schmitz J. *Physical Rehabilitation, Assessment and Treatment.* 2nd ed. Philadelphia: FA Davis; 1988.
25. Lederman, E. *Harmonic Technique.* Edinburgh: Churchill Livingstone; 2000.
26. Bonnard M, Pailhous J. Contribution of proprioceptive information to preferred versus constrained space-time behavior in rhythmical movements. *Exp Brain Res.* 1999;128:568–572.
27. Ramsey SM. Holistic manual therapy techniques. *Prim Care.* 1997;24:759–786.
28. Blackburn J. Trager psychophysical integration—an overview. *J Bodywork Movement Ther.* 2003;7:233–239.
29. Foster KA, Liskin J, Cen S, Abbott A, Armisen V, Globe D, et al. The Trager approach in the treatment of chronic headache: a pilot study. *Altern Ther Health Med.* 2004;10:40–46.
30. Dyson-Hudson TA, Shiflett SC, Kirshblum SC, Bowen JE, Druin EL. Acupuncture and Trager psychophysical integration in the treatment of wheelchair user's shoulder pain in individuals with spinal cord injury. *Arch Phys Med Rehabil.* 2001;82:1038–1046.

31. Whitt PL, MacKinnon J. Trager psychophysical integration: a method to improve chest mobility of patients with chronic lung disease. *Phys Ther.* 1986;66:214–217.

32. Duval C, Lafontaine D, HÈrbert J, Leroux A, Panisset M, Boucher JP. The effect of Trager therapy on the level of evoked stretch responses in patients with Parkinson's disease and rigidity. *J Manipulative Physiol* Ther. 2002;25:455–464.

33. Hill PD, Humenick SS, Tieman B. Maternal activities used to soothe crying of 3-week-old breastfed infants. *J Perinat Educ.* 1997;6:13–20.

34. White-Traut RC, Goldman MBC. Pre-mature infant massage: is it safe? *Pediatr Nurs.* 1988;14:285–289.

35. White-Traut RC, Nelson MN. Maternally administered tactile, auditory, visual, and vestibular stimulation: relationship to later interactions between mother and premature infants. *Res Nurs Health.* 1988;11:31–39.

36. Upledger J, Vredevoogd JD. *Craniosacral Therapy.* Seattle: Eastland Press; 1983.

## Further Reading

Bauer W, Short CL, Bennett GA. The manner of removal of proteins from normal joints. *J Exp Med.* 1933;5:419.

Blackburn J. Trager. Part 2: hooking up: the power of presence in bodywork. *J Bodywork Movement Ther.* 2004;8:114–121.

Blackburn J. Trager. Part 3: at the table. *J Bodywork Movement Ther.* 2004;8:178–188.

Blackburn J. Trager mentastics. Part 4: presence in motion. *J Bodywork Movement Ther.* 2004;8:265–277.

Haynes W. Rolling exercises designed to train the deep spinal muscles. *J Bodywork Movement Ther.* 2003;7:153–164.

Hendricks T. Effects of immobilisation on connective tissue. *J Manual Manipulative Ther.* 1995;3:98–103.

Johnson SK, Frederick J, Kaufman M, Mountjoy B. A controlled investigation of bodywork in multiple sclerosis. *J Altern Complement Med.* 1999;5:237–243.

Korner AF, Guilleminault C, Van den Hoed J, Baldwin RB. Reduction of sleep apnea and bradycardia in preterm infants on oscillating water beds: a controlled polygraphic study. *Pediatrics.* 1978;61:528–533.

Pederson DR. The soothing effect of rocking as determined by the direction and frequency of movement. *Can J Behav Sci.* 1975;7: 237–243.

Rood M. The use of sensory receptors to activate, facilitate, and inhibit motor response, autonomic and somatic, in developmental sequence. In: Sattely C, ed. *Approaches to the Treatment of Patients with Neuromuscular Dysfunction.* Dubuque, IA: William C. Brown; 1962.

Ter Vrugt D, Pederson DR. The effects of vertical rocking frequencies on the arousal level of two-month old infants. *Child Dev.* 1973;44:205–209.

Tolle R. The trager approach. *Massage Ther J.* 2005;44:60–67.

Wyke BD. Articular neurology and manipulative therapy. In: Glasgow EF, Twomey LT, Scull ER, et al, eds. *Aspects of Manipulative Therapy.* Edinburgh: Churchill Livingstone; 1987.

# Chapter 12
## Percussive Techniques

Percussive techniques are those massage techniques that use controlled striking of the body to quickly deform and release tissues. These techniques enhance airway clearance, reduce or increase neuromuscular tone, and increase alertness. This chapter describes the various percussive techniques, how to perform them, and how to apply them in practice sequences. A section on further study includes a discussion of relevant outcomes and evidence, cautions and contraindications, and how to use the techniques in treatment.

### Table 12-1 Summary of Outcomes for Percussive Techniques

| | Technique | | |
| Outcome | Clapping | Tapping | Other Forms of Percussion |
| --- | --- | --- | --- |
| Increased airway clearance/mobilization of secretions | ✓ | ? | ? |
| Increased respiration/gaseous exchange | ✓ | ? | ? |
| Decreased dyspnea due to increased airway clearance | ✓ | ? | ? |
| Pain reduction through hyperstimulation analgesia | P | P | P |
| Systemic and sensory arousal and enhanced alertness | P | P | P |
| Normalized neuromuscular tone in patients with some CNS disorders | ? | P | P |
| Alteration of movement responses in patients with some CNS disorders | ? | P | P |
| Balance of agonist/antagonist function in patients with some CNS disorders | ? | P | P |

✓: the outcome is supported by research summarized in this chapter. P: the outcome is possible. ?: the outcome is debatable (research results are absent or inconsistent).

## Percussion: Foundations

# DEFINITION

Percussion: Repeated rhythmic light striking.[1-11]

# USES

Therapists have used the various forms of percussion to improve **airway clearance**, as **proprioceptive stimulation techniques**, to increase **levels of arousal**, and for **pain** relief.

# PALPATION PRACTICE

1. For all regions of the body, using fingertip palpation and graduated pressure, estimate the thickness of the subcutaneous fatty layer and the superficial and deeper layers of muscle.
2. Using a well-illustrated anatomy text as a reference, draw the position of the lungs and its lobes on a partner who is positioned in prone, supine, side-lying, or any of the **postural drainage** positions shown in Figure 12-14.

| Theory In Practice | |
|---|---|
| **Percussive Techniques** | |
| Patient Profile | A patient who regularly receives massage presents for a lunch hour massage prior to making an important business presentation later in the afternoon. He usually requests deep neuromuscular and connective tissue techniques and deep moist heat to address elevated resting tension and related shortness in the muscles of his back and neck. |
| Subjective Findings | ▪ This patient wants the practitioner to address the usual issues and areas.<br>▪ He does not want to feel drowsy after the massage since he has to perform well later in the afternoon. |
| Objective Findings | ▪ Range of motion: Slightly limited cervical range of motion (less than 10%) related to elevated resting tension. |
| Treatment Approach | ▪ It is possible to address the elevated resting tension and restrictions of range effectively without resorting to techniques that produce marked sedation. For example, avoid the use of heat, deep pressure, sustained specific compression, direct fascial technique, rocking, and working around the sacrum.<br>▪ Your list of techniques might include: skin rolling, the full range of neuromuscular techniques, and shaking. Limit the depth to more superficial layers of tissue, and use a somewhat faster pace than you would normally use, with a stroke rate between one and two strokes per second. Use active stretching techniques such as hold-relax to engage the patient.<br>▪ Finish each region with a couple of minutes of percussion and with superficial fingertip stroking. |

## Critical Thinking Question

Percussion is often incorporated as a part of **stimulating massage**. In what common situations might clients benefit from enhanced alertness?

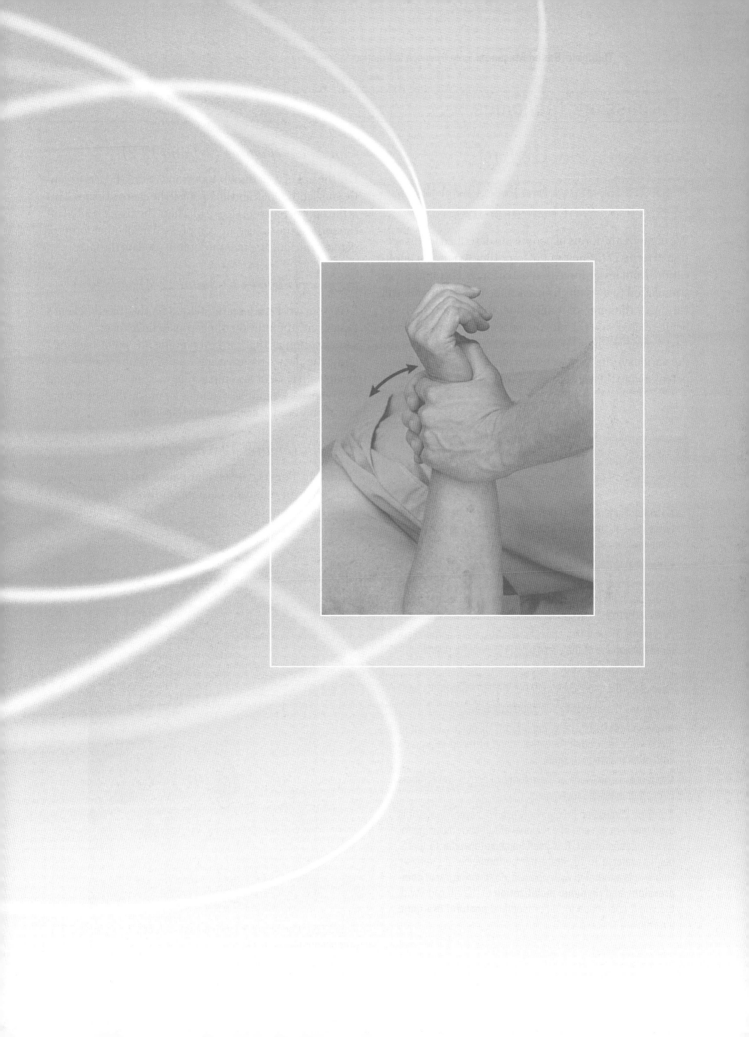

## Percussion: Technique

# MANUAL TECHNIQUE

## Manual Contact Surfaces and Uses of the Forms of Percussion

We organize the forms of percussion described in this section in terms of the amount of force they require for application: from lesser force to greater force. The amount of stimulation that results from each form of percussion will vary with the force of application, the area of the body being treated, and the rate of application. Figures 12-1 to 12-13 show the hand positions and contact surfaces for the various forms of percussion and therapists applying percussion to the various regions of the body.

---

**Box 12-1**    **Components of Percussion**

---

**Contact:** Fingers, fingertip(s), ulnar border of hands, palms, heels, dorsal surface of interphalangeal joints, in various combinations

**Pressure:** Light to heavy

**Engages:** Superficial subcutaneous tissues (lighter forms) to deeper muscle and contained viscera such as the lungs (heavier forms)

**Direction:** The contact and release strokes are perpendicular to the surface of the client's body (except for pounding)

**Amplitude/length:** N/A

**Rate:** 2 to 10 or more cycles per second (Hz) using both hands

**Duration:** 30 seconds to 20 minutes or more

**Intergrades with:** The various forms of percussion intergrade with each other; however, none of these intergrade with other massage techniques.

**Combines with:** None of these forms of percussion combine with other massage techniques.

**Context:** Percussion is commonly used in several ways. It is used briefly at the end of a regional or full-body massage for its stimulating effect. It is used immediately prior to therapeutic exercise to facilitate the performance of exercise. Finally, it is alternated with vibration, rib springing (rapid **compression**), and **rhythmic mobilization** of the rib cage with the client positioned in full or modified **postural drainage** positions.

---

### *Pincement (Figures 12-1 and 12-2)[2]*

Use the tips of your thumb, index, and middle fingers to gently and lightly pinch and lift or pluck the client's tissues. This is the only percussion stroke in which the tissue is lifted off the surface; the tissues are compressed in all other forms of percussion. Pincement is most often used on the face.

### *Tapping (Figures 12-3 and 12-4)[2,6,8–11]*

Keep your wrist and forearm still and gently strike the client's tissues with the individual fingertips or finger pads, using the same motion as that for keyboarding. In "point hacking," strike the client's tissues using your fingertips together as a group with a slight accompanying wrist motion.[1] Tapping and point hacking are also suitable for use on the face and are commonly used in **neuromuscular facilitation**.

### *Hacking (Figures 12-5 and 12-6)*

Hold your fingers, wrists, and palms loosely and facing each other in relatively close opposition. Make contact using the ulnar borders of your 5th finger and hands; one

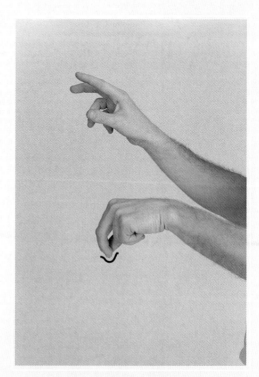

**Figure 12-1** Hand position and contact surfaces for pincement. The practitioner lifts or plucks the tissue upward.

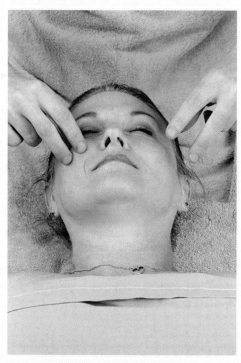

**Figure 12-2**  Pincement performed on the face.

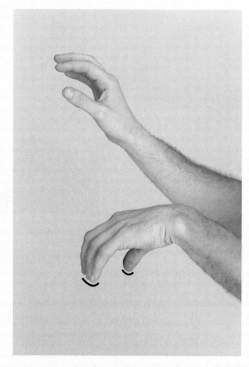

**Figure 12-4**  Hand position and contact surface for point hacking.

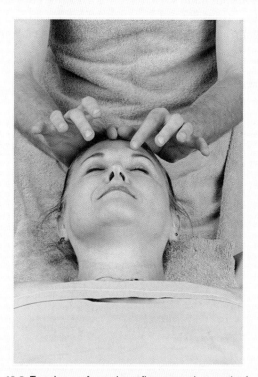

**Figure 12-3**  Tapping performed one finger at a time on the face.

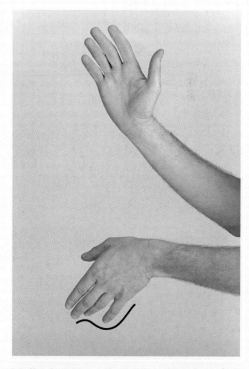

**Figure 12-5**  Hand position and contact surface for hacking.

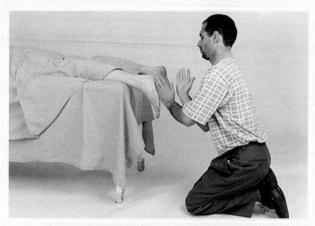

Figure 12-6 Hacking applied to the sole of the foot will gently wake a sleeping client.

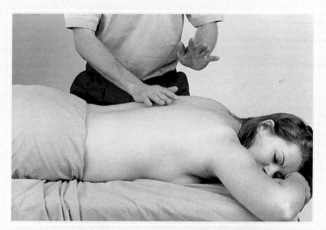

Figure 12-8 Slapping is very stimulating when applied to bare skin. It is suitable for large, flat areas like the back.

author suggested making contact with the posterior surface of the three medial fingers.[6] Alternate hands in order to apply light and rapid strokes.[1] Hacking can be applied to most areas of the body, other than the head, for a mild stimulating effect.

## Slapping or "Splatting" (Figures 12-7 and 12-8)[2,8,11]

With your hand and fingers held loosely, make contact with the entire open palmar surface. This technique is suit-

able for large flat areas, such as the back or thighs, when a more stimulating effect is desired.

## Clapping (Figures 12-9 and 12-10)[1,2,5,6,8–10]

Few sources[2] distinguish between "cupping" and clapping; therefore, this text considers the terms to be equivalent. Position your hand so that it forms a hollow "cupped" surface that traps air and does not deform on impact.[1,4] To cup your hand, flex your metacarpophalangeal joints to

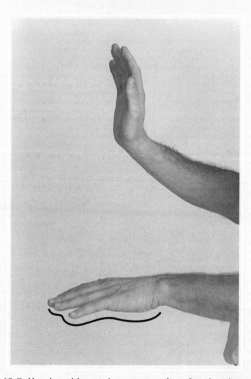

Figure 12-7 Hand position and contact surface for slapping.

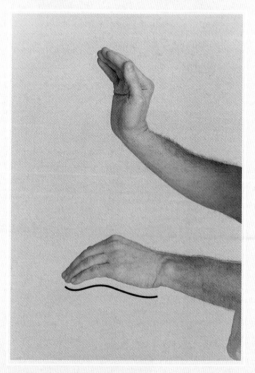

Figure 12-9 Hand position and contact surface for clapping. Contact occurs only around the rim of the hand.

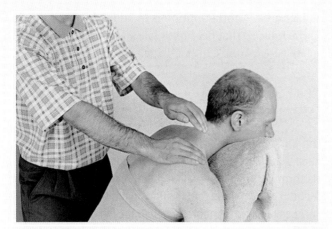

Figure 12-10 Clapping applied to the posterior apical segment of the right lung. ON-LINE VIDEO

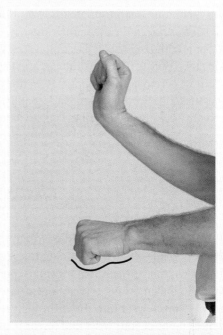

Figure 12-11 Hand position and contact surface for beating.

about 45 degrees, hold your interphalangeal joints in neutral extension, and adduct your fingers and thumb. The degree to which your hand should be cupped will vary with the area of the body that you are treating. For example, your hand should be flatter over flat surfaces, such as the posterior chest, and more cupped to fit curved areas, such as the lateral surfaces of the rib cage.[4] Let your wrist remain as loose as possible and avoid excessive arm movement, since this can cause rapid fatigue. Clapping is the technique of choice when performing **postural drainage** to increase **airway clearance**, and it does not have to be particularly forceful or rapid to be effective for this purpose.[4] You can also use clapping in areas other than the thorax such as over large muscle groups.[1]

## Beating or "Rapping" (Figures 12-11 and 12-12)[1,2,8]

Position your hand in a loose fist and use the heel of your hand and dorsal surface of the interphalangeal joints to percuss larger muscles or even the sacrum. You can use more force when applying beating than clapping because beating is applied over large muscle groups, while clapping is applied over the rib cage where there is less overlying muscle.[1]

## Pounding (Figure 12-13)[1,2,8,10]

Position your hand in a loose fist and use the ulnar surface of your hand as the contact surface.[1] Abduct your elbows, hold your hands near your midline, and apply the strokes in circles that move in the sagittal plane away from your chest and return toward your abdomen as you strike the

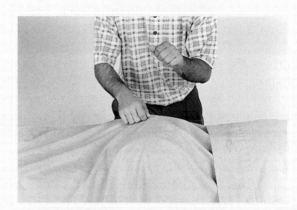

Figure 12-12 Vigorous beating is suitable for large muscles such as the gluteals. ON-LINE VIDEO

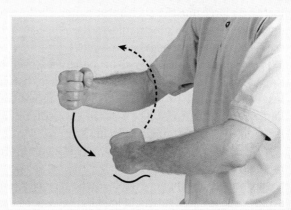

Figure 12-13 Hand position, direction of movement, and contact surface for pounding. ON-LINE VIDEO

client. This technique is appropriate for large, thick muscle groups such as the glutei and hamstrings.

Note: Some authors consider the compressive vibration and shaking used during postural drainage and percussion to be a form of percussion.[5,6] Chapter 9, Neuromuscular Techniques, describes compression, and Chapter 11, Passive Movement Techniques, describes coarse vibration and shaking.

## MANUAL TECHNIQUE FOR ALL FORMS OF PERCUSSION

1. For all forms of percussion, keep your wrist and hand as relaxed as possible while maintaining the position of the chosen contact surface. Light forms of percussion require only small motions of your fingers or wrist. For the heavier forms, generate force through the combined movement of your wrist and forearm, as well as elbow flexion and extension.

2. Make the contact and release strokes quick, light, and even. Use both hands and alternate hands while performing the strokes with a fast, stable rhythm. This rhythm can take considerable practice to achieve. Bear in mind that an even rate of application is more important to achieve than increased speed. Consequently, strive to achieve evenness first, and only then increase the tempo of the application. A rate of 3 to 8 Hz is acceptable when the technique is performed with both hands.

3. The form of percussion and the force with which it is applied must be adjusted to the thickness, type, and sensitivity of the target tissue. Use very light force over the face and areas of unprotected bone. Use moderate force over thinner muscle groups, as in the forearm, or where there is dense fascia. Finally, use the heaviest force over large muscles such as the glutei. The force of application of percussion should also be adjusted to the size, age, and general health of the client.

4. Whenever possible, avoid applying percussion over the same area for more than a few seconds, since this can become irritating to the client. Instead, move your hands through the region of focus in a consistent pattern such as a circle or in parallel lines.[1,4]

5. Apply percussion through a gown, a sheet, or a towel as necessary to reduce irritation.

6. Avoid bony prominences such as the clavicles, and avoid breast tissue. If the client has large breasts, ask her to use her hand to hold breast tissue away from the con-

tact area. Another option is to adjust her position on the table so that her breast falls away from the contact area, for example in side-lying.

## How percussion might work

The cupped shape of the hand used in chest percussion traps air against the rib cage and sets up a vibration that travels through the chest wall and lung tissue.[1] This vibration dislodges the mucus that is stuck in the bronchial tree.[1,8,11] Percussion used for neuromuscular facilitation may achieve an effect by repeatedly stimulating stretch receptors (spindles) within the muscle.[1,8,11] The intense stimulation of percussion may initiate a generalized **sympathetic response** that leads to increased alertness.[8,11] Finally, pain relief may occur through spinal gating.[1,11]

## THERAPIST'S POSITION AND MOVEMENT

1. When treating the limbs and torso, stand at a right angle to the long axis of the tissues to be treated and use a **standing upright posture** or a **wide-stance knee bend** shown in Chapter 6, Preparation and Positioning for Massage (Figures 12-8 and 12-12). Incline or lean toward, or over, the target tissues when applying heavier forms of percussion, such as pounding, or to generate a faster rate of application (Figure 12-6).

2. Hold your elbows partly flexed; the amount of flexion will vary with the form of percussion, area, size of client, and working posture chosen (Figures 12-6, 12-8, 12-12, and 12-13). The power for the strokes of heavier forms of percussion comes from a combination of movements that are performed while the upper arms remain stationary. The primary motion for this stroke is flexion and extension of your wrist, and the secondary motion is a small amount of elbow flexion and extension.

3. Allow your shoulders, elbows, and wrists to remain loose throughout the applications of all percussive techniques.[1,4]

4. During longer applications of percussion (clapping) that address several lung segments (25 to 40 minutes), change positions frequently to minimize the mechanical strain of performing this physically demanding treatment (Figure 12-14).

# BRONCHIAL DRAINAGE

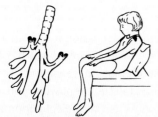

**UPPER LOBES Apical Segments**

Bed or drainage table flat.

Patient leans back on pillow at 30° angle against therapist.

Therapist claps with markedly cupped hand over area between clavicle and top of scapula on each side.

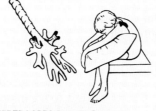

**UPPER LOBES Posterior Segments**

Bed or drainage table flat.

Patient leans over folder pillow at 30° angle.

Therapist stands behind and claps over upper back on both sides.

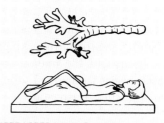

**UPPER LOBES Anterior Segments**

Bed or drainage table flat.

Patient lies on back with pillow under knees.

Therapist claps between clavicle and nipple on each side.

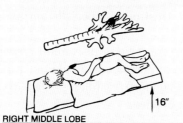

**RIGHT MIDDLE LOBE**

Foot of table or bed elevated 16 inches.

Patient lies head down on left side and rotates ¼ turn backward. Pillow may be placed behind from shoulder to hip. Knees should be flexed.

Therapist claps over right nipple area. In females with breast development or tenderness, use cupped hand with heel of hand under armpit and fingers extending forward beneath the breast.

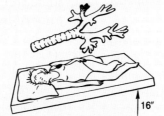

**LEFT UPPER LOBE Lingular Segments**

Foot of table or bed elevated 16 inches.

Patient lies head down on right side and rotates ¼ turn backward. Pillow may be placed behind from shoulder to hip. Knees should be flexed.

Therapist claps with moderately cupped hand over left nipple area. In females with breast development or tenderness, use cupped hand with heel of hand under armpit and fingers extending forward beneath the breast.

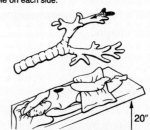

**LOWER LOBES Anterior Basal Segments**

Foot of table or bed elevated 20 inches.

Patient lies on side, head down, pillow under knees.

Therapist claps with slightly cupped hand over lower ribs. (Position shown is for drainage of left anterior basal segment. To drain the right anterior basal segment, patient should lie on his left side in same posture).

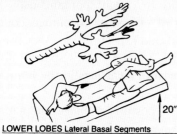

**LOWER LOBES Lateral Basal Segments**

Foot of table or bed elevated 20 inches.

Patient lies on abdomen, head down, then rotates ¼ turn upward. Upper leg is flexed over a pillow for support.

Therapist claps over uppermost portion of lower ribs. (Position shown is for drainage of right lateral basal segment. To drain the left lateral basal segment, patient should lie on his right side in the same posture).

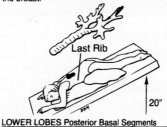

**LOWER LOBES Posterior Basal Segments**

Foot of table or bed elevated 20 inches.

Patient lies on abdomen, head down, with pillow under hips. Therapist claps over lower ribs close to spine on each side.

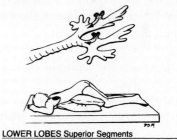

**LOWER LOBES Superior Segments**

Bed or table flat.

Patient lies on abdomen with two pillows under hips.

Therapist claps over middle of back at tip of scapula on either side of spine.

**Figure 12-14** Postural drainage positions for adults. (Reprinted from Rothstein J, Roy S, Wolf S. The Rehabilitation Specialist's Handbook. 3rd ed. Philadelphia: FA Davis; 2004 with permission of FA Davis.)

# PALPATE

Since your hands are in contact with the client's tissues for fractions of a second at a time, detailed palpation is impossible. You can, however, form a general impression of the resiliency (springiness) of the tissues being contacted. This resiliency will vary with the amount of subcutaneous fat, level of **muscle resting tension**, and supporting bony structure that are present in the region.

# OBSERVE

While performing the technique, observe the client and look and listen for the following signs of correct application of the technique.

1. Each form of percussion makes a characteristic sound on impact. For example, on healthy tissue, cupping makes a hollow resonant sound as the trapped air resonates between the cupped hand and the chest wall. If your hand flattens on impact, this sound will not occur, and more importantly, the effect of the technique may not penetrate as deeply into the lung tissue as needed. Bear in mind that the sound of cupping on impact—dull, resonant, or hyperresonant—may not be a reliable method of assessing the health of the client's underlying tissues.[12]
2. During the application of **postural drainage and percussion**, listen to and observe the client's breathing, coughing, and expectoration.[4]
3. During the application of postural drainage and percussion, periodically check the client's face to monitor her comfort level.[4]
4. When applying any percussion stroke for reflex **stimulation**, watch the client for signs of waking, **arousal**, or irritation.

# COMMUNICATION WITH THE CLIENT

Communicate to prepare the client for treatment and to seek feedback on the client's level of comfort during the technique. Following are some examples of statements that you can use.

## In General

1. "I'm going to start the percussion now." Since percussive techniques, even when applied gently, often represent an abrupt change in sensation from other massage techniques, tell the client when you are going to begin percussion. When you select cupping or slapping, you should also prepare the client for the noise of the technique.
2. "Do you feel comfortable?" or "Do you need a break?" Since the application of percussion can be extremely stimulating, ensure that the client is not feeling irritated by the treatment, especially during longer applications.
3. "Does this cause you pain or discomfort anywhere?" The application of percussion should not cause the client pain or discomfort, regardless of the purpose for which it is being applied.[4]

## When Clapping Is Used with Postural Drainage to Enhance Airway Clearance

1. Clients may start to cough spontaneously during the application of clapping. Encourage coughing, forced expiration, and expectoration. Also, provide a suitable receptacle for the client's sputum and use appropriate **Standard Precautions** in the handling of body fluids.
2. A long sequence of postural drainage and percussion (up to 40 min[4]) can be a strenuous intervention for the client, as well as the therapist. Assess the client's comfort and level of fatigue every few minutes.
3. Mucus may continue to move for up to an hour following the application of postural drainage and percussion.[4] Encourage the client to cough and expectorate as required after treatment.

## A Practice Sequence for Percussion

Practice time: Allow 20 minutes per person.
You will not be able to apply percussion continuously throughout this sequence because it is a demanding technique to perform. Use **broad-contact compression** in between the different forms of percussion to allow your hands and arms to rest.

### Prone
The back and gluteals are a good test area. Undrape one side, and let the other side remain draped. You will treat both sides to determine the effect of the draping on the client's experience of the stroke.

To begin, apply a series of broad-contact palmar compression strokes over the entire area for a minute. Apply pincement for a minute. Return to compression for a minute.

Then apply in turn:

- Tapping
- Point hacking
- Hacking
- Slapping
- Cupping
- Beating (apply to gluteals only)
- Pounding (apply to gluteals only)

Alternate palmar compression and the progressively more vigorous forms of percussion. Finish with compression. Solicit feedback from your client about how each form of percussion felt and how the application of percussion differed between the draped and undraped sides.

For additional study: Explore the use of lighter forms of percussion on more densely innervated areas such as the face and hands. How much percussive force is tolerable in each of these areas? Which strokes can and cannot be applied?

## A Practice Sequence for Postural Drainage and Percussion of an Adult

Practice time: Allow 30 minutes per person.
You will need an articulated, tilting treatment table or bed to achieve the elevation required for the various postural drainage positions. If this is not available, you can approximate the positions using eight or more standard pillows.[4,13]

Review any factors in your client's history that would require a reduction in force of application of the percussion (see the Cautions and Contraindications section later in this chapter). Note that positioning for pulmonary drainage in tilted positions with the head down will in itself elevate blood pressure, which is a caution for hypertensive clients.[1,4]

Remember to avoid the scapula, clavicle, and breast tissue. If the client has large breasts, ask her to use her hand to hold breast tissue away from the contact area. Use caution around the floating ribs.

Apply the following cycle of techniques to as many of the segments illustrated in Figure 12-14 as time allows. In a clinical situation, one position should be maintained for 5 or 10 minutes or even longer. You can then apply continuous clapping for 3 to 5 minutes to a small area, followed by vibration and therapeutic breathing exercises. For a practice sequence, you may shorten these times to include a wider selection of positions.

1. Assume a postural drainage position (see Figure 12-14).
2. Apply clapping continuously with a stable rhythm over indicated segment of the lung for 1 or 2 minutes.
   As far as possible, use the cupped hand position and obtain the characteristic resonant sound; this is not always possible for a large-handed therapist. In smaller areas, use only one cupped hand or apply pounding or hacking.
3. Initiate compression and **coarse vibration** at the peak of each deep inspiration and continue them throughout expiration in the following manner. Compress the thorax over the segment as the client begins to exhale. While maintaining this compression, apply coarse vibration throughout the exhalation. Release compression to permit inhalation. In addition, instruct the client to forcibly exhale or vocalize "Ahhh."[8] Instruct the client to expectorate as required.
4. Alternatively, apply repeated rapid compression with a rapid partial release between each compression stroke (rib springing[4]). Instruct the client to forcibly exhale or vocalize "Ahhh" and to expectorate as required.
5. Intersperse rocking using rib contacts, or **rhythmic mobilization** of the rib cage, with the percussion to give both client and therapist a break from the more vigorous technique.

Change positions until you have treated several segments of the lung. At the end of this sequence, position the client in prone and finish with 5 minutes of **sedative** massage. Finish by instructing your client to sit up. Then practice giving instruction for appropriate follow-up care.

## Percussion: Further Study and Practice

## NAMES AND ORIGINS

Other texts often call percussion "**tapotement**."[1-11] Although there is unanimous usage of the equivalent terms percussion and tapotement, different names are often applied to some of the forms of percussion. For example, clapping is sometimes known as "cupping."[1,8,10] The section on manual technique earlier in this chapter gives alternate names for the forms of percussion.

## OUTCOMES AND EVIDENCE

The various forms of percussion have different effects. Clinicians can use them for the treatment of **airway clearance**, as **proprioceptive stimulation** techniques, for increasing **levels of arousal**, and for **pain** relief. Clinicians use percussion, specifically clapping, to mechanically loosen secretions in the lungs and facilitate airway clearance. They frequently use it in clinical conditions that are associated with the production of copious or viscous mucus.[1,4,14] In traditional cardiopulmonary physical therapy, percussion is combined with **postural drainage** and is followed by, or alternated with, vibration of the rib cage or rapid compression and release of the rib cage (called rib "springing" or "shaking").[1,4,14] Postural drainage has its own indications, contraindications, and outcomes.[4] Research suggests that the entire procedure of postural drainage and percussion promotes the movement of mucus in a cephalic direction through the bronchial tree and increases the clearance of sputum,[15-20] with one dissenting opinion.[21] This effect may be more pronounced in conditions in which there are large volumes of sputum.[22,23] The use of postural drainage and percussion may be declining with the advent of many recently developed techniques for airway clearance that use mechanical motion and ventilation.[15-17,24-31]

There are many issues related to whether the measures used in the research on percussion and postural drainage are relevant. For example, recent reviews question the use of the volume of sputum cleared by the client as a valid outcome measure in research on bronchial conditions,[15,32,33] although sputum clearance has been associated with increased client comfort.[16] Other authors consider blood oxygenation to be a more relevant measure of pulmonary function[14,18,32,34]; however, the relationship between improved oxygenation and the clearance of sputum remains unclear.[14,15,35] In addition, the results of research on the effects of postural drainage and percussion on pulmonary function testing are equivocal for several clinical conditions: post-surgically,[36] in critically ill clients with atelectasis,[14,24,37] in mechanically ventilated children,[38] and in chronic bronchitis and bronchiectasis.[15] Percussion remains valuable in the treatment of cystic fibrosis[16,17,39,40] and some rarer pulmonary conditions,[41] although other methods may be equally effective for clearing sputum.[42]

Several massage texts state that percussion stimulates stretch reflexes that facilitate the contraction and shortening of muscle when it is applied to the muscle belly or tendon.[5,8,10] In addition, traditional physical therapy practice, such as the techniques of Bobath and Rood, has applied various forms of percussion, especially tapping, to muscles or tendons to increase neuromuscular tone and facilitate normalized movement patterns in clients with neurological conditions such as spasticity.[43] Other sources, however, suggest that tapping tendons or muscles may inhibit contraction both locally and in synergist muscle groups by stimulating cutaneous receptors.[44,45]

Clinicians consider percussion to have a general stimulating effect that most likely varies with the location, vigor, and duration of its application.[1,2,5,6,8-10] This has been the rationale for applying percussion during **precompetition sports massage** or at the end of sedative massage to increase the client's level of arousal.[2] By contrast, Frownfelter[4] notes that the monotonous rhythm and rate of the application of clapping for extended periods may have a relaxing effect.

Applications of percussion may also have a variety of minor effects. It may produce a local hyperemia.[5,10] As with other massage techniques, percussion produces a transient hyperstimulation analgesia, which may make it suitable for pain relief in neuralgia or amputation.[1] Finally, mechanical percussion does not promote recovery from short-term intense muscular activity.[46] Table 12-1 summarizes the main outcomes for percussion.

### ? Critical Thinking Question

What is the rationale for using percussion to prepare for exercise with clients who have neurological conditions?

## EXAMINING THE EVIDENCE

A recent crossover study[42] of 24 clients with cystic fibrosis compared the effectiveness of **postural drainage and percussion (PDP)** in enhancing airway clearance with the effectiveness of two mechanized alternatives: interpulmonary percussive ventilation and high-frequency chest wall percussion. The main outcome measure was sputum collected during the 30-minute treatments and for 15 minutes after treatment. The researchers judged PDP, as administered in 12 positions, to be equal with the other methods with respect to its ability to enhance short-term airway clearance. Clients showed no significant preference for any of these treatments. This study is thorough, well-described, and repeatable. The authors also discuss the study's limitations, which included a modest sample size and the validity of sputum clearance as an indicator of pulmonary function.

Varekojis SM, Douce FH, Flucke RL, Filbrun DA, Tice JS, McCoy KS, Castile RG. A comparison of the therapeutic effectiveness of and preference for postural drainage and percussion, intrapulmonary percussive ventilation, and high-frequency chest wall compression in hospitalized cystic fibrosis patients. *Respir Care.* 2003;48:24–28.

# CAUTIONS AND CONTRAINDICATIONS

Clinicians need clinical training and supervised practice to master the proper application of percussive techniques. Advanced training may be advisable when dealing with pathological conditions. All of the general and local contraindications noted for massage techniques apply to the use of percussion (see Chapter 3, Clinical Decision Making for Massage). The application of percussive techniques should not cause the client pain or discomfort. Posttreatment erythema and client reports of discomfort are undesirable effects that indicate incorrect application of the technique.[4] A thin layer of fabric, such as a sheet or gown, placed between the clinician's hands and the client's skin can reduce skin sensitivity without substantially reducing the force of the technique.[1,4] There are also several specific contraindications to the use of percussion.

Percussion of the thorax is contraindicated in cases of severe rib fracture, untreated tension pneumothorax, con-firmed or possible coronary thrombosis or pulmonary embolism, unstable cardiac conditions, conditions that are prone to hemorrhage, after chest or spinal surgery,[1,4] and during an acute episode of asthma.[47] The positional changes required for postural drainage may cause increased oxygen demand, carbon dioxide release, blood pressure, and cardiac output.[1,48] Consequently, the head-down position must be used with caution, particularly if clients are hypertensive or have had a head injury.[1,4,49] Percussion used alone can also increase heart rate and blood pressure.[1,34] Notwithstanding these cautions, postural drainage and percussion can be tolerated by acutely ill clients, provided that the procedure is administered within strict guidelines,[1,4,15,49] such as monitoring critically ill clients for hypoxemia and increasing the administration of oxygen.[19] The procedure should only be applied to clients who have pulmonary conditions that are associated with increased amounts of sputum.[19] Finally, although neither postural drainage nor percussion make gastroesophageal reflux worse,[50] avoid treating clients with these techniques after meals.[4]

There are separate contraindications and cautions for the application of percussion in areas other than the thorax. First, clinicians consider even light percussion to be a local contraindication in acute and subacute injuries that are moderate or severe.[1] Clinicians are also are advised to avoid muscles with **spasm**, postexercise cramping, active **trigger points**, or latent trigger points.[1,10,51] In addition, use caution when applying percussion over bony prominences such as the clavicles and vertebral spinous processes. Finally, reduce the force of application of percussion, or avoid using this technique, in areas where muscle tone or bulk are less than normal, over the kidneys, around the floating and lower ribs, around the faces of clients with a history of physical or other abuse, and wherever there is hypersensitivity.[1,2,4,8–10]

## ? Critical Thinking Question

Why should clinicians avoid performing percussion over active or latent trigger points?

# USING PERCUSSION IN TREATMENT

## For Postural Drainage and Percussion

1. There are several approaches to facilitating the thinning and clearance of sputum. If possible, encourage the client to drink water 30 to 60 minutes before the

intervention.[4] Steam inhalation (humidification) can reduce the viscosity of the mucus and may also dilate the bronchioles. **Aerosol therapy** using an ultrasonic nebulizer can assist in liquefying and mobilizing mucus.[4] Prior application of warm moist heat to the client's anterior or posterior thorax may reflexly dilate the bronchioles, if this is appropriate for the client's clinical condition.[52]

2. During postural drainage and percussion, position the client in the sequence of positions for postural drainage (Figure 12-14). Less rigorous, modified postural drainage positions may be as effective as traditional postural drainage positions.[4,37]

3. Intersperse clapping with broad-contact compression and simultaneous vibration of the rib cage.

4. Synchronize vibration with forced expiration, coughing, or audible huffing by the client.[1,4,8]

5. The use of suctioning,[15] methods of modifying mechanical ventilator airflow such as positive expiratory pressure,[17,25,40] and other mechanical devices, such as cyclically inflated pneumatic belts,[25] can be used with clients who have atelectasis or who are critically ill.

## After Performing Postural Drainage and Percussion

1. Encourage the clearance of sputum and rest, as required, for the following hour.[4,26,53]

2. Teach the client techniques for cough stimulation and for effective coughing.[15]

3. The client can benefit from learning exercises for chest-wall mobility, ventilator muscle training, conditioning, reconditioning, neuromuscular relaxation, and postural training.[1,7,17,53]

4. Instruct the client on how to perform self-drainage.[25]

5. Clients may find self-administered chest clapping beneficial, although research has not consistently shown that it enhances the rate of sputum clearance or the level of oxygen saturation.[54]

## For Facilitation and Inhibition of Neuromuscular Tone

1. Use joint traction and approximation, quick stretch, resistance, fine vibration, light touch, and repetitive brushing to increase **neuromuscular tone** and facilitate movement in clients with neurological conditions.[43,55]

2. Specific compression (inhibitory pressure), slow superficial stroking, static contact ("maintained touch"), prolonged cold, and neutral warmth are techniques that can be used to inhibit neuromuscular tone and facilitate movement in clients with neurological conditions.[43,55]

## To Increase Arousal

Machines that produce percussion for general use (e.g., the Thumper®) are available and enjoyed by some clients. Since these produce very vigorous percussion, carefully review contraindications and cautions (e.g., the presence of active or latent trigger points) before their use.

## Clinical Case

## History of Present Illness

A 10-year-old boy with cystic fibrosis who was admitted to an acute care setting with acute bronchitis. His clinical condition has responded to medical management, and he is in the later stages of therapy.

## Subjective

■ Complaints of shortness of breath at rest and during activity
■ Perceived dyspnea measured using the Borg Perceived Exertion Rating Scale[56]

# Objective

## Impairments

- Increased sputum production
- Persistent productive cough
- Impaired/ineffective airway clearance secondary to increased sputum production and ineffective cough and other airway clearance mechanisms
- Increased anterior-posterior diameter of the chest with decreased lateral costal and diaphragmatic expansion of the rib cage during respiration
- Sternal respiratory pattern with accessory muscle use and intercostal indrawing during respiration
- Scattered polyphonic wheezing and crackles throughout the ventilatory cycle audible during auscultation
- Decreased midexpiratory flow rate on spirometric pulmonary function tests
- Hyperinflation, peribronchiolar thickening, flattening of the diaphragm, and bronchiectasis of the upper lobes apparent on chest x-ray

## Functional Limitations

- Ambulation tolerance 50 feet, secondary to shortness of breath
- Inability to complete activities of daily living, such as dressing tasks, without frequent rest periods secondary to shortness of breath
- Poor endurance and decreased levels of oxygen saturation during functional activity

# Analysis

## Treatment Rationale

To enhance airway clearance and facilitate decreased dyspnea and increased rib cage mobility.

| Impairment | Outcomes and Role of Massage |
|---|---|
| Impaired airway clearance | Increased airway clearance |
| | Primary treatment; direct effect of clapping on the mobilization of sputum, especially when used with postural drainage |
| Decreased rib cage mobility | Increased rib cage mobility |
| | Primary treatment; direct effect of massage techniques on reducing chronic shortening of intercostal muscles, accessory muscles of breathing, and diaphragm; direct effect of "rib springing" on increasing the mobility of the sternocostal, costovertebral, and costochondral joints |
| Accessory muscle use | Decreased accessory muscle use |
| | Secondary treatment; accessory muscle use reflects an increased work of breathing[3,4] that is not directly affected by the use of massage techniques; effects of massage techniques that can contribute to decreased accessory muscle use include: reduction of chronic shortening of accessory muscles, increased perceived relaxation, and decreased perceived anxiety |

| Dyspnea | Decreased dyspnea |
| | Secondary treatment; indirect effect of massage on dyspnea through increased perceived relaxation, decreased perceived anxiety, and increased airway clearance |

| *Activity Limitation* | *Functional Outcomes* |
| --- | --- |
| Decreased ambulation | Patient will be able to ambulate 100 feet without a decrease in oxygen saturation and complaints of shortness of breath |
| Shortness of breath with self-care activities | Patient will be able to complete self-care activities, such as dressing, without frequent complaints of shortness of breath |
| Decreased endurance for self-care activities | Patient will demonstrate the use of appropriate energy-conservation techniques during performance of self-care activities and ambulation |

## Plan

| Massage Techniques | Clapping of the thorax with postural drainage |
| --- | --- |
| | Rib springing |
| | Coarse vibration combined with broad-contact compression of the rib cage |
| | Petrissage to anterior and posterior thoracic and cervical muscles |
| | Wringing of the rib cage |
| | Stripping of scalene muscles |
| | Direct fascial techniques on the inferior costal margin and along the intercostal spaces |
| Other Appropriate Techniques and Interventions[57] | Effective coughing techniques |
| | Forced expiration or audible huffing to facilitate airway clearance |
| | Use of a positive expiratory pressure mask |
| | Diaphragmatic breathing exercises |
| | Education in energy-conservation techniques during ambulation and activities of daily living |
| | Graded therapeutic exercise program |
| | Encourage fluid replacement |
| | Review of self-administered postural drainage and mechanical percussion for home program |

## References

1. de Domenico G, Wood EC. *Beard's Massage.* 4th ed. Philadelphia: WB Saunders; 1997.
2. Benjamin PJ, Tappan FM. *Tappan's Handbook of Healing Massage Techniques.* 4th ed. Upper Saddle River, NJ: Pearson Prentice Hall; 2005.
3. Frownfelter DL, Dean E. *Principals and Practice of Cardiopulmonary Physical Therapy.* 3rd ed. St. Louis: CV Mosby; 1996.
4. Frownfelter DL. *Chest Physical Therapy and Pulmonary Rehabilitation: An Interdisciplinary Approach.* Chicago: Year Book; 1987.
5. Holey E, Cook E. *Evidence-Based Therapeutic Massage.* 2nd ed. Edinburgh: Churchill Livingstone; 2003.

6. Hollis M. *Massage for Therapists.* 2nd ed. Oxford, England: Blackwell Science; 1998.

7. American Physical Therapy Association. Guide to Physical Therapist Practice. 2nd ed. Alexandria, VA: American Physical Therapy Association; 1999.

8. Fritz S. *Mosby's Fundamentals of Therapeutic Massage.* 3rd ed. St. Louis: Mosby; 2004.

9. Loving J. *Massage Therapy.* Stamford, CT: Appleton & Lange; 1999.

10. Salvo SG. *Massage Therapy: Principles and Practice.* 2nd ed. Philadelphia: WB Saunders; 2003.

11. Yates J. *A Physician's Guide to Therapeutic Massage.* 3rd ed. Toronto: Curties Overzet, 2004.

12. Soh TS, Soh SC, Ng LL, et al. Inter-rater reliability of percussion note as a respiratory assessment tool. *Physiother Singapore.* 1998;1:9–12.

13. Wood EC, Becker PD. *Beard's Massage.* 3rd ed. Philadelphia: WB Saunders; 1981.

14. Ciesla ND. Chest physical therapy for patients in the intensive care unit. *Phys Ther.* 1996;76:609–625.

15. Jones AP, Rowe BH. Bronchopulmonary hygiene physical therapy in chronic obstructive pulmonary disease and bronchiectasis. *Cochrane Library (Oxford).* 1998;1–3.

16. Ambrosino N, Callegari G, Galloni C, et al. Clinical evaluation of oscillating positive expiratory pressure for enhancing expectoration in diseases other than cystic fibrosis. *Monaldi Arch Chest Dis.* 1995;50:269–275.

17. Thomas J, Cook DJ, Brooks D. Chest physical therapy management of patients with cystic fibrosis. A meta-analysis. *Am J Respir Crit Care Med.* 1995;151:846–850.

18. Gallon A. Evaluation of chest percussion in the treatment of patients with copious sputum production. *Respir Med.* 1991;85:45–51.

19. Connors AF Jr, Hammon WE, Martin RJ, Rogers RM. Chest physical therapy. The immediate effect on oxygenation in acutely ill patients. *Chest.* 1980;78:559–564.

20. Jones A, Rowe BH. Bronchopulmonary hygiene physical therapy in bronchiectasis and chronic obstructive pulmonary disease: a systematic review. *Heart Lung.* 2000;29:125–135.

21. van der Schans CP, Piers DA, Postma DS. Effect of manual percussion on tracheobronchial clearance in patients with chronic airflow obstruction and excessive tracheobronchial secretion. *Thorax.* 1986;41:448–452.

22. Davis K Jr, Johannigman JA, Campbell RS, et al. The acute effects of body position strategies and respiratory therapy in paralyzed patients with acute lung injury. *Crit Care.* 2001;5: 81–87.

23. Fink JB. Positioning versus postural drainage. *Respir Care.* 2002; 47:769–777.

24. Raoof S, Chowdhrey N, Raoof S, et al. Effect of combined kinetic therapy and percussion therapy on the resolution of atelectasis in critically ill patients. *Chest.* 1999;115:1658–1666.

25. Hardy KA, Anderson BD. Noninvasive clearance of airway secretions. *Respir Care Clin North Am.* 1996;2:323–345.

26. McIlwaine MP, Davidson AG. Airway clearance techniques in the treatment of cystic fibrosis. *Curr Opin Pulm Med.* 1996;2: 447–451.

27. Thomas J, DeHueck A, Kleiner M, et al. To vibrate or not to vibrate: usefulness of the mechanical vibrator for clearing bronchial secretions. *Physiother Can.* 1995;47:120–125.

28. Pryor JA. Physiotherapy for airway clearance in adults. *Eur Respir J.* 1999;14:1418–1424.

29. McIlwaine PM, Wong LT, Peacock D, Davidson AG. Long-term comparative trial of conventional postural drainage and percussion versus positive expiratory pressure physiotherapy in the treatment of cystic fibrosis. *J Pediatr.* 1997;131:570–574.

30. Oermann CM, Sockrider MM, Giles D, Sontag MK, Accurso FJ, Castile RG. Comparison of high-frequency chest wall oscillation and oscillating positive expiratory pressure in the home management of cystic fibrosis: a pilot study. *Pediatr Pulmonol.* 2001;32:372–377.

31. Whitman J, Van Beusekom R, Olson S, Worm M, Indihar F. Preliminary evaluation of high-frequency chest compression for secretion clearance in mechanically ventilated patients. *Respir Care.* 1993;38:1081–1087.

32. Dean E. Oxygen transport: a physiologically-based conceptual framework for the practice of cardiopulmonary physiotherapy. *Physiotherapy.* 1994;80:347–355.

33. Hess DR. The evidence for secretion clearance techniques. *Respir Care.* 2001;46:1276–1293.

34. Dallimore K, Jenkins S, Tucker B. Respiratory and cardiovascular responses to manual chest percussion in normal subjects. *Aust J Physiother.* 1998;44:267–274.

35. Dall'Alba PT, Burns YR. The relationship between arterial blood gases and removal of airway secretions in neonates. *Physiother Theory Pract.* 1990;6:107–116.

36. Eales CJ, Barker M, Cubberley NJ. Evaluation of a single chest physiotherapy treatment to post-operative, mechanically ventilated cardiac surgery patients. *Physiother Theory Pract.* 1995; 11:23–28.

37. Stiller K, Jenkins S, Grant R, et al. Acute lobar atelectasis: a comparison of five physiotherapy regimens. *Physiother Theory Pract.* 1996;12:197–209.

38. Krause MF, Hoehn T. Chest physiotherapy in mechanically ventilated children: a review. *Crit Care Med.* 2000;28:1648–1651.

39. Boyd S, Brooks D, Agnew-Coughlin J, Ashwell J. Evaluation of the literature on the effectiveness of physical therapy modalities in the management of children with cystic fibrosis. *Pediatr Phys Ther.* 1994;6:70–74.

40. Langenderfer B. Alternatives to percussion and postural drainage: a review of mucus clearance therapies: percussion and postural drainage, autogenic drainage, positive expiratory pressure, flutter valve, intrapulmonary percussive ventilation, and high-frequency chest compression with the ThAIRapy vest. *J Cardiopulm Rehabil.* 1998;18:283–289.

41. Hammon WE, McCaffree DR, Cucchiara AJ. A comparison of manual to mechanical chest percussion for clearance of alveolar material in patients with pulmonary alveolar proteinosis (phospholipidosis). *Chest.* 1993;103:1409–1412.

42. Varekojis SM, Douce FH, Flucke RL, Filbrun DA, Tice JS, McCoy KS, Castile RG. A comparison of the therapeutic effectiveness of and preference for postural drainage and percussion, intrapulmonary percussive ventilation, and high-frequency chest wall compression in hospitalized cystic fibrosis patients. *Respir Care.* 2003;48:24–28.

43. Griffin JW. Use of proprioceptive stimuli in therapeutic exercise. *Phys Ther.* 1974;54:1072–1079.

44. Lederman E. *Fundamentals of Manual Therapy.* New York: Churchill Livingstone; 1997.

45. Belanger AY, Morin S, Pepin P, et al. Manual muscle tapping decreases H-reflex amplitude in control subjects. *Physiother Can.* 1989;41:192–196.

46. Cafarelli E, Sim J, Carolan B, et al. Vibratory massage and term recovery from muscular fatigue. *Int J Med.* 1990;11: 474–478.

47. Gameros-Gardea RA. Inhalation therapy in asthma. *Rev Alerg Mex.* 1996;43:109–115 (Abstract).

48. Horiuchi K, Jordan D, Cohen D, et al. Insights into the increased oxygen demand during chest physiotherapy. *Crit Care Med.* 1997;25:1347–1351.

49. Imle PC, Mars MP, Ciesla ND, et al. The effect of chest physical therapy on intracranial pressure and cerebral perfusion pressure. *Physiother Can.* 1997;49:48–55.

50. Chen HC, Liu CY, Cheng HF, et al. Chest physiotherapy does not exacerbate gastroesophageal reflux in patients with chronic bronchitis and bronchiectasis. *Chang Keng I Hsueh Tsa Chih.* 1998;21:409–414.

51. Travell JG, Simons DG. Myofascial pain and dysfunction. In: *The Trigger Point Manual, Volume 1.* Baltimore: Williams & Wilkins; 1983.

52. Moor F, Peterson S, Manwell E, et al. *Manual of Hydrotherapy and Massage.* Oshawa, Canada: Pacific Press Publishing; 1964.

53. Kisner C, Colby LA. *Therapeutic Exercise: Foundations and Techniques.* 4th ed. Philadelphia: FA Davis; 2002.

54. Carr J, Pryor JA, Hodson ME. Self chest clapping: patients' views and the effects on oxygen saturation. *Physiotherapy.* 1995;81:753–757.

55. O'Sullivan SB. Strategies to improve motor control. In: O'Sullivan SB, Schmitz J, eds. *Physical Rehabilitation, Assessment and Treatment.* 2nd ed. Philadelphia: FA Davis; 1988.

56. Borg GA. Psychophysical bases of perceived exertion. *Med Sci Sport Exerc.* 1982;14:377–381.

57. Ashwell J, Agnew-Coughlin J, Boyd S, Brooks D. Cystic fibrosis. In: Campbell S, Palisano R, Vander Linden P, eds. *Physical Therapy for Children.* Philadelphia: WB Saunders; 1994.

## *Further Reading*

Blazey S, Jenkins S, Smith R. Rate and force of application of manual chest percussion by physiotherapists. *Aust J Physiother.* 1998;44:257–264.

Chopra SK, Laplin OV, Simmons DH, et al. Effects of hydration and physical therapy on tracheal transport velocity. *Am Rev Respir Dis.* 1977;15:1009–1014.

Clarke SW, Cochrane GM, Webber B. Effects of sputum on pulmonary function. *Thorax.* 1973;28:262.

Egbert LD, Battit GE, Welch CE, Bartlett MK. Reduction of postoperative pain by encouragement and instruction of patients. *N Engl J Med.* 1964;270:825–827.

Hillegass EA, Sadowsky HS. *Essentials of Cardiopulmonary Physical Therapy.* Philadelphia: WB Saunders; 1994.

Hussey JM. Effects of chest physiotherapy for children in intensive care after surgery. *Physiotherapy.* 1992;78:109–113.

Irwin S, Techlin JS. *Cardiopulmonary Physical Therapy.* St. Louis: CV Mosby; 1995.

Kremer H. Continuing education in anesthesia and intensive care at the Limburg St. Vincenz

Hospital. Stimulating respiratory therapy—an alternative to the chemical club. Study of respiratory stimulating cutaneous administration in intensive care patients. *Krankenpfl J.* 2002;40:162–169.

La Grasse P. Still in favor of mechanical vibration. . . "Mechanical massage at the Battle CreekSanitarium." *Massage Ther J.* 2005;43:20.

Mackenzie CG, Imle PC, Ciesla N. *Chest Physiotherapy in the Intensive Care Unit.* 2nd ed. Baltimore: Williams & Wilkins; 1989.

Miller WG. Rehabilitation of patients with chronic obstructive lung disease. *Med Clin North Am.* 1967;5:349.

Oermann CM, Swank PR, Sockrider MM. Validation of an instrument measuring patient satisfaction with chest physiotherapy techniques in cystic fibrosis. *Chest.* 2000;118:92–97.

Opdekamp C. Role of physical therapy in the infant; role of assistive equipment in the physical therapy of patients with cystic fibrosis. *Rev Mal Respir.* 2003;20:S177–S188.

Nguyen HP, Le DL, Tran QM, et al. CHROMASSI: a therapy advice system based on chrono-massage and acupression using the method of ZiWuLiuZhu. *Medinfo.* 1995;8:998.

Perrotta C, Ortiz Z, Roque M. Chest physiotherapy for acute bronchiolitis in paediatric patients between 0 and 24 months old. *Cochrane Database Syst Rev.* 2005;2:CD004873. Petty TL. *Chronic Obstructive Pulmonary Disease.* New York: Marcel Dekker; 1978.

Pham QT, Peslin R, Puchelle E, et al. Respiratory function and the rheological status of bronchial secretions collected by spontaneous expectoration and after physiotherapy. *Bull Physiopathol Respir (Nancy).* 1973;9:292.

Watchie J. *Cardiopulmonary Physical Therapy—A Clinical Manual.* Philadelphia: WB Saunders; 1995.

Webber BA, Pryor JA. *Physiotherapy for Respiratory and Cardiac Problems.* Edinburgh: Churchill Livingstone; 1993.

# Chapter 13

## Sequencing Massage Techniques

This chapter builds on the clinical decision-making model for Outcome-Based Massage and earlier technique chapters by explaining how to create basic sequences of massage techniques. In doing so, it outlines principles for selecting and ordering massage techniques to achieve specific clinical outcomes. Members of different health care professions will include additional nonmassage techniques with these sequences to create interventions and plans of care that fit their scopes of practice.

## Sequencing Massage Techniques: Foundations

### STEPS IN THE SEQUENCING OF MASSAGE TECHNIQUES

A **sequence** of massage techniques is a structured, outcome-based series of massage techniques that make up an **intervention** or a part of an intervention. We use the term "sequence," instead of the term "routine," because the latter implies the use of massage techniques without the required assessment of the client's needs. Sequences of massage techniques should be highly structured, rather than routine or random. The structure of these sequences should reflect the therapists' understanding of the purpose of the techniques they are using and their clients' needs. It should also be consistent with the **principles of design** that address why therapists combine massage techniques in certain sequences; how interventions begin, proceed, and end; and how the constraints of time and location affect the treatment process. In reality, treatment approaches can vary considerably. When presented with the same situation, 10 experienced therapists will design 10 sequences of massage techniques that will have distinct differences and notable similarities.

The five steps in the design of a sequence of massage techniques are:

1. Summarize the **clinical findings** and **outcomes**
2. Select treatment techniques
3. Specify the scope and duration of the sequence of massage techniques
4. Choose a **framing general massage technique**
5. Sequence the chosen massage techniques according to principles.

We suggest that students initially work in small groups to design sequences of massage techniques and record this design process. Although this is a slow process, the critical thinking that is an integral part of the design process will become second nature with repetition. At that point, students will be able to perform much of the design of sequences of massage techniques mentally during the course of the Evaluative and Treatment Planning Phases of the clinical decision-making process.

## Summarize the Clinical Findings and Outcomes

The starting point for the design of any sequence of massage techniques is your summary of clinical findings from the client examination and a succinct statement of the desired outcomes (see Figures 3-1 and 3-2 in Chapter 3, Clinical Decision-Making for Massage). You should prioritize this list of outcomes, in consultation with the client, and then decide which **body structures** and **body functions** you can treat.

## Select Treatment Techniques

Therapists base their selection of treatment techniques on the outcomes they can achieve with each technique. For that reason, you should familiarize yourself with the outcomes for a variety of massage techniques (see Chapters 7 through 12 and Table 13-1). Clearly, not all massage techniques are useful or indicated for all medical conditions. You must also go beyond simply matching techniques to outcomes to consider broader questions related to your client and the context of treatment. These questions can include: "Has my client indicated an interest in wellness?" "What is his overall energy level and emotional state?" "Is there a problem with the function of a particular tissue or structure?" "Is there any ongoing systemic pathological process?" "Does he have pain, and if so, should I treat it directly or can I treat it by addressing the underlying **impairment**?" "Are there restrictions of positioning or draping

that would preclude the use of some massage techniques?" "What are the client's primary treatment goals?" With practice, you can begin to identify a list of potentially useful massage techniques for addressing the client's needs, as answers to these broader questions arise during the course of the Evaluative Phase. You will also identify other treatment techniques that are appropriate for the client's medical condition, impairments, and **functional limitations**. You will then refine your list of massage and other treatment techniques during the **Treatment Planning Phase** (see Chapter 3, Clinical Decision-Making for Massage).

Health care professionals who use massage as one of several treatment modalities have to determine how much emphasis to place on massage techniques in an intervention. In these situations, it may help you to identify soft tissue dysfunction that can impede your treatment of the client's other impairments. Take, for example, the case of a client who presents with a decreased ability to raise his arm, which appears to be secondary to muscle weakness. During the client examination, the therapist determines that the client has an abnormal **scapulohumeral rhythm** and soft tissue restrictions in the scapular region, in addition to muscle weakness. In this situation, both a physical therapist and a massage therapist may consider it more effective to begin by using massage techniques to reduce the soft tissue restrictions in the client's scapular region. Nevertheless, their respective scopes of practice would result in differences in how the intervention would proceed from that point. Both therapists could use some form of **joint play** technique to increase **accessory joint motion**. In this way, they would address the client's soft tissue dysfunction and decreased accessory joint motion in preparation for exercise used to increase muscular performance and joint mobility. The physical therapist may have a greater range of electrotherapeutic modalities, such as neuromuscular electrical stimulation, and physical agents available to integrate into the intervention. Furthermore, as the client improved, the physical therapist would progress her use of advanced therapeutic exercise techniques and functional training to address the client's functional limitations. Finally, both therapists would ensure that education in self-care was an ongoing component of this intervention.

## Specify the Scope and Duration of the Sequence of Massage Techniques

The scope of sequences of massage techniques usually falls into one of two categories: regional sequences or full-body

## Table 13-1 Summary of Outcomes for Massage Techniques

This chart shows the effects and outcomes for the categories of techniques discussed in the Chapters 7 to 12 on massage techniques.

| Effects/Uses | Category of Technique (Chapter) | | | | | |
|---|---|---|---|---|---|---|
| | 7 | 8 | 9 | 10 | 11 | 12 |
| Decreased capsular restriction | ? | ? | P | P | P | ? |
| Increased joint mobility | ? | P | ✓ | ✓ | P | ? |
| Increased joint integrity | ? | ? | P | P | P | ? |
| Increased muscle extensibility | ? | ? | ✓ | ✓ | P | ? |
| Pain reduction | | | | | | |
|   Counterirritant analgesia | ✓ | P | P | P | P | P |
|   Via sedation | ✓ | ✓ | ✓ | P | P | ? |
|   Via treatment of dysfunction | ? | ✓ | ✓ | ✓ | P | P |
| Increased venous return (direct) | ? | P | P | ? | ? | ? |
| Increased lymphatic return (direct) | ? | ✓ | P | ? | ? | ? |
| Decreased joint effusion | ? | ✓ | P | ? | ? | ? |
| Separation/lengthening of fascia | ? | ? | P | ✓ | P | ? |
| Promotion of dense connective tissue remodeling (in chronic stage) | ? | ? | P | P | ? | ? |
| Increased connective tissue mobility | ? | ? | P | P | ? | ? |
| Decreased muscle spasm | P | P | P | ? | ? | ? |
| Decreased resting tension of skeletal muscle | ? | P | P | P | P | ? |
| Decreased trigger point activity | ? | ? | ✓ | P | ? | ? |
| Increased postural awareness | ? | ? | P | P | P | ? |
| Normalized structural alignment | ? | ? | P | P | ? | ? |
| Normalized sensation/reduction of nerve compression | ? | ? | P | P | ? | ? |
| Enhanced muscle performance (secondary effect) | ? | ? | ✓ | ✓ | P | ? |
| Balanced agonist/antagonist function | ? | ? | ✓ | ✓ | P | P |
| Increased rib cage mobility | ? | ? | P | P | P | ? |
| Increased respiration/gaseous exchange | ? | ? | ? | ? | ? | ✓ |
| Increased airway clearance/mobilization of secretions | ? | ? | ? | ? | ✓ | ✓ |
| Decreased dyspnea | ? | ? | P | P | ✓ | ✓ |
| Increased relaxation | ✓ | ✓ | ✓ | ✓ | P | ? |
| Decreased level of cortisol | ✓ | P | ✓ | P | P | ? |
| Systemic sedation | ✓ | ✓ | ✓ | P | P | ? |
| Normalized neuromuscular tone | ✓ | ✓ | P | ? | P | ? |
| Alteration of movement responses | ✓ | ✓ | ✓ | ✓ | ✓ | P |
| Stimulated peristalsis | P | ✓ | P | P | P | ✓ |
| Stimulated immune function | P | P | ✓ | P | P | ? |
| Sensory or systemic arousal and enhanced alertness | P | P | ✓ | P | P | P |
| Promoted weight gain/development | ✓ | ? | ✓ | ? | P | ? |

✓: the outcome is supported by research summarized in this chapter. P: the outcome is possible. ?: the outcome is debatable (research results are absent or inconsistent).

sequences. When you are identifying a region for treatment, treat conventional anatomical regions, as defined by major bony and muscular landmarks, together. In practice, you can make any large adjoining area of a client's body the focus of a regional sequence. Furthermore, you will often treat the client's hands, feet, and face and head as separate regions because of the complexity of those regions. Finally, you can combine regional sequences to address larger areas of the body. Box 13-1 lists body segments that therapists often treat together in sequences of massage techniques.

Your decision on whether the scope of the sequence of massage techniques will be a region or a larger area depends on the client's medical condition, the techniques

| Box 13-1 | **Areas Commonly Treated Together As Regions** |
|---|---|

Face and head
Face, head, and neck (all surfaces)
Head and neck (all surfaces)
Posterior shoulders and neck
Arm and hand
Hand
Abdomen
Abdomen and anterior thorax
Anterior thorax
Anterior thorax, shoulders, and neck
Lateral abdomen and thorax (side-lying)
Back and posterior neck
Back
Lumbar and gluteal areas
Posterior thigh, including gluteals, leg, and foot
Posterior thigh, leg, and foot
Posterior leg and foot
Medial thigh, leg, and foot (side-lying)
Lateral thigh, leg, and foot (side-lying)
Foot

you select, and the amount of time available for the intervention. First, a localized medical condition, such as a **tendinopathy**, **fasciitis**, or **capsular restriction**, requires a regional focus. You will also have to perform a more localized treatment for inflammation when orthopedic lesions are severe (in either the acute or chronic stage). Nevertheless, as the section on agonist-antagonist balance discusses, the use of certain massage techniques, such as neuromuscular techniques, will sometimes necessitate that you broaden the scope of the regional sequence of massage techniques, regardless of the duration of the intervention. When shorter treatment times are the norm within a clinical setting, it is difficult to address the entire body within an intervention, other than by using very general massage techniques. Short, full-body sequences of 20 minutes or less do not permit much time for local treatment. Consequently, this is advisable only when you seek to achieve general outcomes related to the client's level of arousal such as **sedation** or stimulation. When the time available for treatment is short and the outcomes are general, you and the client may still prefer to focus on a region of choice such as the back. Finally, longer treatment times will often permit the integration of a local treatment into the full-body sequence that you are performing.

It is essential for you to specify and adhere to a time for your application of a given regional or full-body sequence. Some therapists object to this approach on the basis that "clock watching" conflicts with the supportive, nurturing nature of a therapeutic intervention or that it inhibits learning. In practice, the contrary is true. Respect for time boundaries reflects a respect for the client and facilitates a respect for the other boundaries that are required for an appropriate client–therapist relationship. Furthermore, the time available for treatment influences all decisions about the number, type, and ordering of the techniques used, even though it may not change the basic emphasis of the intervention. In other words, it is more difficult to design a good sequence of massage techniques without knowing how much time you have available to execute it.

There are some general guidelines for the timing of sequences of massage techniques. Regional sequences can take from 5 to 45 minutes or more to apply, and full-body sequences can require from 15 to 90 minutes or more. Shorter sequences of massage techniques need to address fewer outcomes with fewer techniques in order to be **coherent** and effective. In addition, the outcomes that you can expect to achieve with treatments of shorter duration will vary with your level of experience, the medical condition you are treating, and the massage techniques you are using. Table 13-2 provides some suggested minimum times in which experienced therapists can address discrete tasks within the context of a regional sequence of massage techniques. The amount of time that you allocate to using massage techniques, in relation to the other treatment techniques, will also be consistent with the relative impact of the soft tissue dysfunction on the client's functional level and other factors including your scope of practice and clinical setting. Furthermore, all other factors being equal, when soft tissue dysfunction has a significant impact on the client's functional level, you can justify a greater emphasis on the use of massage techniques.

## Critical Thinking Question

What are the arguments for and against using the same sequence of massage techniques at every session within a client's episode of care?

## Choose a Framing General Technique

"**General**" and "**specific**" are useful, if somewhat imprecise, concepts that summarize several of the defining compo-

| Table 13-2 | Suggested Times for Sequences of Massage Techniques That Seek to Achieve Common Outcomes | |
|---|---|---|
| **Region** | **Outcome** | **Minimum Time (minutes)[a]** |
| Back | Systemic sedation, decreased anxiety | 10–20 |
| Back | Systemic or sensory arousal, enhanced awareness | 5–15 |
| Thorax | Increased airway clearance | 15–45 |
| Thorax | Increased rib cage mobility | 10–30 |
| Limb | Increased lymphatic return | 20–60 |
| Limb | Reduced spasticity | 10–30 |
| Joint | Increased range (one joint) | 5–20 |
| Any | Counterirritant analgesia | 15–45 |
| Any | Decreased trigger point activity | 3–20 |
| Any | Decreased resting level of tone | 5–30 |
| Any | Local fascial lengthening | 3–15 |
| Any | Promotion of tendon remodeling | 2–15 |
| ALL | Deep systemic sedation | 30–60 |

[a]The first figure represents a minimum duration of treatment (less time than this would make it difficult to achieve the outcome consistently). The second figure represents a comfortable length of time; more time can often be used to good effect. These figures assume treatment by an experienced therapist.

nents for massage techniques. General massage techniques[1] engage and provide information about a large area of the body or a large group of tissues. These techniques have a large amplitude, use a broad contact surface (sometimes repeatedly over contiguous areas), and are inherently not localized to a particular area. Some examples of general massage techniques include superficial effleurage, direct fascial technique performed with a broad contact, palmar compression done in a series, and rocking. By contrast, specific massage techniques have smaller amplitudes, use small contact surfaces, and are localized to a specific region. Specific compression and cross-fiber friction are examples of specific techniques. It is a worthwhile exercise to attempt to group massage techniques according to whether they are general or specific. Box 13-2 provides a suggested organization.

### Critical Thinking Question

What other order would you suggest to show the continuum from general to specific for the techniques listed in Box 13-2? What is the relationship between the specificity of a technique and the depth at which it is applied?

Sequences of massage techniques most often consist of a mix of general and specific massage techniques,

---

**Box 13-2** | **General vs. Specific**

The following list orders selected massage techniques from relatively more general (top) to more specific (bottom):

- Rocking
- Superficial stroking
- Superficial effleurage
- Deep effleurage
- Broad-contact direct fascial technique
- Broad-contact myofascial release
- Shaking
- Wringing
- Picking-up
- Superficial lymph drainage technique
- Static contact
- Broad compression
- Squeezing
- Fingertip and thumb kneading
- Skin rolling
- Friction
- Specific compression

although you can use either type of technique by itself. It is unusual to omit a general massage technique in Western systems of massage. On the other hand, Oriental or **Eastern approaches**, such as **Shiatsu**, may consist only of specific compression.[2] Their rationale for massage is very different from that of Western systems (see the discussion of meridian theory in Chapter 9, Neuromuscular Techniques). There are advantages to selecting one general massage technique that you repeat at intervals during the course of the sequence of massage techniques. In this way, this technique becomes the principal palpation tool and serves to frame and connect the other techniques that you use. The repeated use of this general massage technique imparts a sense of structure to the sequence of massage techniques. As Fritz[3] so aptly puts it, this technique can act as the "broth" in which the other, more specific techniques "float." Furthermore, although you can select more than one general massage technique for use in a given sequence, this practice may result in the loss of **coherence** of a sequence of massage techniques. Consequently, you should choose the **framing general massage technique** with the overall outcomes of the intervention in mind. Table 13-3 lists some of the characteristics of general massage techniques that you need to consider before choosing to use them.

## Sequence the Chosen Massage Techniques According to Principles

The next step in designing an effective sequence of massage techniques is to organize the massage techniques according to clearly defined principles. The following is a formal summary of sequencing principles that we have implicitly introduced throughout the chapters on techniques (Chapters 7 to 12) in the sections entitled Manual Technique and in the Context part of the Components boxes.

### Apply General Massage Techniques before Specific Ones[4,5]

You should apply general massage techniques before specific ones for two reasons. First, this approach permits an assessment of the broader manifestations of a local problem. Second, you can use the general massage techniques to affect the client's level of arousal.

When you apply general massage techniques before performing more localized techniques, you obtain a full palpatory scan of the tissues that are mechanically connected to the specific area that may be the focus of your intervention. This allows you to identify imbalances in the tissues adjacent to a local lesion that you may have missed during the client examination. For example, a local lesion can affect antagonist and synergist muscle groups, as well as proximal and distal tissues. This often occurs in predictable patterns that relate to the type of lesion. General treatment over the entire region allows you to assess and address the broader manifestations of the local problem prior to performing a more specific local treatment.

The following example will illustrate this principle. If you are treating a chronic **tendinitis** at the common extensor origin (tennis elbow), you might use the following progression from general to specific massage techniques. You would first apply the general massage techniques to the client's arm, including regional superficial effleurage and broad neuromuscular techniques to reduce the resting

| **Table 13-3** | Characteristics of Some General Massage Techniques | | |
|---|---|---|---|
| **Technique** | **Requires Oil** | **Works Through Sheet** | **Advantages/ Disadvantages** |
| Broad-contact compression in a series | No | Yes | Takes more time but gives information about deeper tissues |
| Myofascial release | No | ±[a] | Takes minutes |
| Rocking | No | ± | Highly sedative but motion may increase pain |
| Superficial stroking | No | Yes | Produces only reflex effects |
| Superficial effleurage | Yes | No | Takes little time |

[a]±: the technique may be applied through the fabric, but this may reduce its effectiveness.

level of tone in the agonist, antagonist, and synergist muscles. You would then apply specific neuromuscular techniques, such as stripping to the agonist muscle, prior to performing cross-fiber friction on the affected tendon. Toward the end of the time you allotted for the sequence, you would reverse the order of massage techniques, from specific to general again. The entire sequence leading up to the friction may take as little as 5 minutes, yet it can still be beneficial.

General massage techniques are ideal for achieving outcomes related to level of arousal. For example, if **relaxation** or **sedation** is among the desired outcomes, then returning to the long flowing strokes of superficial effleurage or the rhythmic undulations of rocking at intervals will enhance the sedative effects you provide throughout the intervention. You can also use more specific massage techniques to address local restrictions within the same intervention. If you proceed too quickly to treating with specific massage techniques or spend too long on these, it may be more difficult for you to achieve and maintain effective relaxation in your client.

The relative amount of time that you will spend using general and specific massage techniques will vary with the outcomes you seek, the time you have available for the intervention, and the mechanical depth that specific massage techniques must achieve (see the section on the progression from superficial to deeper massage techniques in this chapter). For example, a 20-minute full-body intervention, with relaxation as the desired outcome, might consist only of general massage techniques. On the other hand, a 20-minute regional intervention for a chronic orthopedic lesion, which aims to promote remodeling of dense connective tissue, might include 15 minutes of very specific massage techniques.

## Apply Superficial Massage Techniques Before Deeper Ones[1-8]

Superficial massage techniques engage structures near the surface of the client's body, whereas deeper massage techniques engage tissue layers that lie deep to the superficial tissues. The appropriate depth of the massage technique you apply will vary with the client's medical condition. Deeper massage techniques are not necessarily better, and you do not have to engage structures mechanically far below the surface to produce profound or lasting effects.

There are several reasons to begin with the application of superficial massage techniques. Superficial massage techniques allow the client to accommodate to your touch. They also enable you to palpate with your hands in the most relaxed and sensitive position. Finally, some medical conditions can impede your ability to palpate and treat the client's underlying tissues appropriately. For example, when **edema**, which accompanies acute inflammation, and **fibrosis**, which is associated with chronic conditions, occur at the superficial level, they can limit your ability to palpate deeper structures accurately. In these situations, proceed to the first tissue layer at which you can palpate an abnormality, and then treat that layer until the tissue feels normal. At that point, you may increase your pressure to access deeper structures. A useful analogy for this approach to treatment is peeling the layers of an onion.

When the restriction is in multiple layers of muscle or connective tissue, you may not be able to determine the location of the restriction accurately at the beginning of the intervention. Nevertheless, the basic procedure remains the same: proceed gradually through superficial layers to the first palpable restriction, normalize this restriction, and then treat progressively deeper layers of tissue restriction. Regardless of the massage techniques you use, gradually reduce the pressure and briefly re-engage each layer that you previously addressed as you approach the end of the regional sequence. This allows you to reassess any additional effects that your use of deeper massage techniques may have had on the superficial tissues.

Here are some examples of this progression from superficial to deeper massage techniques. If traumatic edema is present, do not attempt to engage structures underlying the local edema with massage techniques until the edema has resolved. Usually within a day of initiating treatment, you can perform superficial reflex techniques on the site of trauma and then superficial fluid techniques to the proximal margin of swelling, as tolerated by the client. After this, return to superficial reflex techniques. During later interventions, use the same basic pattern of treating from superficial to deep to superficial on the site of the lesion as the edema resolves. With each intervention, you should reach progressively deeper tissue layers.

If the client's subcutaneous tissues are normal but a restriction exists in a superficial layer of muscle, you may progress the depth of the massage techniques within a minute or two to include **neuromuscular techniques** that engage this layer. If the difficulty lies in a deeper muscular layer, begin as noted in the previous example, and then engage progressively deeper layers of muscle before you finally engage the layer in which the restriction lies.

You can use **superficial reflex techniques**, such as static contact, superficial stroking, and fine vibration, at any time in an intervention and for virtually any length of time. Therapists often use these techniques at the beginning and end of full-body or regional sequences. You may omit the use of superficial reflex techniques entirely if muscle or connective tissue is the focus of your intervention.

## Coordinate and Repeat the Transitions from General to Specific to General and from Superficial to Deep to Superficial

In practice, you execute the transitions from general to specific to general and from superficial to deep to superficial simultaneously. In other words, begin sequences of massage techniques with general techniques that engage superficial tissues over large areas, and then progress to specific techniques that engage deeper tissues in a succession of smaller areas. You will return to the use of more general and superficial techniques between your treatment of the smaller areas. When time permits, make these transitions in depth and specificity several times during a regional sequence of massage techniques. This strategy permits you to assess the tissue responses continually, and at different depths, throughout the region you are treating. Using these guidelines can reduce the occurrence of agonist-antagonist imbalances that can result from your application of the deep, specific massage techniques needed to treat chronic restrictions in muscle and connective tissue (see later in this chapter).

## Use Principles Related to Enhancing Fluid Return

The following principles are relevant when you specifically seek to enhance lymphatic or venous return. Although these principles are common in classical sequences that emphasize effleurage and petrissage, you can disregard them if you are not attempting to enhance fluid return.

### Use Centripetal Pressure and the Assistance of Gravity When Possible

The use of **centripetal** pressure, with minimal pressure on the return stroke, ensures that the mechanical flow of fluid receives maximal assistance in the direction of its normal return.[3-7,9,10]

### Begin Proximally, Proceed Distally, Return Proximally, and Repeat[2-5,7,9,10]

When the aim of treatment is to increase **lymphatic return** from a region, begin the massage stroke as proximally (close to the heart) as time allows and progressively move in a distal direction until you approach the region. Ensure that the direction of pressure of each stroke is always cen-

tripetal. For the limbs, this requires that you begin at least as proximally as the axillary or inguinal lymph nodes. Repeat this sequence of applying massage techniques from proximal to distal as frequently as the time available for the intervention allows. This approach of beginning treatment proximally creates a proximal reservoir into which you will direct the fluid that is located in the distal region.[10] If the client's lymphatics in a proximal region are not intact, designate an adjacent proximal body segment as the reservoir to which you will direct the fluid from the distal region. For example, this region may be the contralateral side of the client's trunk or ipsilateral side of her chest.

### Maximize the Relaxation of the Proximal Muscle Groups

Mennell[11] noted that deep veins and lymphatics are embedded in skeletal muscle. Consequently, excessive muscular tone can compress the lumen of the deep veins and lymphatics and reduce venous and lymphatic flow. This explains why you reduce the external pressure on the collapsible vessels and passively assist venous and lymphatic return when you ensure that there is maximum pliability of all of the muscles between the heart and the body segment you are draining. If time allows, use neuromuscular and connective tissue techniques to increase the general mobility and muscular relaxation of the muscles of the thorax. In some cases, such as with hand edema secondary to **thoracic outlet syndrome**, addressing mobility and muscular relaxation in the thorax may be your first priority. In practice, you may want to shift your focus quickly to the client's affected limb because of time constraints. Make this decision carefully because addressing proximal regions may be more effective.

The sequencing of massage techniques is often more flexible when you are applying superficial reflex, connective tissue, specific neuromuscular, and passive movement techniques. Note that when circulatory concerns are not the focus of treatment, you may use centrifugal pressure (with the exception of deep centrifugal pressure over incompetent veins or, as some authors suggest, all veins[1,2]), and you may treat distal areas first.

## Coordinate All Transitions

Therapists frequently encounter situations in which the tissues in adjacent body segments, which they wish to engage, lie at different depths. For example, with posttraumatic swelling of the wrist, the application of massage techniques on the immediate site of the injury is contraindicated, minimal, or light, depending on the nature and degree of the injury. In this case, begin a regional sequence of massage techniques for the superficial tissue layers on the proximal portion of the client's arm to enhance superficial lymphatic return. Then gradually move your hands in a distal direction toward the proximal edge of the swelling. Progress to using deeper massage techniques for the deeper tissue layers of the upper arm to relax the client's muscles and enhance the deep lymphatic return from his proximal arm. Then alternate between the proximal application of deeper massage techniques and the distal application of superficial massage techniques, moderating the depth of stroke as you move from one body segment to the other. To complete the intervention, apply superficial massage techniques over the entire portion of the client's limb that you are treating.

### Apply Massage Techniques from the Periphery to the Center of the Region You Are Treating[5]

When a circumscribed area of local pathology is the focus of your intervention, begin with a general sequence of massage techniques to the region. Then gradually apply massage techniques closer to the periphery of the local area of pathology. This strategy permits you to palpate related tissue changes that may occur in areas that are remote from the local region you are treating. Furthermore, it enables you to gradually introduce massage techniques to an area that may show tenderness and other altered responses to touch.

Use the same principle of applying massage techniques from the periphery to the center of the region when you are treating an area of local swelling. In this case, apply massage techniques in a **centrifugal** direction at the periphery of the area of swelling and gradually move toward the center of the area of swelling as the peripheral fluid is absorbed.

### Critical Thinking Question

How would you use the principles for designing sequences of massage techniques to create a sequence to reduce local pain and swelling for a client with an acute-stage ankle sprain?

### Address Agonist, Antagonist, and Synergist Groups

You must be careful to avoid producing an imbalance in the client's myofascial system when you use neuromuscular or connective tissue techniques. This is particularly important if you are applying these massage techniques in small areas,

with a higher force, or for long periods. For example, Simons, Travell, and Simons[12] have noted that releasing trigger points can produce a **reactive tightening**, or cramping, in related muscles and may activate other trigger points. Therapists who use connective tissue techniques also routinely note positional shifts in related body segments in response to the local application of massage techniques.

When you apply deep specific massage techniques locally, without including general massage techniques, clients will commonly experience undesirable responses to the treatment within half an hour to 3 days after the intervention. These responses can include reactive tightening and pain in (a) areas that are immediately proximal or distal to the site that you treated, (b) in antagonist or synergist muscle groups that are located on the same side of an adjacent joint, or (c) in antagonist or synergist muscle groups that lie across a joint. Reactive pain and restrictions can be detrimental to the client's medical condition. In addition, it may worsen until the imbalance caused by treatment resolves or you treat it. To avoid this situation, you must also address the related areas where reactive tightening may occur whenever you include the application of local, deep, specific massage techniques within an intervention. The less experienced therapist can apply general neuromuscular techniques, such as broad-contact compression or petrissage, for this purpose. A very experienced therapist may use a postural assessment to identify relatively shortened areas that require lengthening in order to maintain adequate myofascial balance. Regardless of your level of expertise, you should alert the client to the possibility of these effects of treatment and ensure that the client understands that it is important to let you know if a troublesome shift in pain or symptoms occurs after the intervention. You may also teach the client appropriate stretching exercises to minimize reactive tightening.

In general, the intensity and duration of the application of massage techniques to balance antagonist and synergist muscle groups will vary in direct proportion to the specificity, depth, and duration of the sequence of massage techniques that you perform on the main area of treatment. This part of the intervention might require from 10% to 50% of your designated treatment time. Your ability to identify which antagonist and synergist muscle groups are the most prone to reactive tightening and to judge how long to spend on addressing this issue will improve with experience and, one hopes, with a minimum of client distress.

### Treatment of the Contralateral Side

You may have to treat the client's contralateral side or limb within an intervention that addresses a unilateral lesion. For example, when treating a client with a unilateral **piriformis syndrome**, you may justifiably include petrissage, stripping, and specific compression as the primary massage techniques to lengthen the client's affected piriformis. Nevertheless, you must also treat the client's unaffected gluteals and lateral rotators in order to achieve a balanced bilateral distribution of tension throughout the pelvic musculature. Therapists vary as to whether they apply massage techniques to the contralateral limb before or after their treatment of the client's affected limb. It may be easier for you to judge the depth and intensity of the treatment that is required to achieve balance with the client's contralateral limb after you have treated the affected limb. When you are treating an acute-stage unilateral orthopedic lesion, you may also treat the client's contralateral side as a means of addressing compensations that may arise from altered patterns of muscular use.

### Treatment of the Related Axial Skeleton

If you apply deep specific neuromuscular or connective tissue techniques on one of a client's limbs (even the distal limb), you should also treat the related portion of the axial skeleton with general techniques, even if only briefly. For the lower limbs, apply general petrissage to the lumbar musculature bilaterally, and for the upper limbs, apply general petrissage to the cervical musculature bilaterally. For example, when you treat a client with **DeQuervain's tenosynovitis**, apply superficial effleurage to the client's entire arm, broad-contact petrissage to his upper arm and then to his lower arm, additional specific neuromuscular techniques to his lower arm, friction to the tendons in the region of the anatomical snuff box, and broad-contact petrissage and superficial effleurage to his entire arm. Furthermore, either precede or follow this sequence of massage techniques with the brief application of broad-contact or general petrissage to the client's contralateral arm and cervical musculature (about 25% of the treatment time).

### Critical Thinking Question

Why is it necessary to treat other areas of the client's body when you are treating a local restriction of muscle and connective tissue?

### Sequence Massage Techniques with Other Appropriate Treatment Techniques

You will often use massage techniques in conjunction with other treatment techniques that are relevant to the client's medical condition. This section contains some examples that illustrate how to sequence massage techniques with physical agents and therapeutic exercise.

Do not alter the sequence of the massage techniques when you are coordinating the application of heat and cold with massage techniques. Instead, apply the selected physical agent either before or after the sequence of massage techniques. Do not routinely apply cryotherapy, such as ice or cold packs, before applying massage techniques that use any amount of force. This application can result in a decrease in the client's sensation in the region that you are treating. This decrease in sensation diminishes the client's ability to provide accurate feedback about the tenderness or pain arising from the involved tissues during the sequence of massage techniques. You can use cryotherapy after these massage techniques to reduce the client's symptoms or the consequences of overtreatment. For example, if you believe that you have overtreated a client with friction (which should happen rarely), then it would be appropriate for you to ice the treatment area after the friction. You may also apply cold packs to another body segment concurrently with the sequence of massage techniques. This would be the case if you were treating an acute orthopedic injury, such as a sprained ankle, and used cold packs on the site of the lesion (as it was elevated) while you applied massage techniques proximally to reduce edema.

If you are treating healthy tissues or chronic lesions, you can apply heat either before or after local sequences of massage techniques. When you are treating muscle, apply heat before sequences of massage techniques to relax the muscle, decrease tissue viscosity, and allow easier access to deep tissue layers.[13] If, however, you are using massage techniques to lengthen or stretch dense connective tissue with greater force, then it is not appropriate to apply heat *immediately* before the sequence of massage techniques because this heating may increase the risk of uncontrolled collagenous rupture.[14]

You often perform sequences of massage techniques before you use therapeutic exercise. In this case, the massage techniques prepare the client's tissue for active or resisted exercise by increasing tissue extensibility, improving the balance of agonist/antagonist function, and enhancing the client's level of alertness. You can also use sequences of massage techniques prior to the application of passive exercise, such as stretching or passive range of motion exercises, to enhance the effects of those techniques. A skillful therapist can alternate between massage techniques and passive exercise so that they blend seamlessly throughout the intervention. Finally, in cases in which the client has abnormal neuromuscular tone, you can use massage techniques as proprioceptive stimulation to normalize neuromuscular tone and the client's movement responses in preparation for therapeutic exercise or functional activity.[15]

### Critical Thinking Question

What modalities other than massage are within your scope of practice? What are some of the ways in which you can combine massage techniques with these modalities?

## DESIGN OF REGIONAL SEQUENCES OF MASSAGE TECHNIQUES

Box 13-3 summarizes the steps involved in designing a sequence of massage techniques for a region. Using this approach, you can generate a wide variety of sequences of massage techniques that address different outcomes.

Theory in Practice 13-1 to 13-9 include some simple examples with questions and instructions to guide students and novice therapists in the art of designing sequences of massage techniques. These examples are by no means the only possible sequences; they simply illustrate how you can apply the guidelines discussed in this chapter. Students and novices should not hurry this portion of their training, since the exploration of a variety of different sequences of massage techniques will encourage a flexible, adaptable approach to treatment. Even the design of seemingly simple regional sequences involves considerable reflection and planning on the part of the therapist. Therapists who practice in settings where intervention time is short (10 to 20 minutes) especially need to master the principles of massage design because there is often no extra time in which to address oversights in their planning.

---

**Box 13-3** | **Steps in the Design of Regional Sequences of Massage Techniques**

1. Summarize findings from the client examination.
2. Identify appropriate functional outcomes.
3. Summarize and prioritize outcomes.
4. Choose relevant massage techniques to address the impairments.
5. Assign time for the regional sequence.
6. Choose the framing technique(s).
7. Sequence the massage techniques, keeping in mind:
   - Position of superficial reflex work, if included
   - General to specific to general
   - Superficial to deep to superficial
   - Proximal to distal, if you are working to enhance fluid return
   - Periphery to center, if you are working with circumscribed local pathology
   - Agonist/antagonist/synergist balance, if you are including neuromuscular or connective tissue techniques to release local restriction

Do other regions have to be included? If so, design these sequences and revise the time budget for the intervention.

---

**Theory in Practice 13-1**

### A Short Regional Sequence for the Back[2,6]

Purpose: Preparation of the client's tissues for lumbar joint mobilization techniques and stabilization exercises; does not require removal of the client's clothing

Outcomes: Decreased level of resting tension throughout the muscles of the back, increased muscle extensibility

Time: 10 minutes

Framing General Technique: Broad-contact compression

Techniques and Order of Application:

1. Beginning prone, apply broad-contact compression with your palms systematically. Work bilaterally from the client's upper back to his gluteals.
2. Sustain each compression for 30 seconds or until you feel the tissues begin to soften.
3. Encourage the client to breathe deeply.
4. Apply compression with your forearms to the client's lumbar area, one side at a time, avoiding direct pressure on his spinous processes.
5. Apply compression with your doubled fists to the gluteus medius, one side at a time.
6. Apply specific compression with your doubled thumbs. Focus on the tightest parts of the lumbar erector spinae and gluteus medius. Sustain this as time permits.
7. Finish with a line of palmar compressions down the client's back to the gluteals.

## Theory in Practice 13-2

### A Short Regional Sequence for the Leg[2,6,10]

Purpose: Preparation of a postsurgical (total knee replacement, ligament repair) client's tissues for joint mobilization techniques, deep stretching of knee musculature, and range of motion exercises; does not require removal of the client's clothing

Outcomes: Increased venous return, decreased edema, increased muscle extensibility, decreased level of muscle resting tension, reduction of pain

Time: 10 minutes

Framing General Technique: Broad-contact compression

Techniques and Order of Application:
1. Position the client supine, with her affected thigh elevated at least to 30 degrees and the knee in a loose-packed position.
2. Encourage diaphragmatic breathing.
3. Apply several palmar compressions to the client's upper thorax, synchronized with the client's exhalation.
4. Beginning at the inguinal area, apply broad-contact compression with moderate pressure to the client's tolerance, following a sequence similar to that illustrated in Figure 9-8.
5. Reduce pressure near the client's knee. Do not apply the technique over edema or if the client reports an increase in pain.
6. Repeat the sequence as time allows. Change your emphasis from the central thigh to the lateral thigh and especially to the medial thigh.
7. If the swelling is only on the anterior surface of the client's knee and not behind the knee, then you may continue with gentle muscle squeezing applied to the calf from proximal to distal in a continuation of the same pattern of proximal to distal to proximal.
8. Finish with superficial stroking down the client's entire leg.

## Theory in Practice 13-3

### A Short Regional Sequence for the Neck[2,6]

Purpose: Complementary to joint mobilization techniques, stabilization and postural awareness exercises for a client with a cervical pain and decreased range of motion; does not require removal of the client's clothing

Outcomes: Hyperstimulation analgesia, reduction of trigger point activity, decreased resting tension of skeletal muscle

Time: 10 minutes

Framing General Technique: Superficial effleurage

Techniques and Order of Application:
1. With the client in supine, loosen the client's collar or bare the neck area as much as possible.
2. Using a small amount of nonstaining lotion, perform superficial effleurage bilaterally and then unilaterally on the posterior and lateral surfaces of the client's neck. Increase the depth with each repetition of the stroke in order to engage the client's muscles.
3. Apply several strokes of broad-contact direct fascial technique to the lateral and posterior surfaces of the neck.
4. Use picking-up on the sternocleidomastoid muscles, one side at a time.
5. With your fingertips and thumbs, knead the anterior and posterior muscles of the neck with the client's cervical spine in neutral and rotated positions.
6. Use stripping or ischemic compression to treat trigger points, as time permits, and follow with the appropriate stretches.
7. Finish with superficial effleurage, gentle traction of the cervical spine, and holding of the occiput.

## Theory in Practice 13-4

### A Short Regional Sequence for the Arm

Purpose: Complementary to joint mobilization techniques, electrotherapeutic modalities, and therapeutic exercise for clients with lateral or medial epicondylitis; does not require removal of the client's clothing

Outcomes: Hyperstimulation analgesia, increased connective tissue mobility, decreased resting tension of skeletal muscle, enhanced collagen fiber remodeling

Time: 10 minutes

Framing General Technique: Myofascial release

Techniques and Order of Application:
1. With the client in supine, begin with a myofascial release arm pull.
2. Apply more specific myofascial releases to the anterior deltoid, biceps, and entire extensor group of the forearm.
3. Apply broad-contact compression and muscle squeezing to all muscles of the arm and forearm, with as much pressure as the client can tolerate.
4. Using a small amount of lotion, apply stripping to the client's wrist extensors. If time allows, apply stripping to the wrist flexors as well.

5. Apply 1 to 2 minutes of friction to the most tender point of the tendon.
6. Apply muscle squeezing and broad-contact compression to both arms.
7. Finish with a bilateral arm pull, followed by cervical traction.

---

## Theory in Practice 13-5

ON-LINE VIDEO

### A Regional Sequence for the Abdomen[2,6,16]

Caution: When practicing this sequence, keep in mind that deep abdominal pressure is not advisable immediately preceding or during menstruation because of sensitivity and because local congestion limits the practitioner's ability to palpate. Even light abdominal massage during menstruation may alter the flow and duration of the menses. See detailed discussion of contraindications and cautions in Chapter 3, Clinical Decision Making for Massage.

Outcomes: Stimulated peristalsis, relaxation, decreased resting tension throughout the abdominal musculature

Time: 20–30 minutes

Framing General Technique: Superficial effleurage

Techniques and Order of Application:
1. Static contact applied to navel and occiput
2. Superficial stroking of the abdomen in clockwise circles
3. Effleurage progressing from superficial to deep in clockwise circles
4. Wringing, picking-up, and palmar kneading applied to the entire abdomen
5. Specific kneading and stripping to abdominal muscle (moderate pressure can be used as long as there is a high horizontal component—high shear—to localize the force to the skeletal muscle)
6. Draw knees up to a crook-lying position to slacken abdominal wall
7. Deep specific compression applied in **retrograde** sequence from the sigmoid colon to the iliocecal valve
8. Palmar kneading
9. Wringing
10. Large-amplitude sedative shaking
11. Rocking
12. Static contact at navel and occiput

Make the pace slow and the movements rhythmic. Apply each massage technique for 1 to 2 minutes. After you introduce superficial effleurage, return to it for a few strokes before you add each new massage technique. Switch sides

as required. The application and release of deep specific digital compression must be very slow, and the practitioner must pay close attention to the patient's comfort level. The literature suggests that abdominal massage may have a reflex or mechanical effect on peristalsis.[17–26] Practitioners who use massage techniques extensively have a common perception that abdominal massage will promote colonic emptying. Nevertheless, the opinions about the mechanisms by which this might occur vary, since the nervous control of peristalsis itself is complicated. The following techniques may promote peristalsis:

1. Superficial reflex techniques applied over the abdominal wall
2. Nonspecific neuromuscular techniques that decrease the tone of the skeletal muscle of the abdominal wall and affect intestinal flow via somatovisceral reflexes
3. Deep massage techniques that mechanically stretch the viscera, causing reflex contractions of the smooth muscle of the intestine.
4. Deep specific massage techniques that mechanically assist movement in the direction of the colonic flow (Mennell[11] doubted that this was possible)

With respect to these four possible mechanisms, the prevalent practice is to perform light massage techniques, such as superficial stroking, in the direction of colonic flow. Neuromuscular techniques and connective tissue techniques, such as wringing, can be oriented according to the direction of the muscle fibers you are treating or in any way that causes an effective stretch of the tissues of the abdomen, as long as strokes do not directly oppose the flow in the colon. Finally, perform deep massage techniques that specifically seek to move intestinal contents over the colon with pressure in the direction of peristaltic flow in a retrograde sequence from the sigmoid colon to the iliocecal valve.[1,2,6] The last mechanism presupposes that the skeletal muscle that forms the abdominal wall has been sufficiently relaxed to allow the pressure of the technique to physically engage the viscera. It is important to remember that promoting a generalized **parasympathetic response** is a nonspecific way of facilitating peristalsis. You can do this when you are working on any region.

Further Exercises:
1. Design and practice a 20-minute abdominal sequence with the same aims that you perform through a sheet.
2. Design and practice a similar abdominal sequence that you perform from one or both sides with the patient in side-lying.
3. How might you have accomplished some of the treatment with the patient prone? Consider, for example, what lumbar wringing might achieve.

## Theory in Practice 13-6

### A Regional Sequence for the Leg[2,6,10]

Outcomes: Increased **lymphatic return** from a leg with an intact lymphatic system, relaxation

Restrictions: Administer directly on skin using talc, cornstarch, or chalk as lubricant

Time: 20–30 minutes

Framing General Techniques: Superficial and deep effleurage

Massage Techniques and Order of Application:
1. Position the patient supine with legs elevated 30 to 45 degrees.
2. Instruct patient in deep diaphragmatic breathing.
3. Apply rhythmic palmar compression over the upper ribs for 2 to 3 minutes.
4. Apply superficial effleurage to entire affected leg.
5. Apply superficial lymphatic technique beginning at proximal thigh and then beginning progressively more distal with each new series of strokes, until you reach the foot (repeat ad lib).
6. Apply deep effleurage.
7. Use a series of centripetally moving palmar compressions applied in a pattern similar to that used in the lymphatic technique in Step 5 (i.e., beginning proximally and starting progressively more distal with each new series until the foot is reached) (repeat ad lib).
8. Use passive relaxed movements for all joints, beginning at the hip and proceeding to the ankle.
9. Apply superficial effleurage.

Although this sequence uses few massage techniques, you must repeat them. Frequent repetition is required when moving fluid. In addition, a repetitive rhythm will assist you in achieving sedation. Note that there are two general massage techniques used here: superficial effleurage is interspersed with the superficial lymphatic technique, whereas deep effleurage is interspersed with the compressions. You could use this sequence to drain a localized traumatic edema anywhere in the leg such as an ankle **sprain**, quadriceps **contusion**, or hamstring **strain**. There are several modifications required for doing so: avoid areas of acute tissue damage, reduce the pressure around these areas, avoid pushing fluid through areas of congestion, and perform passive movements only where they do not recreate the patient's pain.

Further Exercises:
1. How would you address the same impairments with massage techniques that use oil as a lubricant? How would you do this without using lubricant?
2. Design and practice a similar sequence that seeks to drain a designated area on the thorax toward the ipsilateral axilla.
3. How would the sequence change if the application of mechanical techniques was a contraindication in the area of the patient's ankle?
4. How would the sequence change to address swelling in the posterior calf (for example, an acute calf contusion or Achilles tendon rupture)?
5. Should you alter the sequence to include other proximal segments or the contralateral leg?

## Theory in Practice 13-7

### A Regional Sequence for the Neck, Head, and Face[2,6]

Outcomes: **Hyperstimulation analgesia**, reduction of trigger point activity, decreased resting tension of skeletal muscle, increased range of motion, relaxation

Restrictions: No lubricant

Time: 20–30 minutes

Framing General Technique: Palmar compression

Massage Techniques and Order of Application: In Supine
1. Palmar superficial stroking
2. Palmar compression done as a series from the top of the neck to the clavicle, unilaterally, then palmar compression to head (repeat with the head rotated to the other side)
3. Muscle squeezing to neck
4. Specific compression on either side of spine and to suboccipital muscles, followed by appropriate stretch
5. Specific compression to sites of upper trapezius and sternocleidomastoid trigger points (use pincer compression for sternocleidomastoid), followed by appropriate stretches
6. Gentle fingertip kneading to face and more vigorous fingertip kneading to scalp
7. Fingertip fascial technique with short strokes to scalp
8. Gentle palmar compression from top of neck toward axilla in several series
9. Superficial stroking throughout with palms and then fingertips

Spend from 2 to 4 minutes on each item. Turn the patient's head frequently, and if necessary, ensure that you support the patient's neck with a small pillow for comfort. Return to the application of palmar compression done as a series from the top of the neck to the axilla between each new massage technique. This sequence with slight changes would be valuable in many cases of muscular tension or trigger point headache

## Theory in Practice 13-8

ON-LINE VIDEO

### A Regional Sequence for the Back[2,6]

Outcomes: Decreased level of resting tension throughout the muscles of the back, increased muscle extensibility, increased mobility of spinal joints and rib cage, reduction of pain, relaxation
> Time: 20–40 minutes
> Framing General Techniques: Superficial and deep effleurage

Techniques and Order of Application:
1. Static contact applied to sacrum and occiput
2. Superficial palmar stroking down spine
3. Effleurage progressing from superficial to deep
4. Wringing, picking-up, palmar kneading applied to the whole back
5. Deep effleurage with forearm; finger and thumb kneading to erector spinae muscles
6. Stripping along erector spinae muscles with elbow
7. Bilateral specific compression along erector spinae muscles—10 locations at 20 seconds per location
8. Palmar kneading
9. Wringing
10. Superficial palmar stroking, becoming progressively slower
11. Static contact at sacrum and occiput

Make the pace slow and your movements rhythmic. Apply each massage technique for 1 to 2 minutes. After you introduce superficial effleurage, return to it for a few strokes before you add each new technique. Switch sides every few minutes. It may exacerbate muscular imbalances if you perform all massage techniques on one side of the client's back before switching. Simply break contact, move around the table, and recommence. Practitioners might use this type of sequence for patients with back pain or tightness associated with prolonged bed rest and in the chronic stage of erector spinae strain or lumbar facet derangement.

Further Exercises:
1. Why might you have to address the extensors of the hip after you perform this sequence? How would you alter the sequence to include these?
2. For similar aims and techniques, how would you adapt this routine for other regions? Practice several of these in a similar time interval.
3. For similar outcomes, how would the selected massage techniques differ for a clothed patient? Design and practice a regional back sequence with this restriction in mind.
4. How would you alter this sequence if there were only 15 minutes available for the intervention? If there were only 10 minutes?

## Theory in Practice 13-9

### A Regional Sequence for the Shoulders

Outcomes: Decreased **resting tension** of skeletal muscle, separation and lengthening of superficial fascial layers, enhanced **muscle performance** (secondary), increased joint mobility
> Restrictions: Use minimal lubricant
> Time: 30+ minutes (to do both shoulders)
> Framing General Technique: Rhythmic mobilization

Massage Techniques and Order of Application:
1. Rhythmic mobilization
2. General, broad-contact neuromuscular technique (compression and squeezing)
3. Myofascial release arm pull through glenohumeral range from neutral to full abduction
4. General direct fascial tissue technique applied with a broad contact and combined with slow active arm and shoulder movements
5. Stripping to rotator cuff muscles, followed by related stretches
6. Rhythmic mobilization

Additional: Split the sequence into the application of techniques with the patient in supine and then prone, or perform the entire sequence with the patient in side-lying (both sides). Apply all massage techniques from midthorax to occiput and distal to the elbow. Include all muscles that produce motion at the glenohumeral joint and the scapulothoracic articulation. Use minimal lubricant; otherwise, there will not be enough drag for the connective tissue work. Return to rhythmic mobilization frequently and ensure that it is not too stimulating. Both shoulders should receive equal time, although in different areas. Usually, the patient's dominant shoulder is tighter anteriorly, and his nondominant shoulder is tighter posteriorly. Get the patient off the table after you complete one side and compare the range and ease of movement between the two shoulders. Once you have completed both shoulders, spend at least 5 minutes to address the neck with conventional stretching, myofascial release, and traction. This would make an acceptable intervention for a **capsular restriction**. If the patient presented with **adhesive capsulitis**, you might add after the stripping: trigger point work (especially to subscapularis[12]), friction to relevant tendons,[27] and joint mobilization.

# DESIGN OF MORE EXTENSIVE SEQUENCES OF MASSAGE TECHNIQUES

The most common example of a more extensive sequence of massage techniques is the "full-body massage" sequence. In its simplest form, a full-body sequence of massage techniques is simply a series of regional sequences performed in a chosen order and covering the entire body. These regional sequences are designed using the guidelines outlined earlier in this chapter, employ similar techniques, and are similar in character. Box 13-4 expands on the steps required for the design of regional sequences so that you can apply these regional sequences to more extensive sequences. The sequences in Theory in Practice 13-10 to 13-13 address the same general outcomes in all regions, with about an equal allocation of time between regions.

If there is a specific condition in one region that requires a different technical approach, then that sequence will differ from the others, and you will need to allocate more time to that sequence. Specifying an order and time

---

| Box 13-4 | **Steps in the Design of More Extensive Sequences of Massage Techniques** |
|---|---|

1. Summarize findings from the client examination.
2. Identify appropriate functional outcomes.
3. Summarize and prioritize outcomes.
4. Choose relevant massage techniques to address the impairments.
5. Assign time for the entire intervention.
6. Choose regions that you will include or exclude.
7. Specify initial times and order for regions.
8. Choose the framing technique(s).
9. Sequence the massage techniques for regional sequences, keeping in mind:
   - Placement of superficial reflex work, if included
   - General to specific to general
   - Superficial to deep to superficial
   - Proximal to distal, if you are working to enhance fluid return
   - Periphery to center, if you are working with circumscribed local pathology
   - Agonist/antagonist/synergist balance, if you are including neuromuscular or connective tissue techniques to release local restriction

If you are including a regional sequence(s) to address a particular condition, do you need to adjust the initial time budget?

---

## A Full-Body Sequence for Stress When You Cannot Remove Clothing

Outcomes: Relaxation, decreased perceived anxiety (and **cortisol** levels), improved immune function, decreased resting tension of skeletal muscle

Restrictions: Patient is clothed

Time: 20, 40, or 60 minutes for all regions

Framing General Techniques: Rocking, broad-contact compression

Beginning prone, apply the following massage techniques in this order in each region:

1. Static contact
2. Rocking
3. Broad-contact compression all over the region (you may synchronize its application on the thorax with the patient's exhalations)
4. Alternate between broad-contact compression and specific compression in areas where muscular tension is higher
5. Intersperse compressions with rocking ad lib
6. Finish each region by returning to rocking and static contact

The more you use compression (especially if it is specific), the greater the decreases in the client's muscle resting tension you will achieve. *It is both possible and useful to learn how to cover all regions in as short an interval as 20 minutes,* although the amount of specific compression that you can include will be very limited. In doing so, ensure that the general character of the sequence remains the same, regardless of the time in which you perform it. Do not increase the speed with which you apply the individual techniques when you have less time for the intervention. Instead, use fewer repetitions and more general techniques. This sequence would be suitable for reducing the effects of stress. You might also incorporate it into longer interventions when anxiety and stress exacerbate primary symptoms in medical conditions such as asthma (between attacks), fibromyalgia, or chronic whiplash injuries.

Further Exercises:

1. Where would you incorporate superficial stroking and muscle squeezing into this sequence?
2. Design and perform a sequence that accomplishes the same aims using lubricant.
3. Design and perform a version of this exercise with the patient in side-lying position (i.e., left side-lying and then right side-lying).

## A Full-Body Sequence to Increase Range of Motion

Outcomes: Generalized increased joint mobility, relaxation
   Restrictions: No lubricant
   Time: 30, 45, or 60 minutes for all regions
   Order of Regions: Various orders are possible; finish with at least 15 minutes on the back, neck, and pelvis
   Framing General Technique: All of the techniques used are general, and you could choose any of them to frame the sequence

Massage Techniques and Order of Application in Each Region:
1. Perform one or two strokes of direct fascial technique with a broad contact.
2. Perform one myofascial stretch with wide hand placement.
3. Stretch associated joints (stretch hands and feet as a unit).

You could use this sequence for a healthy individual who complains of generalized stiffness a day after vigorous physical activity. Sixty minutes would allow you to treat 15 to 20 localized areas that you should distribute evenly throughout the body, unless there is an obvious deficit in range of motion in one joint. Because the chosen massage techniques require time for a viscoelastic response to occur in the patient's tissues, your tempo must be slow, and the pressure should be moderate. The depth of release and the resulting increase of range of motion in any one area will be very small in comparison to what you would achieve if you concentrated the procedure on one or two regions of the body for the entire treatment time. We initially advise students not to concentrate connective tissue technique around one joint because compensations can arise quickly.

Further Exercise:
1. Perform a version of this exercise with the patient in side-lying. Try to foresee and deal with difficulties regarding positioning before you start.

ON-LINE VIDEO

## A Stimulating Full-Body Sequence

Outcomes: Systemic **arousal**, enhanced awareness, marginal decrease in muscle resting tension, increased perceived relaxation
   Restrictions: No lubricant
   Time: 20 or 40 minutes for all regions
   Order of Regions: Supine and prone, head to feet
   Framing General Technique: Coarse running vibration

Massage Techniques and Order of Application in Each Region:
1. Coarse running vibration
2. Shaking
3. Fast rhythmic palmar compression and muscle squeezing (1–2 techniques/second)
4. Light hacking
5. Superficial fingertip stroking (limit the time spent on this last massage technique, or the effect may be too stimulating for the patient)

This sequence has a character similar to that of some precompetition sports sequences of massage techniques, and you might use it to alleviate lethargy and fatigue temporarily. Because of the brisk tempo and relatively short time, the neuromuscular techniques (Step 3) cannot penetrate much below the superficial layers of muscle.

Further Exercises:
1. Outline, and provide a rationale for, a selection of massage techniques and tempo for a precompetition sports situation.
2. For the same outcomes and duration of treatment, how would you alter the sequence if you were to use a lubricant?
3. How short can you make the duration and still have the massage feel **coherent** to the patient?

## A Gentle Full-Body Sequence to Relieve Pain and Maintain Joint Range

Outcomes: Maintain joint mobility and integrity, prevention of capsuloligamentous restrictions, increased lymphatic return, analgesia, relaxation, sensory arousal
   Restrictions: None
   Time: 30–40 minutes for all regions (full body)
   Order of Regions: Supine then prone, head/thorax toward limbs (i.e., proximal to distal)
   Framing General Technique: Superficial effleurage

Massage Techniques and Order of Application in Each Region:
1. At the outset of the intervention, encourage full breathing using both diaphragmatic and costal segments
2. Superficial effleurage progressing deeper to engage superficial muscle layers
3. Gentle wringing and nonspecific kneading

4. Gentle rhythmic mobilization and rocking
5. Passive relaxed movements (no overpressure)
6. Return frequently to, and end with, superficial effleurage

This sequence is similar to the sequence that is traditionally recommended for treating rheumatoid arthritis in the non-inflammatory phase.[27] In particular, this sequence is relatively short in order to prevent fatiguing the patient. As in Theory in Practice 13-7, the depth of massage techniques is limited because of time constraints.

Further Exercises:
1. How might you modify this sequence to address reduced range and complaints of stiffness in the hands?
2. How could you integrate the use of a hot pack into this sequence?
3. If a patient fell asleep during this sequence, what massage techniques—gently applied—could you use to awaken him?

for each regional sequence can help you overcome the problem of being unable to complete your treatment in the available amount of time. Furthermore, you must prioritize the outcomes for a given intervention, since you often have more work than you can accomplish. Clear priorities and precise timing will minimize the likelihood that you will lose focus or get sidetracked.

The practice of including all of the regions of the client's body in an intervention is common for "wellness massage" (general full-body relaxation massage).[1,2,6] The regions that you leave out of an intervention will vary with social norms, your training, and the preferences of your client. Within 45 to 60 minutes, it is often possible to address, at least briefly, each region of the client's body. Since many medical conditions require a more extended local focus, the time constraints of many clinical settings often require that you omit some regions or treat them briefly with general massage techniques. Consequently, it is important that you determine during the initial interview whether the client expects all regions to be included in a longer sequence of massage techniques.

If you practice in a setting where longer interventions (30 to 60 minutes) are possible, you may wish to integrate the specific treatment for a local condition with a more extensive sequence for the entire body. In this situation, you will give the region of focus more time than you would give it in a full-body sequence that has no regional focus. You have two options for allocating treatment time: include all of the remaining regions and shorten the treatment time

proportionally or eliminate some regions so that the final sequence addresses less than the full body (e.g., just the upper body). This approach to the design of sequences of massage techniques may seem reasonable if you have first practiced full-body sequence of massage techniques for wellness. *You should not conceptualize outcome-based interventions that address specified impairments as a full-body sequence for wellness with slight alterations. Often, you must alter a basic full-body sequence so much that the result bears scant resemblance to the general sequences that you perform for relaxation.*

There is no single order in which you must treat regions of the client's body during a full-body sequence of massage techniques.[1-4] You may begin regional sequences at the client's head or feet and then proceed region by region to the other end of the client's body in prone, supine, or side-lying. You will then turn the client and repeat or reverse the order of treatment of the regions. If you have a clear emphasis on one category of technique, then you may face some restrictions to the order in which you can address regions (Table 13-4).

# FULL-BODY SEQUENCES OF MASSAGE TECHNIQUES FOR WELLNESS

## Approaches to Full-Body Massage for Wellness

If you have performed the practice sequences in Chapters 7 to 12 on massage techniques, then you have already carried out a number of different approaches to full-body sequences of massage techniques to achieve specific outcomes. These "one-technique" sequences have limited scope; however, they can be effective and rewarding for both client and therapist. In practice, approaches to full-body massage usually include a greater variety of massage techniques that therapists apply at a consistent rate and rhythm to produce a coherent, structured, sensory experience for the client.

**Classical, or "Swedish," massage**, as it is commonly practiced today, uses mostly superficial fluid and neuromuscular techniques that are applied rhythmically with a broad contact surface and moderate centripetal pressure.[2,6] (The rate of application is quite slow for therapists who are trained in North America and faster for therapists who are trained in Europe.) When performed in this way, classical massage increases the return of lymph, reduces

| Table 13-4 | Suggestions for Ordering Regions When Emphasis Is Placed on Particular Massage Techniques |
|---|---|
| **Emphasized Technique** | **Suggestions for Ordering Regions** |
| Connective tissue | If there is extensive connective tissue work, start and/or end with work around the sacrum and iliac crest |
| Connective tissue, passive movement | Include the axial skeleton (i.e., neck, back, pelvis, sacrum); if there is deep, specific, or extensive work around the lumbar/pelvic region, include at least briefly the lower legs and feet |
| Neuromuscular | If there is deep, specific work on limbs, conclude with the related axial skeleton, i.e., cervical or lumbar area |
| Percussive | Rarely if ever emphasized throughout the body; if concentrated in the thorax for an extended period, finish with sedative reflex technique |
| Superficial fluid | Start on upper thorax and proceed distally to region of focus; work distally from next major proximal set of lymph nodes |
| Superficial reflex | Start and finish with sacrum, occiput, face hands, or feet |

Note: The chapters on individual techniques (Chapters 7 to 12) discuss the basis for most of these suggestions.

the level of muscle resting tension, reduces anxiety, and enhances the client's awareness. This effective approach to the full-body sequence of massage techniques continues to be the archetype for wellness massage in North America.

Increased access to the massage forms of other cultures and the work of modern Western innovators has recently spurred a technical renaissance in the practice of massage. Many of these traditions, or approaches, use a limited spectrum of massage techniques and refine related client examination and palpation skills to a high degree. Table 13-5 summarizes some of these approaches.[1–3,6–9,28] Without trivializing the philosophical differences that exist between these approaches, you can characterize them

as the refined application of specialized massage techniques that results in specific effects and different sensory experiences for the client. When appropriate to the clinical situation and executed with skill, any one of these approaches can produce excellent results.

## Maximizing Relaxation in Wellness Massage

Repair and regeneration of the body and mind occur more effectively when the nervous system is in a parasympathetic state. A central premise of **wellness massage** is that systemic **relaxation** or **sedation** is a desirable outcome in

| Table 13-5 | Characteristic Massage Techniques of Some Popular Massage-Related Approaches[1–3,5–8,20] |
|---|---|
| **Approach, System, or School** | **Characteristic Massage Techniques** |
| Lomilomi | Fast, superficial and deep effleurage and fast, broad neuromuscular technique |
| Manual lymph drainage | Superficial effleurage and superficial lymphatic technique |
| Myofascial Release | Myofascial release, craniosacral techniques |
| Neuromuscular technique | Specific kneading, stripping, specific direct fascial technique |
| Polarity | Static contact and compression |
| Rolfing, Bindegewebsmassage | Direct fascial technique |
| Shiatsu | Compression, specific (ischemic) compression, stretching |
| Therapeutic Touch, Reiki | Static contact |
| Trager | Rocking, and sedative rhythmic mobilization and shaking |

most situations. Another central premise is that reduction of resting tension of skeletal muscle is also usually desirable. These facts are also true when you are applying massage techniques to medical conditions, although other goals related to presenting impairments may be a higher priority for both you and the client.

An important axiom of practice is that *to relax a client, you must be relaxed.* The corollary is equally true: *clients will not relax if you are agitated.* It is as though the physical state of relaxation or tension passes from person to person. Although this axiom is worth remembering, it is very easy to forget in a busy practice. Suggesting that you work from a place of deep calm does not imply that you will show a lack of attention, inquiry, or intention or that you will suspend your capacity for critical thinking. A good therapist is adept at achieving a relaxed, attentive state within herself, while keeping her focus on the objectives of treatment and using precise technique. As discussed in Chapter 6, Preparation and Positioning for Massage, we advise you to practice gentle stretching, conscious breathing, and some ritual of calming the mind throughout the workday, especially in the few minutes preceding a sequence of massage techniques. Using conscious diaphragmatic breathing and controlled repetitive movement with correct body mechanics can also deepen your relaxation when performing massage.

Students and novice therapists often learn how to perform a general full-body sequence of massage techniques for relaxation in an environment that is relatively free of pressure. When faced with the pressures of completing client examinations, handling complex clinical situations, and managing the time constraints of practice, they commonly fail to relax when performing massage techniques. Although the resulting sequence of massage techniques may be technically competent, it may feel somewhat disjointed or ineffective to both therapist and client because it lacks the critical element of relaxation that contributes so much to the experience of both parties.

Box 13-5 summarizes some hints to help you achieve and maintain effective relaxation in your clients. Temper these suggestions with the observation that different techniques will produce deep relaxation from client to client and from day to day. In light of this, you must always monitor the client's subtle body cues and inquire about the client's response to treatment to determine the effectiveness of an intervention to produce deep relaxation.

| Box 13-5 | To Maximize a Client's Relaxation During a Sequence of Massage Techniques |
|---|---|

Prior to touch:
Ensure that the client

- Needs and desires relaxation
- Has expressed expectations and preferences
- Is comfortable
- Is breathing fully but without forcing, using the diaphragm

Ensure that you

- Are breathing fully using your diaphragm
- Have a clear logistical plan for the intervention
- Have a calm mind, free of distracting self-talk
- Are relaxed and free of stress or pain

Ensure that the environment is quiet and as private as possible.

While in contact, ensure that:

- The rate and rhythm of similar strokes is constant
- Pressure transitions within each stroke are smooth
- Transitions from one type of stroke to another are smooth
- Contact is made and broken gently and carefully
- Communication is minimal
- The client is comfortable after each change of position
- YOU DO NOT EVER RUSH OR HURRY

After contact, allow a rest period of 10 to 60 minutes.

## Sequencing Massage Techniques: Further Study and Practice

## ADDRESSING THE EFFECTS OF STRESS

Although there is no direct link between the autonomic nervous system and skeletal muscle, research suggests that a generalized elevation of muscle resting tension is one of the effects of stress and the activation of the sympathetic nervous system.[29,30] As a result, massage techniques that reduce muscle resting tension are valuable for treating the short-term and long-term effects of stress. Since neuromuscular techniques, connective tissue techniques, and movement techniques can all affect the level of resting tension in skeletal muscle, they are obvious choices for returning a client's body to homeostasis after periods of stress.

Addressing the effects of stress by altering the level of resting muscle tension is not the same as producing relaxation, although you may address them with the same massage techniques. If you want to treat stress in otherwise healthy individuals, try to achieve (at least) the following three outcomes: produce relaxation in the client throughout the sequence of massage techniques, decrease the level of resting tension of skeletal muscle, and improve the quality and quantity of movement, since movement is often restricted by stress-related muscular tension. If you only achieve relaxation with your intervention, the client may soon feel no different than he did before the massage intervention. If, however, you also alter the client's level of muscle resting tension and the movement patterns of the skeletal muscles, then the sedative effect will be more long lasting. A good clinician can seamlessly incorporate massage techniques that alternately, or simultaneously, address all of these outcomes, while addressing the other outcomes for the intervention.

For further details about treatment for stress, see Chapter 14, Using Massage to Achieve Clinical Outcomes.

## THE ART OF COHERENCE

In the context of Outcome-Based Massage, **coherence** is the consistent order or structure of an intervention. Coherence is the result of clear and consistent intention(s) on the part of the clinician. Maintaining coherence is relevant in all sequences of massage techniques. It is, however, of particular importance in sequences that last longer than 15 minutes and use a wide variety of massage techniques to address multiple outcomes. Coherent sequences can give a client an overall feeling of being in harmony and balance throughout the sequence of massage techniques and after the intervention. It is easy to imagine an incoherent full-body sequence: vigorous fast shaking on one leg, smooth slow superficial effleurage on the other, similarly mismatched massage techniques on the arms, myofascial release on the back, and light percussion on the face. Other examples of strategies that result in lack of coherence are discussed in Box 13-6.

Earlier in this chapter, we introduced several strategies that can help you to produce coherent massage interventions. The most important of these is your unwavering relaxation around the treatment table. Constant relaxation throughout the sequence conveys a consistency of manner and approach to the client, regardless of the technical content of the intervention. Another strategy for making an intervention coherent is to achieve and maintain a generalized nervous response in the client throughout the intervention.

---

| Box 13-6 | An Unpleasant Experiment: The Incoherent Sequence of Massage Techniques |
| --- | --- |

Time: Allow about 20 minutes

- Prepare for prone or supine.
- Choose massage techniques with conflicting intentions.
- Randomly and rapidly vary rate, rhythm, and pressure.
- Arbitrarily switch back and forth from region to region.
- Ignore your posture: slump or lean in an uncontrolled fashion.
- Talk to the client about whatever crosses your mind.
- It usually takes less than 5 minutes to make an unforgettable point to the person on the table. Once the client stops the exercise, help him or her return to homeostasis with some sedative massage techniques.

---

The desired response is usually relaxation. A third way of increasing the coherence of a sequence of massage techniques is to use the same framing **general technique** (palpatory stroke, connecting stroke) to touch all regions of the client's body during the intervention. When you return to the same technique at intervals during the intervention, you give a sense of sensory regularity to the sequence, which can put the client at ease. When you touch all regions of the client's body, even if only briefly with general strokes, you reinforce a client's sense that you are considering his needs as a whole person, not merely as an instance of an illness or disorder. This is often a crucial and unstated concern when the client has experienced long-standing pain or physical disability. Nevertheless, *it is not how much of the client's body that you touch that is critical but the way in which you touch it.* You can unwittingly reduce coherence when you use too many massage techniques, with a large variation in rate, pressure, and palpatory focus. Box 13-7 summarizes strategies to enhance coherence of full-body sequences of massage techniques

## STUDENT PRACTICE OF FULL-BODY SEQUENCES OF MASSAGE TECHNIQUES

It is quite common for beginning students of massage to be taught one well-choreographed, coherent, generic routine that incorporates a variety of massage techniques (predominantly neuromuscular) according to general principles.[6–9] This approach has both good and bad points. In learning

<table>
<tr><td>Box 13-7</td><td>**Strategies to Enhance Coherence of More Extensive Sequences**</td></tr>
</table>

- Let yourself relax thoroughly and continuously during the sequence of massage techniques.
- Choose a small number of outcomes and stick to them.
- Aim for a generalized nervous response in the client (i.e., sedation or arousal).
- Use the same framing general technique in all regions.
- Maintain consistent rhythm in all regions.
- As far as possible, maintain a comparable rhythm in all massage techniques.
- Use similar (not necessarily identical) massage techniques in all regions.
- Be cautious of overloading a sequence with many different sensations. Practitioners of massage would also be wise to experience or observe the work of good practitioners of the various massage-related approaches listed in Table 13-5. Their methods of practice often artfully demonstrate many of these strategies for enhancing coherence.

the routine, students unconsciously absorb sound principles. By contrast, students often develop a certain rigidity of technical approach that can be detrimental in later clinical practice and that is *very* hard to retrain. It is generally preferable for beginning students and novice clinicians to design and practice a variety of coherent full-body sequences that address different outcomes and have differing durations such as 15-, 30-, 45-, and 60-minute sessions. This practice teaches you mental flexibility and prepares you to handle time-consuming clinical problems without sacrificing the emphasis on treating the whole person, which is the hallmark of good treatment.

Thorough training will enable students to perform a large number of different sequences of massage techniques with a strict observance of the character and duration of each sequence. We caution students against the early development of a particular "style," since this is often a technical limitation in disguise or a projection of personal preference. It is better for you to attempt to master many massage styles and understand how the selected outcomes define the style of any given Outcome-Based Massage intervention.

## References

1. Fritz S. *Mosby's Fundamentals of Therapeutic Massage.* 3rd ed. St. Louis: Mosby; 2004.
2. Benjamin PJ, Tappan FM. *Tappan's Handbook of Healing Massage Techniques.* 4th ed. Upper Saddle River, NJ: Pearson Prentice Hall; 2005.
3. Fritz S. *Fundamentals of Therapeutic Massage.* St Louis: Mosby-Lifeline; 1995.
4. Salvo SG. *Massage Therapy: Principles and Practice.* 2nd ed. Philadelphia: WB Saunders; 2003.
5. Quality Assurance Committee of the College of Massage Therapists of Ontario. *Code of Ethics and Standards of Practice.* Toronto: College of Massage Therapists of Ontario; 2006.
6. de Domenico G, Wood EC. *Beard's Massage.* 4th ed. Philadelphia: WB Saunders; 1997.
7. Holey E, Cook E. *Evidence-Based Therapeutic Massage.* 2nd ed. Edinburgh: Churchill Livingstone; 2003.
8. Beck MJ. *Milady's Theory and Practice of Therapeutic Massage.* 3rd ed. Albany, NY: Milady; 1999.
9. Wood EC, Becker PD. *Beard's Massage.* 3rd ed. Philadelphia: WB Saunders; 1981.
10. Lederman E. *The Science and Practice of Manual Therapy.* 2nd ed. Edinburgh: Churchill Livingstone; 2005.
11. Mennell JB. *Physical Treatment by Movement, Manipulation and Massage.* 5th ed. Philadelphia: Blakiston; 1945.
12. Simons DG, Travell JG, Simons LS. *Myofascial Pain and Dysfunction. The Trigger Point Manual, Volume 1.* 2nd ed. Baltimore: Williams & Wilkins; 1999.
13. Michlovitz S. *Thermal Agents in Rehabilitation.* 3rd ed. Philadelphia: FA Davis; 1996.
14. Cummings GS, Tillman LJ. Remodeling of dense connective tissue in normal adult tissues. In: Currier DP, Nelson RM, eds. *Dynamics of Human Biologic Tissues.* Philadelphia: FA Davis; 1992:45–73.
15. O'Sullivan SB. Strategies to improve motor control. In: O'Sullivan SB, Schmitz J, eds. *Physical Rehabilitation, Assessment and Treatment.* 2nd ed. Philadelphia: FA Davis; 1988.
16. Hollis M. *Massage for Therapists.* 2nd ed. Oxford, England: Blackwell Science; 1998.
17. Kim MA, Sakong JK, Kim EJ, Kim EH, Kim EH. Effect of aromatherapy massage for the relief of constipation in the elderly. *Taehan Kanho Hakhoe Chi.* 2005;35:56–64.
18. Jeon SY, Jung HM. The effects of abdominal meridian massage on constipation among CVA patients. *Taehan Kanho Hakhoe Chi.* 2005;35:135–142.
19. Emly M, Wilson L, Darby J. Abdominal massage for adults with learning disabilities. *Nurs Times.* 2001;97:61–62.
20. Le Blanc-Louvry I, Costaglioli B, Boulon C, Leroi AM, Ducrotte P. Does mechanical massage of the abdominal wall after colectomy reduce postoperative pain and shorten the duration of ileus? Results of a randomized study. *J Gastrointest Surg.* 2002; 6:43–49.
21. Preece J. Introducing abdominal massage in palliative care for the relief of constipation. *Complement Ther Nurs Midwifery.* 2002;8:101–105.
22. Shirreffs CM. Aromatherapy massage for joint pain and constipation in a patient with Guillain Barré. *Complement Ther Nurs Midwifery.* 2001;7:78–83.

23. Ernst E. Abdominal massage therapy for chronic constipation: a systematic review of controlled clinical trials. *Forsch Komplementarmed.* 1999;6:149–151.

24. Emly M. Abdominal massage. *Nurs Times.* 1993;89:34–36.

25. Resende TL, Brocklehurst JC, O'Neill PA. A pilot study on the effect of exercise and abdominal massage on bowel habit in continuing care patients. *Clin Rehabil.* 1993;7:204–209.

26. Klauser AG, Flaschentrager J, Gehrke A, Muller-Lissner SA. Abdominal wall massage; effect on colonic function in healthy volunteers and in patients with chronic constipation. *Z Gastroenterol.* 1992;30:246–251.

27. Wale JO. *Tidy's Massage and Remedial Exercises in Medical and Surgical Conditions.* 11th ed. Bristol: John Wright & Sons; 1968.

28. Stillerman E. *The Encyclopedia of Bodywork.* New York: Facts on File; 1996.

29. Hoehn-Saric R. Psychic and somatic anxiety: worries, somatic symptoms and physiological changes. *Acta Psychiatr Scand Suppl.* 1998;393:32–38.

30. Millensen JR. *Mind Matters: Psychological Medicine in Holistic Practice.* Seattle: Eastland Press; 1995.

## *Further Reading*

American Physical Therapy Association. *Guide to Physical Therapist Practice.* 2nd ed. Alexandria, VA: American Physical Therapy Association; 1999.

Arvedson J. *Medical Gymnastics and Massage in General Practice.* London: JA Churchill; 1930.

Baumgartner AJ. *Massage in Athletics.* Minneapolis: Burgess; 1947.

Beard G. History of massage technique. *Phys Ther Rev.* 1952;32:613–624.

Bohm M. *Massage: Its Principles and Techniques.* Gould E, trans. Philadelphia: JB Lippincott; 1913.

Claire T. Bodywork: *What Type of Massage to Get and How to Get the Most Out of It.* New York: William Morrow; 1995.

Collinge W. *The American Holistic Health Association Complete Guide to Alternative Medicine.* New York: Warner Books; 1996.

Cyriax J. Theory and practice of massage. In: *Textbook of Orthopedic Medicine, Volume 2. Treatment by Manipulation, Massage and Injection.* 11th ed. London: Bailliere Tindall; 1984.

Cyriax JH, Cyriax PJ. *Cyriax' Illustrated Manual of Orthopaedic Medicine.* 2nd ed. Oxford: Butterworth-Heinemann; 1993.

Hoffa A. *Technik der Massage.* Stuttgart: Verlag von Ferdinand Ernke; 1897.

Kellogg JH. *The Art of Massage.* Battle Creek, MI: Modern Medicine Publishing; 1923.

Kellogg JH. *The Art of Massage: A Practical Manual for the Nurse, the Student and the Practitioner.* Battle Creek, MI: Modern Medicine Publishing; 1929.

King RK. *Performance Massage.* Champaign, IL: Human Kinetics; 1993.

Licht S, ed. *Massage, Manipulation and Traction.* Baltimore: Waverly Press; 1960.

Loving J. *Massage Therapy.* Stamford, CT: Appleton & Lange; 1999.

Macias Merlo ML. Abdominal massage: therapy for the control of chronic constipation. *Rev Enferm (Spanish).* 1985;8:16–19.

McMillan M. *Massage and Therapeutic Exercise.* 2nd ed. Philadelphia: WB Saunders; 1925.

Meagher J. *Sports Massage.* Barrytown, NY: Station Hill Press; 1990.

Prosser EM. *A Manual of Massage and Movement.* 2nd ed. London: Faber & Faber; 1941.

Rattray F, Ludwig L. *Clinical Massage Therapy.* Toronto: Talus Inc.; 2000.

Seyle H. History and present status of the stress concept. In: Goldberger L, Breznitz S, eds. *Handbook of Stress: Theoretical and Clinical Aspects.* New York: Macmillan; 1982.

Seyle H. *The Physiology and Pathology of Exposure to Stress.* Montreal: Acta; 1950.

Tappan FM. *Healing Massage Techniques.* Norwalk, CT: Appleton & Lange; 1988.

Tidy NM. *Massage and Remedial Exercises.* London: John Wright; 1932.

Westland G. Massage as a therapeutic tool, parts 1 and 2. *Br J Occup Ther.* 1993;56:129–134, 177–180.

Yates J. *A Physician's Guide to Therapeutic Massage.* 3rd ed. Toronto: Curties Overzet; 2004.

Ylinen J, Cash M. *Sports Massage.* London: Stanley Paul; 1980.

Zhang Y, Zhang YL, Cheng YQ. Clinical observation of constipation due to deficiency of vital energy treated by massage and finger pressure methods. *Chung Hua Hu Li Tsa Chih (Chinese).* 1996;31:97–98.

# Chapter 14

# Using Massage to Achieve Clinical Outcomes

The foundation for Outcome-Based Massage is the growing body of research that suggests the merits of massage for **wellness** and the treatment of an increasing number of medical conditions.[1–9] In Outcome-Based Massage, therapists use an iterative four-phase clinical decision-making process (Evaluative, Treatment Planning, Treatment, and Discharge phases) to create effective **interventions** that use massage techniques to achieve specified clinical outcomes. The first section of this chapter provides practical guidelines for developing and progressing interventions for wellness and the treatment of **impairments** that use massage techniques to achieve specific clinical outcomes. The later sections outline examples of interventions and progressions that achieve outcomes related to a variety of impairments.

## Guidelines for Developing and Progressing Interventions for Wellness and the Treatment of Impairments

## THE ROLE OF IMPAIRMENTS AND PATHOPHYSIOLOGY IN TREATMENT PLANNING

Historically, in "medical massage," the use of massage to treat medical conditions, therapists have applied standard treatment regimens that are specified for each medical condition.[1,9] By contrast, Outcome-Based Massage suggests that therapists recognize that clients with medical conditions present with related **impairments**, secondary to **pathophysiology**, that therapists must assess and treat.[10,11] In other words, rather than applying a standard treatment regimen for a medical condition, therapists using Outcome-Based Massage can treat clients with the same medical condition differently. Their treatment for each client will depend on the client's presenting impairments, the **outcomes** that reflect those impairments, and the client's stated treatment goals. Therapists using Outcome-Based Massage also use information on the client's impairments to guide their decisions on massage techniques, treatment progression, **contraindications** to treatment, and special treatment considerations. To illustrate Outcome-Based Massage, this chapter provides examples of interventions for specific impairments that we developed using this approach. Therapists can combine interventions that treat individual impairments within a **plan of care** in order to address each client's unique clinical presentation and goals.

# COMBINING INTERVENTIONS FOR MULTIPLE BODY STRUCTURES AND FUNCTIONS

Few clients present for treatment with a single impairment or wellness goal. Consequently, therapists typically have to address multiple impairments or wellness goals within a single intervention.[1,11] In doing so, they must combine interventions for different impairments and body structures into a single plan of care. The following guidelines can assist therapists in selecting and combining interventions for differing impairments and body structures. Therapists can incorporate these guidelines into the clinical decision-making steps outlined in the Chapter 3, Clinical Decision Making for Massage, and Chapter 5, Client Examination for Massage.

## Guidelines for Combining Interventions for Different Impairments and Wellness Goals

1. List all of the client's impairments and wellness goals that you plan to address within your plan of care.
2. Consider the **contraindications** and **cautions** to treatment for each impairment, wellness goal, and massage technique. You may have to exclude some techniques from the intervention entirely or modify how you apply them locally based on these contraindications and cautions. Each technique you choose for the final list of techniques must be *safe for all* of the client's impairments. Furthermore, each technique you choose must be *effective for at least one* of the client's impairments or wellness goals. At times, the final plan of care may not be the most effective treatment for a given impairment because the preferred treatment technique is contraindicated by for one of the client's other impairments or wellness goals.
3. The relative priority of impairments or wellness goals will guide your choice and progression of techniques. Give priority to impairments that are more severe (greater grade) and that cause other impairments. In addition, consider the client's priorities for care. You can give a prioritized impairment or wellness goal more emphasis by:

- Treating it first in the series of interventions
- Treating it first in each intervention
- Selecting the majority of treatment techniques in the plan of care to address it
- Allotting more time to address it during each intervention

4. If you assign impairments or wellness goals equal priority, decide whether you will treat them simultaneously or sequentially within each intervention and within the episode of care as a whole.

# PROGRESSION OF INTERVENTIONS

## Progression of Interventions for Medical Conditions

The treatment of a client's medical condition **progresses** through stages that reflect the clinical course and **prognosis** of that condition and client. Therapists can use information from several sources to guide treatment progression. These sources include practice guidelines, findings from the client examination, and clinical experience.

Professions often establish broad **practice guidelines** for the treatment of medical conditions to provide therapists with a general framework for planning and progressing interventions. These condition-specific practice guidelines and professional practice guidelines outline a general guide to prognoses, expected numbers of visits per episode of care, **outcome measures**, and relevant types of intervention for a range of medical conditions. We use the American Physical Therapy Association's *Guide to Physical Therapist Practice*[10] as the example for this chapter. At the time of printing, we were unable to locate a comparable, systematic, national set of practice guidelines for a wide range of medical conditions written specifically for massage therapists. Table 14-1 contains an excerpt of the practice guidelines for physical therapy interventions for selected musculoskeletal and neurological disorders.[10] The American Physical Therapy Association did not develop these guidelines for a therapist who uses massage therapy techniques extensively; they assume the use of other clinical techniques as primary modalities. Furthermore, these guidelines are for situations in which therapists are addressing a broader range of impairments and **functional limitations** in their interventions than those that are specific to the use of massage techniques. Consequently, the number of massage-based interventions would be lower for a physical therapist than it would be for a massage therapist who is treating the same condition.

| Table 14-1 | Duration of Physical Therapy Regimens and Expected Number of Visits for Selected Orthopedic and Neurological Conditions | |
|---|---|---|
| **Condition** | **Duration of Expected Physical Therapy Regimen** | **Number of Visits** |
| Tendinitis, bursitis, fasciitis | 8–16 weeks | 6–24 |
| Postural conditions | 12 months | 6–20 |
| Sprain/strain/dislocation | 2–16 weeks | 3–21 |
| Uncomplicated joint arthroplasty | 6 months | 12–60 |
| Disk herniation | 1–6 months | 8–24 |
| Cerebrovascular accident (stroke) | Until maximum independence is achieved | 10–60 |
| Peripheral nerve injury | 4–8 months | 12–56 |

Data from American Physical Therapy Association. *Guide to Physical Therapist Practice.* 2nd ed. Alexandria, VA: American Physical Therapy Association; 1999.

In reality, the appropriate number of interventions using massage techniques will also vary with other factors, including the cause, severity, acuity, and complexity of the client's medical condition; the use of complementary modalities; and the client's overall health status and age. For this reason, therapists should try to avoid using a standard plan of care for all clients with a given medical condition. Instead, they need to remain outcome-based in their practices and tailor the progression of massage and other techniques within a given **episode of care** to the client's presenting impairments, functional limitations, and wellness goals. This will involve monitoring the client's progression from one stage of recovery to the next by assessing changes in his impairments and functional limitations, rather than by determining the amount of time that has elapsed since the onset of his medical condition. At each stage, the therapist should modify the plan of care so that it remains consistent with the client's current impairments and functional limitations.

Therapists' ability to progress interventions effectively can improve with appropriate clinical experience. They can use their observations of clients' responses to treatment and the typical course of medical conditions as a foundation on which to base their decisions about treatment progression. Furthermore, novice therapists and students can use the consistent application of the clinical decision-making process and principles of Outcome-Based Massage, preferably in collaboration with an experienced therapist, to enhance their skill in progressing interventions.

## Progression of Wellness Interventions

The development of interventions that include or focus on wellness-related outcomes follows a similar process to the one outlined earlier. Prior to embarking on a wellness intervention, it is very important that therapists first identify any impairments that are present. Often clients who request **wellness interventions** present with impairments, such as **stress**, **altered body image**, **postural conditions**, **elevated resting tension**, **latent trigger points**, and reduced active range of motion. Prior to initiating the wellness intervention, therapists will need to discuss, evaluate, and treat those impairments, as appropriate within their scope of practice, using the guidelines described in this chapter. Once therapists have distinguished between impairments and wellness-related outcomes, then they can use the clinical decision-making process (see Chapter 3, Clinical Decision-Making for Massage) to guide their development and progression of the wellness intervention.

During the client examination, therapists identify wellness goals that are of ongoing importance to the client. These wellness goals can include enhancing muscle and general **relaxation**, optimizing **ease of movement**, and achieving optimal mental focus. Based on the examination findings, therapists negotiate reasonable long- and short-term outcomes for each wellness goal through careful dialogue with the client. Through ongoing client re-examination, therapists obtain information on the changes in the client's body structures and functions or functional status that signal the need for progression of the wellness intervention. They also modify or redirect the plan of care so that it remains consistent with the client's current status and moves the client towards the next set of outcomes. In this way, therapists use an iterative clinical decision-making process to facilitate the client's ongoing progress towards his wellness outcomes.

In contrast to the treatment of medical conditions, there is a lack of practice guidelines for the duration of treatment and the number of visits for wellness goals. Furthermore, the required number of sessions will vary with a variety of factors including the number and nature of identified issues, the complexity of the client's wellness outcomes, the presence and treatment of underlying or related impairments, and the client's overall health status and age. Moreover, wellness interventions often (and should) include a significant educational component. Consequently, the client's willingness and capacity to learn and implement **lifestyle** changes can affect the duration of treatment.

Therapists should not omit the four-phase clinical decision-making process (Evaluative, Treatment Planning,

Treatment, and Discharge) when they provide wellness interventions. Furthermore, they should not make a wellness plan of care open-ended. As with interventions for medical conditions, the treatment process should lead to **discharge**. If a wellness client seeks ongoing treatment for legitimate reasons, therapists can follow one plan of care to its completion and then begin another phase of treatment with a formal client re-examination. This enables the client and therapist to consider what they have achieved with each plan of care and avoids the trap of exploiting the client by scheduling an undetermined number of interventions that have an ill-defined purpose.

### Critical Thinking Question

How does the process of developing interventions to address impairments (**medical massage**) differ from the process for developing interventions to address wellness goals? How are they similar?

# DISCHARGE

If clinicians follow the principles for progressing interventions outlined in this and other chapters, then the transition from the Treatment Phase to the Discharge Phase will be gradual and imperceptible. Chapter 3, Clinical Decision Making for Massage, and Chapter 4, Interpersonal and Ethical Issues for Massage, outline the steps that clinicians follow to prepare their clients physically and psychologically for discharge. Some additional clinical issues are worthy of mention. As clinicians identify the resolution of the client's impairments through ongoing re-examinations, they can progress their use of techniques that address the client's functional limitations, such as functional training, as their scope of practice permits. Finally, as discharge approaches, clinicians will ensure that they address the client's needs for self-care education, equipment, and referrals to other health care professionals and services, and other needs that lie within their scope of practice.

## Interventions for Impairments: Foundations

The following examples of interventions for impairments consider both traditional approaches to practice and the growing body of evidence for massage techniques. Although they have undergone peer review by practicing therapists, teachers, and students, we have not subjected them to the extensive review that would lead us to consider them **practice guidelines**. For all of these suggested interventions, bear in mind that clients may present with other impairments or medical conditions that will have their own set of cautions and contraindications for treatment.

# INTERVENTIONS FOR PSYCHONEUROIMMUNO-LOGICAL IMPAIRMENTS

## Stress: Impaired Ability to Relax, General Adaptation Syndrome–Early Stages

### Relevant Outcomes
- Reduced stress or distress (in a wide variety of situations)[12,13–72]
- Improved ability to relax
- Improved adaptability to stress[73]
- Improved behaviour[42,72,74–78]
- Improved immune function[3,5,17,18,20,24,30,34,38,44,79–82]

### Clinical Relevance

The literature suggests that **stress** contributes to a large percentage of medical conditions.[83–85] In addition, posttraumatic stress and **posttraumatic stress disorder** often follow traumatic experiences.[86–88] Furthermore, many otherwise-healthy clients complain of too much stress or an impaired ability to relax. Reduced stress and associated outcomes are important considerations for clients with depressed immune function.[3,5,18,24,30,34,38,44,80–82]

### Treatment Considerations

At the outset of treatment, determine the stage of the **general adaptation syndrome**[89–91] at which the client presents. This step is important because a client at later stages of the general adaptation syndrome, who is approaching **exhaustion** or "burnout," will involve more cautions and contraindications to treatment than a client at the earlier stages of **alarm** or resistance. Determine whether the client has a diagnosis of **clinical depression**, an **anxiety disorder**, or other psychiatric condition. In addition, ensure that you have a thorough understanding of any physical symptoms associated with his condition, the current management of his condition, and other health care professionals involved in his care. Consult with other treating health care professionals if you have any concerns regarding treatment. Furthermore, regardless of whether or not the client has a psychiatric condition, consider referring him to his physician if his stress levels and physical symptoms do not improve with treatment. Finally, be conscious and supportive of the fact that a client's habits and thought processes will have a profound influence their ability to deal with stress.[84]

## Guidelines for Using Massage Techniques

- First, prepare yourself so that *you* are fully relaxed.
- Ensure that the treatment area is warm, quiet, and softly lit.
- Speak in a quiet voice.
- Offer the client a choice of several types of relaxing music[92] (yours or his own) or silence.
- Position the client for maximum comfort.
- You can use almost any massage technique for **sedative** or relaxation massage[4] including: superficial reflex,[41,93] superficial fluid,[94] neuromuscular, connective tissue, and passive movement techniques.[95] In addition, small amounts of percussion may be appropriate for some clients. Well-performed rocking is possibly the most sedative of all massage techniques.[96]
- Sedative massage is typically fairly slow, rhythmic, and predictable. When performing repetitive petrissage, try using a stroke rate of 50 to 70 cycles per minute.[97]
- Many clients who have experienced massage prefer moderate or deep work.[98] They may find superficial work irritating[9] because it does not address their muscular tension. Solicit honest feedback about treatment depth and match the depth of your work to the client's needs.
- Ensure that your application of techniques is not causing pain (around 3/10 to 5/10 maximum on the self-reported pain scale) even when you are performing **neuromuscular** or **connective tissue techniques** on deeper structures.
- There are several key locations for treatment. Since the hands, feet, and head (including face and ears) are high-tension areas, which are highly innervated, include them in treatment unless you are short of time.[21,36,39,43,56,64,74,99-103] The cranium and sacrum contain **parasympathetic** outflow that you can affect manually[104,105] with prolonged holding of these areas or prolonged repetitive palmar stroking from occiput to sacrum. Deep gluteal work, especially around

the sacral and iliac attachments, can also be highly effective. Furthermore, any techniques that you perform along the axial skeleton may produce reflex **autonomic** effects as a result of inhibition of **sympathetic** activity[106,107] or facilitation of parasympathetic activity.[3]

- Treatment times that are longer than 30 minutes probably produce much greater sedative responses.[4] Treatment times under 15 minutes may be less effective.[46]
- **Aromatherapy** oils added to the carrier lubricant (at a rate of 5 to 20 drops per 50 ml of carrier)[108] may improve relaxation.[32,33,66,108,109] Sedative oils include: melissa, valerian, neroli, passion flower, orange flower, petitgrain, and lavender.[108]
- You can integrate treatment for other impairments into this basic approach for relaxation, and by doing so, you may increase the sedative effects further. For example, you can treat **adaptive shortening** of muscle and connective tissue, trigger points, and elevated resting tension in the shoulder muscles within this treatment framework for relaxation.

## Complementary Modalities

You can use the following complementary modalities during an intervention for relaxation.

- **Diaphragmatic breathing** and relaxation techniques, such as **guided awareness**, **progressive muscle relaxation**, autogenic training, imagery, and meditation, make an excellent beginning or end to an intervention.[21,110] You can also use them concurrently with massage techniques depending on the context. If you do not feel confident in your ability to guide clients in these relaxation techniques, you can obtain recorded instructions for clients to use in the clinic or at home.[111,112]
- **Passive movements** and prolonged, gentle **stretching** are appropriate.
- Systemic heat (steam, sauna, whirlpool, or bath) in the range of warm to hot[113] is sedative and is an excellent prelude to the massage if it is available.[113,114] You can also use systemic heat followed by a cool rinse or plunge. Furthermore, a local application of moist heat (hydrocollator or thermophore) is an appropriate alternative to full-body heat.
- Stress management education is also helpful.[73]

Between interventions, clients can use any of the complementary modalities listed above and the following:

- Moderate active exercise such as walking
- Movement systems that emphasize relaxation and awareness such as **Feldenkrais**, **Tai Chi**, or **Hatha yoga**

## General Adaptation Syndrome–Later Stages

### Relevant Outcomes
- Recovery of autonomic **homeostasis**

### Clinical Relevance
Clients who are approaching the third stage of the general adaptation syndrome, which involves exhaustion, disintegration, or burnout, are a distinct subset of the clients with this condition. They may be experiencing a serious health crisis that requires stress leave from work, medical treatment, or hospitalization.[89]

### Treatment Considerations
Ongoing management by a physician and referral to other relevant health care providers is essential.

### Guidelines for Using Massage Techniques
- Be conservative in the number and level of stimulation of all techniques.
- Offer shorter treatment sessions, 20 to 30 minutes long, consisting of light, gentle techniques including **reflex techniques**, superficial effleurage, light (at most, moderate-depth) neuromuscular techniques.
- Cause no pain.
- Carefully monitor the effects of treatment, both during and after treatment.
- Progress the intervention to include the techniques we described for clients with earlier stages of the general adaptation syndrome as the client shows less **fatigue** and improved tolerance of treatment.

### Complementary Modalities
- Suggest simple nonvigorous exercise, such as walking, within the client's tolerance.
- Modify the systemic hydrotherapy procedures that are suggested for early stages of the general adaptation syndrome to techniques of moderate duration that use warmth[113] without contrast or only mild contrast. Local warmth to tolerance is acceptable.

### Critical Thinking Question
How does treatment differ for early and later stages of the general adaptation syndrome?

**EXAMINING THE EVIDENCE**

In 2004, a group of psychologists from the University of Illinois published a landmark meta-analysis of massage therapy research.[4] Rigorous search and selection criteria yielded 37 studies with 1802 participants, including 795 who received massage. The authors examine single-dose effects of massage on **state anxiety**, negative mood, pain, **cortisol level**, blood pressure, and heart rate. They found that massage treatments had statistically significant effects on state anxiety, blood pressure, and heart rate. They also found that massage treatments had statistically significant multiple-dose effects on **trait anxiety**, **depression**, and delayed onset of pain. The authors discussed these results in the context of common theories on the effects of massage techniques. They proposed that some effects of massage techniques may be due to positive expectations of client and therapist and from their interpersonal contact, rather than the particular technique used or the site to which it is applied. This is similar to some of the findings on psychotherapy. This hypothesis may explain general outcomes related to psychoneuroimmunology and pain but may not be valid for the specific effects of massage techniques on physiological impairments such as trigger points or scar tissue.

Moyer CA, Rounds J, Hannum JW. A meta-analysis of massage therapy research. *Psychol Bull.* 2004;130:3–18.

## Insomnia, Reduced or Disturbed Sleep

### Relevant Outcomes
- Improved pattern and quality of sleep[5,19,23,33,48,49,111,115–126]
- Improved duration of sleep[49,116,119,127–129]

### Clinical Relevance
Disturbed sleep is a common symptom of stress. In addition, disturbed sleep often accompanies serious or terminal diseases, surgery (both before and after), hospitalization,[129] chronic pain, depression, and addiction.[128,130]

### Treatment Considerations
Prior to initiating treatment, discuss the cause of the client's sleep disturbance. Stress, clinical depression, addiction, **chronic pain**, and disease all have their own cautions for

treatment. Most of these underlying conditions necessitate referral to the client's physician.

## Guidelines for Using Massage Techniques

■ All of the massage strategies described for the treatment of stress are appropriate.

## Complementary Modalities

■ All of the complementary techniques described for the treatment of stress are appropriate.

■ Clients may need to retrain poor sleep habits by reducing stimulation in the evening, developing a ritual for use prior to retiring, faithfully maintaining a regular sleep time, and avoiding daytime naps.

■ Immediately before retiring, the client can use any of the following:
  ■ Gentle stretching (especially of the posterior surface of the body)
  ■ Diaphragmatic breathing and relaxation exercises[45,110]
  ■ A warm, not hot, bath with or without the addition of relaxing essential oils such as lavender, chamomile, cypress, juniper, neroli, marjoram, and melissa[108,109,113,114,131]
  ■ A cold abdominal wash[113,114]
  ■ An abdominal heating compress[113,114]

# Fatigue, Lethargy, Suboptimal Arousal

## Relevant Outcomes
■ Decreased fatigue[13,47,69,103,132–136]
■ Increased **arousal**
■ Preparedness for activity

## Clinical Relevance
Uncomplicated fatigue typically results from stress or lack of sleep. Fatigue is also a symptom of medical conditions such as anemia, thyroid conditions, convalescence, rheumatoid arthritis and related systemic connective tissue diseases, cancer, and depressive psychiatric conditions. At the other end of the clinical continuum, increased arousal is often a requirement for optimal performance in athletic and artistic performance. These related impairments all share a treatment approach that seeks to heighten arousal through physical stimulation.

## Treatment Considerations
Prior to initiating treatment for a client who presents with fatigue, ensure that you understand the cause of the client's fatigue. If there is no obvious cause for prolonged fatigue or if you have any concerns about associated systemic or psychiatric conditions, consult with the client's physician. If the client's fatigue is associated with a psychiatric condition, consult with the client's physician or other treating health care professionals and monitor for any signs of self-destructive behavior. Up to a point, therapists can use massage techniques to counteract uncomplicated fatigue. Nevertheless, the best course of action for the client may be to obtain more sleep.

## Guidelines for Using Massage Techniques

■ Traditionally, massage techniques to counteract fatigue are fast-paced, light, and rhythmic.[1,98] The pace and depth of **stimulating massage** techniques are generally similar to the pace and depth of **precompetition sports massage** techniques.[137] Many studies that reported reduced fatigue after massage techniques did not, however, use this approach. Nonetheless, be cautious when you apply sedative techniques to any client who reports a low energy level.

■ Make the treatment duration short. For example, take 20 minutes for all or most of the body.

■ Useful techniques for stimulation include superficial stroking, effleurage, broad-contact compression, petrissage, coarse vibration, nonsedative shaking, and percussion. Avoid techniques that require a slower pace, such as fascial work, and techniques that may cause discomfort, such as trigger point release.

■ Your depth of penetration will be superficial as a result of the faster pace of treatment.

## Complementary Modalities

■ You can perform hydrotherapy techniques that use cold, contrast, and friction (rubbing with an abrasive cloth or brush), before or after the treatment. Match the vigor of the technique to the client's tolerance. Some examples of techniques in ascending order of vigor are: **dry brushing**, cold wash, **salt glow**, **cold mitten friction**, and high-contrast alternating temperature percussion jet ('blitzguss').[113,114,138] You can modify the strength of the stimulation of a technique by increasing or decreasing the area of the client's body to which you apply it. These techniques may have additional beneficial effects on immune function.[139]

■ Instruct the client in the use of brisk, aerobic exercise, within her tolerance, between interventions.

# INTERVENTIONS FOR IMPAIRMENTS RELATED TO PAIN

## Before Treating Pain

During the evaluative phase, obtain the answers to the following important questions.

1. *Are there any contraindications or cautions that necessitate referral to another health care professional?*
   Pain that is severe, of sudden onset, unfamiliar to the client, and associated with systemic or neurological symptoms, or that is unrelated to activity are "**red flags**" that suggest that you should immediately refer the client to a physician for further investigation.
2. *Is the pain acute pain or chronic pain?*
   Acute **nociceptive pain** is usually, but not always, associated with the acute stage of a medical condition. **Chronic pain** and **chronic pain syndromes** may not be associated with readily apparent physical signs. You can further distinguish between the categories of pain summarized in Box 14-1.
3. *What is causing the pain(s)?*
   Surprisingly, therapists often overlook this issue. Use client examination techniques to identify the structure(s) that is the source of pain. Although massage techniques may reduce the perception of pain from an

unidentified cause, through **hyperstimulation analgesia** or **sedation**, direct treatment of the cause(s) of pain is preferable, whenever possible.

During the treatment planning phase, try to answer the following questions:

1. *Is any cause of the pain an impairment that you can treat directly with massage techniques?*
   Use appropriate massage techniques to treat the impairments that cause the client's pain, such as **edema**, reduced mobility of connective tissue, elevated resting tension, spasm, and trigger points, directly.
2. *Is hyperstimulation analgesia appropriate?*
   Another strategy for reducing pain is to use massage techniques for hyperstimulation analgesia or counterirritant analgesia. For example, prolonged mechanical vibration will reduce pain in the same dermatome as the site of application[141] (see information on mechanical vibration in Chapter 7, Superficial Reflex Techniques). You can also use heat, cold, and active exercises to achieve this effect.
3. *Is sedation the only strategy for reducing pain when using massage techniques?*
   The least specific approach to managing pain with massage techniques is to use massage techniques to relax or sedate the client in order to change her perception of pain. An example of this is when therapists use massage techniques to modify a client's perception of cancer pain.

| Box 14-1 | Categories of Pain and Examples (adapted from Wittink and Michel[140]) | |
|---|---|---|
| **Category** | **Example** | |
| Acute nociceptive pain | Acute inflammation; a recent orthopedic injury | |
| Subacute nociceptive pain | A partly healed orthopedic injury | |
| Recurrent acute nociceptive pain | A flare up of rheumatoid arthritis | |
| Ongoing acute pain with ongoing nociception | An uncontrolled neoplasm | |
| **Intractable** chronic (greater than 6 months) nonmalignant pain with nociception | **Radiculopathy** from an unoperated disk lesion; some chronic stage inflammatory conditions that have not fully healed | |
| Intractable nonmalignant chronic (greater than 6 months) pain without nociception | Idiopathic chronic low back pain | |
| Many clients who present for treatment fall into the last two categories. | | |

Pain may *contribute* to impairments, such as elevated resting tension and trigger points. Address those associated impairments with massage techniques if this is appropriate.

## Acute Nociceptive Pain

### Relevant Outcomes
- Reduction of pain[3,13,17,25,27,32,37,46,48,54,55,58,60,63,64,68,70,101,120,134,135,141–177]
- Analgesia

### Clinical Relevance
This category of pain is relevant to acute injuries, trauma, and a variety of systemic illnesses.

### Treatment Considerations
When you are treating acute nociceptive pain, be aware of **red flags** that require immediate referral to a physician. In addition, determine the type of pain your client is reporting: acute nociceptive pain, recurrent episodes of acute nociceptive pain, nociceptive pain associated with the **chronic stage of inflammation**, **chronic pain** due to other causes, pain that is associated with **chronic pain syndrome**, or **myofascial pain**. Communicate with, and refer to, other health professionals as needed to clarify the client's type of pain. Furthermore, if the client's acute nociceptive pain is the result of a systemic illness, then consider the relevant contraindications and cautions listed in Table 3-2 (see Chapter 3, Clinical Decision Making for Massage).

### Guidelines for Using Massage Techniques
- If tissues are in the acute stage of inflammation, as a result of a recent orthopedic injury:
  - Ensure that the client has received appropriate medical management.
  - Treat the impairments that are causing the client's pain, such as edema and muscle spasm, using the approaches discussed in the relevant sections of this chapter.
  - Depending on the **grade of injury**, the client may not tolerate touch on or near the site of acute injuries. Do not cause pain or increase the client's pain.
  - You may achieve hyperstimulation or counterirritant analgesia by applying superficial reflex or neuromuscular techniques away from the site of injury, on the related dermatome or myotome, or on the contralateral side.[13,121,144] Note that a recent **meta-**

**analysis** disputed the mechanism of hyperstimulation analgesia (gate control theory) and concluded that the immediate effects of massage techniques on pain were not significant.[4]
- In addition, techniques to enhance relaxation can decrease the client's perception of pain.
- If you cannot address the cause of the client's pain directly with massage techniques, for example with acute nociceptive pain associated with cancer,[13,18,20,25,29,32,37,48,64,103,117,133–135,144,154,162,169,173,174,178–189] ensure that the client has appropriate medical management and pay careful attention to the cautions and contraindications related to her particular condition. Once you have done so, use general massage techniques at a tolerable depth to achieve systemic relaxation and hyperstimulation analgesia. Bear in mind that these clients may have other causes of pain, such as trigger points, that you can treat directly with massage techniques.

### Complementary Modalities
- Elevate the client's limb and use cold hydrotherapy for acute-stage inflammation in orthopedic conditions.
- You can use heat, cold, and contrast to achieve hyperstimulation analgesia through spinal gating.
- Use systemic or local heat to achieve sedation.
- To produce hyperstimulation analgesia, use passive movements, joint traction, and joint mobilization techniques on, or around, the damaged structures. Base your treatment on the client's tolerance, relevant contraindications, and your scope of practice.

### Critical Thinking Question
Which strategies for treating pain would be most appropriate for the different categories of pain listed in Box 14-1?

## INTERVENTIONS FOR CIRCULATORY IMPAIRMENTS

## Impaired Venous Return, Impaired Lymphatic Return, Edema, Lymphedema

### Relevant Outcomes
- Improved venous return[190,191]
- Improved lymphatic return
- Reduced edema or lymphedema[117,184,191–200]

## Clinical Relevance

This chapter groups impaired venous return, impaired lymphatic return, edema, and lymphedema together because you use a similar treatment approach for these impairments. These impairments can be associated with a variety of medical conditions, including dependent edema, acute inflammation caused by trauma, varicose veins, chronic venous insufficiency, varicose or venous ulcers, lymphedema secondary to radiation or surgery, cardiomyopathy, and congestive heart failure.

## Treatment Considerations

Note that many of the medical conditions associated with these impairments have their own cautions and contraindications related to the client's medical and pharmaceutical management. In addition to those specific issues, consider the following cautions. Treat traumatic edema according to its stage and clinical presentation[201,202] (see the discussion of inflammation in this chapter). Work gently on or around areas of dystrophic skin. Avoid the immediate vicinity of varicose ulcers and varicose veins.[1,8] *Do not treat clients with congestive heart failure without consulting the supervising physician because increasing fluid return may compromise the client's cardiac function.*[203] Finally, therapists cannot use massage techniques to resolve some forms of lymphedema, such as those due to protein deficiency.[94]

## Guidelines for Using Massage Techniques and Complementary Modalities

- Refer to Chapter 7, Superficial Reflex Techniques, and Chapter 13, Sequencing Massage Techniques, for details of the principles of increasing fluid return and clinical examples. The general treatment approach is to begin treatment proximally, move contact distally,[95] and then repeat this procedure several times or more. Use **centripetal** pressure throughout the treatment.
- Interventions to increase fluid return often consist of only modern or only classical technique, and this may be preferable. It is best not to combine modern techniques (superficial lymph drainage technique or **manual lymph drainage**) and classical techniques (superficial effleurage and petrissage) within a given intervention, unless you are experienced in the use of both approaches.
- Therapists who are familiar with both modern and classical techniques may evaluate the effects of the following combination. Instruct the client in deep diaphragmatic breathing, and encourage this throughout the intervention. Begin with the manual lymph drainage **terminus stroke**[94] and follow this with broad-contact compression performed on the client's upper rib cage.[204] Within the region of edema,

begin proximally and superficially with one or both superficial techniques, applying them using the basic pattern of proximal to distal to proximal. Then proceed slowly to the application of deep effleurage and petrissage with the pattern of proximal to distal to proximal. Finally, perform one or both superficial techniques again. Throughout the entire sequence, alternate your contact back and forth from proximal to distal areas repeatedly, and then return periodically to either terminus or compression of the rib cage.

- Elevated muscle resting tension and connective tissue tightness may exert pressure on vessels and restrict fluid return. Therapists may, therefore, consider treating these impairments.

## Complementary Modalities

- Use positioning and passive movement to assist fluid return.[1,191,205]
- Use joint traction and accessory joint movements to facilitate nutrition of an effused joint.[202,205]
- Muscle contraction is a major cause of lymphatic return; choose from a variety of active exercises according to the client's condition and level of activity.[206,207] Exercises and compression bandages[191,207] may provide most of the benefit of **complex decongestive therapy** in cases of lymphedema.[184,194,195,208,209]
- Clients can use compression pumps[191] and cylindrical rollers[210] for self-massage to promote lymph drainage.
- Use cold hydrotherapy to treat traumatic edema in the acute stage of injury or inflammation and hot hydrotherapy to treat traumatic edema in the chronic stage of injury or inflammation. In these situations, apply hydrotherapy as baths, compresses, or packs.[113,114]

### ? Critical Thinking Question

You are using superficial fluid techniques to increase fluid return. In which direction would you orient your strokes: proximal to distal or distal to proximal? Would your pressure be centripetal or centrifugal? Explain your answers.

# INTERVENTIONS FOR RESPIRATORY IMPAIRMENTS

## Impaired Airway Clearance

### Relevant Outcomes

- Improved airway clearance[211–213]
- Decreased congestion[214]

## Clinical Relevance

Impaired **airway clearance** is associated with pulmonary conditions such as chronic obstructive pulmonary disease, chronic bronchitis, emphysema, asthma, cystic fibrosis, pneumonia, recovery from surgery, and the common cold.

## Treatment Considerations

All or the conditions listed above, except for the common cold, require medical and pharmaceutical management that make it important for you to consider cautions and contraindications to treatment.[215] Decreased airway clearance occurs in conjunction with other respiratory impairments discussed later in this chapter.

Percussion of the thorax is contraindicated in cases of severe rib fracture, untreated tension pneumothorax, confirmed or possible coronary thrombosis or pulmonary embolism, unstable cardiac conditions, conditions that are prone to haemorrhage, after chest or spinal surgery, and during an acute episode of asthma. The positional changes required for **postural drainage** may cause increased oxygen demand, carbon dioxide release, altered blood pressure, and cardiac output. Consequently, therapists must use the head-down position with caution, particularly if clients are hypertensive or have had a head injury. Percussion used alone can also increase heart rate and blood pressure.[216]

## Guidelines for Using Massage Techniques

The standard treatment approach is postural drainage and percussion, although the effectiveness of this procedure is often debated.[211,213,217] Position the client in the relevant postural drainage position. Then apply clapping, rib-springing, rhythmic mobilization, and coarse vibration combined with compression to the related portion of the rib cage (see Chapter 11, Passive Movement Techniques). Encourage the client to exhale forcibly, cough, and expectorate during and following treatment. You may have to teach the client how to initiate a cough.[202] Collect the client's sputum and dispose of it using **Standard Precautions**.[218] An entire sequence may take 50 to 60 minutes or longer. You may choose to drain only a subset of the client's lobes in one particular session.

## Complementary Modalities

- Instruct the client to drink water before and after postural drainage and percussion.
- Immediately precede postural drainage and percussion with a bronchial steam or a bronchial steam with the addition of five drops of eucalyptus or peppermint oil[108] or commercially available products.
- A deep moist heat on the back or front (avoiding the precordium) is an alternative to bronchial steam.[113]

- You can adapt this entire procedure for home use, using percussion administered by a caregiver or even self-clapping administered by the client.
- Effective mechanical alternatives to postural drainage and percussion used in hospitals include intrapulmonary percussive ventilation and high-frequency chest wall compression.[211]

# Elevated Resting Tension of Respiratory Muscles

## Relevant Outcomes

- Decreased resting tension in respiratory muscles
- Reduced muscle tone

## Clinical Relevance

What follows is a specialized version of the treatment for elevated resting tension described elsewhere in this chapter. We include it here because it is an important adjunct to treatment for respiratory conditions, such as chronic obstructive pulmonary disease, asthma, and cystic fibrosis, in which client's inspiration is prolonged and labored. You can also use this treatment for clients on bed rest and athletes competing in aerobic or endurance events.

## Treatment Considerations

The respiratory muscles that are affected include the scalenes, sternocleidomastoid, and the diaphragm. Learn to recognize the **trigger point** referral patterns for these muscles, since these trigger points are a common occurrence (see Chapter 9, Neuromuscular Techniques). Treat trigger points and other coexisting impairments, such as stress and adaptive shortening of the affected muscle(s), at the same time as your treatment for the primary impairment. Note that some of the medical conditions associated with **hypertrophic** respiratory muscles have their own cautions and contraindications related to the client's medical and pharmaceutical management.

## Guidelines for Using Massage Techniques

Use specific neuromuscular and connective tissue techniques for the scalenes, sternocleidomastoid, and diaphragm. If necessary, review the general descriptions of petrissage, stripping, specific compression, myofascial release, and direct fascial technique in Chapter 9, Neuromuscular Techniques, and Chapter 10, Connective Tissue Techniques, as well as Figures 9-10, 9-20, 9-23, 9-29, 10-2, 10-9, and 10-16 and other texts that have regional atlases of techniques.[219–222]

### Complementary Modalities

- Relevant therapeutic exercise includes stretching of the scalenes and sternocleidomastoid muscles.
- Client education on diaphragmatic breathing and other breathing exercises is essential.[112,202]
- Educate clients on the roles of the diaphragm, scalenes, sternocleidomastoid, and abdominal muscles during normal and forced inspiration and expiration.
- Therapists may find progressive aerobic exercise useful for some conditions.

# INTERVENTIONS FOR IMPAIRMENTS RELATED TO MUSCLE

## Unnecessary Muscle Tension

### Relevant Outcomes

- Voluntary release of unnecessary muscle tension
- Improved awareness of unnecessary muscle tension

### Clinical Relevance

Unnecessary muscle tension is a very common cause or result of elevated resting tension in response to situational stress (see the sections on stress in this chapter).

### Treatment Considerations

There are no contraindications associated with this impairment. Two issues to explore prior to treatment are situations in the client's life that may be contributing to situational stress and the client's medications, which may affect muscle resting tension.[215]

### Guidelines for Using Massage Techniques

- Begin with complementary techniques for increasing the client's awareness of unnecessary tension outlined in this section.
- Follow the general approach for a relaxing treatment outlined in the section on stress.
- Once a client has released unnecessary tension, apply the massage techniques that can reduce resting tension (see Elevated Resting Tension section later in this chapter). Whenever a palpable change in resting tension occurs, bring this change to the client's attention to familiarize her with the feeling of her muscles being relaxed and loose.
- The process of facilitating release of unnecessary tension and then decreasing resting tension to a level that

makes an impression on the client is a lengthy one. It may take several 1-hour sessions for a given region and up to several months of treatment before your client can recognize and start to change the physical and mental habits that lead her to tense her muscles in stressful situations.[84,223] If your client undergoes a period of increased stress, you may have to spend one or more sessions refreshing her previously acquired awareness of decreased muscle tension.

### Complementary Modalities

- At the beginning of treatment, clients may not be aware of unnecessary muscle tension. Sometimes simply lifting a limb or placing your hand on an area for up to a minute will be sufficient for a client to realize that she is unnecessarily contracting a muscle. If this does not work, then direct her attention to the area of unnecessary muscle tension with comments such as: "Are you aware that you are holding on here?" "Are you aware of tension here?" "Can you find a way to let this tension go?" Be wary of using language, such as directive commands, that suggests that effort on the client's part is required because the opposite is true.
- Passive movement techniques (see Chapter 11, Passive Movement Techniques) often assist the client in releasing unnecessary muscle tension.

## Elevated Resting Tension

### Relevant Outcomes

- Reduced resting tension[224]

### Clinical Relevance

Elevated resting tension of skeletal muscle is one of the most common reasons that people seek treatment with massage techniques. This impairment is associated with several medical conditions and activities, such as stress,[223] athletic performance, overuse injuries, orthopedic injuries, postural malalignment, trigger points, **fibromyalgia**, arthritis, and connective tissue diseases.

### Treatment Considerations

Prior to beginning treatment to decrease muscle resting tension, ensure that the client has released **unnecessary muscle tension**, using the approach described for that impairment. Resting tension is a complex phenomenon that has passive (material) and active (contractile) components (see Understanding Muscle Resting Tension section in Chapter 5, Client Examination for Massage). Consequently, you need to assess the degree and quality of elevated resting tension in normally innervated muscle using palpation and highly developed manual skills. In addition, identify the cautions and contraindications for the client's medical condition.

### Guidelines for Using Massage Techniques

- Use massage techniques that **engage** muscle and related fascia, especially neuromuscular techniques, connective tissue techniques, and passive movement techniques. *When applying neuromuscular techniques, such as petrissage and stripping, you must engage the layer of muscle in which you wish to change resting tension.*
- Connective tissue techniques, such as myofascial release and direct fascial release, have a local effect on resting tension. In addition, because of the interconnected nature of the fascial layers, they may also have regional effects.
- Using soothing techniques, such as rocking, to achieve a general sedative effect may produce a marginal systemic decrease in muscle resting tension.

### Complementary Modalities

- Heat, either local or systemic, temporarily reduces resting tension.[113,225]
- Systematic stretching also reduces resting tension.[202]
- Aerobic and strength training exercises generally raise muscle resting tension, at least temporarily. Postexercise stretching may counteract this effect.

### Critical Thinking Question

What are the similarities and differences between unnecessary resting tension and elevated resting tension? How would your treatment approaches for these two impairments differ?

## Trigger Points, Myofascial Pain

### Relevant Outcomes

- Decreased trigger point activity[191,226–228]
- Decreased myofascial pain[229,230]
- Increased range of motion[231]

### Treatment Considerations

Myofascial pain can be excruciating. Therefore, you must respect the client's pain during examination and treatment. Trigger points can mimic visceral disease, such as a heart attack,[230] and result in unusual pain referrals and symptoms that seem unrelated to activity.[232,233] In the case of trauma or repetitive strain, finding the exact mecha-

nism of injury can help you identify the muscle(s) with trigger points.

Pain referral patterns for single trigger points correspond to diagrams such as Figure 9-45. Referrals that are commonly seen in a clinical practice include trapezius, sternocleidomastoid, iliocostalis, longissimus, scalenes, pectoralis major and minor, splenius capitus and cervicis, subscapularis, infraspinatus, gluteus medius, tensor fascia lata, hamstrings, quadriceps, tibialis anterior, and tibialis posterior. Table 14-2 describes common myofascial pain syndromes. When a client has multiple trigger points, the referral patterns combine in an overlapping fashion. As a result, the client may perceive a wider distribution of pain that does not correspond to any one trigger point referral map. Identify key trigger points because their treatment may eliminate the need to treat the satellite trigger points.[230] In addition, identify perpetuating factors, as far as possible.

You may have to distinguish between the tender points of fibromyalgia and trigger points.[234] The tender points of fibromyalgia are not trigger points. In addition, the diagnosis of fibromyalgia requires the presence of at least 11 specific tender points and an associated sleep disturbance. Nevertheless, clients with fibromyalgia may also have trigger points that may respond favorably to treatment.[136]

### Guidelines for Using Massage Techniques

- Treatment by any method seeks to restore full, painfree range of motion.
- Stripping and specific compression (trigger point pressure release) are massage techniques designed to treat trigger points (see Chapter 9, Neuromuscular Techniques). You may precede and follow these techniques with regional massage techniques, which include petrissage, myofascial release, or direct fascial technique applied with a broad contact surface.
- Identify and treat primary trigger points first, if possible, since their treatment will reduce symptoms in satellites. Identify and treat all trigger points in a functional unit including agonists, antagonists, and synergists.[230]

### Complementary Modalities

- Follow massage techniques for trigger point release immediately with passive movement through the full range of motion of that muscle (do not overstretch), active movement through the full range of motion, and the application of moist heat.[229,230]
- Moist heat before treatment or by itself is beneficial.[235]
- Since ice packs will increase the activity of trigger points, do not use them on or around trigger points unless you are treating an acute orthopedic injury. Once the acute

## Table 14-2    Myofascial Pain Syndromes[229,230]

Trigger points contribute to pain and dysfunction of virtually all soft tissue injuries such as sprains, repetitive strain injuries, and fractures. However, they can appear on their own, as trigger point syndromes or myofascial pain syndromes. Some myofascial pain syndromes are common enough to have names of their own. Following is a list of conditions in which trigger points are either the sole cause of pain or a major factor in the condition.

| Syndrome | Trigger Points Involved |
|---|---|
| Tension headache | Five common causes of tension headache are trigger points in:<br>■ upper trapezius<br>■ sternocleidomastoid<br>■ splenius capitis and cervicis<br>■ suboccipitals<br>■ temporalis |
| Temporomandibular joint dysfunction | Temporomandibular joint dysfunction may involve actual joint pathology, or it can be due to trigger point activity in the lateral pterygoid, with secondary involvement of the medial pterygoid, masseter, and temporalis |
| Frozen shoulder | Frozen shoulder is a clinical term that may involve fibrosis of the glenohumeral capsule (adhesive capsulitis); it may also be due to trigger points in subscapularis, with secondary involvement of the other rotator cuff muscles |
| Thoracic outlet syndrome | Thoracic outlet syndrome is often caused by entrapment of the trunks of the brachial plexus in between the anterior and medial scalenes or underneath pectoralis minor; trigger points in these muscles may also contribute to the client's pain |
| Trigger finger | This syndrome may involve trigger points in the long finger flexors of the forearm |
| Weeder's thumb | This syndrome may involve trigger points in opponens pollicis |
| Lumbago or back pain | "Lumbago" is an archaic term for lower back pain that has many causes and requires differential assessment; lower back pain can be caused solely by trigger points in the gluteus medius, spinal extensors (erector spinae and multifidi), or psoas, with additional involvement of quadratus lumborum |
| Pseudosciatica | Travell and Simons use this term to refer to an imitation of lumbar **radiculopathy** caused by trigger points in gluteus minimus |
| Piriformis syndrome | This complex syndrome, which may involve entrapment of the sciatic nerve in piriformis, can be caused or perpetuated by trigger points in the piriformis and the other lateral rotators |
| Entrapment syndromes | An entrapment syndrome involves continuous pressure on a peripheral nerve or trunk that causes a **neurapraxia**, with resulting neurological symptoms; an example of an entrapment syndrome that is caused by trigger points is thoracic outlet syndrome; there are many other less common examples detailed in longer texts[229,230] |

stage of an injury has resolved, treat the trigger points as described earlier in this chapter. Use ice in the context of the very specific "ice-and-stretch" protocol described in other texts.[230]

■ Use gentle stretching or the combination of stretching after PNF techniques (agonist contract, hold-relax, and rhythmic stabilization) or postisometric relaxation.[230] When you are using stretching, ensure that you orient the stretch along the affected muscle fibers and avoid producing pain in a related joint (a "positive stretch sign").[228]

■ **Strain-counterstrain** (**positional release**) and high-velocity, low-amplitude techniques maybe of value.[236]

■ For self-care, teach clients a protocol that includes local heat, self-massage, self-stripping, self-compression with a small firm ball, and stretching (or hold-relax), followed by full active range of motion.[235]

■ When teaching self-compression with a ball, limit the treatment time to a few 30-second applications, followed by the appropriate stretch and heat. Clients are prone to overdo self-compression because it feels good; this can cause **reactive cramping** or unbalance the function around a joint. If a client reports that he has to compress a muscle frequently to maintain relief, then conduct a client re-examination to identify factors that are perpetuating the trigger points.

# INTERVENTIONS FOR CONNECTIVE TISSUE IMPAIRMENTS

## Decreased Connective Tissue Mobility

This category includes impairments in which poor tissue modeling compromises normal connective tissue mobility such as **adhesions**, **scarring**, decreased mobility of skin and/or fascia, **fascial restrictions**, and **contractures**. Therapists use a similar treatment approach for this group of impairments.

### Relevant Outcomes

- Increased mobility of connective tissue, including decreased adhesions, improved mobility of scar tissue, increased mobility of skin and fascia, reduced fascial restriction, and reduced contracture[237]
- Increased range of motion[238,239]

### Clinical Relevance

There are several possible causes of decreased connective tissue mobility. First, it often occurs during the chronic stage of inflammatory repair and is, therefore, relevant for orthopedic injuries such as fractures and sprains, various types of arthritis, inflammatory connective tissue diseases, trauma, surgery, and burns. Second, decreased connective tissue mobility can be the result of prolonged periods of reduced mobility that is associated with illness or hospitalization. Finally, it is associated with postural conditions in the form of adaptive tissue shortening. Microscarring and a reduced capacity to adjust to loads may be associated with **repetitive strain injuries** such as **tendinitis** and **tendinosis**.[201]

### Treatment Considerations

Cautions and contraindications for the techniques that therapists use to treat connective tissue restriction include malignancy, cellulitis, fever, systemic or local infection, acute circulatory conditions, osteomyelitis, aneurysm, obstructive edema, acute rheumatoid arthritis, open wounds, sutures, hematomas, healing fractures, osteoporosis, anticoagulant therapy, advanced diabetes, and hypersensitivity of the skin.[240] Prior to treating decreased connective tissue mobility, *ensure that the client has no signs of local acute inflammation.* Some orthopedic conditions, such as repeated sprains or rheumatoid arthritis, may involve joint laxity or instability. Do not treat these joints with techniques that attempt to lengthen the already lengthened or weakened

connective tissue. Finally, do not treat any area of connective tissue in isolation; local treatment will have a systemic effect that will facilitate postural changes.

### Guidelines for Using Massage Techniques

- Skin rolling, myofascial release, direct fascial technique, and friction (see Chapter 10, Connective Tissue Techniques) are the main techniques for treating decreased connective tissue mobility.[221,222,241-245] When a large amount of tissue is affected, as with postural adaptive shortening or contracture of a large joint, use broad surfaces and more general techniques. These include myofascial release with widely positioned hands and direct fascial techniques delivered with the forearm. To treat smaller amounts of tissue, for example localized fibrosis within a tendon[246] or a capsule,[238] use specific techniques such as friction applied with fingers or thumb(s). In addition, you may find petrissage and stripping beneficial if you apply them slowly and with sufficient drag; avoiding the use of too much oil will enable you to achieve this.
- When multiple layers of tissue are affected, begin at the surface and progress treatment through the restrictions in deeper layers.
- Early-stage treatment of burns, to prevent or reduce the formation of scar tissue, involves highly specialized protocols that are beyond the scope of this text.[237,247] Box 14-2 outlines some "scar techniques" that may be appropriate for use on *mature* scar tissue.
- **Rhythmic mobilization** applied *after* the treatment of connective tissue may enhance the client's movement patterns.
- Myofascial trigger points often coexist with many varieties of connective tissue restriction.[229,230,248-250] See guidelines for treatment of trigger points presented earlier in this chapter and in Chapter 9, Neuromuscular Techniques, in the sections on stripping and specific compression.
- If connective tissue restriction is associated with poor posture, refer to the section on adaptive shortening later in this chapter.
- Monitor the treatment effects, before and after treatment, using a postural scan.
- Long-lasting lengthening of connective tissue happens quickly, provided that you use the correct technique. In fact, with some conditions, you can see positive treatment effects within several minutes. Consequently, small, uncomplicated, and recently matured scars may respond in a single session. Longstanding conditions will require several local treatment sessions to achieve lasting change, as well as more general treatments to

---

**Box 14-2**     **Scar Techniques for Mature Scars**

So-called "scar techniques" that are used to model a *mature* scar are simply examples of all the connective tissue techniques previously described in detail in Chapter 10, Connective Tissue Techniques. Apply these in an orderly sequence that begins with light pressure to engage superficial layers and then proceeds to engage deeper layers of restriction. Remember that the area of reduced mobility often extends far to the sides of a visible scar and far below the surface.

**Skin rolling.** Grasp and roll the skin and subcutaneous fascia along like a wave. Vary the lifting force and direction of the stroke during repeated passes. Use this as an introductory technique and to periodically assess the mobility of the superficial tissues as treatment proceeds.[201]

**Myofascial release.** Using fingertip or palmar contact, take the slack out of the skin and subcutaneous tissues.[201] Then hold this position, without gliding, for 90 seconds or longer while **creep** occurs. Increase pressure with successive applications to engage the deeper tissue layers. Vary the direction of the force. Use two-handed releases with widely positioned hands if the restriction affects a large area.

**Direct fascial technique.** Use one or two slowly gliding digits to bow the scar tissue into a C shape or an S shape[9,201] or make the stroke follow a J pattern.[244] Use your grouped fingers or your entire palm if the restriction affects a large area.

**Friction.** Use friction, applied with your fingertips or thumbs on very dense hard areas, until palpable softening occurs. Orient strokes transverse or parallel to the scar or use circles.[201] Use a broad surface such your palm for a large restriction.

---

address compensations that exist throughout the client's body. Widespread fascial restriction, which is seen with postural conditions, can take more than 15 hours of treatment.

### Complementary Modalities

- Use stretching exercises within the full range of motion.[202]
- Use higher grade **joint mobilization** if adhesions affect the joint capsule.[201,202]
- Use active exercises, within the full range of motion, after you have restored muscle length. Both stretching and active exercises are also effective within the client's self-care program.
- Follow changes in alignment with postural awareness exercises (see Decreased Postural and Kinesthetic Awareness, later in this chapter).
- Consider therapeutic exercise for increasing muscle performance (strength, endurance, power) once you have restored mobility.[247]
- Local heat is appropriate before massage techniques (allow several minutes to elapse before applying connective tissue techniques) or stretching. Before you apply heat, ensure that there are no signs of acute inflammation.

# INTERVENTIONS FOR POSTURAL IMPAIRMENTS

## Postural Malalignment due to Bony Deformity

### Relevant Outcomes

- Improved postural alignment

### Clinical Relevance

Bony deformity, such as small hemipelvis or true leg-length discrepancy, may play a role in hyperkyphosis, hyperlordosis, and scoliosis.[229] Systemic conditions like Scheuermann's disease, tuberculosis of the spine, and bone cancer may also cause or contribute to postural conditions.

### Treatment Considerations

Refer the client to an appropriate health care professional for correction of bony asymmetry with orthotics, prosthetics, or surgery.

### Guidelines for Using Massage Techniques

- If possible, do not attempt to treat tissue contractures or adaptive shortening until the client has had his underlying bony malalignment corrected.
- Use neuromuscular or connective tissue techniques at a moderate depth, as required for symptomatic pain relief in areas of elevated resting tension and trigger points.[251]
- After correction of the bony malalignment, treat adaptive shortening, adaptive lengthening, and decreased postural awareness using massage techniques described in the relevant sections of this chapter.

### Complementary Modalities

- After correction of the bony malalignment, use complementary modalities for adaptive shorting, adaptive lengthening, and decreased postural awareness as described in the relevant sections of this chapter.

## Adaptive Shortening with Impaired Balance of Agonist/Antagonist Muscle Function

### Relevant Outcomes

- Increased extensibility of muscle and fascia
- Improved balance of agonist/antagonist muscle function
- Improved postural alignment[252]

### Clinical Relevance

Adaptive shortening of soft tissues may be associated with hyperkyphosis, hyperlordosis, scoliosis, iliotibial band contracture, valgus knee structure, patellofemoral syndrome, and pes planus.[1,2,202]

### Treatment Considerations

Before you begin an intervention for adaptive shortening, ensure that it is not the result of asymmetrical bone structure, such as a true leg-length discrepancy[251] or small hemipelvis. If that is the case, consult the earlier section on postural deformity for a modified approach. Study at length the relationships between fascial planes and layers that anatomy texts describe.[253] Be aware that releasing shortened structures can result in fairly quick changes in the client's postural alignment. Those changes may, in turn, change the mechanical load on other structures and result in a change in the client's symptoms.

### Guidelines for Using Massage Techniques

- With postural conditions, the client's pain is frequently the result of a stretch on the antagonist muscles that oppose the shortened myofascial units. One standard approach to treatment is to *treat shortened structures first.*[254] If the client's pain is severe, you may choose to treat the lengthened structures first or concurrently with those that show adaptive shortening.
- Connective tissue techniques are the methods of choice for treating adaptive shortening.[220–222,244] Neuromuscular techniques are less effective but useful (see the Outcomes and Evidence section for Petrissage in Chapter 9, Neuromuscular Techniques). Neither superficial reflex nor superficial fluid techniques engage the relevant tissue layers of muscle and associated fascia. Furthermore, passive movement and percussive techniques do not subject the tissues to sufficient **drag**. Note that myofascial release and direct fascial technique require sustained horizontal traction force along layers to lengthen the fascia (see Chapter 10, Connective Tissue Techniques). Use specific compression and stripping,[252] since adaptively shortened structures often contain trigger points.[229,230,255] Finally, passive movement techniques, such as rhythmic mobilization, applied *after* connective tissue and neuromuscular techniques can help to restore more expansive movement patterns.[95]
- Assess the client's posture before and after interventions with a postural scan. Record treatment effects carefully.
- Box 14-3 presents a simple protocol for treating adaptive shortening.

### Complementary Modalities

- Local heat is appropriate before massage techniques or stretching. Allow several minutes to elapse before applying connective tissue techniques.
- Use therapeutic exercise for stretching the shortened tissues.[202]
- Use active exercises within the full range of motion after you have restored muscle length.
- Include both stretching and active exercises in the client's self-care program.
- Therapeutic exercise to improve muscle performance is essential; consult texts on therapeutic exercise for details.[202]
- Follow changes in postural alignment with postural awareness exercises (see Chapter 6, Preparation and Positioning for Massage).

| Box 14-3 | A Simple Massage Protocol to Treat Adaptive Shortening |
|---|---|

Following is a simple protocol that you can use to structure a single session of 30, 45, or 60 minutes to treat adaptive shortening.

1. Perform a **postural scan**.
2. Choose a target group of muscles that shows adaptive shortening.
3. Briefly apply broad, general direct fascial technique or myofascial release *to the region*.
4. Lengthen the target group of muscles with specific connective tissue techniques and then stretch them.
5. Treat the entire region with neuromuscular techniques, such as petrissage, and then rhythmic mobilization.
6. Address the opposite side similarly, following Steps 3 to 5.
7. Address the related axial skeleton with broad connective tissue techniques and neuromuscular techniques such as petrissage.
8. Be sure to include the paraspinal and neck musculature as in Step 7, if only briefly.
9. Monitor changes with a postural scan.
10. Guide the client through standing aligned posture, as described in Chapter 6, Preparation and Positioning for Massage.

Progress this intervention by choosing a different group of adaptively shortened muscles at each session.

### Critical Thinking Question

In interventions that address postural conditions, why treat shortened areas earlier in the intervention?

# INTERVENTIONS FOR IMPAIRMENTS RELATED TO INFLAMMATION

## Acute-Stage Inflammation

### Relevant Outcomes
- Reduced signs and symptoms of inflammation, such as reduced edema
- Reduced pain
- Increased active range of motion

### Clinical Relevance
Acute inflammation can be associated with a variety of orthopedic medical conditions, including musculoskeletal trauma, repetitive strain injuries, and osteoarthritis. It also occurs after surgery. Finally, it can accompany various systemic conditions such as rheumatoid arthritis and related connective tissue diseases.

### Treatment Considerations
Prior to treating traumatic orthopedic injuries, ensure that the client's anatomical structures are stable. If you are in doubt, refer the client for medical assessment and management. When inflammation is secondary to a repetitive strain injury, identify the causal activity and find out if the client can reduce or cease that activity. When inflammation is associated with osteoarthritis or any systemic disease, understand how the client's medical and pharmacological management affects his inflammatory process, pain, edema, and spasm.

### Guidelines for Using Massage Techniques
Acute inflammation is not an impairment; instead, it is a physiological process that is associated with a *group* of impairments including primarily edema, acute nociceptive pain, and spasm. This section reviews the treatment approaches for the primary impairments associated with inflammation and includes an example of how to combine treatment techniques within a single intervention.

*Initial Treatment*
- First, treat any edema that is present because resolution of the edema will also reduce pain.
- You can use several techniques to facilitate the resolution of edema. Apply broad-contact compression or superficial lymph drainage (**terminus stroke**) to the junction of common lymphatic duct and vena cava in the thorax. Apply superficial fluid techniques proximal to the site of inflammation (working distally to the peripheral margin of swelling) repetitively for 20 minutes or more to drain edema (see Chapter 8, Superficial Fluid Techniques). Apply neuromuscular techniques proximally to open the deep lymphatic drainage.
- To inhibit spasm, apply very gentle petrissage and gentle specific compression to unaffected portions of muscles that pass through the inflamed area (see the section on spasm in this chapter).
- To inhibit pain, apply superficial reflex techniques as tolerated to the site. When the client's lesion is more severe and local touch is contraindicated, you can achieve counterirritant analgesia by applying these techniques

proximally in the related dermatome, to antagonist muscle groups, or even to the contralateral side.

- There may be a variety of other impairments away from the site of injury, such as reduced active range of motion, elevated resting tension, and trigger points, which respond to the appropriate massage techniques (see the sections on range of motion, elevated resting tension, and trigger points). When working away from the side of the edema, do not attempt to push fluid through a congested area, and avoid placing excessive mechanical stress on the remote sections of structures that pass through the injury site.

### Progression of Massage Techniques through the Subacute Stage

- Apply superficial fluid techniques closer to the center of the site of the injury as the edema lessens and local sensitivity at the site of the injury declines. In addition, once the local edema has resolved, increase the pressure of the massage technique through the superficial tissues to engage the investing layer of the deep fascia and then the superficial muscular layers. Introduce light neuromuscular and connective tissue techniques and small-amplitude passive movement techniques to apply a stress to the newly deposited connective tissue elements.
- You can treat off-site impairments somewhat more aggressively in the subacute stage than you could in the acute stage, as long as you keep the relevant cautions in mind.

### Complementary Modalities

#### Initial Treatment

- To treat edema, elevate the body segment 30 to 45 degrees and apply an ice pack. Ice promotes **retrostasis**, provides anesthesia, and reduces spasm.[113,225]
- Encourage *deep* diaphragmatic breathing.
- To inhibit pain in the region of a stable joint, use passive movements and gentle joint mobilization techniques, as the client's tolerance and your scope of practice permit.[202]
- To maintain muscle performance, have the client perform isometric muscle contractions of the muscles that pass through the inflamed area, within his level of tolerance.
- Educate the client about the nature of his condition, the requirement for rest, and the use of elevation, ice, compressive bandages, and assistive devices such as splints or crutches.[202]

## Chronic-Stage Inflammation

### Relevant Outcomes

- Reduced signs and symptoms of inflammation, such as improved connective tissue modeling, reduced pain, and full active range of motion

### Clinical Relevance

The chronic stage of inflammation can be associated with a variety of conditions, including trauma, orthopedic injuries, repetitive strain injuries, surgery, osteoarthritis, rheumatoid arthritis, and related connective tissue diseases.

### Treatment Considerations

Assess how chronic or subacute injuries are progressing with treatment on the following dimensions. Determine whether the treatment was appropriate and successful. Confirm the clinical stage of the injury based on findings from the client examination.[201,202] Ensure that reinjury has not exacerbated the acute stage of an orthopedic condition. Finally, when inflammation is associated with osteoarthritis or any systemic disease, understand how the client's medical and pharmacological management affects his inflammatory process, pain, and other symptoms.

### Guidelines for Using Massage Techniques

- Chronic inflammation is not an impairment; instead, it is a physiological process with a *group* of associated impairments, which differ from those associated with acute inflammation. The main impairments that occur at the site of inflammation are the result of poor connective tissue modeling during the repair process. These impairments include adhesions, scarring, consolidated edema, fascial restriction, and abnormal density and reduced mobility of connective tissue structures. You can treat all of these impairments in a similar manner using connective tissue and neuromuscular techniques.
- If you are continuing an intervention in which you addressed the acute stage of the client's inflammatory process, gradually increase the force with which you apply neuromuscular and connective tissue techniques at the site of injury. You will not need to use more than moderate force because your use of massage techniques in the earlier stages of healing would promote adequate tissue modeling. The entire progression of massage techniques on the site of injury from the acute stage through the chronic stage might take 4 or more weeks for a second- or third-degree injury.
- The intervention will differ on sites of old injuries that were inadequately treated or not treated at all and

when there is longstanding musculoskeletal pain after an injury.

*Progression When the Client Presents with Longstanding Chronic-stage Tissue Restrictions*

■ In this case, you may have to use some force and persistence over several interventions to progress through the restrictions that exist in the different layers of muscle and connective tissue. Furthermore, compensatory changes and multiple sources of pain may complicate your progression of the client's intervention.

### Compensatory Changes

■ **Compensatory changes** in the musculoskeletal system that develop in response to local damage, such as restrictions in mobility, movement, and coordination, complicate chronic injuries.[256] The severity and extent of these compensatory changes often reflect the severity of the original tissue damage and the amount of time that has elapsed since the injury. A client's complaints of chronic impairments that had an insidious onset may be the result of these compensatory changes. Furthermore, the client may be unaware of the causal relationship between a forgotten injury and his current complaints.

■ Begin treatment by locating and addressing the layers of restriction *at the original site of injury.* You must also identify and treat shortening in soft tissue that has arisen as a mechanical consequence of the original injury in order to achieve a satisfactory resolution of the client's impairments and associated functional limitations. Unraveling the compensatory patterns[256] associated with a chronic injury may take more time than your treatment of the original injury.

### Multiple Sources of Pain

■ The client may present with multiple sources of local and referred pain in his muscles, fascia, and joints because longstanding chronic conditions can result in the development of widespread restrictions in multiple layers of soft tissue.[256] As a result, you may find it impossible to identify any one tissue or structure as the primary focus of your treatment.

■ In this situation, consider performing several interventions of progressively deeper neuromuscular and connective tissue techniques at the outset of treatment in order to reduce the tension in the superficial layers of muscle and connective tissue throughout the body. This strategy may reduce both compensatory changes and multiple sources of pain. As you progressively reduce the tension in

the superficial and deeper tissue layers, the client may experience a succession of both familiar and unfamiliar symptoms that endure for days or weeks. The end result is that you, and the client, will probably be able to identify one tissue or structure as the primary focus of treatment.

### A Strategy for Achieving Adequate Depth in the Treatment of Chronic Lesions

■ Inexperienced therapists often attempt to cover too wide an area with too general a focus when they are treating chronic lesions. As a result, their treatment fails because they have not worked deeply enough in any one area. The application of specific deep massage techniques is indispensable but time consuming. A single area, such as the shoulder, can take anywhere from 30 to 90 minutes to treat. When you need to use deep, specific massage techniques extensively, subdivide the client's body into smaller manageable areas and schedule the treatment of these areas for two or more consecutive sessions.

■ Ensure that you include **general massage** techniques and address the client's antagonist and synergist muscle groups to minimize the potential for imbalances in the client's myofascial system.

### Complementary Modalities

■ Complementary techniques for chronic inflammation include all forms of stretching, joint traction, and joint mobilization.

■ Poor strength and endurance associated with chronic inflammatory processes respond to progressive strengthening and aerobic exercise.

### Critical Thinking Question

What are the similarities and differences between your treatment approach for acute-stage inflammation and chronic-stage inflammation?

# INTERVENTIONS RELATED TO IMPAIRMENTS IN RANGE OF MOTION

## Reduced Active Range of Motion

### Treatment Considerations

Reduced active range of motion is a common impairment *that you must treat by addressing one or more causal impairments or conditions.* It is extremely important for you to identify the underlying cause(s) of the reduction in range of motion before you begin treatment. Any of the following impairments or conditions can cause the client to exhibit reduced active range of motion:

- Adaptive shortening
- Joint or bone malformation
- Inflammation (trauma and surgery are two very common causes)
- Mechanical instability (from a fracture or ruptured structure)
- Scar tissue, connective tissue shortening, and adhesions
- Pain (pain itself is often secondary to other impairments)
- Trigger points
- Increased muscle resting tension
- Muscle spasm
- Muscle weakness
- General deconditioning (if severe)
- Edema
- Spastic paralysis
- Flaccid paralysis
- Rigidity
- Atrophy (due to disuse or abnormal innervation)

See the guidelines for treating many of these impairments in relevant sections of this chapter.

# INTERVENTIONS FOR NEUROLOGICAL IMPAIRMENTS

Neurological impairments require more advanced approaches to treatment, which we describe in Interventions for Impairments: Further Study and Practice.

---

## Theory In Practice:

### Juggling Many Impairments

#### Patient Profile

Your patient is a successful 50-year-old architect who currently works part-time due to family obligations and health issues. Her family doctor diagnosed fibromyalgia 1 year ago after she experienced several years of progressive pain. A neurologist also recently diagnosed carpal tunnel syndrome. She sought treatment for help managing the pain and fatigue associated with **fibromyalgia**.

#### Clinical Findings

Subjective:

- Her main complaints are widespread constant musculo-skeletal pain, stiffness, and frequent whole-head headaches.
- Pain: Her baseline VAS pain level is about 3/10, and this frequently rises to 6 or 7/10. Pain interrupts her sleep several times a night.
- Paresthesia: She rates the tingling pain in her right wrist as less important; it bothers her only after long periods of computer drafting and occasionally wakes her up at night.
- Fatigue: She also complains of fatigue, which limits her ability to work and to participate in recreational activities with her family.
- Sleep: She sleeps in the fetal position.

Objective:

- Posture: Hyperkyphosis, an anterior head posture, and an upper-crossed syndrome.
- Observation: There is no obvious swelling anywhere in the upper limbs.
- Range of Motion: Cervical range of motion is limited in a capsular pattern; side flexion and rotations are equally limited, extension is limited.
- Neurological Tests: Cervical range of motion does not reproduce hand paresthesia. Thoracic outlet tests on both sides show absent pulses without reproducing hand symptoms. Carpal tunnel tests, such as Phalen's, reproduce tingling in the hand on the right side after 15 seconds.
- Palpation: Tender points associated with fibromyalgia. There are numerous trigger points and hard, indurated areas throughout her musculature.

#### Treatment Approach

- The list of this patient's impairments is long and includes: stress, interrupted sleep, fatigue, altered body image, acute nociceptive pain, chronic pain, probable deconditioning, elevated resting tension, trigger points, adaptive shortening and lengthening, and decreased postural awareness.
- In developing your plan of care, review the treatment considerations and guidelines for massage techniques associated with these impairments. For example, her potential for fatigue requires an approach that is gentle and not taxing.
- Initially, it may be useful to limit treatment to 30 minutes and apply massage techniques with light to moderate pressure. Once you learn how she responds to treat-

ment, you will likely be able to increase both the length and depth of treatment. Within this framework, you can attempt the full range of massage techniques, including all neuromuscular and connective tissue techniques.

- Areas of priority include the head, anterior and posterior neck, anterior chest, arms, and back. You will not be able to address all of these in depth in each session. Consequently, you will have to schedule particular areas of focus for the first 5 or 10 sessions, while reserving some time in each session to address areas of concern that arise on the day of treatment. If possible, include the whole body each session, even if briefly. You can accomplish this with the skillful use of rocking and other general techniques.

- Given the likelihood that she has developed a chronic pain syndrome, encourage her to consult service organizations, such as the local Fibromyalgia Society, and other health care professionals.

- For initial homecare, teach stretching, especially of the neck and upper body, relaxation techniques such as diaphragmatic breathing, and walking within her tolerance. She may find a nighttime wrist splint helpful.

- You can progress this intervention by increasing the pressure and duration of massage techniques to her tolerance. Progress her homecare program by increasing the variety of techniques that you use to address the different impairments.

- Conduct a thorough re-examination of this patient (and of all patients with chronic conditions) at the end of every period for which you have set an outcome, for example, every 6 to 8 weeks. At each re-examination, revisit the outcomes and priorities you have established for this patient and, if necessary, draft a new plan of care (see Chapter 3, Clinical Decision Making for Massage). Discharge this patient when she has achieved all of the outcomes in her plan of care for that episode of care.

## Interventions for Impairments: Further Study and Practice

# INTERVENTIONS FOR PSYCHONEUROIMMUNO-LOGICAL IMPAIRMENTS

## Altered Body Image

### Relevant Outcomes
- Improved body image[53,67,128,257–259]

### Clinical Relevance
**Altered body image** may be a relevant impairment for clients with eating disorders,[53] depression,[128] serious or life-threatening diseases, cancer,[258,260,261] mastectomy,[257] surgery, amputation, disfigurement through trauma or burns, stroke, aging, history of physical or sexual abuse,[87,259,262,263] and posttraumatic stress disorder.[88,264]

### Treatment Considerations
Each condition listed above, with the exception of uncomplicated aging, requires appropriate medical and/or psychiatric management. Refer to and consult with other health care professionals as the client's condition requires.[128]

### Guidelines for Using Massage Techniques and Complementary Modalities
- When you are treating clients with altered body image, your approach to the client and her issues are more important than the massage techniques that you use.[88] In particular, provide support, understanding, clear communication with the client, and very careful attention to consent.

- When you apply massage techniques, include as much of the client's body as the relevant contraindications and cautions permit. In addition, treat affected and unaffected areas during the same treatment.

- These clients may have avoided touching an injured or painful area or a surgical site for a long period of time, even years. You may have to treat these areas in stages, beginning with static contact on adjacent areas and gradually moving towards the site.

- Use general massage strokes to cover entire regions and promote relaxation.

- Use guided awareness and static contact to focus the client's attention on areas that are relevant to her presenting issues.
- The relatively rare phenomenon of **somatoemotional release** is more likely to happen when a client has experienced trauma.[86] Box 14-4 suggests basic guidelines for working with clients who experience somatoemotional release during interventions.
- Consider structuring interventions in three parts that sequentially aim to establish trust and safety, allow the client to explore sensation, and obtain healthy closure.[88] Consult the details of this process in Chapter 4, Interpersonal and Ethical Issues for Massage.

---

| Box 14-4 | **When a Client Experiences Emotional Release** |
|---|---|

Here are some guidelines for entry-level clinicians to use when clients experience emotional release during the intervention.[86,96,264,265]

**DO**

1. Honor emotional release without encouraging it. Be open to observing it.
2. Let a client who is experiencing a release know that the phenomenon is normal. Briefly explain **tissue memory** and **touch-triggered memory**.
3. Ask him if he wants you to stop working or to take your hands off his body.
4. Relax while you allow the release to take its normal course, often less than 10 minutes.
5. Encourage the client to acknowledge what has happened.
6. Offer the client the opportunity to talk about the experience, without pressuring him to do so.
7. **Ground** the client at the intervention's end with sedative work on the sacrum and feet.
8. Have on hand a pamphlet that explains what touch-triggered memory is. Be prepared to refer to it, if this seems appropriate.
9. Ensure that the client is able to drive or to use public transit before he leaves.

**DO NOT**

1. Move the focus of the intervention to the area where the release is centered.
2. Pressure the client to give details about "what is going on."
3. Engage in or make any attempt to interpret emotional content.
4. Leave the client alone until he indicates that he is ready.

---

# INTERVENTIONS FOR IMPAIRMENTS RELATED TO PAIN

## Chronic Pain, Chronic Pain Syndromes

### Relevant Outcomes

- Increased functional activity[140,266]
- Analgesia[16,267,268]
- Decreased depression

### Treatment Considerations

- *The primary outcome is improved functional activity* when you are treating clients with chronic pain and chronic pain syndromes. While the reduction of pain is desirable, it does not always occur and, consequently, is not always the measure of a successful treatment.
- Be aware of **red flags** that require immediate referral to a physician. In addition, follow the guidelines in this chapter for determining the client's type of pain.
- Chronic pain is a distinct, complex medical condition that requires an interdisciplinary approach to treatment.[140,269] Treatment, especially of **chronic pain syndrome**, does not depend primarily on the treatment of other impairments, such as edema or muscle tension, although such treatment may be useful.
- Clients with chronic pain may show unusual patterns of pain behavior and are often clinically depressed.[270] Consequently, if a client presents with a diagnosis of chronic pain or you suspect that this may be her diagnosis, communicate with or refer her to a physician for appropriate treatment.
- Be conscious of the client's potential for dependency on your interventions.[271]
- Be aware that the client's expectations about massage techniques may affect their treatment outcomes.[266]

### Critical Thinking Question

What are the similarities and differences between your outcomes and treatment approaches for acute nociceptive pain and chronic pain syndrome?

### Guidelines for Using Massage Techniques

- *Ensure that you have addressed all treatable causes of pain.*
- Explore the use of *all* massage techniques, since they are potentially useful.

- Progress from superficial to deep massage techniques within the client's tolerance.

## Complementary Modalities

- Machines that produce 100-Hz vibration are inexpensive. Clinicians can easily incorporate them into massage interventions without sacrificing hands-on time. They are also good for homecare.
- **TENS** relieves many kinds of pain,[272–278] and clients can self-administer this modality.
- Clients may find self-massage useful.
- All hydrotherapy methods are potentially useful, including: local hot and cold packs, whirlpool, whirlpool followed by cold shower, percussion douche,[113,114,279] and longer interventions designed to promote autonomic homeostasis.[141,279]
- Encourage aerobic exercise to prevent or reduce deconditioning.
- Use stretching, diaphragmatic breathing, relaxation training, and specific visualization methods for helping clients cope with pain.[110]
- Adapt as many techniques as possible for self-care. Emphasize self-care that improves the client's level of functional activity and independence.

# INTERVENTIONS FOR CIRCULATORY IMPAIRMENTS

## Impaired Arterial Supply

### Relevant Outcomes

- Improved arterial supply[127,280–283]
- Improved tissue oxygenation

### Treatment Considerations

Clients who present with local impairment of their arterial supply may also have an associated cardiovascular disease that has specific cautions and contraindications. In addition, applying heat to the extremities is often contraindicated in clients with impaired arterial supply (e.g., diabetics) because local heating may increase the metabolic demand of the tissues beyond what the circulatory system can supply[138] and, consequently, result in tissue damage. In this situation, some clinicians also believe that **circulatory massage** techniques are contraindicated,[203] although it is unclear how much massage techniques can increase arterial supply (see the Outcomes and Evidence section for Petrissage in Chapter 9, Neuromuscular Techniques). Finally, both heat and mas-

sage techniques may be contraindications for clients with diabetes due to the reduced sensation associated with diabetic neuropathy.

### Guidelines for Using Massage Techniques

- Current research is not consistent about whether any massage technique will significantly increase arterial supply.[3,127,281,282,284–289] It is unlikely that superficial reflex techniques increase arterial supply. The authors suspect that massage techniques, such as broad-contact compression and petrissage, are limited in their ability to produce this effect unless the clinician's manual technique is extremely precise. For example, hyperemia following tapotement may only indicate a change in **perfusion**, rather than an overall increase in the volume of blood going through the tissues.[290]
- Exponents of European schools of medical massage describe reflex circulatory effects, which can be achieved through precise, studied application of various neuromuscular and connective tissue techniques.[106,107,291]
- Repetitive mechanical compression devices may increase blood supply[291] as well as return.

### Complementary Modalities

- Exercise, especially aerobic exercise, is the most effective method of increasing arterial supply.
- Local heat increases arterial supply.[225] Clinicians can use it in healthy clients, although it may be contraindicated in those with advanced circulatory disease or diabetes.[203]
- A short cold wash or a heat treatment applied proximally over a supplying artery may be useful in clients for whom a heat treatment in the affected region is contraindicated.[113,138]

# INTERVENTIONS FOR RESPIRATORY IMPAIRMENTS

## Chest Wall Tightness

### Relevant Outcomes

- Increased chest wall mobility

### Treatment Considerations

This impairment is associated with impairments or medical conditions that result in restricted breathing, such as stress, postural malalignment such as scoliosis and kyphosis, trigger points in certain muscles, respiratory conditions such as emphysema, and prolonged bed rest or inactivity. Because treatment involves the use of pressure on the client's chest wall, identify whether mechanical massage techniques are contraindicated for the client's condition. This would be the case for osteoporosis, osteomalacia, chest wounds, or a flail chest. Note that longstanding postural dysfunction or organ pathology, such as barrel chest in emphysema, may limit improvements in chest wall mobility.

### Guidelines for Using Massage Techniques

■ The first phase of treatment involves freeing restrictions in the muscles and connective tissue superficial to the ribs. Work with the client in side-lying, supine, and prone. In each position, apply general neuromuscular and connective tissue techniques, such as wringing and the myofascial release arm pull, to muscles of the trunk from the pubis/sacrum to the clavicle.[179]

■ Apply specific neuromuscular techniques and connective tissue techniques to all the intercostal spaces. Systematically work your fingertips or thumbs ("stripping" or "rib-raking") *into* the intercostal spaces and around the clavicle and costal arch. This specific work may take you 1 or 2 hours, and you may have to split it between several interventions.

■ After you have freed restrictions in muscle or connective tissue, apply rhythmic mobilization ("rib-springing"), rib compressions, and rocking to the rib cage.

### Complementary Modalities

■ Stretching and facilitated stretching to the thorax increase thoracic mobility.[202]

■ For self-care, teach your client a combination of controlled deep breathing and stretching exercises of the large muscle groups of the thorax, such as the pectorals and spinal extensors.

■ Systemic or regional application of heat can precede massage techniques or exercise.

■ **Hatha yoga** is an appropriate home practice for people with chest wall tightness.

## Abnormal or Altered Breathing Patterns

### Relevant Outcomes

■ Improved or normalized breathing patterns

### Clinical Relevance

A less than optimal breathing pattern, with an overuse of accessory muscles of inspiration and an underuse of the diaphragm, occurs frequently in the general population. In addition, altered breathing patterns are associated with multiple impairments and medical conditions that restrict breathing, including stress, postural malalignment, trigger points in certain muscles, respiratory conditions, the use of tobacco, and prolonged bed rest or inactivity.

### Treatment Considerations

Begin your treatment by identifying the abnormalities in your client's breathing pattern. Determine whether she presents with a "paradoxical" breathing pattern, in which the abdominal diameter decreases during inspiration.[229] In addition, understand how your client's medical condition or impairments contribute to her abnormal breathing pattern.

### Guidelines for Using Massage Techniques

■ Treat your client's other respiratory impairments, such as chest wall tightness and elevated resting tension of respiratory muscles, with relevant massage techniques prior to initiating education on normal respiration.

### Complementary Modalities

■ Education is the main approach to normalizing clients' breathing patterns. First, help your client develop an awareness of his current pattern of breathing. Have him place his hands on specified structures (scalenes, sternocleidomastoid, and the chest and abdominal walls) to monitor them for muscular contraction or shifts in position during inspiration and expiration. Looking in a mirror may also help the client to become familiar with his current habits of breathing. Once he has grasped these concepts, teach him how to perform diaphragmatic breathing and how to notice the difference between this breathing pattern and upper chest breathing and lateral costal breathing.[202]

■ Diaphragm strengthening (breathing with weights, "sandbag breathing")[202,293] can be extremely important in respiratory diseases.[202]

■ Improved postural awareness may facilitate a normalized breathing pattern.

## INTERVENTIONS FOR IMPAIRMENTS RELATED TO MUSCLE

## Muscle Spasm

### Relevant Outcomes

■ Reduced muscle spasm[294]

## Clinical Relevance

Muscle spasm is associated with spasmodic **torticollis**, traumatic orthopedic injuries, disk lesions and other conditions that compress nerves or nerve roots, athletic performance, acute visceral conditions such as appendicitis, arterial disorders including intermittent claudication, and pregnancy. It can also be the side effect of some medications, such as lithium, and the result of nutritional deficiencies. Exposure to cold, dehydration, pre-existing trigger points, and postural imbalance exacerbate muscle spasm.

## Treatment Considerations

If you client presents with acute muscle spasm, attempt to find the cause of the spasm since this may require a referral to a physician, as in the case of recent trauma or metabolic imbalance in a runner. Furthermore, your assessment of the acuity of the client's condition can guide your approach to treatment.

## Guidelines for Using Massage Techniques and Complementary Modalities

- Do not stretch a muscle that is in extreme spasm.
- Incorporate all techniques for relaxation, such as diaphragmatic breathing and relaxing or sedative massage techniques, away from the site of spasm.
- On the site of spasm, attempt the following ordered progression of techniques, while ensuring that you *do not increase your client's pain*. Perform all techniques within the client's tolerance.
  1. Contract the antagonist. This activity moves the muscle in spasm into a lengthened position. Repeat this active lengthening between other techniques.
  2. Apply specific compression and cross-fiber petrissage on the attachments of the muscle. Combine these with active movement within the client's tolerance.[241,294]
  3. Apply specific compression, using your thumbs to drag the two attachments of the muscle in spasm towards the muscle belly ("muscle approximation").[218]
  4. Use superficial reflex techniques such as superficial stroking (caution with fine vibration) on site.
  5. Apply gentle petrissage on site.
  6. Have the client perform gentle stretching.
  7. Use hold-relax techniques that engage the muscle.
  8. Use strain-counterstrain or positional release techniques.[295]
  9. Adapt Techniques 1, 5, 6, and 7 above for self-care.
- Apply heat or cold based on the stage of the client's medical condition and his response to treatment.
- Strengthening the client's antagonist muscles may be an appropriate long-term goal.

# Muscle Weakness Associated with Reduced Resting Tension or Neuromuscular Tone

## Relevant Outcomes

- Increased **strength** and **power**

## Clinical Relevance

Weakness can occur after trauma, orthopedic injury, surgery, illness, and bed rest. It is also a common result of inactivity in the elderly. Furthermore, muscle weakness can be associated with neurological conditions such as Parkinson's disease and hemiplegia.

## Treatment Considerations

Before initiating treatment, determine the cause of the client's weakness and relevant cautions and contraindications. It is also important for you to distinguish between weakness, **fatigue**, and deconditioning. For example, some clients with neurological conditions, such as Parkinson's disease or hemiplegia, present with weakness that is secondary to other impairments that affect movement, such as **spasticity**.

## Guidelines for Using Massage Techniques and Complementary Modalities

- There are no massage techniques that you can use to increase muscle strength in normally innervated tissues.
- Therapeutic exercise is the primary treatment technique that you can use to treat muscle weakness in normally innervated tissues.
- Regular application of massage techniques may indirectly improve strength in clients with neurological problems such as carpal tunnel syndrome, spinal cord injury, and multiple sclerosis.[31,70,102] Physical therapy texts describe facilitation techniques (see following Complementary Modalities section) that may produce short-term increases in an abnormally innervated muscle's ability to contract.[296] Use these techniques immediately *prior to exercise* to facilitate the contraction of a weakened muscle.
- Clinicians often use regional or general massage techniques to prepare client's muscles for exercise in athletic settings.[137]

## Complementary Modalities

- Use therapeutic exercise for increasing muscle performance. The full range of strengthening methods is described in numerous texts on therapeutic exercise.[202,297,298]

- Joint traction and approximation, quick stretch, fine vibration, light touch, and repetitive stroking ("brushing") can be used to increase neuromuscular tone and facilitate movement.[296]
- Short applications of cold may stimulate arousal and indirectly facilitate resistance exercise.[225]
- Conversely, prolonged heat and prolonged cold temporarily reduce strength.[225]

# INTERVENTIONS FOR CONNECTIVE TISSUE IMPAIRMENTS

## Restriction of Joint Capsule or Ligaments

### Relevant Outcomes

- Increased mobility of joint capsule or ligaments[299]

### Clinical Relevance

Restrictions of the joint capsule or ligaments accompany capsulitis, adhesive capsulitis, osteoarthritis, inflammatory arthritic conditions, and systemic connective tissue diseases, such as lupus, where there is joint involvement.

### Treatment Considerations

Prior to treating decreased connective tissue mobility, *ensure that the client has no signs of* **acute inflammation**. Some orthopedic conditions, such as repeated sprains or rheumatoid arthritis, may involve joint laxity or instability. Do not treat these joints with techniques that attempt to lengthen the already lengthened or weakened connective tissue.

### Guidelines for Using Massage Techniques

- This impairment is a special case of impairment of decreased connective tissue mobility.
- Apply general connective tissue techniques to all fascial layers that cross the client's joint. The most beneficial approach may be the application of specific techniques, such as friction, to the affected ligament(s) or capsule.[300]

### Complementary Modalities

- In addition to hydrotherapy and exercises mentioned for decreased mobility of connective tissue, use joint traction and joint mobilization techniques to mobilize the joint capsule,[201,202] as your scope of practice permits.

## Hypermobility (Laxity) of Joint Capsule or Ligaments

### Relevant Outcomes

- Increased joint integrity
- Increased joint stability

### Clinical Relevance

Ligament or capsular laxity can be secondary to repeated joint dislocations and sprains, trauma, inflammatory arthritic conditions, systemic connective tissue disorders, pregnancy, and occupations that place a chronic load on particular joints such as dance or gymnastics.

### Treatment Considerations

When treating ligament or capsular laxity, consider any cautions and contraindications stemming from the client's medical condition such as pain level and medications. If a joint seems unstable or at risk for repeated dislocation or sprain, stabilize it with taping techniques, as your scope of practice permits, and refer your client to her physician if appropriate.

### Guidelines for Using Massage Techniques

- *No massage technique will tighten overstretched or weakened connective tissue.* Therapeutic exercise is the primary treatment modality.
- During the application of massage techniques, avoid positions of instability or capsular stretch. Avoid performing connective tissue techniques or aggressive neuromuscular techniques on the site of laxity. When only one side of a joint is lax, as is the case with repeated inversion sprains of the ankle, cautious application of connective tissue techniques to the shortened side of the joint may facilitate functional activity.
- Do not attempt to decrease the resting tension in the muscles that cross the joint, since these may be acting to stabilize the joint in the absence of other support. In cases of **functional instability**, general massage techniques may facilitate awareness of movement and posture, as described in the section on postural impairments.

### Complementary Modalities

- You can use therapeutic exercise to enhance muscle performance and control to stabilize the joint during active movement. In the early stages of treatment, select therapeutic exercises in the midrange and avoid the extreme ends of range. Numerous texts on therapeutic exercise detail appropriate stabilization protocols.[201,202]

- Include postural awareness training for cases of functional instability.

# INTERVENTIONS FOR POSTURAL IMPAIRMENTS

## Adaptive Lengthening with Stretch Weakness[202] and Impaired Balance of Agonist/Antagonist Muscle Function

### Relevant Outcomes
- Increased strength
- Improved balance of agonist/antagonist muscle function
- Improved postural alignment

### Clinical Relevance
Whenever one group of muscles adapts by shortening, the antagonist group adapts by lengthening. Adaptive lengthening may be associated with hyperkyphosis, hyperlordosis, scoliosis, iliotibial band contracture, valgus knee structure, patellofemoral syndrome, and pes planus.[202]

### Treatment Considerations
When muscles and fascia lengthen adaptively, they must function in a lengthened position, which puts them at a mechanical disadvantage. As a result, they cannot develop maximum contractile force.[202] These muscles exhibit what is termed stretch weakness and are subject to fatigue, **spasm**, and **myofascial trigger points**. *Do not lengthen these muscles further* with vigorously applied connective tissue or neuromuscular techniques.

### Guidelines for Using Massage Techniques
- First, treat adaptively shortened structures as described in the Adaptive Shortening with Impaired Balance of Agonist/Antagonist Muscle Function section.
- *None of the massage techniques affect weakness in normally innervated tissues.* Use various muscle performance exercises[202,297,298] to strengthen the lengthened muscles.
- Percussion may produce a marginal and transient increase in tone in abnormally innervated tissue. There is, however, no basis for using percussion on lengthened muscles with normal innervation (see Outcomes and Evidence sections for percussive techniques in Chapter 12, Percussive Techniques).

- Adaptively lengthened muscles often contain taut bands and trigger points,[249,255] which applications of percussion may irritate. Furthermore, these trigger points may be satellites that will resolve once you have treated the adaptively shortened antagonists.[230,301,302] If they do not resolve, treat them with ischemic compression and short stripping strokes.

### Complementary Modalities
- Increase muscle performance with appropriate therapeutic exercise.[202]
- Use moist heat, gentle stretch, and active range of motion after the massage techniques for treating trigger points.[230]

## Decreased Postural or Kinesthetic Awareness

### Relevant Outcomes
- Improved postural awareness

### Clinical Relevance
Decreased postural awareness is associated with hyperkyphosis, hyperlordosis, scoliosis, and other postural conditions.[202]

### Treatment Considerations
Decreased postural awareness often accompanies postural misalignment due to adaptive muscle shortening and lengthening. Occasionally, a decreased postural awareness, a "postural fault," will be the client's only presenting postural impairment.[202]

### Guidelines for Using Massage Techniques
- Massage techniques help to increase body awareness in a general sense.[303-305]
- When adaptively shortened areas lengthen quickly during treatment, the client may immediately notice changes as soon as he stands. Nevertheless, no massage technique by itself can produce a lasting increase in a client's postural *awareness* without some guidance by the clinician.
- Our clinical experience suggests that applying deep massage techniques to the client's feet, immediately prior to the client standing at the end of an intervention, may help the client adapt to and integrate postural changes that have occurred as a result of connective tissue or neuromuscular techniques.

### Complementary Modalities

■ Postural exercises accompanied by verbal and tactile cues are the primary treatment method for increasing postural awareness.[202] During these exercises, position or guide the client's body into a better alignment, and help the client to recognize this improved alignment. The client may then hold this position for a short period to develop muscular control.

■ Do not instruct clients to practice postural exercises for extended periods since this may lead to an undesirable increase in muscular tension. It is better to suggest exercises that the client practices for up to 10 minutes once or twice a day. Over time, the client will gradually acquire improved postural habits during daily activities.

■ Some examples of simple postural exercises are:

1. The client lies in an aligned position on the treatment table. Passively position the client in the best alignment possible and have the client maintain this position for 10 minutes or longer. This works well as a prelude to the following exercises.

2. Use standing aligned posture and seated aligned posture as described in Chapter 6, Preparation and Positioning for Massage. Floor-length mirrors in your clinical setting and the client's home facilitate self-monitoring in these exercises. The client can also perform seated aligned posture while sitting on a Swiss ball.

3. Pelvic tilt. Teach this in progressively more difficult positions: supine with the knees up (crook-lying), full supine, standing with the back and back of the pelvis against a wall for reference, and lastly, free-standing.[222]

# INTERVENTIONS FOR NEUROLOGICAL IMPAIRMENTS

## Spasticity, Spastic Paralysis

### Relevant Outcomes

■ Reduction of spasticity[102,224]
■ Improved or normalized movement patterns[306]

### Clinical Relevance

Spasticity is associated with cerebrovascular accidents, cerebral palsy, multiple sclerosis, traumatic brain injuries, and other neurological conditions.

### Treatment Considerations

Spasticity is the result of central nervous system (CNS) damage. Although the body does not replace destroyed upper motor neurons, the nervous system is capable of neuroplasticity, which is physical change in response to stimulus and activity. Neuroplasticity is the mechanism that supports clinicians' treatments for re-educating movement patterns following CNS damage. Even with diagnostic imaging, clinicians cannot be certain about the extent of a client's CNS damage and cannot predict the client's capacity for regaining function. Consequently, clinicians assist clients to regain and maintain as much function as possible.

The treatment of neurological conditions is complex and beyond the scope of this text. The role of massage techniques in the treatment of spasticity focuses on the modulation of **neuromuscular tone** and the treatment of secondary impairments, such as contractures, fatigue, trigger points, and altered body image. The following are examples of the secondary impairments associated with neurological conditions. Clients with multiple sclerosis may also present with fatigue, incoordination, and trigger points; clients with severe spasticity may also have contractures. Furthermore, clients with neurological conditions may also present with deficits in communication that make education and informed consent a concern. Finally, clients may have functional limitations that require guidelines for client safety.

### Guidelines for Using Massage Techniques

■ The treatment described in this section is for spasticity. Consult the suggested practices described elsewhere in this chapter for the treatment of coexisting impairments.

■ Position the client so that the muscle groups you are going to treat are not stretched.[307]

■ Limbs with spastic muscles are sensitive to sudden stretch and need slow, smooth handling.

■ Begin with muscle groups with less spasticity and contracture when you are treating your client's extremities.[307] Begin proximally on the limb, by treating the large joints, and proceed distally, to smaller joints, as the spasticity around the proximal joints releases. Appropriate massage techniques include slow, fairly deep,[1] continuous and rhythmic[307] effleurage, kneading,[1] and broad-contact compression.[308] Combine these techniques with slow, smooth range of motion and stretching; specific compression and friction at the origins and insertions of spastic muscles[307]; stripping; and gentle rhythmic mobilization.[9] In addition, use superficial stroking down the related axial skeleton and down the affected limb itself.

■ Apply gentle tapping to the stretched muscle groups that oppose the spastic muscles immediately prior to exercise in order to facilitate contraction and active movement.[296]

■ One author suggests limiting the treatment time to less than 30 minutes.[307]

## Complementary Modalities

■ Since stress exacerbates spasticity, use a sedative approach to treatment that incorporates diaphragmatic breathing and other relaxation techniques.

■ Use slow, controlled, and prolonged active and passive stretching.[1,9] Perform stretching with a gentle pumping action, if appropriate.[307]

■ Systemic heat, to promote relaxation, and local deep moist heat, to reduce resting tension of muscle, may be useful adjuncts to treatment, provided that the client does not have multiple sclerosis.[203]

## Flaccidity, Flaccid Paralysis

### Relevant Outcomes

■ Maintenance of the integrity of denervated tissue

■ Prevention or reduction of complications of flaccid paralysis[309]

### Clinical Relevance

Flaccid paralysis is associated with neurological conditions such as polio, postpolio syndrome, and peripheral neuropathies that result from prolonged nerve compression or nerve injury. It also occurs in cases of compression **neurapraxia** such as lumbar radiculopathy, thoracic outlet syndrome, carpal tunnel syndrome, and trigger point compression syndromes.

### Treatment Considerations

Consider the following issues when you are treating flaccid paralysis. First, the location and severity of your client's lesion will dictate his level of muscle function. If your client underwent surgical repair of a peripheral nerve, his prognosis will depend on his postsurgical course and the rate of nerve regrowth. Second, if the client's tissues have been denervated for any length of time and are fragile, you will need to use light pressure during treatment.[1] Flaccid areas may also have

impaired sensation and are subject to the contraindications for that impairment. Finally, your focus of treatment may be on associated impairments, such as edema, weakness, or contracture in the unopposed antagonists.[1]

### Guidelines for Using Massage Techniques

■ Use the traditional approach to using massage techniques for flaccid tissue of superficial, relatively stimulating techniques, which you apply with little force and without drag on the client's tissues.[1]

■ Treat the antagonist muscles that have normal innervation with moderate-pressure neuromuscular techniques, which you perform with minimal drag on the client's denervated tissues.

■ While you are waiting for nerve regeneration, it may be more important for you to treat associated edema and contracture.[1] The sections on edema and contracture in this chapter describe relevant treatment guidelines for those impairments.

■ It may be possible to use massage techniques to reduce pressure on a nerve or nerve root that is causing or contributing to paralysis. For example, you may be able to use massage techniques to:

1. Reduce lumbar spasm that increases compression on a lumbar nerve root in a disk herniation.

2. Decrease resting tension of the scalenes and pectoralis minor, which causes compression on a brachial plexus root in thoracic outlet syndrome.

3. Reduce edema and fascial restrictions that contribute to the compression of the median nerve in a carpal tunnel syndrome.

4. Eliminate trigger point activity that contributes to some peripheral nerve compression neurapraxias.

### Complementary Modalities

■ Use passive and active-assistive exercise if your client lacks the strength to perform active range of motion.

■ Progress to active-assisted, active, and resisted exercise as the client's motor function returns.

## References

1. Wale JO. *Tidy's Massage and Remedial Exercises.* 11th ed. Bristol: John Wright and Sons Ltd.; 1968.
2. Thomson A, Skinner A, Piercy J. *Tidy's Physiotherapy.* 12th ed. Oxford, England: Butterworth Heinemann; 1991.
3. Field TM. Massage therapy effects. *Am Psychol.* 1998;53: 1270–1281.
4. Moyer CA, Rounds J, Hannum JW. A meta-analysis of massage therapy research. *Psychol Bull.* 2004;130:3–18.
5. Field T. Massage therapy. *Med Clin North Am.* 2002;86: 163–171.
6. Field T. *Massage Therapy Research.* 1st ed. Edinburgh: Churchill Livingstone Elsevier; 2006.
7. Rich, G. *Massage Therapy: The Evidence for Practice.* 1st ed. Edinburgh: Mosby; 2002.

8. MacDonald G. *Massage for the Hospital Patient and Medically Frail Client.* 1st ed. Philadelphia: Lippincott Williams and Wilkins; 2005.

9. Rattray F, Ludwig L. *Clinical Massage Therapy.* Toronto: Talus Incorporated; 2000.

10. American Physical Therapy Association. *Guide to Physical Therapist Practice.* 2nd ed. Alexandria, VA: American Physical Therapy Association; 1999.

11. Goodman CC, Boissonnault WG, Fuller KS. *Pathology: Implications for the Physical Therapist.* 2nd ed. Philadelphia: Saunders; 2003.

12. Reader M, Young R, Connor JP. Massage therapy improves the management of alcohol withdrawal syndrome. *J Altern Complement Med.* 2005;11:311–313.

13. Post-White J, Kinney ME, Savik K, Gau JB, Wilcox C, Lerner I. Therapeutic massage and healing touch improve symptoms in cancer. *Integr Cancer Ther.* 2003;2:332–344.

14. Phipps SP. Reduction of distress associated with paediatric bone marrow transplant: complementary health promotion interventions. *Pediatr Rehabil.* 2002;5:223–234.

15. McRee LD, Noble S, Pasvogel A. Using massage and music therapy to improve postoperative outcomes. *AORN J.* 2003;78:433–442,445–447.

16. Hernandez-Reif M, Field T, Krasnegor J, Theakston H. Lower back pain is reduced and range of motion increased after massage therapy. *Int J Neurosci.* 2001;106:131–145.

17. Hernandez-Reif M, Field T, Ironson G, et al. Natural killer cells and lymphocytes increase in women with breast cancer following massage therapy. *Int J Neurosci.* 2005;115:495–510.

18. Hernandez-Reif M, Ironson G, Field T, et al. Breast cancer patients have improved immune and neuroendocrine functions following massage therapy. *J Psychosom Res.* 2004;57:45–52.

19. Hernandez-Reif M, Field T, Largie S, et al. Parkinson's disease symptoms are differentially affected by massage therapy vs. progressive muscle relaxation: a pilot study. *J Bodywork Movement Ther.* 2002;6:177–182.

20. Hernandez-Reif M, Field T, Ironson G, et al. Natural killer cells and lymphocytes increase in women with breast cancer following massage therapy. *Int J Neurosci.* 2005;115:495–510.

21. Hattan J, King L, Griffiths P. The impact of foot massage and guided relaxation following cardiac surgery: a randomized controlled trial. *J Adv Nurs.* 2002;37:199–207.

22. Dicker A. Using Bowen therapy to improve staff health. *Aust J Holist Nurs.* 2001;8:38–42.

23. Cullen LA, Barlow JH. A training and support programme for caregivers of children with disabilities: an exploratory study. *Patient Educ Couns.* 2004;55:203–209.

24. Boylan M. Massage boosts immunity in breast cancer patients. *J Aust Trad Med Soc.* 2005;11:59–62.

25. Chu JJ. Managing cancer symptoms with massage therapy. *Am J Nurs.* 2005;105:72G–72H.

26. Doellman D. Ease a child's anxiety during PICC insertion—without sedation. *Nursing.* 2005;35:68–68.

27. Chang MY, Wang SY, Chen CH. Effects of massage on pain and anxiety during labour: a randomized controlled trial in Taiwan. *J Adv Nurs.* 2002;38:68–73.

28. Chang M, Chen CH, Huang KF. A comparison of massage effects on labor pain using the McGill Pain Questionnaire. J Nurs Res. 2006;14:190–197.

29. Clifford P. Outcome based treatment planning for clients with cancer. *J Soft Tissue Manipulation.* 2003;11:3–12.

30. Diego MA, Field T, Hernandez-Reif M, Shaw K, Friedman L, Ironson G. HIV adolescents show improved immune function following massage therapy. *Int J Neurosci.* 2001;106:35–45.

31. Diego MA, Field T, Hernandez-Reif M, et al. Spinal cord patients benefit from massage therapy. *Int J Neurosci.* 2002;112:133–142.

32. Fellowes D, Barnes K, Wilkinson S. Aromatherapy and massage for symptom relief in patients with cancer. *Cochrane Database Syst Rev.* 2004;2:CD002287.

33. Field T. Massage and aroma therapy. *Int J Cosmetic Sci.* 2004;26:169–170.

34. Field T, Cullen C, Diego M, et al. Leukemia immune changes following massage therapy. *J Bodywork Movement Ther.* 2001;5:271–274.

35. Field T, Delage J, Hernandez-Reif M. Movement and massage therapy reduce fibromyalgia pain. *J Bodywork Movement Ther.* 2003;7:49–52.

36. Oh HJ, Park JS. Effects of hand massage and hand holding on the anxiety in patients with local infiltration anesthesia. *Taehan Kanho Hakhoe Chi.* 2004;34:924–933.

37. Sola I, Thompson E, Subirana M, Lopez C, Pascual A. Non-invasive interventions for improving well-being and quality of life in patients with lung cancer. *Cochrane Database Syst Rev.* 2004;4:CD004282.

38. Baskwill A, Kilty M, Hamilton A, Atkinson H. Massage therapy positively impacts quality of life for HIV+ individuals. *J Soft Tissue Manipulation.* 2003;11:4–6.

39. Kober A, Scheck T, Schubert B, et al. Auricular acupressure as a treatment for anxiety in prehospital transport settings. *Anesthesiology.* 2003;98:1328–1332.

40. Rakel B, Barr JO. Physical modalities in chronic pain management. *Nurs Clin North Am.* 2003;38:477–494.

41. Research: Reiki induces relaxation, liminal state of awareness. *Massage Magazine.* 2002;129.

42. Diego MA, Field T, Hernandez-Reif M, et al. Aggressive adolescents benefit from massage therapy. *Adolescence.* 2002;37:597–607.

43. Jirayingmongkol P, Chantein S, Phengchomjan N, Bhanggananda N. The effect of foot massage with biofeedback: a pilot study to enhance health promotion. *Nurs Health Sci.* 2002;4:A4.

44. Lovas JM, Craig AR, Raison RL, Weston KM, Segal YD, Markus MR. The effects of massage therapy on the human immune response in healthy adults. *J Bodywork Movement Ther.* 2002;6:143–150.

45. Mamtani R, Cimino A. A primer of complementary and alternative medicine and its relevance in the treatment of mental health problems. *Psychiatr Q.* 2002;73:367–381.

46. Okvat HA, Oz MC, Ting W, Namerow PB. Massage therapy for patients undergoing cardiac catheterization. *Altern Ther Health Med.* 2002;8:68–70,72,74–75.

47. Rexilius SJ, Mundt C, Erickson Megel M, Agrawal S. Therapeutic effects of massage therapy and handling touch on caregivers of patients undergoing autologous hematopoietic stem cell transplant. *Oncol Nurs Forum.* 2002;29:E35–E44.

48. Smith MC, Kemp J, Hemphill L, Vojir CP. Outcomes of therapeutic massage for hospitalized cancer patients. *J Nurs Scholarsh.* 2002;34:257–262.

49. Field T. Fibromyalgia pain and substance P decrease and sleep improves after massage therapy. *J Clin Rheumatol.* 2002; 8:72–76.

50. Williamson J, White A, Hart A, Ernst E. Randomised controlled trial of reflexology for menopausal symptoms. *BJOG.* 2002;109:1050–1055.

51. Brady LH, Henry K, Luth JF 2nd, Casper-Bruett KK. The effects of shiatsu on lower back pain. *J Holist Nurs.* 2001;19:57–70.

52. Hadfield N. The role of aromatherapy massage in reducing anxiety in patients with malignant brain tumours. *Int J Palliat Nurs.* 2001;7:279–285.

53. Hart S, Field T, Hernandez-Reif M, et al. Anorexia nervosa symptoms are reduced by massage therapy. *Eat Disord.* 2001; 9:289–299.

54. Hernandez-Reif M, Field T, Krasnegor J, Theakston H. Lower back pain is reduced and range of motion increased after massage therapy. *Int J Neurosci.* 2001;106:131–145.

55. Hernandez-Reif M, Field T, Largie S, et al. Children's distress during burn treatment is reduced by massage therapy. *J Burn Care Rehabil.* 2001;22:191–195.

56. Kim MS, Cho KS, Woo H, Kim JH. Effects of hand massage on anxiety in cataract surgery using local anesthesia. *J Cataract Refract Surg.* 2001;27:884–890.

57. Cooke B, Ernst E. Aromatherapy: a systematic review. *Br J Gen Pract.* 2000;50:493–496.

58. Fischer RL, Bianculli KW, Sehdev H, Hediger ML. Does light pressure effleurage reduce pain and anxiety associated with genetic amniocentesis? A randomized clinical trial. *J Matern Fetal Med.* 2000;9:294–297.

59. Hernandez-Reif M, Field T, Krasnegor J, Theakston H, Hossain Z, Burman I. High blood pressure and associated symptoms were reduced by massage therapy. *J Bodywork Movement Ther.* 2000;4:31–38.

60. Hernandez-Reif M, Martinez A, Field T, Quintero O, Hart S, Burman I. Premenstrual symptoms are relieved by massage therapy. *J Psychosom Obstet Gynaecol.* 2000;21:9–15.

61. Petry JJ. Surgery and complementary therapies: a review. *Altern Ther Health Med.* 2000;6:64–74.

62. Preyde M. Effectiveness of massage therapy for subacute low-back pain: a randomized controlled trial. *CMAJ.* 2000;162:1815–1820.

63. Richards KC, Gibson R, Overton-McCoy AL. Effects of massage in acute and critical care. *AACN Clin Issues.* 2000;11:77–96.

64. Stephenson NL, Weinrich SP, Tavakoli AS. The effects of foot reflexology on anxiety and pain in patients with breast and lung cancer. *Oncol Nurs Forum.* 2000;27:67–72.

65. Zeitlin D, Keller SE, Shiflett SC, Schleifer SJ, Bartlett JA. Immunological effects of massage therapy during academic stress. *Psychosom Med.* 2000;62:83–84.

66. Wilkinson S, Aldridge J, Salmon I, Cain E, Wilson B. An evaluation of aromatherapy massage in palliative care. *Palliat Med.* 1999;13:409–417.

67. Hernandez-Reif M, Field T, Fielt T, Theakston H. Multiple sclerosis patients benefit from massage therapy. *J Bodywork Movement Ther.* 1998;2:168–174.

68. Field T, Hernandez-Reif M, Taylor S, Quintino O, Burman I. Labor pain is reduced by massage therapy. *J Psychosom Obstet Gynaecol.* 1997;18:286–291.

69. Field T, Quintino O, Henteleff T, Wells-Keife L, Delvecchio-Feinberg G. Job stress reduction therapies. *Altern Ther Health Med.* 1997;3:54–56.

70. Field T, Diego M, Cullen C, et al. Carpal tunnel syndrome symptoms are lessened following massage therapy. *J Bodywork Movement Ther.* 2004;8:9–14.

71. Field T, Diego MA, Hernandez-Reif M, Schanberg S, Kuhn C. Massage therapy effects on depressed pregnant women. *J Psychosom Obstet Gynaecol.* 2004;25:115–122.

72. Field T, Pickens J, Prodromidis M, et al. Targeting adolescent mothers with depressive symptoms for early intervention. *Adolescence.* 2000;35:381–414.

73. Haraldsson K, Fridlund B, Baigi A, Marklund B. The self-reported health condition of women after their participation in a stress management programme: a pilot study. *Health Social Care Commun.* 2005;13:224–230.

74. Remington R. Calming music and hand massage with agitated elderly. *Nurs Res.* 2002;51:317–323.

75. Rowe M, Alfred D. The effectiveness of slow-stroke massage in diffusing agitated behaviors in individuals with Alzheimer's disease. *J Gerontol Nurs.* 1999;25:22–34.

76. Field T. Violence and touch deprivation in adolescents. *Adolescence.* 2002;37:735–749.

77. Field TM, Quintino O, Hernandez-Reif M, Koslovsky G. Adolescents with attention deficit hyperactivity disorder benefit from massage therapy. *Adolescence.* 1998;33:103–108.

78. Khilnani S, Field T, Hernandez-Reif M, Schanberg S. Massage therapy improves mood and behavior of students with attention-deficit/hyperactivity disorder. *Adolescence.* 2003;38:623–638.

79. Henrickson M. Clinical outcomes and patient perceptions of acupuncture and/or massage therapies in HIV-infected individuals. *AIDS Care.* 2001;13:743–748.

80. Shor-Posner G, Miguez MJ, Hernandez-Reif M, Perez-Then E, Fletcher M. Massage treatment in HIV-1 infected Dominican children: a preliminary report on the efficacy of massage therapy to preserve the immune system in children without antiretroviral medication. *J Altern Complement Med.* 2004;10:1093–1095.

81. Goodfellow LM. The effects of therapeutic back massage on psychophysiologic variables and immune function in spouses of patients with cancer. *Nurs Res.* 2003;52:318–328.

82. Birk TJ, McGrady A, MacArthur RD, Khuder S. The effects of massage therapy alone and in combination with other complementary therapies on immune system measures and quality of life in human immunodeficiency virus. *J Altern Complement Med.* 2000;6:405–414.

83. The relation of stress and psychiatric illnesses to coronary heart disease. *Acta Psychiatr Scand.* 2006;113:241–244.

84. Brosschot JF, Pieper S, Thayer JF. Expanding stress theory: prolonged activation and perseverative cognition. *Psychoneuroendocrinology.* 2005;30:1043–1049.

85. Shepshelovich D, Shoenfeld Y. Prediction and prevention of autoimmune diseases: additional aspects of the mosaic of autoimmunity. *Lupus.* 2006;15:183–190.

86. Heller DP, Heller L. Somatic experiencing in the treatment of automobile accident trauma. *J Soft Tissue Manipulation.* 2003;11:7–11.

87. Price C. Characteristics of women seeking body-oriented therapy as an adjunct to psychotherapy during recovery from childhood sexual abuse. *J Bodywork Movement Ther.* 2004; 8:35–42.

88. Fitch P, Dryden T. Recovering body and soul from post-traumatic stress disorder. *Massage Ther J.* 2000;39:40–45.

89. Leidy NK. A physiologic analysis of stress and chronic illness. *J Adv Nurs.* 1989;14:868–876.

90. Selye H. Stress and the reduction of distress. *J S C Med Assoc.* 1979;75:562–566.

91. Selye H. Forty years of stress research: principal remaining problems and misconceptions. *Can Med Assoc J.* 1976;115:53–56.

92. McCaffrey R, Locsin RC. Music listening as a nursing intervention: a symphony of practice. *Holist Nurs Pract.* 2002;16:70–77.

93. Brooks WW, Conrad CH, Nedder AP, Bing OH, Slawsky MT. Thoracic massage permits use of echocardiography in unanesthetized rats. *Comp Med.* 2003;53:288–292.

94. Foldi M, Strosenreuther R. *Foundations of Manual Lymph Drainage.* 3rd ed. St. Louis: Elsevier Mosby; 2005.

95. Lederman E. *Harmonic Technique.* Edinburgh: Churchill Livingstone; 2000.

96. Andrade CK, Clifford PC. *Outcome-Based Massage.* Baltimore: Lippincott Williams & Wilkins; 2001.

97. Hendrickson T. *Massage for Orthopedic Conditions.* Baltimore: Lippincott Williams & Wilkins; 2003.

98. Research: Moderate-pressure massage increases relaxation. *Massage Magazine.* 2004:154.

99. Lens epithelial cell outgrowth studied. *Rev Ophthalmol.* 2001;8:65.

100. Pattillo MM. Therapeutic and healing foot care: a healthy feet clinic for older adults. *J Gerontol Nurs.* 2004;30:25–32.

101. Wang HL, Keck JF. Foot and hand massage as an intervention for postoperative pain. *Pain Manag Nurs.* 2004;5:59–65.

102. Siev-Ner I, Gamus D, Lerner-Geva L, Achiron A. Reflexology treatment relieves symptoms of multiple sclerosis: a randomized controlled study. *Mult Scler.* 2003;9:356–361.

103. Kohara H, Miyauchi T, Suehiro Y, Ueoka H, Takeyama H, Morita T. Combined modality treatment of aromatherapy, footsoak, and reflexology relieves fatigue in patients with cancer. *J Palliat Med.* 2004;7:791–796.

104. Cottingham JT, Porges SW, Lyon T. Effects of soft tissue mobilization (rolfing pelvic lift) on parasympathetic tone in two age groups. *Phys Ther.* 1988;68:352–356.

105. Cottingham JT, Porges SW, Richmond K. Shifts in pelvic inclination angle and parasympathetic tone produced by rolfing soft tissue manipulation. *Phys Ther.* 1988;68:1364–1370.

106. Turchaninov R. *Therapeutic Massage: A Scientific Approach.* Phoenix, AZ: Aesculapius Books; 2000.

107. Turchaninov R. *Medical Massage.* 2nd ed. Phoenix, AZ: Aesculapius Books; 2006.

108. Price S, Price L. *Aromatherapy for Health Professionals.* 2nd ed. Edinburgh: Churchill Livingstone; 1999.

109. Lee SY. The effect of lavender aromatherapy on cognitive function, emotion, and aggressive behavior of elderly with dementia. *Taehan Kanho Hakhoe Chi.* 2005;35:303–312.

110. Payne RA. *Relaxation Techniques.* 3rd ed. Edinburgh: Elsevier Churchill Livingstone; 2005.

111. Hanley J, Stirling P, Brown C. Randomised controlled trial of therapeutic massage in the management of stress. *Br J Gen Pract.* 2003;53:20–25.

112. Bay E. *Empowered Breathing.* Toronto: The Relaxation Response Ltd; audiotape.

113. Nikola RJ. *Creatures of Water.* 3rd ed. Salt Lake City: Europa Therapeutic; 1997.

114. Fowlie L. *Heat and Cold as Therapy.* Toronto: Curties-Overzet Publications; 2006.

115. Escalona A, Field T, Singer-Strunck R, Cullen C, Hartshorn K. Brief report: improvements in the behavior of children with autism following massage therapy. *J Autism Dev Disord.* 2001;31:513–516.

116. Tsay SL, Rong JR, Lin PF. Acupoints massage in improving the quality of sleep and quality of life in patients with end-stage renal disease. *J Adv Nurs.* 2003;42:134–142.

117. Williams AF, Vadgama A, Franks PJ, Mortimer PS. A randomized controlled crossover study of manual lymphatic drainage therapy in women with breast cancer-related lymphedema. *Eur J Cancer Care (Engl).* 2002;11:254–261.

118. Field T, Hernandez-Reif M, Diego M, Feijo L, Vera Y, Gil K. Massage therapy by parents improves early growth and development. *Infant Behav Dev.* 2004;27:435–442.

119. Shen P. Two hundred cases of insomnia treated by otopoint pressure plus acupuncture. *J Tradit Chin Med.* 2004;24:168–169.

120. Soden K, Vincent K, Craske S, Lucas C, Ashley S. A randomized controlled trial of aromatherapy massage in a hospice setting. *Palliat Med.* 2004;18:87–92.

121. Weze C, Leathard HL, Stevens G. Evaluation of healing by gentle touch for the treatment of musculoskeletal disorders. *Am J Public Health.* 2004;94:50–52.

122. Dieter JN, Field T, Hernandez-Reif M, Emory EK, Redzepi M. Stable preterm infants gain more weight and sleep less after five days of massage therapy. *J Pediatr Psychol.* 2003;28:403–411.

123. Wang XH, Yuan YD, Wang BF. Clinical observation on effect of auricular acupoint pressing in treating sleep apnea syndrome. *Zhongguo Zhong Xi Yi Jie He Za Zhi.* 2003;23:747–749.

124. Barlow J, Cullen L. Increasing touch between parents and children with disabilities: preliminary results from a new programme. *J Fam Health Care.* 2002;12:7–9.

125. Ferber SG, Laudon M, Kuint J, Weller A, Zisapel N. Massage therapy by mothers enhances the adjustment of circadian rhythms to the nocturnal period in full-term infants. *J Dev Behav Pediatr.* 2002;23:410–415.

126. Tsay SL, Chen ML. Acupressure and quality of sleep in patients with end-stage renal disease—a randomized controlled trial. *Int J Nurs Stud.* 2003;40:1–7.

127. Agarwal KN, Gupta A, Pushkarna R, Bhargava SK, Faridi MM, Prabhu MK. Effects of massage and use of oil on growth, blood flow and sleep pattern in infants. *Indian J Med Res.* 2000;112:212–217.

128. Cassar M. The application of massage in psychogenic disorders. *Positive Health.* 2004:45–45.

129. Richards K, Nagel C, Markie M, Elwell J, Barone C. Use of complementary and alternative therapies to promote sleep in critically ill patients. *Crit Care Nurs Clin North Am.* 2003;15:329–340.

130. Cassar M. *Handbook of Clinical Massage.* 2nd ed. Edinburgh: Churchill Livingstone; 2004.

131. Field T, Diego M, Hernandez-Reif M, et al. Lavender fragrance cleansing gel effects on relaxation. *Int J Neurosci.* 2005;115:207–222.

132. Cho YC, Tsay SL. The effect of acupressure with massage on fatigue and depression in patients with end-stage renal disease. *J Nurs Res.* 2004;12:51–59.

133. Yang JH. The effects of foot reflexology on nausea, vomiting and fatigue of breast cancer patients undergoing chemotherapy. *Taehan Kanho Hakhoe Chi.* 2005;35:177–185.

134. Cassileth BR, Vickers AJ. Massage therapy for symptom control: outcome study at a major cancer center. *J Pain Symptom Manage.* 2004;28:244–249.

135. Deng G, Cassileth BR, Yeung KS. Complementary therapies for cancer-related symptoms. *J Support Oncol.* 2004;2:419–426.

136. Offenbacher M, Stucki G. Physical therapy in the treatment of fibromyalgia. *Scand J Rheumatol Suppl.* 2000;113:78–85.

137. Archer P. *Therapeutic Massage in Athletics.* Philadelphia: Lippincott Williams & Wilkins; 2007.

138. Thrash AT, Thrash C. *Home Remedies.* Seale, AL: Thrash Publications; 1981.

139. Iwama H, Akama Y. Skin rubdown with a dry towel activates natural killer cells in bedridden old patients. *Med Sci Monit.* 2002;8:CR611–CR615.

140. Wittink H, Michel TH, eds. *Chronic Pain Management for Physical Therapists.* 2nd ed. Boston: Butterworth Heinemann; 2002.

141. Roy EA, Hollins M, Maixner W. Reduction of TMD pain by high-frequency vibration: a spatial and temporal analysis. *Pain.* 2003;101:267–274.

142. van den Dolder PA, Roberts DL. A trial into the effectiveness of soft tissue massage in the treatment of shoulder pain. *Aust J Physiother.* 2003;49:183–188.

143. Bag B, Karabulut N. Pain-relieving factors in migraine and tension-type headache. *Int J Clin Pract.* 2005;59:760–763.

144. Cook CAL, Guerrerio JK, Slater VE. Healing touch and quality of life in women receiving radiation treatment for cancer: a randomized controlled trial. *Altern Ther Health Med.* 2004;10:34–41.

145. Bodhise PB, Dejoie M, Brandon Z, Simpkins S, Ballas SK. Non-pharmacologic management of sickle cell pain. *Hematology.* 2004;9:235–237.

146. Huntley AL, Coon JT, Ernst E. Complementary and alternative medicine for labor pain: a systematic review. *Am J Obstet Gynecol.* 2004;191:36–44.

147. Norrbrink Budh C, Lundeberg T. Non-pharmacological pain-relieving therapies in individuals with spinal cord injury: a patient perspective. *Complement Ther Med.* 2004;12:189–197.

148. Simkin P, Bolding A. Update on nonpharmacologic approaches to relieve labor pain and prevent suffering. *J Midwifery Womens Health.* 2004;49:489–504.

149. Yildirim G, Sahin NH. The effect of breathing and skin stimulation techniques on labour pain perception of Turkish women. *Pain Res Manag.* 2004;9:183–187.

150. Chung UL, Hung LC, Kuo SC, Huang CL. Effects of LI4 and BL 67 acupressure on labor pain and uterine contractions in the first stage of labor. *J Nurs Res.* 2003;11:251–260.

151. Dudley G, McGrath KN, Pheley AM. Length of stay and medication use in hysterectomy patients treated with a single massage treatment. *J Bodywork Movement Ther.* 2003;7:222–227.

152. Piotrowski MM, Paterson C, Mitchinson A, Kim HM, Kirsh M, Hinshaw DB. Massage as adjuvant therapy in the management of acute postoperative pain: a preliminary study in men. *J Am Coll Surg.* 2003;197:1037–1046.

153. Sakurai M, Suleman MI, Morioka N, Akca O, Sessler DI. Minute sphere acupressure does not reduce postoperative pain or morphine consumption. *Anesth Analg.* 2003;96:493–497.

154. Stephenson N, Dalton JA, Carlson J. The effect of foot reflexology on pain in patients with metastatic cancer. *Appl Nurs Res.* 2003;16:284–286.

155. Stephenson NL, Dalton JA. Using reflexology for pain management. A review. *J Holist Nurs.* 2003;21:179–191.

156. Taylor AG, Galper DI, Taylor P, et al. Effects of adjunctive Swedish massage and vibration therapy on short-term postoperative outcomes: a randomized, controlled trial. *J Altern Complement Med.* 2003;9:77–89.

157. Bellieni CV, Bagnoli F, Perrone S, et al. Effect of multisensory stimulation on analgesia in term neonates: a randomized controlled trial. *Pediatr Res.* 2002;51:460–463.

158. Dryden T, Menard MB, Hunter W. The effect of a single massage on pain sensation and pain unpleasantness. *J Soft Tissue Manipulation.* 2002;10:20–22.

159. Le Blanc-Louvry I, Costaglioli B, Boulon C, Leroi AM, Ducrotte P. Does mechanical massage of the abdominal wall after colectomy reduce postoperative pain and shorten the duration of ileus? Results of a randomized study. *J Gastrointest Surg.* 2002;6:43–49.

160. Lemstra M, Stewart B, Olszynski WP. Effectiveness of multidisciplinary intervention in the treatment of migraine: a randomized clinical trial. *Headache.* 2002;42:845–854.

161. Akbayrak T, Citak I, Demirturk F, Akarcali I. Manual therapy and pain changes in patients with migraine—an open pilot study. *Adv Physiother.* 2001;3:49–54.

162. Billhult A, Dahlberg K. A meaningful relief from suffering experiences of massage in cancer care. *Cancer Nurs.* 2001;24:180–184.

163. Gentz BA. Alternative therapies for the management of pain in labor and delivery. *Clin Obstet Gynecol.* 2001;44:704–732.

164. Kim J, Jang S, Kim Y, Lee S, Song J. Developing CD-ROM based multimedia digital textbook of san-yin-jiao (SP-6) pressure for reducing the labor pain and shortening the labor time. *Medinfo.* 2001;10:1038–1041.

165. Kubsch SM, Neveau T, Vandertie K. Effect of cutaneous stimulation on pain reduction in emergency department patients. *Accid Emerg Nurs.* 2001;9:143–151.

166. Shirreffs CM. Aromatherapy massage for joint pain and constipation in a patient with Guillain-Barré. *Complement Ther Nurs Midwifery.* 2001;7:78–83.

167. Field T, Peck M 2nd, et al. Postburn itching, pain, and psychological symptoms are reduced with massage therapy. *J Burn Care Rehabil.* 2000;21:189–193.

168. Gallagher G, Rae CP, Kinsella J. Treatment of pain in severe burns. *Am J Clin Dermatol.* 2000;1:329–335.

169. Grealish L, Lomasney A, Whiteman B. Foot massage. A nursing intervention to modify the distressing symptoms of pain and nausea in patients hospitalized with cancer. *Cancer Nurs.* 2000;23:237–243.

170. Kubsch SM, Neveau T, Vandertie K. Effect of cutaneous stimulation on pain reduction in emergency department patients. *Complement Ther Nurs Midwifery.* 2000;6:25–32.

171. Pan CX, Morrison RS, Ness J, Fugh-Berman A, Leipzig RM. Complementary and alternative medicine in the management of pain, dyspnea, and nausea and vomiting near the end of life. A systematic review. *J Pain Symptom Manage.* 2000;20:374–387.

172. Uher EM, Vacariu G, Schneider B, Fialka V. Comparison of manual lymph drainage with physical therapy in complex regional pain syndrome, type I. A comparative randomized controlled therapy study. *Wien Klin Wochenschr.* 2000;112:133–137.

173. Wilkie DJ, Kampbell J, Cutshall S, et al. Effects of massage on pain intensity, analgesics and quality of life in patients with cancer pain: a pilot study of a randomized clinical trial conducted within hospice care delivery. *Hosp J.* 2000;15:31–53.

174. Sellick SM, Zaza C. Critical review of 5 nonpharmacologic strategies for managing cancer pain. *Cancer Prev Control.* 1998;2:7–14.

175. Apostle-Mitchell M, MacDonald G. An innovative approach to pain management in critical care: therapeutic touch. *Off J Can Assoc Crit Care Nurs.* 1997;8:19–22.

176. Barnes J. Myofascial release in treatment of thoracic outlet syndrome. *J Bodywork Movement Ther.* 1996;1:53–57.

177. Goffaux-Dogniez C, Vanfraechem-Raway R, Verbanck P. Appraisal of treatment of the trigger points associated with relaxation to treat chronic headache in the adult: relationship with anxiety and stress adaptation strategies. *Encephale.* 2003; 29:377–390.

178. Gray RA. The use of massage therapy in palliative care. *Complement Ther Nurs Midwifery.* 2000;6:77–82.

179. Crawford JS, Simpson J, Crawford P. Myofascial release provides symptomatic relief from chest wall tenderness occasionally seen following lumpectomy and radiation in breast cancer patients. *Int J Radiat Oncol Biol Phys.* 1996;34:1188–1189.

180. Szuba A. Literature watch. The addition of manual lymph drainage to compression therapy for breast cancer related lymphedema: a randomized controlled trial. *Lymphat Res Biol.* 2005;3:36–41.

181. Yates JS, Mustian KM, Morrow GR, et al. Prevalence of complementary and alternative medicine use in cancer patients during treatment. *Support Care Cancer.* 2005;13:806–811.

182. Roy L. Massage therapy for people with cancer: a practitioner's experience. *Positive Health.* 2004:48–50.

183. Klein J, Griffiths P. Acupressure for nausea and vomiting in cancer patients receiving chemotherapy. *Br J Community Nurs.* 2004;9:383–388.

184. McNeely ML, Magee DJ, Lees AW, Bagnall KM, Haykowsky M, Hanson J. The addition of manual lymph drainage to compression therapy for breast cancer related lymphedema: a randomized controlled trial. *Breast Cancer Res Treat.* 2004;86:95–106.

185. Shin YH, Kim TI, Shin MS, Juon HS. Effect of acupressure on nausea and vomiting during chemotherapy cycle for Korean postoperative stomach cancer patients. *Cancer Nurs.* 2004;27:267–274.

186. Wilcock A, Manderson C, Weller R, et al. Does aromatherapy massage benefit patients with cancer attending a specialist palliative care day centre? *Palliat Med.* 2004;18:287–290.

187. Dunwoody L, Smyth A, Davidson R. Cancer patients' experiences and evaluations of aromatherapy massage in palliative care. *Int J Palliat Nurs.* 2002;8:497–504.

188. Gecsedi RA. Massage therapy for patients with cancer. *Clin J Oncol Nurs.* 2002;6:52–54.

189. Robin K. Pediatric cancer patients turn to alternative therapies. *HerbalGram.* 2002:13.

190. Gwilt M, Athis J. Treating venous leg ulceration with complementary therapy. *Community Nurse.* 2000;6:51–53.

191. Felty CL, Rooke TW. Compression therapy for chronic venous insufficiency. *Semin Vasc Surg.* 2005;18:36–40.

192. Kessler T, de Bruin E, Brunner F, Vienne P, Kissling R. Effect of manual lymph drainage after hindfoot operations. *Physiother Res Int.* 2003;8:101–110.

193. Haren K, Backman C, Wiberg M. Effect of manual lymph drainage as described by Vodder on oedema of the hand after fracture of the distal radius: a prospective clinical study. *Scand J Plast Reconstr Surg Hand Surg.* 2000;34:367–372.

194. Andersen L, Højris I, Erlandsen M, Andersen J. Treatment of breast-cancer-related lymphedema with or without manual lymphatic drainage: a randomized study. *Acta Oncol.* 2000; 39:399–405.

195. Badger C, Preston N, Seers K, Mortimer P. Physical therapies for reducing and controlling lymphoedema of the limbs. *Cochrane Database Syst Rev.* 2004;4:CD003141.

196. Campisi C, Boccardo F, Casaccia M. Post-mastectomy lymphedema: surgical therapy. *Ann Ital Chir.* 2002;73:473–478.

197. Campisi C, Boccardo F, Zilli A, et al. Lymphedema secondary to breast cancer treatment: possibility of diagnostic and therapeutic prevention. *Ann Ital Chir.* 2002;73:4931498.

198. Casley-Smith JR. Changes in the microcirculation at the superficial and deeper levels in lymphoedema: the effects and results of massage, compression, exercise and benzopyrones on these levels during treatment. *Clin Hemorheol Microcirc.* 2000;23:335–343.

199. Kasseroller RG, Schrauzer GN. Treatment of secondary lymphedema of the arm with physical decongestive therapy and sodium selenite: a review. *Am J Ther.* 2000;7:273–279.

200. Kriederman B, Myloyde T, Bernas M, et al. Limb volume reduction after physical treatment by compression and/or massage in a rodent model of peripheral lymphedema. *Lymphology.* 2002;35:23–27.

201. Hertling D, Kessler RM. *Management of Common Musculoskeletal Disorders.* 4th ed. Philadelphia: Lippincott Williams & Wilkins; 2006.

202. Kisner CK, Colby LA. *Therapeutic Exercise: Foundations and Techniques.* 4th ed. Philadelphia: FA Davis; 2002.

203. Werner R. *A Massage Therapist Guide to Pathology.* 2nd ed. Philadelphia: Lippincott Williams & Wilkins; 2002.

204. Dery MA, Yonuschot G, Winterson BJ. The effects of manually applied intermittent pulsation pressure to rat ventral thorax on lymph transport. *Lymphology.* 2000;33:58–61.

205. Lederman E. *The Science and Practice of Manual Therapy.* 2nd ed. Edinburgh: Elsevier Churchill Livingstone; 2005.

206. Petermans J, Zicot M. Musculo-venous pump in the elderly. *J Mal Vasc.* 1994;19:115–118.

207. Kelly DG. *A Primer on Lymphedema.* Upper Saddle River, NJ: Prentice Hall; 2002.

208. Harris SR, Hugi MR, Olivotto IA, Levine M, Steering Committee for Clinical Practice Guidelines for the Care and Treatment of Breast Cancer. Clinical practice guidelines for the care and treatment of breast cancer: 11. Lymphedema. *CMAJ.* 2001; 164:191–199.

209. Johansson K, Albertsson M, Ingvar C, Ekdahl C. Effects of compression bandaging with or without manual lymph drainage treatment in patients with postoperative arm lymphedema. *Lymphology.* 1999;32:103–110.

210. de Godoy JM, Batigalia F, de Godoy MF. Preliminary evaluation of a new, more simplified physiotherapy technique for lymphatic drainage. *Lymphology.* 2002;35:91–93.

211. Varekojis SM, Douce FH, Flucke RL, et al. A comparison of the therapeutic effectiveness of and preference for postural drainage and percussion, intrapulmonary percussive ventilation, and

high-frequency chest wall compression in hospitalized cystic fibrosis patients. *Respir Care*. 2003;48:24–28.

212. Oermann CM, Sockrider MM, Giles D, Sontag MK, Accurso FJ, Castile RG. Comparison of high-frequency chest wall oscillation and oscillating positive expiratory pressure in the home management of cystic fibrosis: a pilot study. *Pediatr Pulmonol*. 2001;32:372–377.

213. Fink JB. Positioning versus postural drainage. *Respir Care*. 2002;47:769–777.

214. Maa SH, Sun MF, Hsu KH, et al. Effect of acupuncture or acupressure on quality of life of patients with chronic obstructive asthma: a pilot study. *J Altern Complement Med*. 2003;9:659–670.

215. Persad R. *Massage Therapy and Medications*. Toronto: Curties-Overzet Publications; 2001.

216. de Domenico G, Wood EC. *Beard's Massage*. 5th ed. Philadelphia: WB Saunders; 1997.

217. Hess DR. The evidence for secretion clearance techniques. *Respir Care*. 2001;46:1276–1293.

218. Fritz S. *Fundamentals of Therapeutic Massage*. 3rd ed. St. Louis: Mosby; 2004.

219. Clay JH, Pounds DM. *Basic Clinical Massage Therapy*. Philadelphia: Lippincott Williams & Wilkins; 2003.

220. Cantu RI, Grodin AJ. *Myofascial Manipulation: Theory and Clinical Application*. 2nd ed. Gaithersburg, MD: Aspen Publishers; 2001.

221. Stanborough M. *Direct Release Myofascial Technique*. Edinburgh: Churchill Livingstone; 2004.

222. Smith J. *Structural Bodywork*. Edinburgh: Churchill Livingstone; 2005.

223. Lundberg U. Muscle tension. *J Soft Tissue Manipulation*. 2006;13:3–9.

224. Hernandez-Reif M, Field T, Largie S, et al. Cerebral palsy symptoms in children decreased following massage therapy. *Early Child Dev Care*. 2005;175:445–456.

225. Michlovitz SL. *Thermal Agents in Rehabilitation*. 3rd ed. Philadelphia: FA Davis; 1996.

226. Hou CR, Tsai LC, Cheng KF, Chung KC, Hong CZ. Immediate effects of various physical therapeutic modalities on cervical myofascial pain and trigger-point sensitivity. *Arch Phys Med Rehabil*. 2002;83:1406–1414.

227. Archer PA. Three clinical sports massage approaches for treating injured athletes. *Athletic Ther Today*. 2001;6:14–20.

228. Kostopoulos D, Rizopoulos K. *The Manual of Trigger Point and Myofascial Therapy*. Thorofare, NJ: Slack Inc; 2001.

229. Travell JG, Simons DG. *Myofascial Pain and Dysfunction: The Trigger Point Manual. Volume 2*. Baltimore: Williams & Wilkins; 1992.

230. Simons DG, Travell JG, Simons LS. *Myofascial Pain and Dysfunction: The Trigger Point Manual. Volume 1*. 2nd ed. Baltimore: Williams & Wilkins; 1999.

231. Lucas KR, Polus BI, Rich PA. Latent myofascial trigger points: their effects on muscle activation and movement efficiency. *J Bodywork Movement Ther*. 2004;8:160–166.

232. Weiss JM. Pelvic floor myofascial trigger points: manual therapy for interstitial cystitis and the urgency-frequency syndrome. *J Urol*. 2001;166:2226–2231.

233. Delaney JPA, Leong KS, Watkins A, Brodie D. The short-term effects of myofascial trigger point massage therapy on cardiac autonomic tone in healthy subjects. *J Adv Nurs*. 2002;37:364–371.

234. Simons DG, Mense S. Understanding and measurement of muscle tone as related to clinical muscle pain. *Pain*. 1998;75:1–17.

235. Michelotti A, Steenks MH, Farella M, Parisini F. Short-term effects of physiotherapy versus counseling for the treatment of myofascial pain of the jaw muscles. *J Oral Rehabil*. 2002; 29:874.

236. McPartland JM. Travell trigger points: molecular and osteopathic perspectives. *J Am Osteopath Assoc*. 2004;104:244–249.

237. Rochet JM, Zaoui A. Burn scars: rehabilitation and skin care. *Rev Prat*. 2002;52:2258–2263.

238. Guler-Uysal F, Kozanoglu E. Comparison of the early response to two methods of rehabilitation in adhesive capsulitis. *Swiss Med Wkly*. 2004;134:353–358.

239. Wies J. Treatment of eight patients with frozen shoulder: a case study series. *J Bodywork Movement Ther*. 2005;9:58–64.

240. Barnes JF. Myofascial release. In: Hammer WI, ed. *Functional Soft Tissue Examination and Treatment by Manual Methods*. 2nd ed. Gaithersburg, MD: Aspen; 1999:533–548.

241. Sefton J. Myofascial release for athletic trainers, part 3: specific techniques. *Athletic Ther Today*. 2004;9:40–41.

242. Smith FR. Causes of and treatment options for abnormal scar tissue. *J Wound Care*. 2005;14:49–52.

243. Brosseau L, Casimiro L, Milne S, et al. Deep transverse friction massage for treating tendinitis. *Cochrane Database Syst Rev*. 2002;4:CD003528.

244. Mannheim C. *The Myofascial Release Manual*. 3rd ed. Thorofare, NJ: Slack Inc; 2001.

245. Sefton J. Myofascial release for athletic trainers, part 2: guidelines and techniques. *Athletic Ther Today*. 2004;9:52–53.

246. Boisaubert B, Brousse C, Zaoui A, Montigny JP. Nonsurgical treatment of tennis elbow. *Ann Readapt Med Phys*. 2004;47: 346–355.

247. Roques C. Massage applied to scars. *Wound Repair Regen*. 2002;10:126–128.

248. Davies C. Self-treatment of lateral epicondylitis (tennis elbow): trigger point therapy for triceps and extensor muscles. *J Bodywork Movement Ther*. 2003;7:165–172.

249. Gerwin RD. A review of myofascial pain and fibromyalgia: factors that promote their persistence. *Acupunct Med*. 2005;23: 121–134.

250. Fredericson M, Guillet M. Quick solutions for iliotibial band syndrome. *Phys Sportsmed*. 2000;28:53.

251. Alexander D. Myofascial therapy response: leg length inequality. *J Bodywork Movement Ther*. 1999;3:191–197.

252. Hawes MC, Brooks WJ. Reversal of the signs and symptoms of moderately severe idiopathic scoliosis in response to physical methods. *Stud Health Technol Inform*. 2002;91:365–368.

253. Myers T. *Anatomy Trains: Myofascial Meridians for Manual and Movement Therapists*. Edinburgh: Churchill Livingstone; 2001.

254. Kisner C, Colby LA. *Therapeutic Exercise: Foundations and Techniques*. 3rd ed. Philadelphia: FA Davis Company; 1990.

255. Moore MK. Upper crossed syndrome and its relationship to cervicogenic headache. *J Manipulative Physiol Ther*. 2004;27: 414–420.

256. Alexander D. Unravelling compensatory patterns. *J Soft Tissue Manipulation*. 2005;12:6–12.

257. Bredin M. Mastectomy, body image and therapeutic massage: a qualitative study of women's experience. *J Adv Nurs*. 1999;29: 1113–1120.

258. van der Riet P. Massaged embodiment of cancer patients. *Aust J Holist Nurs.* 1999;6:4–13.

259. Price C. Body-oriented therapy as an adjunct to psychotherapy in childhood abuse recovery: a case study. *J Bodywork Movement Ther.* 2002;6:228–236.

260. van der Riet P. Ethereal embodiment of cancer patients. *Aust J Holist Nurs.* 1999;6:20–27.

261. van der Riet P. The sexual embodiment of the cancer patient. *Nurs Inq.* 1998;5:248–257.

262. Healing triumphs over domestic violence. *Massage Bodywork.* 2001;16:17.

263. Mattsson M, Wikman M, Dahlgren L, Mattsson B, Armelius K. Body awareness therapy with sexually abused women. Part 2: evaluation of body awareness in a group setting. *J Bodywork Movement Ther.* 1998;2:38–45.

264. Fitch P. Creating sound treatment plans for complex conditions. *J Soft Tissue Manipulation.* 2002;10:3–7.

265. Erickson S. How to understand tissue memory and its implications. *Massage Ther J.* 2003;42:70–77.

266. Kalauokalani D, Cherkin DC, Sherman KJ, Koepsell TD, Deyo RA. Lessons from a trial of acupuncture and massage for low back pain: patient expectations and treatment effects. *Spine.* 2001;26:1418–1424.

267. Hsieh LL, Kuo CH, Yen MF, Chen TH. A randomized controlled clinical trial for low back pain treated by acupressure and physical therapy. *Prev Med.* 2004;39:168–176.

268. Quinn C, Chandler C, Moraska A. Massage therapy and frequency of chronic tension headaches. *Am J Public Health.* 2002;92:1657–1661.

269. Main CJ, Spanswick CC. *Pain Management: An Interdisciplinary Approach.* 1st ed. Edinburgh: Churchill Livingston; 2000.

270. Fitch P. Massage strategies for depressed clients. *Massage Ther J.* 2003;42:58–67.

271. Geisbrecht D. Third party series: credibility, accountability and third party payers. *The Body Politic.* 2004;2:7–9.

272. Amole Khadilkar. Transcutaneous electrical nerve stimulation for the treatment of chronic low back pain: a systematic review. *Spine.* 2005;30:2657–2666.

273. Barker R, Lang T, Steinlechner B, et al. Transcutaneous electrical nerve stimulation as prehospital emergency interventional care: treating acute pelvic pain in young women. *Neuromodulation.* 2006;9:136–142.

274. Brosseau L, Yonge K, Marchand S, et al. Efficacy of transcutaneous electrical nerve stimulation for osteoarthritis of the lower extremities: a meta-analysis. *Phys Ther Rev.* 2004;9:213–233.

275. King EW, Audette K, Athman GA, Nguyen HOX, Sluka KA, Fairbanks CA. Transcutaneous electrical nerve stimulation activates peripherally located alpha-2A adrenergic receptors. *Pain.* 2005;115:364–373.

276. Miller L, Mattison P, Paul L, Wood L. The effects of transcutaneous electrical nerve stimulation on spasticity. *Phys Ther Rev.* 2005;10:201–208.

277. Resende MA, Sabino GG, Cândido CRM, Pereira LSM, Francischi JN. Local transcutaneous electrical stimulation (TENS) effects in experimental inflammatory edema and pain. *Eur J Pharmacol.* 2004;504:217–222.

278. Sarzi-Puttini P, Cimmino MA, Scarpa R, et al. Osteoarthritis: an overview of the disease and its treatment strategies. *Semin Arthritis Rheum.* 2005;35:1–10.

279. Bruggeman W. *Kneipp Vademecum Pro Medico.* Wurzburg, Germany: Sebastian Kneipp Publications; 1982.

280. Sabir'ianov AR, Sabir'ianova ES, Epishev VV. Trends in slow wave variability of the central circulation in healthy individuals in response to massage of the collar cervical region. *Vopr Kurortol Fizioter Lech Fiz Kult.* 2004;6:13–15.

281. Liu Y, Xu S, Yan J, et al. Capillary blood flow with dynamical change of tissue pressure caused by exterior force. *Sheng Wu Yi Xue Gong Cheng Xue Za Zhi.* 2004;21:699–703.

282. Tsarev AI, Ezhova VA, Kunitsyna LA, Slovesnov SV, Chukreeva LN, Kolesnikova EI. Aromamassage of the cervical collar region in the combined treatment of patients with atherosclerotic dyscirculatory encephalopathy. *Vopr Kurortol Fizioter Lech Fiz Kult.* 2004;5:6–7.

283. Drust B, Atkinson G, Gregson W, French D, Binningsley D. The effects of massage on intra muscular temperature in the vastus lateralis in humans. *Int J Sports Med.* 2003;24:395–399.

284. Hinds T, McEwan I, Perkes J, Dawson E, Ball D, George K. Effects of massage on limb and skin blood flow after quadriceps exercise. *Med Sci Sports Exerc.* 2004;36:1308–1313.

285. Mur E, Schmidseder J, Egger I, et al. Influence of reflex zone therapy of the feet on intestinal blood flow measured by color Doppler sonography. *Forsch Komplementarmed Klass Naturheilkd.* 2001;8:86–89.

286. Martin NA, Zoeller RF. The comparative effects of sports massage, active recovery, and rest in promoting blood lactate. *J Athl Train.* 1998;33:30–35.

287. Perle SM. Effleurage massage, muscle blood flow and long-term post-exercise strength recovery. *J Sports Chiropractic Rehabil.* 1996;10:102.

288. Robertson A, Watt JM, Galloway SDR. Effects of leg massage on recovery from high intensity cycling exercise. *Br J Sports Med.* 2004;38:173–176.

289. Kniazeva TA, Minenkov AA, Kul'chitskaia DB, Apkhanova TV. Effect of physiotherapy on the microcirculation in patients with lymphedema of lower extremities. *Vopr Kurortol Fizioter Lech Fiz Kult.* 2003;1:30–32.

290. Morhenn VB. Firm stroking of human skin leads to vasodilatation possibly due to the release of substance P. *J Dermatol Sci.* 2000;22:138–144.

291. Turchaninov R, Prilutsky B. Massage therapy: a beneficial tool in treating fibromyalgia. *Massage Bodywork.* 2004;19:82–93.

292. Allegra C, Bartolo M Jr, Martocchia R. Therapeutic effects of vascupump treatment patients with Fontaine stage II B arteriopathy. *Minerva Cardioangiol.* 2001;49:189–195.

293. Alexander D, ed. *Massage Therapy Self Care Manual.* Ottawa, Ontario; 2005.

294. Vaughn BF. Integrated strategies for treatment of spasmodic torticollis. *J Bodywork Movement Ther.* 2003;7:142–147.

295. Wheeler L. Advanced strain counterstrain. *Massage Ther J.* 2005;43:84–95.

296. O'Sullivan SB. Strategies to improve motor control. In: O'Sullivan SB, Schmitz J, eds. *Physical Rehabilitation, Assessment and Treatment.* 2nd ed. Philadelphia: FA Davis; 1988.

297. Bandy WD, Sanders B. *Therapeutic Exercise: Techniques for Intervention.* Baltimore: Lippincott, Williams & Wilkins; 2001.

298. Nyland J. *Clinical Decision in Therapeutic Exercise.* Upper Saddle River, NJ: Pearson Prentice Hall; 2006.

299. Jurgel J, Rannama L, Gapeyeva H, Ereline J, Kolts I, Paasuke M. Shoulder function in patients with frozen shoulder before and after 4-week rehabilitation. *Medicina (Kaunas).* 2005;41:30–38.

300. Lowe W. *Orthopedic Massage.* Edinburgh: Mosby; 2003.

301. Simons DG, Mense S. Diagnosis and therapy of myofascial trigger points. *Schmerz.* 2003;17:419–424.

302. Simons DG. Understanding effective treatments of myofascial trigger points. *J Bodywork Movement Ther.* 2002;6:81–88.

303. Gyllensten AL, Hansson L, Ekdahl C. Patient experiences of basic body awareness therapy and the relationship with the physiotherapist. *J Bodywork Movement Ther.* 2003;7:173–183.

304. Fitch P. Depression: how massage therapy can help. *J Soft Tissue Manipulation.* 2002;10:5–12.

305. Henriksen M, Højrup A, Lund H, Christensen L, Danneskiold-Samsøe B, Bliddal H. The effect of stimulating massage of thigh muscles on knee joint position sense. *Adv Physiother.* 2004;6:29–36.

306. Zhou XJ, Zheng K. Treatment of 140 cerebral palsied children with a combined method based on traditional Chinese medicine (TCM) and Western medicine. *J Zhejiang Univ Sci B.* 2005;6:57–60.

307. Wine ZK. Russian medical massage: massage for spasticity. *Massage Magazine.* 1996;1:80–84

308. Tips for working with paralysis, other disabilities. *Massage Bodywork.* 2000;15:30.

309. Wang XH, Zhang LM, Han M, Zhang KQ, Jiang JJ. Treatment of Bell's palsy with combination of traditional Chinese medicine and Western medicine. *Hua Xi Kou Qiang Yi Xue Za Zhi.* 2004;22:211–213.

# Glossary

**Abnormal connective tissue density:** Irregular connective tissue remodeling that occurs during the consolidation and maturation stages of connective tissue healing.

**Accessory joint motion:** The range of motion within synovial and secondary cartilaginous joints that is not under voluntary control and can, therefore, only be obtained passively by the clinician. These motions, also known as joint play movements, are essential for full and pain-free active range of motion.

**Active exercise:** Exercise that is performed voluntarily without assistance.

**Active listening:** To restate a speaker's thoughts and feelings in the listener's own words; also known as paraphrasing. It is an effective way to clarify client desires or goals.

**Active range of motion:** The amount of joint motion that can be achieved by the client during the performance of unassisted voluntary joint motion.

**Active Release®:** A soft tissue system developed by chiropractor Michael Leahy for treatment of chronic and repetitive strain injuries. Active Release protocols for individual muscles combine simultaneous active or passive movement with application of specific and deep neuromuscular techniques.

**Active trigger point:** A trigger point that refers pain in a characteristic pattern whether the muscle in which it is located is working or at rest.

**Acupoint:** In Traditional Chinese Medicine and related systems, a point on a meridian that can be stimulated by various methods to achieve complex effects on physiological function that are usually manifested in areas that are remote to the point of application.

**Acupressure:** A type of massage that uses specific compression to stimulate acupoints and meridians to achieve complex effects on physiological function that are usually manifested in areas that are remote to the point of application.

**Acupuncture:** A technique for treating disease or pain or by inserting into the skin at specific points needles that are then twirled, heated, or subjected to weak electrical current. In Traditional Chinese Medicine, acupuncture is used to treat a wide range of medical conditions, but its use in the West is usually confined to treatment of pain.

**Acute pain:** Pain provoked by noxious stimulation produced by injury and/or disease with unpleasant sensory and emotional experiences (see Pain).

**Acute stage (of inflammation):** The early response to tissue damage marked by local vasodilation and the influx of white blood cells. Acute inflammation is suggested in orthopedic practice when the client complains of diffuse pain that is felt at rest and made worse by movement.

**Adherence:** The extent to which clients follow the instructions for care that they negotiate with their health care providers.

**Adhesions:** A binding together with dense connective tissue of tissues that normally glide or move in relation to each other, with resultant loss of mobility. Like scars, adhesions may result from the replacement of normal tissue that has been destroyed by burn, wound, surgery, radiation, or disease with connective tissue.

**Adhesive capsulitis:** Inflammation and fibrosis of the shoulder joint capsule that causes painfully limited range of motion.

**Aerosol therapy:** The use of medicated mists to treat respiratory conditions.

**Agonist/antagonist balance:** The ability of opposing groups of muscles to reciprocally contract and lengthen through the full range of active movement.

**AIDS:** Acquired immunodeficiency syndrome; caused by infection with the human immunodeficiency virus (HIV).

**Airway clearance:** Ability to move pulmonary secretions effectively through the use of normal mechanisms of cough and the mucociliary escalator.

**Alarm phase:** The first phase of the general adaptation syndrome or nonspecific response to stress described by Hans Selye (1907–1982). It consists of nervous and endocrine responses to mobilize the organism for "flight or fight."

**Alexander, F. Mathias:** (1869–1955) An Australian actor who developed a system of movement training in response to difficulties he experienced in on-stage performance.

**Alexander technique:** A method of retraining movement that is taught by certified instructors in one-on-one guided sessions. Alexander technique emphasizes coordinated, easy, balanced movement performed with an aligned, elongated spine.

**Algometer:** A device that measures tissue sensitivity to pressure.

**Aligned:** Arranged in a line. A well-aligned spine tends towards shallow, even curves and bilateral symmetry.

**Altered body image:** A change in the way a person perceives his or her body, as happens in eating disorders or after disfiguring accidents.

**Amplitude of technique:** An indication of the size of the area that is covered by a technique.

**Analgesia:** Pain relief.

**Anatomical barrier in soft tissue:** The final resistance to normal tissue range of motion that is provided by bone, ligament, or soft tissue. Motion beyond the anatomical barrier results in tissue damage.

**Anatomy Train:** A continuous, connected, linear myofascial pathway that runs through the body. Eleven such pathways have been described in detail by Thomas Myers in the book, *Anatomy Trains.*

**Antalgic:** Literally, against pain. With an antalgic gait, the stance phase on the painful side is shortened.

**Anxiety:** A state of uneasiness, apprehension, or dread accompanied by physical symptoms such as restlessness, muscle tension, rapid heart rate, and difficulty breathing.

**Anxiety disorders:** A group of related mental illnesses that involve severe anxiety in response to stress.

**Armoring:** Myofascial hardness associated with chronically elevated muscle resting tension.

**Aromatherapy:** The use of essential oils distilled from plants to affect mood or to treat impairments or conditions. The fragrant oils are inhaled or diluted in carrier oil and applied during massage.

**Arousal:** The process of awaking or stimulating.

**Arterial supply:** The volume of oxygenated blood carried by arteries that reaches a given structure.

**Attention:** The clinician's capacity to focus on the sensory information that he or she receives primarily, but not exclusively, through his or her hands.

**Automobilization:** Joint mobilization performed by a client on him or herself.

**Autonomic balance:** Appropriate, healthy functioning of the sympathetic and parasympathetic branches of the autonomic nervous system.

**Autonomic phenomena:** Disturbances of the autonomic nervous system, such as vertigo, that may accompany myofascial trigger points in particular muscles.

**Barnes, John F.:** (1939–) American physical therapist who has contributed to the development of Myofascial Release and taught it extensively in workshops. Basic theory and technique related to this approach are presented in Chapter 10, Connective Tissue Techniques.

**Barrier-release phenomenon:** The therapist engages the tissue barrier at the point at which the therapist palpates a resistance to tissue motion. If the therapist sustains the pressure on the tissue barrier, a "release" may occur after a latency period that will vary with the nature and state of health of the tissue. This release results in a reduction of the resistance that will enable the therapist to move the tissue beyond the location of the original barrier without increasing the pressure of palpation.

**Best research evidence:** The best available clinical, client-centered research that examines the accuracy, safety, and efficacy of diagnostic and assessment tests, prognosis markers, and therapeutic interventions.

**Biofeedback:** A technique for training a person to influence autonomic body processes. Using information supplied from monitoring devices, the subject learns to control basic parameters, such as heart rate, and then to influence related activities such as blood pressure.

**Body functions:** The physiological functions of the anatomical systems of the body.

**Body image:** How a person mentally perceives his or her own body.

**Body structures:** The various anatomical structures and systems of the body.

**Bodywork:** A contemporary term that embraces massage and related approaches that contact or move the client's tissues to achieve educational or therapeutic effects.

**Boundary violations:** When the therapist crosses the ethical and interpersonal limits that have been established for the therapeutic relationship with the client.

**Box kneading:** A two-handed form of kneading in which the hands are positioned so that they are diametrically opposed on a limb, then compress toward each other, and then move proximally. This stroke is recommended to increase fluid return.

**Broad-contact compression:** A nongliding neuromuscular technique, delivered with a broad contact surface, that engages the client's muscle with the pressure and release of the stroke administered perpendicular to the surface of the client's body.

**Broad-contact kneading:** A gliding petrissage technique performed in circles or ellipses with a large contact surface such as the palm.

**Burnout:** A condition resulting from chronic stress that is characterized by physical and emotional exhaustion and is sometimes accompanied by clinical depression or illness.

**Bursitis:** Inflammation of a bursa.

**Cadence:** Rhythm.

**Capsular laxity:** Anatomical or pathological lengthening of the joint capsule.

**Capsular restriction:** Anatomical or pathological shortening of the joint capsule.

**Capsulitis and synovitis:** Inflammation of the joint capsule and associated internal ligaments and of the synovium.

**Case-control study:** A study in which researchers identify individuals who have similar outcomes and examine their history to determine if they received the same intervention.

**Case report:** A type of descriptive research that presents an accurate, brief, and clear narrative report of a single instance or event in a systematic format.

**Case series:** A summary of findings on a group of participants with similar characteristics or who received the same intervention without reference to findings on a control group.

**Caution:** A sign, symptom, evaluation, or diagnosis that directs the clinician to be prepared to modify a given procedure in order to reduce the risks associated with its application.

**Center of gravity:** The point in the center of an object, where the object's mass behaves as if it were concentrated. The center of gravity of the upright adult human is anterior to the S2.

**Centrifugal:** 1. Directed away from the heart or distally. 2. Opposed to the direction of venous and/or lymphatic return. 3. Directed away from an area of local pathology.

**Centripetal:** Directed towards the heart or proximally.

**Chaitow, Leon:** British osteopath and naturopath and editor of the *Journal of Bodywork and Movement Therapies* who has written extensively on manual therapy and natural healing.

**Chest wall:** All the structures in the thorax and outside the lungs that move during breathing, including the ribs, intercostal muscles, diaphragm, fascia, and skin.

**Chest wall mobility:** The ability of the chest wall and its component structures and tissues to move freely.

**Chi (Qi):** In Traditional Chinese Medicine, life force or energy. Chi circulates through the body in well-defined cycles through conduits or channels called meridians.

**Chronic inflammation:** See Chronic stage (of inflammation).

**Chronic obstructive pulmonary disease:** A pulmonary disorder that is characterized by the presence of increased airway resistance.

**Chronic pain:** Pain that persists beyond the usual course of healing of an acute disease or beyond the reasonable time in which the injury is expected to heal. Some authors define chronic pain in terms of duration of pain, with a lower limit of duration ranging from 6 weeks to 6 months; others define chronic pain in terms of an increasing dissociation from the physical etiology and increasing affective and cognitive dimensions of pain.

**Chronic pain syndrome:** A clinical syndrome in which clients present with high levels of pain that is chronic in duration, functional impairment, and depression.

**Chronic restrictive pulmonary disease:** A pulmonary disorder that is characterized by the restriction of lung expansion, such as interstitial fibrosis.

**Chronic stage (of inflammation):** The later response to tissue damage, marked by consolidation and maturation of collagen in scar tissue. Chronic inflammation is suggested in orthopedic practice when the client complains of localized pain that is felt only during specific movements, in a small part of the range or at the end range.

**Chronic stress:** A prolonged and heightened state of arousal that has negative physiological and psychological consequences.

**Circulatory massage:** The use of massage techniques, such as superficial effleurage and petrissage, to increase regional or systemic venous and lymphatic return or arterial supply.

**Clapping:** A form of percussion that is used to mechanically loosen secretions in the lungs and to facilitate airway clearance.

**Classical massage, or classic massage:** See Swedish massage.

**Client-centered care:** This approach to care looks beyond the mere delivery of services to the client to include advocacy, empowerment, respect for the client's autonomy, and the client's participation in decision making. When a therapist commits to client-centered care, the client and therapist share the decision-making about how the intervention will proceed.

**Client examination:** The systematic collection of information on the client's health status and clinical condition through history taking, a general systems review, and tests and measures.

**Client values:** The unique preferences, goals, and expectations that each client brings to the therapeutic relationship.

**Clinical care:** Therapists provide clinical care to their clients as they conduct their examinations and interventions.

**Clinical competence to treat:** The therapist's clinical training permits him or her to treat a given client's condition.

**Clinical decision-making:** The process by which clinicians synthesize and analyze information on their clients' conditions and use the results of their analysis to formulate and progress a therapeutic intervention for their clients. Also known as clinical reasoning and clinical problem-solving.

**Clinical decision-making model:** A framework that demonstrates a process by which therapists can synthesize and analyze information on their clients' conditions and use the results of their analysis to formulate and progress a therapeutic intervention for their clients.

**Clinical depression:** A mood disorder characterized by sadness, despair, or apathy that is severe enough to affect a person's ability to perform activities of daily living and to fulfill social roles.

**Clinical experience:** The experience that a therapist acquires by treating clients in clinical settings. Clinical experience (expertise), best research evidence, and patient values are the components of evidence-based practice.

**Clinical expertise:** The therapist's ability to use his or her clinical skills and past experience to identify each client's unique health status and the potential risks and benefits of interventions that he or she could use in each case.

**Clinical findings:** The results of tests and measures and the lists of impairments, body structures and functions, functional limitations, activity limitations, and limitations in participation with which the client presents.

**Clinical hypothesis:** The clinician's hypothesis about the client's key clinical problems.

**Clinical indication:** A sign, symptom, evaluation, or diagnosis that directs the clinician to apply a certain procedure.

**Clinical problem:** The client's presenting issues related to the impairments or functional limitations he or she is experiencing as a result of his or her medical condition.

**Clinical problem list:** A summary of the client's impairments and functional limitations that will be addressed within the plan of care.

**Clinical stage of inflammation:** The clinician's judgment of the stage of inflammation of an injury made by evaluating the severity of the client's symptoms and the results of tests such as range of motion.

**Clonus:** A cyclical, spasmodic hyperactivity of antagonistic muscles that occurs at a regular frequency in response to a quick stretch stimulus.

**Coarse vibration:** A form of vibration that has an amplitude of 1 cm or more and that intergrades with shaking.

**Cochrane Database of Systematic Reviews:** A collection of systematic reviews and meta-analyses that rigorously summarize and interpret the results of high-quality medical research, usually randomized controlled trials.

**Cognitive Transactional Model of Stress:** Lazarus and Folkman's model of stress as the condition that results when a person's interactions with his environment leads him to perceive a discrepancy between the demands of the situation and the resources of the person's biological, psychological, or social systems.

**Cogwheel rigidity:** A ratchet-like response to passive movement, alternating between giving way and resistance.

**Coherence:** Consistent order and structure of a massage sequence or intervention that results from clear and consistent intention(s) on the part of the therapist.

**Cohort study:** A study that follows the outcomes of a group of participants who researchers identify as having received the intervention and a group with similar characteristics who did not.

**Cold mitten friction:** An application of cold water with friction of a coarse towel or sponge that acts as a tonic. A full body application takes 20–30 minutes.

**Cold pack:** A container filled with cold water, frozen gel, or crushed ice that is applied locally to relieve pain or reduce edema.

**Collagen:** An important structural protein of connective tissue that combines into fibers whose great tensile strength reinforces ligaments, tendons, fascia, and cartilage.

**Collagen cross-link:** A chemical bond between adjacent fibers of collagen that reduces mobility of the fibers with respect to each other. Frequency of cross-links increases with age, injury, and immobility and can restrict mobility of the tissue as a whole.

**Combines with:** When one technique is said to "combine" with another, it means that the two techniques may be executed simultaneously.

**Compartment syndrome:** Elevation of fluid pressure within a closed fascial compartment that is caused by trauma or repetitive exercise such as running. Reduced perfusion can result in hypoxia, nerve damage, and muscle necrosis.

**Compensatory changes:** Changes in biomechanics that accumulate progressively throughout the body after an injury as a result of pain or the effects of scar tissue.

**Compensatory strategy:** A technique that is used as a means of compensating for an impairment that is not amenable to active treatment.

**Complementary treatment techniques:** Techniques that therapists use as an adjunct to the primary treatment techniques. In the case of massage treatments, the primary treatment technique would be massage techniques, and other techniques would be used in a complementary manner.

**Complex decongestive therapy (also known as complex or complete decongestive physiotherapy, CDT, or CDP):** A treatment regimen for lymphedema that includes massage, bandaging or compression garments, specific exercises, and education on hygiene.

**Complex regional pain syndrome:** A condition in which people present with persistent, severe pain and/or allodynia (painful response to non-painful stimulus), dystrophic changes, and vasomotor dysfunction as a result of an unstable sympathetic nervous system following an injury or surgery to an extremity.

**Compression:** Any force that is oriented in a manner so that its effect is to shorten or compact a tissue or structure.

**Compression garment:** An elastic sleeve or similar garment that is meant to cover a region and exert pressure on it to prevent or reduce the accumulation of edema.

**Conceptual framework:** A set of empirical generalizations that provides a means of organizing and integrating observations about a specific set of behaviors that one observes in a particular setting.

**Conceptual model:** A diagram that shows the proposed causal linkages among a set of concepts that the individual believes to be related to a particular health problem.

**Congruency:** The point at which a therapist and client are in agreement on process, action, and effect. It also may refer to the therapist's inward integrity being represented in outward action and word.

**Connective tissue:** Tissues that consist of several different types of cells, such as fibroblasts and fat cells, and elastin and collagen fibers embedded in a matrix of gelatinous material, the consistency of which varies in response to many factors. Nerves, blood vessels, lymph vessels, myofibrils, and organs are found within connective tissue.

**Connective tissue disease (CTD):** A group of diseases that affect connective tissues such as muscle, cartilage, tendon, or skin. They are often autoimmune and inflammatory in nature. Examples include systemic lupus erythematosus, rheumatoid arthritis, Sjögren's syndrome, scleroderma, and mixed connective tissue disease.

**Connective tissue massage (CTM):** A system of massage developed by Elizabeth Dicke and popular in Europe in which connective tissue techniques are applied in precise sequences to the skin and superficial fascial layers to elicit specific physiological reflex effects.

**Connective tissue matrix:** The intercellular portion of connective tissue that contains protein-based fibers and ground substance.

**Connective tissue techniques:** Massage techniques that palpate, lengthen, and promote remodeling of connective tissue.

**Connective tissue zones:** Specific areas of muscle and related fascia of the back that exhibit increased tone in response to visceral pathology. According to the theory of Connective Tissue Massage, manipulating a zone associated with an organ will reflexly improve the function of that organ.

**Consent:** See Informed consent.

**Consolidated edema:** Edema in the chronic stage, where inflammatory exudate has been replaced with dense fibrous connective tissue.

**Consolidation:** Combining or grouping into a single unit.

**Contact surface:** The portion of the clinician's hand or arm that is used to execute the stroke.

**Context:** A brief description of how a massage technique is conventionally sequenced in relation to other techniques.

**Contractile tissue:** Muscle, with its enveloping fascial layers, associated tendon(s), and periosteal attachments.

**Contracture:** A permanent muscular shortening due to a variety of physiological changes in muscle, such as fibrosis or loss of muscular balance.

**Contraindication:** A sign, symptom, evaluation, or diagnosis that directs the therapist to avoid applying a certain procedure.

**Controlled lean posture:** An inclined, aligned posture used to efficiently transfer the clinician's body weight to the client in a controlled manner.

**Contusion:** A bruise.

**Cortisol:** A hormone (hydrocortisone) produced by the adrenal cortex. It has multiple physiological effects that counteract the effects of stress.

**Countertransference:** Occurs when the therapist projects feelings onto a client that are unconscious, unprocessed, or unexpressed or idealizes the client in some way.

**Cranial (craniosacral) rhythm:** A subtle, palpable rhythm that occurs 6–14 times a minute and is caused by rhythmic flow of cerebrospinal fluid through the central nervous system.

**Craniosacral Therapy:** Involves assessing and adjusting the movement of the cerebrospinal fluid (CSF), which can become restricted by trauma and stress. Practitioners apply gentle and subtle manipulations to skull, spine, diaphragm, and fascia. Craniosacral therapy originated with osteopath William Sutherland and has been further developed by osteopath John Upledger.

**Creep:** Viscoelastic stretch of connective tissue that occurs when it is subjected to sustained tension and that is palpable.

**Crepitus:** A vibration of variable fineness that is associated with roughened gliding surfaces of a tendon or its sheath or of the articulating surfaces of a joint. Crepitus can sometimes be heard, as well as palpated.

**Cross-link:** See Collagen cross-link.

**Cutaneous reflex:** An involuntary response caused by stimulation of receptors in the skin.

**Cyriax, James H.:** (1904–1985) British orthopedic surgeon and author of an influential textbook of orthopedics that is still in print. Cyriax popularized range of motion testing to identify orthopedic conditions and the use of cross-fiber friction to treat many overuse conditions.

**Decerebrate rigidity:** Rigidity that occurs as a result of brainstem lesions. It presents clinically as sustained contraction and posturing of the trunk and lower limbs in extension.

**Decorticate rigidity:** Rigidity that occurs as a result of brainstem lesions. It presents clinically as sustained contraction and posturing of the trunk and lower limbs in extension and the upper limbs in flexion.

**Deep effleurage:** A general gliding manipulation performed with long strokes and moderate-to-heavy centripetal pressure that deforms superficial or deep layers of muscle.

**Deep fascia:** Connective tissue layer that lies immediately superficial to, or between, muscle fibers. The primary functions of the deep fascia are to allow muscles to move freely, to carry nerve and blood vessels, to fill the space between muscles, and to provide an origin for muscles.

**Deep tissue massage:** An imprecise term that suggests that connective tissue and/or neuromuscular techniques are being applied with enough force to deform myofascial tissue that lies beneath the investing layer of the deep fascia.

**Deform:** To change shape.

**Deformation:** The change in shape of a tissue or structure when it is subjected to pressure.

**Delayed-onset muscle soreness (DOMS):** Muscle soreness felt 24–72 hours after vigorous or unaccustomed exercise, probably caused by microtearing in the muscle fibers.

**Dependent edema:** An increase in extracellular fluid volume that is localized in a dependent area, such as a limb.

**Depression:** See Clinical depression.

**DeQuervain's tenosynovitis:** Overuse inflammation of the tendon and/or synovial sheath of the extensor pollicis brevis and abductor pollicis longus muscles.

**Dermatomal pain:** Pain in the pattern of a dermatome. Injury of a dorsal root may result in sensory loss in the skin or may be felt as a burning or electric pain.

**Dermatome:** An area of skin supplied by one dorsal nerve root.

**Dermis:** The first layer of connective tissue.

**Diagnosis:** The process and result of analyzing and organizing the findings from the client examination into clusters or syndromes.

**Diaphragmatic breathing:** An exercise that trains the client to consciously use the diaphragm during breathing.

**Dicke, Elizabeth:** German physiotherapist who developed connective tissue massage (Bindegewebsmassage) in the 1930s in response to personal illness.

**Direct:** In the context of connective tissue techniques, direct means that the therapist directs the force of the technique toward, and then through, the primary tissue restriction. This is in contrast to indirect techniques in which the therapist applies the force, or moves the client, away from the fascial barrier or restriction of motion.

**Direct effect:** A direct therapeutic effect

**Direct fascial technique:** A slow, gliding connective tissue technique that applies a moderate, sustained tensional force to the superficial fascia or to the deep fascia and associated muscle. It results in palpable viscoelastic lengthening and plastic deformation of the fascia.

**Direct inhibitory pressure:** Specific compression applied to a tendon as a means of inhibiting the tone of the related muscle for a short period of time.

**Direction of technique:** The direction of the applied force. The direction given in the description of techniques is the direction in which the greatest force is applied during the pressure phase of the stroke.

**Disability:** When an individual is unable to perform his or her socially defined tasks, activities, or roles to the expected level.

**Disablement Model:** An extension of the medical model that broadened the therapist's approach to examination, evaluation, and treatment to encompass the client's functional limitations and disability, as well as his or her presenting impairments.

**Discharge:** The transition of the client from the therapist's care to self-care or to treatment by another therapist.

**Discharge Phase:** The final phase of the clinical decision-making process that involves the transition of the client from the therapist's care to self-care or to treatment by another therapist.

**Discrimination:** The clinician's ability to distinguish fine gradations of sensory information.

**Dislocation (luxation):** The displacement of a bone from its normal position in a joint.

**Dissociation:** An impaired perception of reality often accompanied by a numbing of emotions or a disconnecting from the present. A client who is dissociated may appear to exhibit a profound apathy or inability to make decisions or initiate movements or actions. The client may be unaware of the present, of sounds and activities around them, or of the perception of pain.

**Distraction:** See Traction.

**Drag:** 1. Tensile force, stretching force, or traction force exerted along a single tissue layer. 2. Inherent tissue resistance to such force.

**Drainage technique:** Any massage technique or related technique, such as elevation of a limb, that increases the return flow of lymph or venous blood.

**Draping:** The process by which the clinician covers and uncovers portions of the client's body during treatment, while maintaining modesty and respecting appropriate client–clinician boundaries.

**Dry brushing:** Systematic brushing of the skin with a (natural) bristle brush, administered as a tonic, to exfoliate, and to stimulate skin metabolism.

**Dual relationships:** When the professional and social roles and interactions between two people overlap. This may occur when therapists treat family members, friends, or colleagues. Dual relationships are not necessarily wrong or unethical, but they can present uncomfortable situations or conflicts of interest for the therapist and client.

**Duration of technique:** An estimate of a reasonable length of time for which a single technique may have to be applied by a competent clinician to begin to achieve the specified outcomes.

**Dyspnea:** Shortness of breath, labored or difficult breathing, or uncomfortable awareness of one's breathing.

**Ease of movement:** Movement that is comfortable and that requires minimal effort.

**Eastern-influenced massage systems:** Massage systems originating in Asia that are based on radically different conceptual models of body processes than those used in Western medicine, such as energy (Chi) and meridians. Examples of Eastern approaches are Shiatsu, Amma, Thai massage, acupressure, and Jin Shin Do.

**Ectomorph:** A person with a build that is lean, slender, and sparsely muscled.

**Edema:** An accumulation of fluid in cells, tissues, or serous cavities. Edema has four main causes: increased permeability of capillaries, decreased plasma protein osmotic pressure, increased pressure in capillaries and venules, and lymphatic flow obstruction.

**Effleurage:** A group of general gliding manipulations performed with centripetal pressure and varying pressures.

**Effusion:** Excessive fluid in the joint capsule, indicating irritation or inflammation of the synovium.

**Elastic:** Capable of returning to original size and shape after being stretched or deformed.

**Elastic barrier in soft tissue:** The resistance that the clinician feels at the end of the passive range of motion of the tissue when she is taking the "slack" out of the tissue.

**Elastic deformation:** Deformation in response to applied force that disappears after the force is removed; spring-like behavior.

**Elastic recoil:** The return towards original size and shape demonstrated by elastic substances.

**Elastic stretch:** Stretch that disappears after the tensile force is removed.

**Electromyography (EMG):** A technique for recording the electrical (physiological) activity of muscles at rest and while contracting.

**Electronic muscle stimulation (EMS):** A modality where electric impulses are applied externally to muscle to make it contract.

**Elevated resting tension:** Increase in firmness to palpation of muscles at rest.

**Endangerment sites:** Areas of the human body over which the use of direct or sustained pressure is contraindicated.

**End feel:** (1) The qualities of motion or resistance to motion that the clinician palpates in the joint at the end of passive range of motion. (2) For massage techniques, end feel is the quality of resistance to further movement that is perceived by the practitioner at the end of the massage stroke. End feel is related to tissue constituents such as fat, connective tissue (scar tissue), muscle, etc.

**Endomorph:** A person with a build where the trunk is ample and rounded, with a high percentage of body fat.

**Endorphins:** A group of peptide neurotransmitters produced in the brain that act to reduce pain by binding to opiate receptor sites.

**Energetic approaches:** Approaches, such as Therapeutic Touch or Reiki, that use the simple forms of touch to manipulate the energy field or magnetic field of the client's body. See also Eastern approaches to massage.

**Engage:** To enter into contact with. In this text, a tissue is said to be "engaged" during a technique if it is significantly deformed during the technique's application.

**Entrainment:** The alteration of a biological rhythm in response to an external stimulus.

**Entrapment neuropathy:** Nerve compression that can result from bony deformity or muscle and connective tissue shortening and inflammation associated with trigger point activity, fascial restrictions, overuse syndromes, and other clinical conditions.

**Episode of care:** A series of interventions from initial visit to discharge within a single period that a client receives for a specific condition.

**Epithelium:** A layer of closely packed columnar or squamous cells that have little intercellular material between them.

**Ergonomic:** Related to the design and use of workplace equipment that enhances worker wellness.

**Evaluation:** The synthesis of the information from the client examination.

**Evaluative Phase:** The steps in the Evaluative Phase revolve around formulating and confirming a clinical hypothesis about the client's clinical problem or wellness goals.

**Evidence:** Information on clinical care that researchers and therapists collect in a systematic manner.

**Evidence-based medicine (EBM):** The integration of best research evidence with clinical expertise and client values.

**Evidence-based practice:** The integration of best research evidence with clinical expertise and client values to treat individual clients.

**Evidence house:** An approach proposed by Jonas that includes many kinds of rigorous research methods, rather than Sackett's hierarchical model. Jonas suggests that including a variety of research methodologies, such as qualitative research methods, can provide a more balanced and complete picture of what constitutes massage and how it works.

**Examination:** The collection of information on the client's health status and clinical condition through history taking, a general systems review, and tests and measures.

**Exercise tolerance:** The ability to perform cardiopulmonary work.

**Exhaustion phase:** The third and final phase of the general adaptation syndrome or nonspecific response to stress described by Hans Selye (1907–1982). It is characterized by physical and emotional exhaustion and is sometimes accompanied by illness.

**Explicit memory:** The verbal, narrative memory that derives from the hippocampus and that is evoked when a person relates a story.

**Extensibility:** Ability to extend or lengthen.

**Facilitated segment:** A spinal segment whose joints are dysfunctional as a result of visceral imbalance or pathology. Muscles adjacent to the facilitated segment show elevated resting tension and may be edematous or fibrotic. See also Connective tissue zone and Viscerosomatic reflex.

**Fascia:** A tough fibrous membrane composed of dense connective tissue. Superficial fascia contains fat, nerves, and blood vessels and joins the skin to the underlying layer. Deep fascia supports and separates the muscles. Subserous fascia lies between the deep fascia and the body cavities.

**Fascial binding:** See Fascial restrictions.

**Fascial restrictions:** The loss of mobility of one fascial layer with respect to another because of the loss of fluid consistency of ground substance and development of collagenous cross-links. Fascial restrictions can result from repair of tissue damage and from prolonged immobility.

**Fascial sheath:** An envelope of fascia that surrounds another structure, for example a muscle.

**Fascial splinting:** Regional thickening and hardening of fascia in response to increased biomechanical load.

**Fasciculations:** Localized, subconscious muscle contractions that result from the contraction of the muscle cells innervated by a single motor axon and thus do not involve the entire muscle.

**Fasciitis:** Inflammation of fascia.

**Fatigue:** Extreme tiredness or exhaustion; decreased capacity for physical or mental work.

**Feldenkrais Method:** A system, developed by Moshe Feldenkrais (1904–1984), that teaches mindful movement and efficient patterns for functional activities. Instruction by certified practitioners occurs in individual or group settings.

**Fibromyalgia:** A chronic rheumatic syndrome characterized by widespread musculoskeletal pain, the presence of specific tender points, severe fatigue, and sleep disturbances.

**Fibroplasia:** The phase of wound repair when fibroblasts grow and form new extracellular matrix and collagen. Fibroplasia occurs after the inflammatory phase and before the remodeling phase.

**Fibrosed edema:** See Consolidated edema.

**Fibrosis:** Formation of (excess) fibrous connective tissue during the process repair.

**Fibrositic deposit or nodule:** An outdated term used to describe hard pea-sized deposits in muscle and connective tissue that would now probably be recognized as myofascial trigger points.

**Fine vibration:** A superficial reflex technique in which a fast, oscillating or trembling movement is produced on the client's skin that results in minimal deformation of subcutaneous tissues.

**Flexibility:** The ability to bend without breaking.

**Fluidotherapy:** The application of warmed cellulose particles suspended in forced dry air to heat an injured body part prior to exercise.

**Force of palpation:** The direction and manner in which manual strength is applied to tissues during palpation that results in tissues being compressed, stretched, sheared, bent, and twisted.

**Fracture:** Interruption in the continuity of a bone.

**Framework:** The manner in which the intervention is delivered including timing, location, appointment setting, common responses, payment, and issues of confidentiality. It also describes the ethical foundations for decision-making to which the therapist commits. When a therapist's framework is clear to a client, then the client may appreciate the client roles and expectations as well as what the therapist is able to do.

**Framing general massage technique:** A general massage technique that is repeated at intervals during the course of a massage sequence. A framing technique serves as the principal palpation tool, connects the other techniques used, and imparts a sense of structure to the sequence.

**Fremitus:** A pulmonary vibration that a clinician can palpate over the rib cage as the client speaks or vocalizes.

**Friction:** 1. A repetitive, specific, nongliding, connective tissue technique that produces movement between the fibers of dense connective tissue, increasing tissue extensibility. 2. Historically, the term "friction" has a broad, ambiguous usage that has embraced virtually any manner of rubbing between two surfaces.

**Fulling:** A form of broad-contact kneading in which the hands compress down and away from each other to spread or broaden the muscle belly and then lift the muscle up on the return stroke.

**Functional instability:** Instability of a joint under load.

**Functional limitation:** A restriction of the individual's ability to execute a task or action in an ideal situation.

**Functional outcome:** The outcome that is related to the client's functional limitation.

**Galvanic stimulation:** See Electronic muscle stimulation.

**Gate theory of pain:** The widely quoted theory, first proposed by Melzack and Wall in the 1960s, that proposes that perception of painful stimuli in higher brain centers can be inhibited by stimulation of large fiber afferents.

**General adaptation syndrome:** The nonspecific response to stress first described by Austro-Canadian endocrinologist Hans Selye (1907–1982). It consists of three sequential psychoneuroimmulogical phases termed alarm, resistance, and exhaustion.

**General massage (general full-body massage):** Massage that includes all regions of the body. General massage commonly takes 60–90 minutes to perform but can be completed in as little as 15 minutes.

**General technique:** A technique that is applied to an entire region or a larger portion of the body or applied using a broad surface such as the palm, or both.

**Glide:** Movement of the clinician's hand across the client's skin.

**Grade of injury:** Severity of injury. An orthopedic injury may be assigned a numerical grade of 1, 2, or 3 to represent a mild, moderate, or severe injury.

**Grounding:** A practitioner's awareness of his or her contact and connection with the earth. The posture and alignment exercises described in Chapter 6 increase this awareness.

**Ground substance:** See Matrix.

**Guided awareness:** A technique where the therapist guides the client to focus his or her awareness on a body part or process.

**Hatha yoga:** As practiced in the West, Hatha yoga is usually the exercise of performing various postures, called asanas. Traditional Indian Hatha yoga is a comprehensive discipline that includes moral guidelines, asanas, breathing exercises, and meditation.

**Healing Touch:** An energetic approach similar to Therapeutic Touch and Reiki. Practitioners use the simplest form of touch to manipulate the energy field or magnetic field of the client's body.

**Health:** A dynamic process that encompasses multiple domains, including the individual's physical, emotional, social, and intellectual dimensions. In addition, some definitions of health address the individual's ability to fulfill his or her social roles and respond to environmental stressors.

**Health-related quality of life:** The objective and subjective dimensions of an individual's ability to function in, and derive satisfaction from, a variety of social roles in the presence of impaired health status.

**Holding:** See Unnecessary muscle tension.

**Homeostasis:** The state of internal stable equilibrium that is maintained by healthy living organisms in response to external and internal changes.

**Hospice:** A facility or organization that provides palliative care and physical, spiritual, emotional, and economic support for the terminally ill and their families.

**Hot pack:** A container filled with hot water, gel, or clay that is applied locally to increase circulation and produce analgesia.

**H-reflex:** A measure of spinal reflex (motoneuron) excitability that is based on the time required for a stimulus applied to a sensory nerve to travel to the spinal cord and return down the motor nerve. The H-reflex is increased in conditions of spastic paralysis.

**Hyaluronic acid:** A glycosaminoglycan found in the extracellular matrix of connective tissues that contributes to the lubricating qualities of synovial fluid and cartilage.

**Hydration:** The bonding of water molecules to another compound.

**Hyperarousal:** An abnormally heightened state of arousal.

**Hyperemia:** An increase in the amount of blood flowing through a body part, indicated by redness. Hyperemia can be caused by massage and by applications of heat or cold.

**Hyperreflexia:** Exaggerated deep tendon reflexes.

**Hypersensitivity:** This is the sudden painful, jolting, ticklish, or uncomfortable reaction that a client has when touched by the therapist. Hypersensitivity may be caused by an old, unresolved injury or trauma or as a result of chronic protection, overuse, or postural dysfunction.

**Hyperstimulation analgesia:** Pain relief that occurs as a result solely of somatic sensory stimulation in the form of heat, cold, touch, vibration, or movement. See Gate Theory of Pain.

**Hypertonia:** A general term used to refer to muscle tone that is above normal resting levels, regardless of the mechanism for the increase in tone.

**Hypertrophy:** Increase in the size of an organ or structure, usually due to growth of individual cells rather than an increased number of cells.

**Hypotonia:** A general term used to refer to muscle tone that is below normal resting levels, regardless of the mechanism for the decrease in tone.

**Ice massage (cryomassage):** Superficial massage with ice, a cold pack, or an instrument performed locally to reduce pain and inflammation.

**Identification:** The clinician's ability to distinguish between healthy and dysfunctional tissue states and to identify tissues and structures and their responses to applied force.

**Impairment:** A loss or abnormality of the affected individual's body structures or functions that occurs as a result of the initial or subsequent pathophysiology.

**Impairment-related outcome:** The outcome that is related to the impairment of the client's body structure or function.

**Implicit memory (tissue memory):** The nonnarrative, non-verbal, and sensory-motor memory that is typically recorded in the amygdala. When implicit memory is evoked, a client will feel as if the memory is happening in the present.

**Indication:** A sign, symptom, evaluation, or diagnosis that directs the therapist to apply a certain procedure.

**Indirect:** Techniques in which the therapist applies the force, or moves the client, away from the fascial barrier or restriction of motion.

**Indurated:** Hardened.

**Inertial resistance:** The resistance of an object to applied force that depends on its mass.

**Inert tissues:** Tissues that do not contract, for example, ligament, capsule, and nerve.

**Infant massage:** A modified form of classical massage designed for infants. Infant massage improves infant development and parent–child bonding and can be used to treat colic.

**Informed consent:** Obtaining clear and informed consent for treatment from a client involves ensuring that the client understands the intent and direction of therapy. This process requires that the therapist explain exactly what he or she is going to do and how he or she will achieve the specified outcomes. It also requires that the client hears and understands the therapist's explanation, since clients who do not hear the explanation may agree without understanding what the therapist means.

**Inquiring touch:** Intelligent Touch is inquiring touch. A good clinician is constantly asking questions, and the use of massage is no exception to this requirement. The use of inquiring touch does not imply that the clinician's touch feels tentative to the client or that it lack firmness when required.

**Intelligent Touch:** The learned skills essential for successful clinical use of massage: attention and concentration, discrimination, identification, inquiry, and intention.

**Interferential current:** The crossing of two independent medium frequency electrical currents to create a different frequency current at the point of intersection of the two currents. This is used to stimulate large impulse fibers and interferes with the transmission of pain messages at the spinal cord level.

**Intergrades with:** To merge gradually one into another. When one technique is said to "intergrade" with another, the two techniques can be performed consecutively and will merge gradually one into another since there are intermediate hybrid forms of the technique that lie between and resemble both techniques.

**International Classification of Functioning, Disability and Health:** A model that presents human function, health, and disability as an interaction between the individual, the disease process, and the environment in which the individual lives.

**Interstitial fluid pressure:** Pressure that is caused by the amount of fluid in the interstitium or intercellular spaces. The interstitial fluid pressure reflects the degree of hydration of the tissue, and the forces that govern it are described in Starling's Law.

**Intervention:** 1. A single instance during which a clinician delivers care to the client. 2. A technique or series of techniques that are used to address a client's impairments or wellness goals.

**Intractable:** Unresponsive to treatment.

**Investing layer of the deep fascia:** Dense connective tissue layer that lies between the superficial fascia and muscle.

**Ischemic compression:** See Specific compression and Trigger point pressure release.

**Joint integrity:** The extent to which a joint conforms to the expected anatomical and biomechanical norms.

**Joint manipulation:** A high-grade joint mobilization.

**Joint mobilization:** A technique in which therapists apply controlled, graded force to produce accessory joint motions (joint play) in order to restore altered biomechanics (i.e., to restore normal joint play) of the target joint to reduce pain and improve range of motion.

**Joint play:** Small movements that occur between synovial joint surfaces that are necessary for normal joint functioning during range of motion. These motions can be produced by the therapist in a passive client, but they are not under voluntary control and cannot be performed actively by the client.

**Joint position sense:** Ability to accurately locate a joint in space using only proprioceptive information (i.e., when blindfolded).

**Joint range of motion:** The capacity of the joint to move within the anatomical or physiological range of motion that is available at that joint based on its arthrokinematics and the ability of the periarticular connective tissue to deform. Range of motion reflects the function of the contractile, nervous, inert, and bony tissues and the client's willingness to perform a movement.

**Jump sign:** Pain behavior, such as wincing and attempted withdrawal, that a client shows when a trigger point is compressed.

**Kellogg, J. H.:** (1852–1943) American medical doctor who ran the Battle Creek Sanitarium, a health resort that emphasized vegetarian meals, enemas, and exercise. Kellogg wrote well-known texts on massage and hydrotherapy and started a company to market whole-grain cereals.

**Key signs:** The results of tests and measures that are characteristic for any given orthopedic condition.

**Key trigger point:** A trigger point that is responsible for activating one or more satellite trigger points. Inactivation of a key trigger point will inactivate its associated satellites.

**Kinetic chain:** The series of joints that connect the bones of the upper limb or the lower limb.

**Kneading:** A gliding neuromuscular technique, performed in circles or ellipses, that repeatedly compresses superficial tissues and muscle against underlying structures and releases them. See also Petrissage.

**Lactate:** The byproduct of anaerobic glycolysis that accumulates in muscles during intense exercise. Accumulation of lactate is no longer believed to be responsible for delayed-onset muscle soreness.

**Latent trigger points:** Trigger points that are not painful in and of themselves unless they are being palpated.

**Lead pipe rigidity:** Constant resistance to passive movement.

**Lederman, Eyal:** British osteopath and author of several books and articles on manual therapy.

**Legal right to treat:** The therapist's scope of practice permits him or her to treat a given client's condition.

**Level of arousal:** Level of alertness.

**Levels of evidence:** A hierarchy of research designs created by Sackett et al. that ranks several different types of studies. Studies at the top of the hierarchy provide the strongest evidence of a cause-and-effect relationship between the intervention and the outcome and vice versa.

**Life Events Model of Stress:** Holmes and Rahe's model of stress that examined the nature and consequences of negative life events and proposed that interpersonal stressors are predictive of increases in disease activity.

**Lifelong learning:** The philosophy that learning is required throughout the lifespan of a professional career.

**Lifestyle:** The way a person (or a group) lives, including attitudes, values, worldview, patterns of social relations, consumption, entertainment, and dress.

**Lift/lifting:** Lifting of the tissues perpendicularly off the surface of the body, as occurs with some forms of petrissage like picking-up.

**Ligament insufficiency:** Anatomical or pathological shortening of the capsular ligament.

**Ligament laxity:** Anatomic or pathologic lengthening of the capsular ligament.

**Lipoma:** A benign fatty tumor.

**Local reflex signs:** An effect observed in a particular region that is mediated by the nervous system. Examples are discoloration of the skin (blanching or flushing) or more general autonomic responses such as sweating and nausea.

**Lomilomi:** A traditional shamanic massage form from Hawaii that is done to heal and to mark life passages. Lomilomi uses repetitive centripetal elongated gliding strokes, and sessions last for 2 hours or longer.

**Long-axis traction:** Traction in which force is applied parallel to the length of a limb.

**Lubricant:** A substance, such as oil, that a therapist uses to control the amount of glide, friction, and drag that occurs between his or her moving hands and the client's skin.

**Lunge:** A movement used during massage, in which the therapist slowly shifts her body weight onto her forward leg by bending that knee and straightening the back leg, while keeping her torso perfectly poised and upright.

**Lunge and lean:** A movement used during massage in which the therapist inclines her body forward (leans) as she shifts her weight onto her forward leg during a lunge.

**Lunge and reach:** A movement used during massage in which the therapist extends both arms straight ahead at navel level as she shifts weight onto her forward leg during a lunge.

**Lymphatic return:** The volume of lymph returned to the venous system through the lymphatic vessels.

**Lymph drainage techniques:** See Drainage techniques.

**Lymphedema:** Accumulation of abnormal amounts of lymph fluid and associated swelling of subcutaneous tissues that result from the obstruction, destruction, or hypoplasia of lymph vessels.

**Manual lymph drainage (MLD):** Comprehensive massage systems designed to enhance lymphatic return (e.g., Vodder, Leduc). These systems may incorporate various massage techniques but often rely extensively on what is termed in this text as superficial lymph drainage technique. MLD also uses other massage techniques, such as petrissage and direct fascial technique, to address consolidated edema associated with chronic conditions.

**Matrix (extracellular matrix):** The portion of connective tissue found between the cells. It includes proteoglycans, matrix proteins, and water, but not protein fibers such as collagen.

**Maturation (of connective tissue):** The last period of the chronic stage of inflammation (from the 2nd month to a year after injury), when collagen turnover declines and the scar tissue becomes mostly fibrous.

**Mechanical effects of massage:** Effects that are caused by physically moving the tissues by compression, tension (stretch), shearing, bending, or twisting.

**Mechanical techniques:** Massage techniques that compress, stretch, shear, bend, or twist the tissues.

**Mechanoreceptor:** A receptor for information about movement, tension, pressure, or touch.

**Medical massage:** The use of massage to treat medical conditions.

**Medical Model:** Clinical model that focused on measuring and treating the client's presenting impairments without a specific consideration of the client's other personal factors.

**Mennell, James Beaver:** (1880–1957) A British doctor who taught medical massage at St. Thomas's Hospital in London from 1912 to 1935 and wrote an influential text-book on the subject. Mennell's experiences treating the wounded of World War I convinced him first hand of the efficacy of medical massage.

**Meridian:** In Traditional Chinese Medicine, a conduit or channel through which energy (qi, chi, ch'i) circulates through the body in well-defined cycles.

**Mesomorph:** A person with a build that is well-muscled.

**Meta-analysis:** A form of research in which the results of different, similar studies are pooled and analyzed.

**Mobilization:** See Joint mobilization.

**Modality:** Any therapeutic technique. Some examples of physical modalities include hot packs, cryotherapy, ultra-violet radiation, TENS, traction, acupuncture, massage, joint mobilization, and therapeutic exercise.

**Model:** 1. A framework or system of ideas used to explain the workings of the world. 2. A diagram that represents an idea, phenomena, or relationship between variables.

**Moist heat:** Superficial heat that is accompanied by a small amount of steam, such as is obtained from a hydro-collator hot pack or thermophore.

**Motoneuron (motor neuron) excitability:** See H-reflex.

**Motor point:** The place where a motor neuron enters a muscle.

**Muscle endurance:** A muscle's ability to contract, or maintain torque, over a number of contractions or a period of time. Conversely, fatigue is inability to maintain torque, or the loss of power, over time.

**Muscle energy techniques:** Osteopathic techniques in which the patient contracts a muscle in one of a number of ways to promote its relaxation. The patient's position and the duration, direction, and force of the contraction are controlled and gently resisted by the practitioner.

**Muscle extensibility:** The ability of a muscle and its associated fascia to undergo lengthening deformation during the movement of a joint through its anatomic range.

**Muscle integrity:** The extent to which a muscle conforms to the expected anatomical and biomechanical norms.

**Muscle performance:** A muscle's capacity to do work based on its length, tension, and velocity. Neurological stimulus, fuel storage, fuel delivery, and balance, timing, and sequencing of muscle contraction influence integrated muscle performance.

**Muscle power:** Work produced by a muscle per unit of time (strength × speed).

**Muscle resting tension:** The firmness to palpation at rest observed in muscles with normal innervation. Traditionally, muscle resting tension has been described as resulting from the physiological properties of muscle, such as viscosity, elasticity, and plasticity, rather than from motor unit firing.

**Muscle spasm:** Involuntary contraction of a muscle that results in increased muscular tension and shortness that cannot be released voluntarily.

**Muscle squeezing:** A petrissage technique in which one or both hands are used to grasp, lift, and squeeze a muscle, muscle group, or body segment without glide.

**Muscle strain or tear:** Lesion or inflammation of muscle fibers that can occur in response to trauma.

**Muscle strength:** The force or torque produced by a muscle or group of muscles to overcome a resistance during a maximum voluntary contraction.

**Muscle tone:** Resting tension and responsiveness of muscles to passive elongation or stretch.

**Myofascial balance:** Appropriate distribution of tension throughout the connective tissues of the myofascial network. Good myofascial balance promotes upright posture and efficiency and ease of movement.

**Myofascial network:** The muscles and associated connective tissues (tendons, aponeuroses, and fascia) of the locomotor system. This network forms part of a greater system that includes all the structural connective tissues of the body.

**Myofascial pain syndrome:** The sensory, motor, and autonomic symptoms caused by myofascial trigger points.

**Myofascial release:** 1. A connective tissue technique that combines nongliding fascial traction with varying amounts of orthopedic stretch and that results in palpable viscoelastic lengthening and plastic deformation of the fascia. 2. A system of treatment that uses the myofascial release technique in conjunction with craniosacral, osteopathic, and other soft tissue techniques.

**Myofascial trigger point:** A hyperirritable spot in skeletal muscle that is associated with a hypersensitive palpable nodule in a taut band. The area is painful on compression and can give rise to a variety of symptoms, such as referred pain, referred tenderness, motor dysfunction, and autonomic phenomena.

**Myofascial unit:** One muscle and its associated tendons, aponeuroses, and fascial wrappings.

**Myotatic unit:** A functional unit of an agonist and its antagonist muscles.

**Myotherapy:** A method of treating myofascial trigger points, popularized by Bonnie Prudden, that uses specific compression and active exercise to restore full, pain-free movement to muscles.

**Myotomal pain:** Pain in a myotome, or a group of muscles that are supplied by one nerve root.

**Nerve entrapment:** Compression of a peripheral nerve or nerve root.

**Neurapraxia:** Loss of nerve conduction due to compression, without structural change in the axon.

**Neurogenic pain:** Pain that results from noninflammatory dysfunction of the peripheral or central nervous system that does not involve nociceptor stimulation or trauma.

**Neuromuscular facilitation:** The application of techniques, such as tapping and quick stretch, to strengthen the contraction of a muscle. These techniques are often applied immediately prior to exercise for clients who have CNS disorders.

**Neuromuscular inhibition:** The application of massage techniques, such as static contact, or other techniques, such as prolonged cold, to reduce the strength of contraction or tone of a muscle. These techniques are often applied immediately prior to exercise for clients who have CNS disorders.

**Neuromuscular Technique (NMT):** As defined by Chaitow and others, a complex massage system that includes specific finger and thumb techniques that resemble stripping and direct fascial technique.

**Neuromuscular techniques:** Massage techniques that palpate muscle, affect the level of resting tension of muscles, and have additional psychoneuroimmunological effects.

**Neuromuscular tone:** Muscle resting tension and responsiveness of muscles to passive elongation or stretch.

**Nociception:** The stimulus of pain receptors and the resulting transmission of information about pain to the central nervous system (CNS). Nociceptive information can be modulated in the CNS so that the resulting perception of pain is heightened or reduced.

**Nociceptive pain:** Sensitization of peripheral nociceptors as a result of injury to a muscle or a joint that causes increased release of neurotransmitters in the dorsal horn of the spinal cord. The sensitized dorsal horn neurons demonstrate increased background activity, increased receptive field size, and increased responses to peripherally applied stimuli.

**Nongliding:** A technique in which no movement occurs of the hand relative to the skin.

**Nonmyofascial trigger point:** A hyperirritable spot in scar tissue, fascia, periosteum, ligament, or joint capsule that is associated with a hypersensitive palpable nodule in a taut band.

**Nonspecific (treatment) effects:** Positive treatment effects that are not caused by the specific action of the intervention, but rather are due to a subject's expectations of benefit. Placebo response.

**Numeric rating scale:** A numeric scale that clients use to rate the intensity of pain or other subjective symptoms. Zero represents no pain, and 10 represents the worst pain imaginable or previously experienced. The client makes the rating verbally or using a visual scale such as the Visual Analog Scale.

**Object of palpation:** The chosen portion of the sensory field on which the clinician focuses attention during palpation. The object being palpated is not necessarily a physical object; instead, it may be a characteristic, such as temperature, or a phenomenon, such as resistance to movement.

**Osteopathy:** 1. A branch of medicine that uses manual therapy, in addition to other treatment techniques such as medication and surgery, to treat the full range of conditions. A central tenet of osteopathy is that good structural relationships will positively influence function. 2. A form of alternative therapy that uses a variety of manual techniques, such as craniosacral technique, to treat the musculoskeletal system.

**Outcome-Based Massage:** The use of a systematic clinical decision-making process and a defined process for identifying outcomes, selecting techniques based on the evidence, and applying those techniques using effective psychomotor skills.

**Outcome for body structure and function:** The outcome that is related to the impairment of the client's body structure or function.

**Outcome measure:** A variable that is measured in order to gauge the client's progress towards an outcome.

**Outcome or Outcome of care:** The result of a single intervention or of all of the interventions in the plan of care as a whole.

**Overpressure:** With respect to massage techniques, an increase of manual pressure applied to a particular structure, such as a group of lymph nodes, often at the end of a stroke.

**Overtreatment:** Application of techniques for too long a time or with too much force, so that undesirable consequences occur.

**Oxytocin:** A neurotransmitter hormone that stimulates uterine contractions during labor and the production of milk.

**Pain:** An unpleasant sensation associated with actual or potential tissue damage that is mediated by specific nerve fibers to the brain where its conscious appreciation may be modified by various factors.

**Pain scale:** A verbal or visual analog scale that rates a client's experience of pain with numbers from 0 (no pain) to 10 (worst pain ever experienced).

**Palliative care:** Any form of medical care or treatment that aims to alleviate symptoms without curing.

**Palpation:** A method of examination in which the therapist uses the hands and fingers to gather information about the location, size, shape, firmness, temperature, and sensitivity of tissues and structures.

**Parasympathetic:** The branch of the autonomic nervous system with efferent fibers that exit through several cranial nerves and the 2nd to 4th sacral nerves. It slows the heart rate, increases intestinal secretion and peristalsis, constricts bronchioles, and is associated with a general relaxation response of the organism—"rest and digest."

**Parasympathetic response:** See Parasympathetic.

**Parkinsonian rigidity:** Rigidity that occurs as a result of basal ganglia lesions. It presents clinically as a tight contraction of both agonist and antagonist muscles throughout the movement (lead pipe rigidity).

**Passive movement techniques:** Massage techniques that primarily palpate the movement of tissues and structures and result in the repetitive movement of soft tissue masses over the underlying structure(s) with varying degrees of joint motion.

**Passive range of motion:** The amount of joint motion available when an examiner moves a joint through its anatomical or physiological range, without assistance from the client, while the client is relaxed.

**Passive relaxed movements:** See Passive range of motion.

**Pathophysiology:** Physiological changes that occur as a result of a medical condition.

**Peer supervisor:** When therapists are confused by some aspect of the therapeutic process, it is recommended that they consult an experienced peer or supervisor who may assist them in sorting out the problem. This approach to self-care helps therapists to avoid ethical dilemmas and to ensure that they have sufficient resources to help them provide appropriate care.

**Percussion, or percussive techniques:** Massage techniques that deform and release tissues quickly through controlled, repeated, rhythmic, light striking.

**Perfusion:** Local circulation of blood through a specific tissue or organ.

**Petrissage:** A group of related neuromuscular techniques that repetitively compress, shear, and release muscle tissue with varying amounts of drag, lift, and glide.

**Physiological barrier in soft tissue:** The resistance that determines the range of motion of soft tissue that is available under normal conditions. In other words, the range of motion of the tissue lies between the two physiological barriers, with the least amount of resistance being apparent at the midrange.

**Physiological Model of Stress:** Hans Selye's model of stress that is based on the interaction of the adrenal cortex and the neuroendocrine and immune systems during stress. Stress in this model is defined as the body's automatic response ("fight or flight") to a demand that is placed on it.

**Picking-up:** A one-handed or two-handed gliding petrissage technique in which muscle is lifted and squeezed between the fingers and the abducted thumb.

**Piriformis syndrome:** A syndrome of posterolateral hip and leg pain caused by a tight piriformis. This may in turn cause sacroiliac joint dysfunction and sciatic nerve entrapment.

**Pitting edema:** Edema that retains the indentation produced by the pressure of palpation.

**Placebo:** An intervention that is known not to actively cause specific treatment effects and that is used to replace a specified intervention. It is often used in research.

**Plan of care:** The systematic set of therapeutic techniques selected by the clinician to achieve the identified outcomes or wellness goals for a client.

**Plastic deformation:** Deformation in response to applied force that remains after the force is removed; putty-like behavior.

**Pliability:** The inherent quality of tissue that refers to the ease with which it is bent, twisted, sheared, elongated, or compressed.

**Polarity therapy:** An energetic approach developed by Randolph Stone, D.O., D.C., N.D. (1890–1981), that uses static contact to treat blockages in the biomagnetic field of the body.

**Positional release:** A group of related osteopathic techniques that relieve tension and pain in muscles through positioning and gentle sustained pressure.

**Positioning:** The alignment and support of the client's body by the clinician in preparation for the application of massage.

**Postintervention pain/soreness:** Pain that arises after an intervention. When due to massage, it may be due to mild inflammation caused by work that is done too quickly, activation of a latent trigger point, or a shift in tension related to postural rebalancing.

**Postisometric relaxation (PIR):** A technique developed by Karel Lewit, M.D., where the client contracts a tense muscle isometrically against resistance and then relaxes completely as the therapist takes up the slack.

**Posttraumatic stress disorder:** Severe psychological distress that develops after events in which a person is a witness to or exposed to the threat of death or serious injury. Disabling symptoms may include recurrent memories, fears, feelings of helplessness, rage, and avoidance behavior.

**Postural awareness:** See Posture.

**Postural condition:** Any condition of impaired or deficient posture, such as hyperlordosis, hyperkyphosis, scoliosis, and upper and lower cross syndromes. Postural conditions involve (at least) the impairments of adaptive shortening, adaptive lengthening, and impaired postural awareness.

**Postural drainage:** The use of positioning to promote the movement of bronchial secretions through the lungs; conventionally used in conjunction with percussion.

**Postural drainage and percussion (PDP):** The use of postural drainage and clapping (cupping) to mechanically loosen secretions in the lungs and facilitate airway clearance. Clapping is followed by, or alternated with, rapid compression and release of the rib cage.

**Postural exercise:** Any exercise (e.g., stretching, strengthening, or awareness) that is designed to improve posture.

**Postural imbalance:** Lack of balanced length and strength that is seen between agonist and antagonist groups of muscles in postural conditions.

**Postural malalignment:** Abnormal joint alignment caused by soft tissue imbalance or deformity within a bone.

**Postural scan:** A test in which the therapist observes the client's body structure for alignment, symmetry, and muscular balance. A postural scan is performed with the client standing and viewed from the front, back, and both sides.

**Postural tone:** The development of muscular tension in skeletal muscles that participate in maintaining the positions of different parts of the skeleton. The cerebellum regulates postural tone. Unlike muscle resting tension, constant muscle activation is required for the maintenance of postural tone, and the self-sustained firing of motor neurons may reduce the need for prolonged synaptic input in this situation.

**Postural weakness:** Weakness that is seen in muscles that show adaptive lengthening in postural conditions.

**Posture:** The positioning and alignment of the skeleton and associated soft tissues in relation to gravity, the center of mass, and the base of support of the body.

**Power:** See Muscle power.

**Power stroke:** That portion of a circular or elliptical massage technique where pressure is applied to the client's tissues, usually by pushing the hand away from the body and adding some amount of body weight; contrasted with return stroke.

**Practice guidelines:** Broad guidelines for the treatment of medical conditions that provide therapists with a general framework for planning and progressing interventions. These condition-specific practice guidelines and professional practice guidelines outline a general guide to prognoses, expected numbers of visits per episode of care, outcome measures, and relevant types of intervention for a range of medical conditions.

**Precompetition sports massage:** Sports massage performed up to 24-hours before competition, which seeks to enhance arousal and awareness, while promoting relaxation of skeletal muscle.

**Pressure of technique:** The amount of force per unit area of contact surface that the clinician applies.

**Pressure stroke:** See Power stroke.

**Pretest–posttest design:** An experimental research design in which subjects are tested before and after the intervention period.

**Prevention:** A clinical approach that focuses on impeding the development of impairments and medical conditions, rather than treating them after they occur.

**Primary impairment:** Any loss or abnormality of the client's body structures or functions that occurs as a result of the pathophysiology of a medical condition.

**Primary research:** The original research conducted by therapists or researchers. Types of primary research include: clinical trials, surveys, ethnographies, and a variety of other research designs.

**Primary source:** A source that directly documents the primary research, which is the original research conducted by therapists or researchers. Primary sources are typically professional journals, conference presentations, and, occasionally, text books.

**Principles of (sequence) design:** Principles for selecting and ordering massage techniques to achieve specific clinical outcomes.

**Process of care:** The manner in which care is delivered, and the activities that take place within and between the clinician and the client. This encompasses the interpersonal aspects of the client–clinician interaction and the technical aspects of how the clinician provides care.

**Prognosis:** The process of predicting the client's level and timing of improvement.

**Progression:** Incremental changes in the techniques used to treat a client's clinical condition or address the client's wellness goals. Stages of progression reflect the clinical course and prognosis for a given condition and client. Therapists can use information from several sources to guide treatment progression. These sources include practice guidelines, findings from the client examination, and clinical experience.

**Progressive relaxation:** A method to reduce stress and train muscular relaxation developed by Edmund Jacobsen in the 1920s. The client alternately tenses and relaxes groups of muscles sequentially throughout the body.

**Proprioception:** Awareness of position, weight, and movement of the body as a whole and of its parts in relation to each other.

**Proprioceptive neuromuscular facilitation (PNF):** Developed in the 1940s by Dr. Kabat and physical therapists Margaret Knott and Dorothy Voss, is a method of increasing range of motion, strength, endurance, joint stability, and motor control through the stimulation of proprioceptors. Techniques include Hold-Relax, Rhythmic Initiation, Slow Reversal, and Rhythmic Stabilization.

**Proprioceptive palpation:** A form of palpation in which the clinician uses proprioceptive sense to gauge how the client's compressed tissues are deforming under the application of the clinician's body weight.

**Proprioceptive stimulation techniques:** The application of massage techniques, such as tapping, or other techniques, such as quick stretch, to strengthen the contraction of muscle; often done immediately prior to exercise for clients who have CNS disorders.

**Psychoneuroimmunology:** The science that studies the relationships between the nervous, endocrine, and immune systems and how these relationships affect behavior.

**Pulse:** Periodic, regular expansion and contraction of arterial walls in response to the fluid wave caused by contraction of the heart.

**Qi:** See Chi.

**Qualitative research:** Research that uses the collection and analysis of word-based experiential and observational data, rather than numbers. Qualitative research assumes that people define reality.

**Quality of life:** See Health-related quality of life.

**Quantitative research:** Research that uses the collection and analysis of numerical data. The underlying assumption in quantitative research is that there is a reality that exists independently of people.

**Radicular pain:** Pain that is felt in a dermatome, myotome, or sclerotome because of direct involvement of a spinal nerve or nerve root. Also known as nerve root pain.

**Radiculopathy:** Pathology of a nerve root that commonly produces radicular pain.

**Randomized clinical trial (RCT):** A clinical trial whose participants have been randomly allocated to treatment and control groups. RCTs are highly ranked in the hierarchy of quantitative research methods. Sometimes called a randomized controlled trial.

**Rate of technique:** An indication of how fast the force is applied. The rate may describe the speed of the movement of the clinician's hand over the client's skin (distance per second), the frequency of repetitions of a described technique (repetitions per second), or both.

**Reactive cramping/tightening:** The undesirable elevation of resting tension in a massaged muscle group or its antagonist that may appear shortly after treatment. It indicates activation of a latent trigger point or a shift in tension related to postural rebalancing.

**Reactive hyperemia:** Hyperemia that is caused by short applications of cold.

**Recovery:** The improvement in the client's impairments that are the result of a medical condition.

**Red flag:** A sign or symptom that indicates the presence of a condition requiring immediate medical attention.

**Re-examination:** Ongoing repetition of the examination process to determine the client's progress towards his or her clinical or wellness goals.

**Referred pain:** Pain that is felt at another part of the body that is at a distance from the tissues that have caused it because the referred site is supplied by the same or adjacent neural segments.

**Referred tenderness:** Tenderness to palpation that is felt at another part of the body that is at a distance from the tissues that have caused it because the referred site is supplied by the same or adjacent neural segments.

**Reflex effect:** An effect where functional change is mediated by the nervous system (as opposed to a mechanical effect).

**Reflex sympathetic dystrophy (RSD):** See Complex regional pain syndrome.

**Reflex technique:** A massage technique whose effects are largely or solely reflex effects.

**Reflexology:** A system of manual treatment that applies specific compression to reflex points in the foot or hand to normalize function in distant body segments or organs.

**Reiki:** An energetic approach similar to Therapeutic Touch and Healing Touch. Practitioners use the simplest form of touch to manipulate the energy field or magnetic field of the client's body.

**Relaxation:** 1. The process of releasing mental or physical tension. 2. A state of low mental or physical tension. See Parasympathetic.

**Repetitive strain injury (repetitive motion trauma, cumulative trauma syndrome):** Damage to muscles, tendons, or nerves in the upper body that is caused by the sustained postures and repetitive movements such as keyboarding.

**Research competency:** The ability to conduct research.

**Research literacy:** The ability to find, understand, and critically evaluate research evidence for application in professional practice.

**Resilience:** The inherent quality of tissue that restores original form after deformation by applied force.

**Resistance:** The inherent quality of tissue that counteracts the tendency of applied force to produce movement of the tissue.

**Respiratory rhythm:** Periodic, regular movement of the chest wall that occurs during breathing.

**Resting tension of muscle:** See Muscle resting tension.

**Restorative sleep:** Restful sleep that is conducive to health. Sleep disturbances from various causes may alter sleep architecture, so that sleep occurs but does not have its normal restorative effects.

**Restrictive, or pathological barriers, in soft tissue:** Barriers that are observed when soft tissue dysfunction is present. They can be located anywhere between the normal physiological barriers, can limit the available range of motion within the tissues, and can alter the position of the midrange. A restrictive barrier will change the quality of the movement and the "feel" at the end of the tissue range of motion. This is analogous to the abnormal end feels observed in joints.

**Retrograde:** Proceeding backwards from the endpoint. In the case of abdominal massage, if a technique is applied in a retrograde order, it means that the technique is applied first over the sigmoid colon, then the descending colon, then the transverse colon, and lastly over the ascending colon.

**Retrostasis:** Pushing of excess fluid away from an area of the body due to vasoconstriction caused by local application of cold for more than 10 minutes.

**Return stroke:** The portion of a circular or elliptical massage technique where the hand glides to its original position with little or no pressure.

**Rhythmic mobilization:** A technique in which entire structures are repetitively moved, resulting in the movement of soft tissue over bone and the movement of related joints and internal organs.

**Rib cage mobility:** The capacity of the rib cage to move within the available anatomical range of motion during respiration, based on the arthrokinematics of the joints of the rib cage and the thoracic spine, and the ability of the periarticular connective tissue to deform.

**Rigidity:** Increased muscular tone that results from brainstem or basal ganglia lesions. Rigidity involves a uniformly increased resistance in both agonist and antagonist muscles, resulting in stiff, immovable body parts, independent of the velocity of the stretch stimulus.

**Rocking:** A technique in which gentle, repetitive oscillation of the body is produced by repeatedly pushing the pelvis or torso from a midline resting position into lateral deviation and then allowing it to return.

**Rolf, Ida P.:** (1896–1979) American biochemist, originator of Structural Integration and Rolfing, and author of the text *On the Integration of Human Structures*. Dr. Rolf was an influential innovator; for example, she likely introduced both the use of the elbow and forearm as a contact surface and the simultaneous use of massage and active movement.

**Rolfing (The Rolf Method of Structural Integration):** The massage-related approach developed by Ida Rolf combines the following features: the aim of lengthening and balancing the myofascial network to improve posture and movement, an emphasis on connective tissue techniques, a series of 10 sessions, and the use of movement and postural awareness exercises.

**Salt glow:** An application of wet salt to the client's skin with rubbing. A full-body application takes 20–30 minutes, acts as a tonic, and strongly stimulates peripheral circulation.

**Satellite trigger point:** A trigger point that is activated by a key trigger point by being in its area of referral or by being its antagonist or synergist.

**Scanning, or stroking, palpation:** Palpation that moves relatively quickly over a large area. Therapists use this when they want to collect information from a wide area.

**Scapulohumeral rhythm:** The ratio between glenohumeral motion and scapulothoracic motion during shoulder abduction. The normal ratio is 2 degrees of glenohumeral motion for 1 degree of scapulothoracic motion, after 20 degrees.

**Scar:** The fibrous tissue that replaces normal tissues that have been destroyed by a burn, wound, surgery, radiation, or disease.

**Sclerotomal pain:** Pain in a sclerotome, an area of bone or fascia innervated by one segmental nerve root.

**Seated aligned posture:** A posture used during massage, in which the therapist sits upright in a relaxed manner, while requiring his or her awareness of his or her pelvis contacting the chair.

**Secondary effect:** An indirect therapeutic effect.

**Secondary impairments:** Any loss or abnormality of the client's body structures or functions that occurs as a result of the primary impairments.

**Secondary research:** Studies that summarize and draw conclusions from primary research studies. Examples are nonsystematic literature reviews, systematic literature reviews, and meta-analyses.

**Secondary source:** A summary of the information presented in a primary source. Secondary sources can include secondary research studies, such as literature reviews and meta-analyses. Other secondary sources are textbooks, the popular media, the Internet, professional courses, and professional journals.

**Sedation:** The process of calming or allaying nervous excitement. See Relaxation.

**Segmental vertebral dysfunction:** Abnormal movement of the joints in a contiguous section of the spine that often involves adjacent areas of hyper- and hypomobility.

**Self-care activities:** Any actions that clients perform on their own behalf to promote wellness or treat impairments.

**Self-mobilization:** See Automobilization.

**Shoulder separation:** An injury in which the acromioclavicular and coracoclavicular ligaments are torn.

**Sequence:** A structured, outcome-based series or succession of massage techniques that comprise an intervention or a part of an intervention.

**Serotonin:** A widely spread neurotransmitter, 5-hydroxytryptamine, that is involved in depression, appetite, nausea, intestinal motility, sleep cycles, and obsessive compulsive disorders.

**Shaking:** A passive movement technique in which soft tissue, primarily muscle, is repetitively moved back and forth over the underlying bone, with minimal joint movement.

**Sham:** A type of placebo treatment that mimics the form of the actual treatment without actively causing specific treatment effects.

**Shear/shearing:** Deformation that involves sliding of adjacent layers over each other.

**Shiatsu:** A complex Japanese system of massage, based on the meridian system, that makes extensive use of specific compression.

**Simons, Dr. David:** American medical doctor and coauthor with Dr. Janet Travell of both volumes of *Myofascial Pain and Dysfunction*, the first and most authoritative text reference about trigger points.

**Skin:** A layer of epithelium, the epidermis, and the dermis.

**Skin rolling:** A gliding connective tissue technique in which tissue superficial to the investing layer of deep fascia is grasped, continuously lifted, and rolled over underlying tissues in a wave-like motion.

**Slow-stroke back rub:** A light massage of short duration, often performed by nursing staff in hospitals, and the subject of numerous clinical trials.

**Societal limitations:** Those limitations to an individual's level of function that can be attributed to physical or attitudinal barriers in society.

**Soft tissue:** Pliable tissue such as muscle, tendon, fascia, ligament, synovial capsule, cartilage, and nerve.

**Soft tissue dysfunction:** Abnormal function of soft tissues, such as muscle, tendon, fascia, ligament, synovial capsule, cartilage, and nerve, due to impairment or pathophysiology.

**Soft tissue range of motion:** Available range of motion of soft tissue that is analogous to the range of motion available in joints. Within this range of motion, normal soft tissue has three barriers or resistances that can limit movement.

**Solid edema:** See Consolidated edema.

**Somatoemotional release:** 1. The phenomenon of emotional release that occurs in response to a touch therapy and manifests as sighs, crying, laughing, muscle twitches, or anger. 2. A service-marked method of the Upledger Institute that teaches the techniques and skills required to deal with this phenomenon.

**Somatovisceral reflex:** A reflex in which touch, pressure, or thermal stimulation applied to musculoskeletal tissues affects visceral function.

**Spasm:** A sudden, involuntary contraction of skeletal or smooth muscle that causes increased tension in the muscle and often pain. Spasms of skeletal muscle are accompanied by motor neuron firing.

**Spasticity:** Increased muscular tone that results from an upper motor neuron lesion that may or may not be associated with reflex hyperexcitability. Spastic muscle exhibits velocity-dependent increase in tonic stretch reflexes. The quicker the stretch is, the more pronounced the resistance of the spastic muscle.

**Specific compression:** A nongliding neuromuscular technique in which pressure is applied to the target tissue with a specific contact surface in a direction that is perpendicular to the target tissue.

**Specific kneading:** A gliding petrissage technique performed in circles or ellipses and delivered with a small contact surface such as the thumb.

**Specific technique:** A technique that is applied to a localized area, applied with a small contact surface, or both.

**Sports massage:** Massage performed on athletes performed before, between, or after events, for the purpose of preparation, recovery, maintenance, or rehabilitation.

**Sprain:** Overstretching, partial tearing, or complete tearing of a ligament due to trauma.

**Spray and stretch:** A method of inactivating trigger points in which skin overlying the muscle and area of referral is cooled with vapocoolant spray while the muscle is simultaneously stretched. The alternative ice and stretch method has a similar effect but avoids the use of chemicals that damage the ozone layer.

**Standard (Universal) Precautions:** A set of procedures designed to prevent the spread of infectious diseases that describes how to handle blood, serous fluids, and any material that has come in contact with them. These precautions include handwashing and wearing protective equipment such as gloves, masks, and gowns.

**Standing aligned posture:** A posture used during massage in which the therapist stands upright in a relaxed manner while refining her awareness of her feet contacting the ground.

**Standing controlled lean:** A movement used during massage in which the therapist leans forward from the lunge position to contact the client and transfers some of his or her weight to the client in a controlled manner.

**Standing upright posture:** See Standing aligned posture.

**State anxiety:** A measure that represents a person's experience of anxiety at a given moment in time. It is opposed to trait anxiety, which measures anxiety as a more enduring character trait.

**Static contact:** A superficial reflex technique in which the clinician's hands contact the client's body without motion and with minimal force.

**Static palpation:** Palpation that involves no movement of the palpating hand and is best suited for palpating moving phenomena such as pulse or respiratory rhythm.

**Stiffness:** Resistance to applied forces; rigidity.

**Stimulating massage:** Massage that is quick paced and performed to decrease fatigue, increase arousal, or prepare for activity.

**Stimulation:** Sensory input.

**Strain:** Trauma to a muscle and/or its tendon from overstretching or violent contraction. There may be tearing of fibers with a palpable depression in the muscle.

**Strain-counterstrain:** See Positional release.

**Strength:** The maximum force that a muscle or muscle group can produce against resistance.

**Stress:** Any physical, physiological, or psychological stimulus that disrupts homeostasis.

**Stress response:** The individual's cognitive, physiological, affective, or behavioral response to the stressor or stress-causing agent.

**Stripping:** A slow, specific, gliding, neuromuscular technique that is applied from the origin of a muscle to its insertion for the purpose of reducing the activity of trigger points.

**Stroke volume (cardiac stroke volume):** The amount of blood pumped by the left ventricle of the heart in one contraction.

**Structural Integration:** A generic term for the massage systems descended from the work of Ida Rolf, whose practitioners use connective tissue techniques and education to realign clients' bodies in a series of 10 or more interventions.

**Structure of care:** The human, physical, and financial resources that are available for the delivery of care.

**Substance P:** A peptide neurotransmitter that is involved in the regulation of depression, anxiety, and pain and in the body's response to stress and noxious stimuli.

**Superficial effleurage:** A gliding manipulation performed with light centripetal pressure that deforms subcutaneous tissue down to the investing layer of the deep fascia.

**Superficial fascia:** Connective tissue layer that is deep to the skin that houses fat and water; that provides a path for nerves and vessels; and that may contain, in certain areas of the body, striated muscle that controls the movement of the skin, such as the platysma muscle.

**Superficial fluid techniques:** Massage techniques that are applied to tissues superficial to muscle that increase the return flow of lymph and possibly venous blood.

**Superficial lymph drainage technique:** A nongliding technique performed in the direction of lymphatic flow using short, rhythmical strokes with light pressure that deforms subcutaneous tissue without engaging muscle.

**Superficial reflex techniques:** Massage techniques that palpate the skin and primarily affect level of arousal, autonomic balance, and the perception of pain.

**Superficial stroking:** A superficial reflex technique that involves unidirectional pressureless gliding over the client's skin with minimal deformation of subcutaneous tissues; usually applied over large areas.

**Supports:** Objects such as pillows and bolsters that are used to make the client more comfortable, stable, or accessible during massage.

**Swedish massage:** A system of massage, consolidated by Per Henrik Ling (1776–1839), that includes effleurage, petrissage, friction, tapotement, and shaking (or vibration). It is one of the technical foundations for Outcome-Based Massage.

**Swelling:** An abnormal enlargement of a segment of the body.

**Sympathetic response:** A response caused by activating the sympathetic division of the autonomic nervous system, whose efferent fibers exit through the thoracolumbar spinal nerves. Effects include increased heart rate, vasoconstriction in the skin and viscera, vasodilation in skeletal muscle, dilation of bronchioles, and secretion of epinephrine and norepinephrine.

**Systematic review:** A type of secondary research that evaluates findings from individual studies and combines these findings using statistical techniques.

**Systemic connective tissue disorders:** See Connective tissue disease.

**Tai Chi:** An oriental movement discipline, which is related to martial arts, in which choreographed sequences of slow dance-like movements are practiced to develop awareness, flexibility, strength, and poise.

**Tapotement:** See Percussion.

**Taut band:** A group of tense muscle fibers that extend from a trigger point to the muscle's attachments and that will twitch when the trigger point is palpated.

**Taxonomy:** System of classification.

**T-bar:** A T-shaped instrument that is gripped in the hand and used to perform massage techniques to reduce hand strain.

**Tendinitis:** Inflammation of the peritendinous tissues that can occur in response to repetitive mechanical trauma.

**Tendinopathy:** Pathology of a tendon.

**Tendinosis:** Unlike tendinitis, which is an inflammatory condition, tendinosis refers to common overuse conditions of a tendon with a histopathology that is consistent with a noninflammatory, degenerative process of unclear etiology.

**TENS (transcutaneous electrical nerve stimulation):** The application of mild electrical stimulation to electrodes attached to the skin for analgesia.

**Tension, or tensile force:** Any force that is so oriented that its effect is to lengthen a tissue or structure.

**Terminus stroke (MLD):** A stroke applied just above the clavicle that milks the junctions of the right lymphatic and thoracic ducts with the subclavian veins. This stroke begins a drainage sequence for any region of the body.

**Thai massage:** An Eastern massage approach performed with the client clothed and lying on the floor that makes extensive use of specific compression along meridians and passive stretching.

**Theory:** An organized set of facts that explains the relationships between a group of observed phenomena.

**Therapeutic contract:** The agreement between therapist and client as to what goals are to be addressed, how the therapy will proceed, and what is expected of each person.

**Therapeutic effects:** The effects produced by a technique that are used to achieve clinical outcomes. A massage technique can produce multiple therapeutic effects. These may occur locally, only on the site of manipulation, or generally throughout the client's body. The therapeutic effects of massage techniques fall into six categories: mechanical, physiological, psychological, reflex, psychoneuroimmunological, and "energetic."

**Therapeutic rapport:** A relationship of mutual trust and sympathy between a therapist and client.

**Therapeutic relationship:** The therapeutic relationship is the trust relationship that forms between a client and a therapist where the needs of the client, the ethical considerations of the therapist, and the boundaries of what is possible contain and frame the outcomes of care.

**Therapeutic Touch:** An energetic approach developed by Delores Kreiger, RN, in the 1970s. Practitioners use the simplest form of touch and may also move their hands above the surface of the body to manipulate the energy field or magnetic field of the client's body.

**Therapeutic ultrasound:** A treatment modality in which high-frequency sound waves are used to treat musculoskeletal injuries. Effects may be due to warming of tissues, increased blood flow, and stimulation of healing.

**Thixotropy:** The property of some colloids by which they become more fluid when subjected to movement or heat and less fluid when subjected to stasis or cold.

**Thoracic outlet (compression) syndrome (TOS):** A group of conditions caused by compression of the subclavian vessels and trunks of the brachial plexus in the region(s) of the clavicle, the first rib, and the anterior scalene and pectoralis minor muscles. Symptoms may include pain, swelling, and neurological symptoms in the upper limb.

**Tissue memory:** This occurs when a client is touched by a therapist in a way that reminds the client of another earlier and often significant life experience. A cascade of emotional and biochemical responses occur within the client that may cause concern, fear, or bewilderment for the client.

**Tissues engaged by technique:** The target tissues or layers of tissue to which the clinician directs the pressure of the stroke and that are mechanically deformed by application of the technique.

**Tone:** See Muscle tone.

**Torticollis:** A condition in which the head is tilted toward one side and rotated towards the opposite side. It may be congenital or caused by unilateral spasm or trigger points in the sternocleidomastoid.

**Touch Research Institute (University of Miami):** The Touch Research Institute was formally established in 1992 by Tiffany Field, Ph.D., at the University of Miami School of Medicine. Since that time, numerous researchers there have published dozens of articles investigating the effects of massage on a variety of population groups and clinical conditions.

**Touch-triggered memory:** A memory that is triggered by touch. See implicit memory and somato-emotional release.

**Traction:** A sustained pulling force. Manual traction is commonly applied to separate joint surfaces or oriented parallel to the long axis of a limb.

**Traditional Chinese Medicine (TCM):** An ancient, vast, and sophisticated system of philosophy, clinical theory, and practice that has come to the attention of the West in recent decades primarily because of the evidence for the analgesic effects of acupuncture. Fundamental to the system of Chinese medicine are several interrelated concepts that have no parallel concepts in Western medicine. In Chinese medicine, energy (chi) circulates through the body in well-defined cycles through conduits or channels called meridians.

**Trager Method of Psychophysical Integration:** A method of passive rocking and rhythmic mobilization that teaches awareness of relaxation, ease, lightness, and freedom of movement developed by Dr. Milton Trager. Table work is supplemented with dance-like active movements taught to clients for home use to achieve the same ends.

**Trait anxiety:** A measure of anxiety as an enduring character trait. It is opposed to state anxiety, which measures a person's experience of anxiety at a given moment in time.

**Transcutaneous electrical nerve stimulation:** See TENS.

**Transference:** Occurs when a client idealizes and projects feelings onto the therapist that are unconscious, unprocessed, or unexpressed. When unresolved feelings or childhood issues are "transferred" onto the therapist, then a client is said to be experiencing transference.

**Transitional stroke:** A massage stroke that is used between regions or between techniques that take more time. Superficial effleurage and superficial stroking are commonly used transitional strokes.

**Traumatic edema:** Edema that results from trauma.

**Travell, Dr. Janet:** (1901–1997) American medical doctor, and senior coauthor with Dr. David Simons of both volumes of *Myofascial Pain and Dysfunction*, the first and most authoritative text reference about trigger points.

**Treatment:** 1. A clinical intervention that is directed to an impairment in the client's body structure or function. 2. A series of interventions that make up an episode of care.

**Treatment of impairments:** Treatment when the aim is to reduce the impairments associated with medical conditions.

**Treatment Phase:** The Treatment Phase is an ongoing cycle of treatment, re-examination, and treatment progression that begins after the therapist completes the plan of care.

**Treatment Planning Phase:** The steps in the Treatment Planning Phase involve identifying body structures and functions that are appropriate for treatment and selecting treatment techniques that will produce improvements in the client's impairments in body structures and functions, functional limitations, or overall wellness.

**Tremors:** Rhythmic movements of a joint that result from involuntary contractions of antagonist and agonist muscle groups.

**Trigger point:** See Myofascial trigger point.

**Trigger point pain:** Referred pain that arises in a trigger point but is felt at a distance that is often entirely remote from its source. The pattern of referred pain is diagnostic of the site of origin. The distribution of referred trigger point pain rarely coincides entirely with the distribution of a peripheral nerve or dermatomal segment.

**Trigger point pressure release:** Sustained specific compression applied to a trigger point to reduce its activity.

**Trigger point syndrome:** See Myofascial pain syndrome.

**Trophic changes:** Changes in local tissue health usually due to interruption of peripheral nerve supply to an area.

**Twitch response:** A transient reflex contraction of the muscles fibers in the taut band that contains a trigger point, caused by palpation of the trigger point.

**Ultrasound:** See Therapeutic ultrasound.

**Unnecessary muscle tension:** Unwitting muscular contraction or muscle tension that is under voluntary control.

**Upledger, John:** American osteopathic physician and author of numerous texts on craniosacral and related therapies. He is the founder of the Upledger Institute in Florida, which offers training in a wide variety of manual therapies.

**Upper-cross syndrome:** A postural syndrome in which the pectorals, upper trapezius, and levator scapulae tighten and shorten, while the rhomboids, serratus anterior, middle and lower trapezius, and deep neck flexors weaken.

**Varicosities:** Enlarged twisted veins that are commonly found on the legs.

**VAS (visual analog scale):** A scale that clients use to rate the intensity of pain or other subjective symptoms. The client marks the rating on a 10-cm line with descriptors at each end.

**Venous insufficiency (venous stasis):** Reduced return flow of venous blood usually from the lower limb that is caused by incompetent valves and venous hypertension.

**Venous return:** The volume of blood returned to the heart through the veins.

**Venous ulcer:** A slow-healing ulcer associated with impaired venous return that is usually located above the medial malleolus.

**Vestibular reflex:** A reflex that depends on sensory information from the labyrinth of the ear.

**Visceral pain:** Pain in areas of the viscera that are supplied by a nerve root.

**Viscerosomatic reflex:** A reflex in which visceral dysfunction affects the function of musculoskeletal tissues. See Connective tissue zone.

**Viscoelastic:** Showing both viscous/plastic and elastic behavior. For a viscoelastic stretch, some of the length that the tissue gains during the stretch will remain when one releases the tensile force.

**Viscoelastic deformation:** Deformation in response to applied force that partially remains after the force is removed; viscoelastic deformation combines spring-like and putty-like behavior.

**Viscosity, or fluid viscosity:** The property of fluids and semifluids that offers resistance to flow, i.e., stickiness.

**Vodder, Emil:** Originator in the 1920s and 1930s of what later became the Vodder method of Manual Lymph Drainage. There are now numerous lymphatic drainage schools that have been influenced to some degree by the Vodder method.

**Wellness:** A state of being that encompassing both a balance of "mind, body, and spirit" and an individuals' self-

perception of their well-being, which is distinct from their state of "health."

**Wellness behavior:** Personal factors that play a central role in wellness, such as self-nurturance, healthy lifestyles, readiness for change, and perceived health.

**Wellness goals:** Clinical goals for optimizing clients' body structures and functions to enhance their levels of wellness.

**Wellness Interactions Model:** A model that shows an ongoing interaction between a person, wellness, and the person's environment. In this model, an individual's level of wellness can affect any aspect of his or her person at any point in life, and vice versa. At the same time, that individual exists within an environment in which the barriers and facilitators to wellness will influence his or her level of wellness.

**Wellness intervention:** A systematic application of therapeutic techniques to achieve a client's wellness goals, rather than the improvement of impairments.

**Wellness massage:** General massage to achieve wellness goals, in which the main outcomes are commonly the reduction of anxiety, stress response, and muscle resting tension.

**Whole systems research:** An approach for examining the complex interrelationship between the specific and nonspecific effects of a massage intervention or a massage practice as a whole.

**Wide-stance knee bend:** A posture and movement used during massage in which the therapist stands with widely placed feet and then flexes and extends the knees to lower and raise the upright torso in relation to the floor.

**Wringing:** A petrissage technique in which muscle is lifted and sheared between contact surfaces that are moving in opposite directions.

**Yin and yang:** In Traditional Chinese Medicine, the two basic qualities of energy. Yin energy, metaphorically described as "female" and "negative," is ascending and is associated with hollow organs such as the stomach. Yang energy, metaphorically characterized as "male" and "positive," is descending and is associated with solid organs such as the liver. Health is conceptualized as a dynamic balance between yin and yang energy flowing in precise diurnal patterns through the various meridians.

# Index

Page numbers in *italics* designate figures; page numbers followed by "t" or "b" designate tables and boxes, respectively; *see also* cross-references designate related topics or more detailed subtopic lists.